made INCREDIBLY EASY!®

Critical Care Nursing

Adapted for the UK by

Lee R. Cutler, RN, BSc(Hons) MA(ED)

Consultant Nurse, Critical Care, Doncaster & Bassetlaw Hospitals NHS Foundation Trust; Honorary Senior Lecturer, The University of Sheffield; Associate Teaching Fellow, Sheffield Hallam University
and

Judith M. Cutler, RN, DipN, Dip Crit Care, BA(Hons), PGDipEd

Clinical Nurse Educator, Critical Care, Doncaster & Bassetlaw Hospitals NHS Foundation Trust

First UK Editi

...uwer | Lippincott Williams & Wilkins

...imore • New York • London
...g Kong • Sydney • Tokyo

Staff

Director, Global Publishing
Cathy Peck

Production Director
Chris Curtis

Acquisitions Editor
Rachel Hendrick

Academic Marketing Executive
Alison Major

Proofreader
Laura Maguire

Illustrator
Bot Roda

Text and Cover Design
Designers Collective

Printed and bound by RR Donnelley.China
Typeset by MPS Limited, A Macmillan Company.

For information, write to Lippincott Williams & Wilkins, 250 Waterloo Road, London SE1 8RD.

British Library Cataloguing in Publication Data. A catalogue record for this book is available from the British Library.

ISBN-13: 978-1-901831-11-5
ISBN-10: 1-901831-11-6

CCMIE1stUKed011209-060215

Contents

Acknowledgements

Contributors to the UK edition

Rachael Mander, RN, BMedSci, PGDip Crit Care
Staff Nurse in Critical Care, Sheffield Teaching Hospitals NHS
Foundation Trust

Reviewers of the UK edition

Sharon Coad, RN, BSc, PG Dip Ad Ed, Dip HSW
Lecturer and School Lead Critical Care, Department of Nursing,
University of Nottingham

Maria Kiesel, RGN, BSc (Hons) MSc
Senior Lecturer, Department of Health Professions—Trauma and
Critical Care, Birmingham City University

**Nerys Brick, RN, Dip (HE), BSc (Hons) (Nurs), MSc (Renal),
ENB 998, N04, 136, PGCLT (HE) (NMC)**
Senior Lecturer, Adult Nursing and Critical Care, Canterbury Christ
Church University

Debbie Field, RGN, BSc, MSc PhD
Senior Nurse, Lane Fox Respiratory Unit, Guys and St Thomas'
Foundation Trust London

Rachel Swinglehurst, MSc, BSc, PGCE, RGN
University Tutor, Swansea University

Amelia Williamson, RGN, MSc, PGCE (HE)
Lecturer, School of Nursing, University of Birmingham

Foreword to the UK edition

Critically ill patients are not just to be found in critical care units but throughout the wards and departments of acute hospitals. Nurses and other health care professionals will be faced with caring for these patients and meeting the challenges this brings.

To put it simply: critical care nursing isn't easy! New research findings and innovative technology propel treatment at a rapid pace; as such, nursing practice in critical care continues to become more complex. Nurses are required to deliver sophisticated care plans that are underpinned by evidenced-based guidelines. However, at the same time, this needs to be balanced with a holistic and caring approach to the critically ill and their families.

Critical Care Nursing Made Incredibly Easy! (First UK edition) is an excellent and comprehensive resource for a range of nurses: the student nurse who needs resources to aid in learning; the novice nurse who's jumping into a complex practice area; the experienced nurse who's exploring new facets of health care; and the seasoned professional who's searching for novel approaches. This book serves to enhance learning, helping nurses coordinate care to all patients in the critical care unit as well as those who may have deteriorated within another acute ward or department in the hospital.

This well-organised book offers a wealth of tools to guide the nurse attempting to develop critical care knowledge and skills, thus making learning about critical care nursing incredibly easy!

The first chapter presents an overview of the critical care team's responsibilities and the importance of a team approach. The next chapter deals with holistic care issues, and includes information on cultural considerations, pain management, ethical and legal factors and effective communication techniques.

Subsequent chapters are arranged by body system and include a system overview, assessment techniques, diagnostic tests, treatments and common disorders. This edition includes updated clinical information with expanded sections on haemodynamics, sepsis and trauma.

Clever use of graphics is a hallmark of this book. Incorporated in the text are detailed illustrations, highly organised tables and easy-to-read charts. These materials help to clarify complex issues, suggest strategies for comprehending scientific concepts and supply guidelines for providing care for more than 100 critical illness-related disorders. Throughout the text, the role of the nurse as a patient advocate is supported and encouraged.

The cartoons that appear throughout the book are a reminder to the reader that perspective is vital and that humour can be essential to survival in critical care. In addition, icons draw your attention to important issues:

Weighing the evidence—highlights research that guides practice

Senior moments—identifies areas in which older age could impact the nurse's care

Take charge!—focuses on potentially lethal situations and steps to take when they occur

Advice from the experts—offers tips and tricks for nurses and key troubleshooting techniques

Lee R. Cutler, RN, BSc(Hons) MA(ED)
Consultant Nurse, Critical Care, Doncaster & Bassetlaw Hospitals NHS Foundation Trust Honorary Senior Lecturer, The University of Sheffield; Associate Teaching Fellow, Sheffield Hallam University

Judith M. Cutler, RN, DipN, Dip Crit Care, BA(Hons), PGDipEd
Clinical Nurse Educator, Critical Care, Doncaster & Bassetlaw Hospitals NHS Foundation Trust

Contributors and consultants to the US edition

Katrina D. Allen, RN, MSN, CCRN
Nursing Faculty (ADN Program)
Faulkner State Community College
Bay Minette, AL

Jesus Casida, RN, PhD(C), CCRN, APN, C
Assistant Professor
Seton Hall University College of Nursing
Department of Adult Health Nursing
South Orange, NJ

James S. Davis IV, RN, BSN
Clinical Leader
Abington (PA) Memorial Hospital
Abington, PA

Melissa Fiegenbaum, RN, CFRN, NREMT-P
Flight Nurse
PHI Air Medical
Lexington, KY

Susan Simmons Holcomb, PhD, ARNP, BC
Family Nurse Practitioner
Walk-In Health Care of Olathe (KS)
Quivira Family Care
Overland Park, KS

Timothy L. Hudson, RN, BSN, MS, MED, CAN, CCRN, CHE
Chief Nurse, 274th Forward Surgical Team
US Army
Fort Bragg, NC

Todd Isbell, RN, BSN, CCRN-CSC
Director, Critical Care
Mountain View Hospital
Las Vegas, NV

Jill Johnson, RN, MSN, CCRN, CEN, CFRN
Staff Nurse
St Joseph Hospital
Lexington, KY

Karen J. Knight-Frank, RN, MS, CCNS, CCRN
Clinical Nurse Specialist
San Joaquin General Hospital
French Camp, CA

JoAnne Konick-McMahan, RN, MSN, CCRN
Staff Nurse
Harrisburg (PA) Hospital (Pinnacle Health System)
Toxicology, Progressive Care, Respiratory Unit
Harrisburg, PA

Kay Luft, RN, MSN, CCRN
Assistant Professor
Saint Luke's College
Kansas City, MO

Gwendolyn R. Pugh, RN, BA, MSN, CCRN
Staff Nurse
Columbus (GA) Regional Medical Center
Columbus, GA

Susan M. Raymond, MSN, CCRN, ACNP
Chief, Critical Care Nursing
Madigan Army Medical Center
Fort Lewis, WA

Doris J. Rosenow, PhD, CCRN, CNS
Associate Professor
Texas A&M International University
Canseco School of Nursing
Laredo

Just the facts

In this chapter, you'll learn:

♦ roles and responsibilities of the critical care nurse

♦ education for critical care nurses

♦ ways to work with a multidisciplinary team

♦ ways to incorporate clinical tools and best practices into your care.

What is critical care nursing?

Critical care nursing is the delivery of specialised care to critically ill patients or patients with the potential to become critically ill—that is, those who have or are susceptible to life-threatening illnesses or injuries. Such patients may be unstable, have complex needs and require intensive and vigilant nursing care. The Department of Health categorises acute hospital patient care into levels from 0 to 3:

• Level 0 is normal acute ward care.

• Level 1 is acute ward care with the input of critical care specialists, e.g. outreach. This may be required because of recent discharge from a critical care unit or because the patient's condition or therapy/equipment used in their care means increased intervention is needed.

• Level 2 is high dependency care for patients requiring an increased level of monitoring owing to their condition or potential for deterioration or patients with single organ failure/support. Nurse to patient ratios for this level of care are usually one nurse to two patients.

• Level 3 is intensive care for patients with two or more organ failure/support or requiring mechanical ventilation. Nurse to patient ratios for this level of care are usually one nurse to one patient.

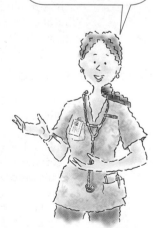

As a critical care nurse, you'll see the most critically ill or injured patients—those who are unstable, have complex needs and require intensive and vigilant nursing care.

Illnesses and injuries commonly seen in patients on critical care units, either separate level 2 and 3 facilities or combined units, include:
• traumatic injuries from such events as road traffic accidents, falls and assaults
• cardiovascular disorders, such as heart failure and acute coronary syndromes (unstable angina and myocardial infarction [MI])
• elective surgeries, such as abdominal aortic aneurysm repair and carotid endarterectomy
• emergency surgeries, such as bowel perforation and neurosurgery
• neurological disorders, such as hypoxic brain damage and subarachnoid haemorrhage
• respiratory disorders, such as acute respiratory failure and pulmonary embolism
• GI and hepatic disorders, such as acute pancreatitis, acute upper GI bleeding and acute liver failure
• renal disorders, such as acute and chronic renal failure
• cancers, such as lung, oesophageal and gastric cancer
• shock caused by hypovolaemia, sepsis and cardiogenic events (such as after MI).

Meet the critical care nurse

Critical care nurses are responsible for making sure that critically ill patients and members of their families receive close attention and the best care possible.

What do you do?

Critical care nurses fill many roles in the critical care and hospital setting, such as staff nurses, sisters, charge nurses, nurse-educators, nurse-managers, clinical nurse specialists, advanced nurse practitioners (ANPs), nurse consultants and outreach nurses. (See *Role call*, page 3.)

Where do you work?

Critical care nurses work wherever critically ill patients are found, including:
• adult, paediatric and neonatal intensive care units (ICUs) and high dependency units (HDUs), or combined critical care units caring for both level 2 and level 3 patients
• coronary care units
• cardiothoracic/neurosurgical/burns/liver units
• accident and emergency departments
• postanaesthesia/postoperative care units
• general wards as part of an 'outreach' team (providing care to patients and education to staff caring for patients with complex care needs, potential to deteriorate or recently discharged from a critical care unit).

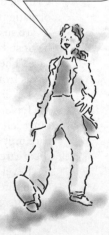

Put your best foot forward and strive to deliver the best care possible to patients and their families.

Role call

By filling various nursing and management roles, a critical care nurse helps promote optimum health, prevent illness, and aid coping with illness or death. Here are various capacities in which a critical care nurse may function.

Staff nurse

- Makes independent assessments
- Plans and implements patient care
- Provides direct nursing care
- Makes clinical observations and executes interventions
- Administers medications and treatments
- Promotes activities of daily living

Nurse-educator

- Assesses learning needs of the staff and students; plans and implements teaching strategies to meet those needs
- Evaluates effectiveness of teaching
- Educates peers and colleagues
- Develops educational resources
- Possesses excellent interpersonal skills

Nurse-manager

- Acts as an administrative representative of the unit
- Ensures that effective and quality nursing care is provided in a timely and fiscally sound environment
- Manages staff and personnel issues, e.g. recruitment and retention, sickness and absence

Clinical nurse specialist

- Participates in education and direct patient care
- Consults with patients and family members

- Collaborates with other nurses and health care team members to deliver high quality care

Advanced nurse practitioner

- Provides expert nursing care to patients and families; can function independently
- Undertakes roles previously carried out by the medical team
- May cover the critical care unit in the absence of a doctor

Nurse consultant

- Provides expert nursing care to patients and families; can function independently
- May obtain histories and conduct physical examinations
- Orders laboratory and diagnostic tests and interprets results
- Promotes evidence-based practice
- Implements new initiatives
- Counsels and educates patients and families
- Conducts audit/research studies
- Serves as a consultant for critical care across the hospital/wider nursing community

Outreach nurse

- Provides care around the hospital to deteriorating or complex patients, or patients recently discharged from critical care
- Educates staff around the hospital to care for seriously ill patients
- Audits practices around the hospital related to critical illness
- Assists in patient rehabilitation following discharge from a critical care unit

What makes you special?

As a nurse who specialises in critical care, you accept a wide range of responsibilities, including:
- being an advocate
- using sound clinical judgment
- demonstrating caring practices

- collaborating with a multidisciplinary team
- demonstrating an understanding of cultural diversity
- providing patient and family teaching.

Advocacy

An advocate is a person who works on another person's behalf. As a patient advocate, you should address the concerns of family members and the community whenever possible.

    As an advocate, the critical care nurse is responsible for:

- protecting the patient's rights
- assisting the patient in the decision-making process by providing education and support
- negotiating with other members of the health care team on behalf of the patient and their family
- keeping the patient and their family informed about the care plan
- advocating for flexible visitation to suit the needs of the patient and family on the critical care unit
- respecting and supporting the patient's decisions
- serving as a liaison between the patient and their family and other members of the health care team
- respecting the values and cultures of the patient
- acting in the patient's best interests.

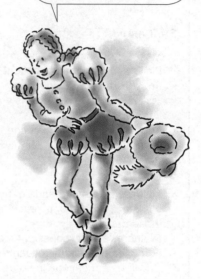

A critical care nurse is perfect for many roles. S/he can act as a nurse-manager, a nurse-educator or another type of specialist.

Stuck in the middle

Being a patient advocate can sometimes cause conflict between you and other members of the health care team. For example, when mechanical ventilation is required because of a patient's deteriorating respiratory function, you may need to relay to the medical team the patient's request to decline this treatment.

    It may also cause conflict between your professional duty and the patient's personal values. For example, the patient may be a Jehovah's Witness and refuse a blood transfusion. In this case, you should consult your hospital's policies and procedures.

One role of the critical care nurse is liaison between the patient and their family and the health care team.

Clinical judgment

A critical care nurse needs to exercise clinical judgment. To develop sound clinical judgment, you need critical thinking skills. Critical thinking is a complex mixture of knowledge, intuition, logic, common sense and experience.

Why be critical?

Critical thinking fosters understanding of issues and enables you to quickly find answers to difficult questions. It isn't a trial-and-error method, yet it isn't strictly a scientific problem-solving method, either.

Critical thinking enhances your ability to identify a patient's needs. It also enables you to use sound clinical decision-making and to determine which nursing actions best meet a patient's needs.

Developing critical thinking skills

Critical thinking skills improve with increasing clinical experience and theoretical knowledge. The best way for you to develop critical thinking skills is by asking questions and learning.

Always asking questions

The first question you should find the answer to is 'What's the patient's diagnosis?' If it's a diagnosis with which you aren't familiar, look it up and read about it. Find the answers to such questions as these:
- What are the signs and symptoms?
- What's the usual cause?
- What complications can occur?

In addition to finding the answers to diagnosis-related questions, also be sure to find out:
- What are the patient's physical examination findings?
- What laboratory and diagnostic tests are necessary?
- Does the patient have any risk factors? If so, are they significant? What interventions would minimise those risk factors?
- What are the possible complications? What type of monitoring is needed to watch for complications?
- What are the usual medications and treatments for the patient's condition? (If you aren't familiar with the medications or treatments, look them up in a reliable source or consult a colleague.)
- How is this diagnosis affecting the patient and their family (physically, mentally, psychologically, emotionally, socially and culturally)?

Critical thinking and the nursing process

Critical thinking skills are necessary when applying the nursing process—assessment, planning, intervention and evaluation—and making patient care decisions.

Step 1: Assessment

To obtain assessment data:
- ask relevant questions
- use patient history, clinical assessment, monitoring, diagnostic tests and investigations to answer your questions

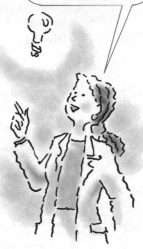

Here's a thought! Critical thinking fosters understanding and enables us to solve difficult problems.

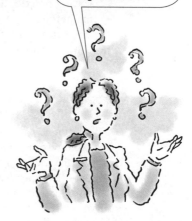

Part of being a critical thinker is asking the right questions and digging to find the right answers.

- validate evidence or data that has been collected
- identify present and potential concerns.

Then be sure to analyse the assessment data and determine the nursing diagnoses. To do this, you must interpret the collected data and identify gaps. For example, if laboratory values are missing, call to obtain test results or request a test that wasn't performed.

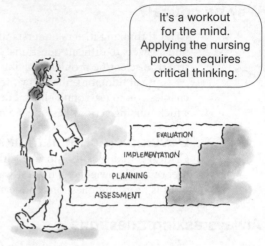

It's a workout for the mind. Applying the nursing process requires critical thinking.

Step 2: Planning

During the planning stage, critical thinking skills come in handy when considering how the patient is expected to achieve goals. During this stage, consider the consequences of planned interventions. This is also the time to set priorities of care for the patient.

Step 3: Implementation

During the implementation stage, use critical thinking to involve the patient and other members of the health care team in implementing the care plan.

Step 4: Evaluation

During the evaluation stage, use critical thinking to continually reassess, modify and individualise care. Evaluation enables you to assess the patient's responses and determine whether expected outcomes have been met.

Caring practice

Caring practice is the use of a therapeutic and compassionate environment to focus on the patient's needs. Although care is based on standards and protocols, it must also be individualised to each patient.

Caring practice also involves:
- maintaining a safe environment
- interacting with the patient and their family in a compassionate and respectful manner throughout the critical care stay
- supporting the patient and their family in end-of-life issues and decisions.

Critical care nurses are usually chief coordinators of a collaborative team of highly skilled professionals—pretty impressive, huh?

Collaboration

Collaboration allows a health care team to use all available resources for the patient. A critical care nurse is part of a multidisciplinary team in which each person contributes expertise. The collaborative goal is to optimise patient outcomes. As a nurse, you may often serve as the coordinator of such collaborative teams. Multidisciplinary teamwork is discussed in more depth later in this chapter.

Cultural diversity

Culture is defined as the way people live and how they behave in a social group. This behaviour is learnt and passed on from generation to generation. Acknowledging and respecting patients' diverse cultural beliefs is a necessary part of high quality care.

Keep an open mind

A critical care nurse is expected to demonstrate awareness and sensitivity towards a patient's religion, lifestyle, family makeup, socioeconomic status, age, gender and values. Be sure to assess cultural factors and concerns and integrate them into the care plan.

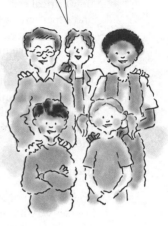

> Cultural awareness and sensitivity ... it's all part of the patient equation in delivering high quality care.

Education

As an educator, a critical care nurse is the facilitator of patient, family and staff education. Patient education involves teaching patients and their families about:
• the patient's illness
• the importance of managing comorbidities (such as diabetes, arthritis and hypertension)
• diagnostic and laboratory testing
• planned surgical procedures, including preoperative and postoperative expectations
• instructions on specific patient care, such as wound care and range-of-motion exercises.

Staff as students

Critical care nurses also commonly serve as staff educators. Examples of staff teaching topics you may need to address include:
• how to use new equipment
• how to interpret diagnostic test results
• how to administer a new medication.

> Critical care nurses are teachers, too. Their students include patients, family members and other staff.

Becoming a critical care nurse

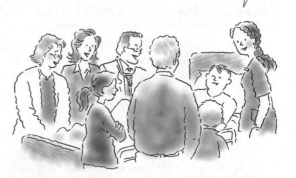

Most nursing students are only briefly exposed to critical care nursing. Much of the training required to become a critical care nurse is learned on the job.

Learning by doing

On-the-job training is central to gaining the extensive skills required by a critical care nurse. There are several ways to become trained as a critical care nurse.

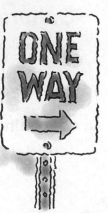

One way...

Your hospital may provide a competency-based orientation programme for new critical care nurses. In a programme such as this, you gain knowledge and experience while working on the critical care unit and a *preceptor* (a staff nurse with specialised training in critical care nursing) provides guidance. Part of this orientation will usually include a supernumerary period.

An orientation period allows the nurse time to acquire knowledge and the technical skills needed to work in the critical care environment. Such technical skills include working with equipment, such as cardiac monitoring systems, mechanical ventilators and haemodynamic monitoring devices. The nurse must also understand the principles of safe practice and the actions of the various critical care medications she gives.

...or another

Your hospital or local university may provide a critical care course. Such courses vary in duration from 6 months to 1 year. The courses usually consist of classroom lectures and clinical exposure to the critical care environment. They normally provide a formal critical care qualification as well as academic credit.

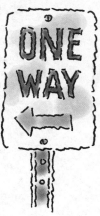

...and even further

A teaching and assessing qualification as well as possession of a variety of expanded roles (such as arterial sampling, IV administration, venepuncture, cannulation and defibrillation) and a formal critical care qualification are usually required for progression to senior positions. Evidence of continuous development in skills and knowledge is required for all staff as part of Nursing and Midwifery Council (NMC) professional registration.

Nursing responsibilities

As a critical care nurse, you're responsible for all parts of the nursing process: assessing, planning, implementing and evaluating care of critically ill patients. Remember that each of these steps gives you an opportunity to exercise your critical thinking skills.

Assessment

Critical care nursing requires that you constantly assess the patient for subtle changes in condition and monitor all equipment being used. Caring for critically ill patients may involve the use of such highly specialised equipment as cardiac monitors, haemodynamic monitoring devices, intra-aortic balloon pumps, haemofiltration machines and ICP monitoring devices. As part of the patient assessment, you also assess the patient's physical and psychological status and interpret laboratory data. Identifying that a patient is either deteriorating or improving is an important part of assessment.

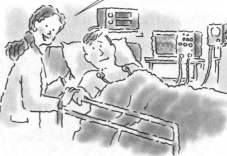

Critical care assessment involves constantly evaluating the patient's condition and monitoring equipment.

Planning

Planning requires you to consider the patient's psychological and physiological needs and set realistic patient goals. The result is an individualised care plan for your patient. To ensure safe passage through the critical care environment, you must also anticipate changes in the patient's condition. For example, for a patient admitted with a diagnosis of MI, you should monitor cardiac rhythm and anticipate rhythm changes. If an arrhythmia, such as a complete heart block, develops the treatment plan may need to be changed and new goals established. The nature of critical illness means that the plan must constantly be adapted to the patient's changing condition according to your assessment findings.

What's the problem?

In planning, be sure to address present and potential problems, such as:
- pain
- decreasing level of consciousness
- infection
- respiratory failure
- sputum retention
- cardiac arrhythmias
- altered haemodynamic states
- impaired physical mobility
- impaired skin integrity
- deficient fluid volume
- constipation
- delirium, sleep deprivation
- anxiety.

amongst many others. ...

Implementation

As a nurse, you must implement specific interventions to address existing and potential patient problems.

A call to intervene

Examples of interventions related to the cardiovascular system include:
- monitoring and treating cardiac arrhythmias
- assessing haemodynamic parameters, such as pulmonary artery pressure, central venous pressure and cardiac output
- titrating vasoactive infusions
- assessing organ perfusion
- monitoring responses to therapy.

There's more in store

Some other common interventions are:
- repositioning the patient to maintain joint and body functions, and promote tissue viability, lung expansion and sputum clearance
- performing hygiene measures to reduce infection, prevent skin breakdown and maintain patient comfort
- assisting the patient with coughing and deep-breathing exercises to prevent pulmonary complications.

Evaluation

It's necessary for you to continually evaluate a patient's response to interventions. Use such evaluations to change your plan of care as needed to make sure that your patient continues to progress towards achieving the set outcomes.

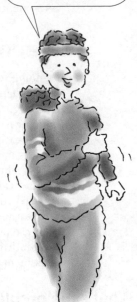

No time to stop! The wide range of interventions I perform really keeps me on the go!

Multidisciplinary teamwork

Nurses working with critically ill patients commonly collaborate with a multidisciplinary team of health care professionals. The team approach enables caregivers to better meet the diverse needs of individual patients.

The goal is holism

The goal of collaboration is to provide effective and comprehensive (holistic) care. Holistic care addresses the biological, psychological, social and spiritual dimensions of a person.

Team huddle

A multidisciplinary team providing direct patient care may consist of many professionals. Members commonly include:
- registered nurses
- doctors

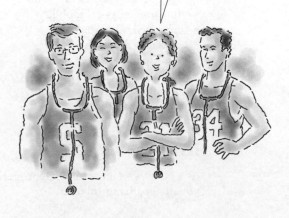

Everyone on the health care team contributes expertise. The goal is to provide effective holistic care.

- health care assistants/health care support workers/assistant practitioners
- operating department practitioners (ODPs)
- advanced nurse practitioner (ANP) (such as clinical nurse specialists and nurse practitioners)
- physiotherapists
- microbiologist and infection control team
- dieticians
- pharmacists
- administrative/clerical staff. (See *Meet the team*).

Working with registered nurses

Teamwork is essential in the stressful environment of critical care. The critical care nurse needs to work well with the other professional registered nurses on the unit.

Meet the team

Various members of the multidisciplinary team have collaborative relationships with critical care nurses. Here are some examples.

Health care assistant/health care support worker/assistant practitioners

- Provides direct patient care to critically ill patients under supervision of a registered nurse (for assistant practitioners this role is further developed after significant critical care training)
- Assists registered nurse in admitting, transferring and discharging patients
- Maintains stock levels and carries out cleaning duties
- Assists with equipment maintenance

Operating department practitioners (ODPs)

- May work on the critical care unit in a role similar to a registered nurse after additional critical care training
- Act as an assistant to the anaesthetic medical team, facilitating safe patient transfers and procedures such as endotracheal intubations
- May perform a technical role for equipment maintenance, preparation and purchasing

Physiotherapist

- Assesses muscle groups and mobility and improves motor function of critically ill patients
- Assesses respiratory status and function and aims to improve respiratory condition

- Develops specialised care plan and provides care based on the patient's functional abilities and the disease process or physical injury
- Facilitates rehabilitation as patient condition improves

Pharmacist

- Assesses patient medication, ensuring availability and highlighting incompatibilities
- Acts as resource to nursing and medical staff regarding drug actions, side effects and administration
- Develops drug policies for critical care
- Obtains appropriate parenteral feed according to patient needs

Speech therapist

- Assesses the critically ill patient's ability to swallow and develops a care plan with appropriate interventions
- Teaches techniques for dealing with swallowing impairment, communication methods for those with aphasia and techniques to assist with auditory processing difficulties

Wound/ostomy/continence nurse

- Assesses, monitors and makes recommendations to the practitioner regarding the patient's skin integrity, wound management or bowel and bladder issues
- Helps to develop a treatment plan

(continued)

Meet the team (continued)

Dietician

- Monitors a critically ill patient's dietary intake
- Assesses the patient's daily caloric intake and reports deviations
- Devises meal plans and enteral feeding regimes to meet the practitioner-recommended needs for the patient
- Recommends dietary interventions

Pastoral caregiver

- Has title dependent on religious links, e.g. chaplain, priest, imam
- Meets patient's and family's spiritual and religious needs
- Provides support and empathy to the patient and their family
- Delivers patient's last rites (post death rituals) as appropriate

Microbiologist and infection control team

- Educate staff on infection prevention, infection control, infection screening and antibiotic therapy
- Monitor infection rates and investigate infections

Administrative/clerical staff

- Maintain patient's notes and associated unit documentation and records
- Collect data and input for audit purposes
- Perform secretarial and receptionist roles

Supporting each other

It's important to have a colleague to look to for moral support, physical assistance with a patient and problem solving. No one person has all the answers but, together, nurses have a better chance of solving any problem.

Working with doctors

Patients in critical care rarely have only one doctor. Most have an admitting doctor, and daily care is provided by a team of anaesthetic staff with critical care training. Referral to medical specialists may be required, such as:
- a cardiologist
- a neurologist
- a nephrologist
- a haematologist.

In addition, in most hospitals, you will also interact on a regular basis with medical students, junior doctors and trainees who are under the direction of the consultant.

Coordinated efforts

Having a good professional working relationship with doctors involved in patient care is essential. In many cases, a nurse coordinates patient care amongst the many different specialists.

Teamwork requires a lot of coordination! It's so groovy when everything comes together.

Short and sweet

Because a doctor spends only a short period with each patient, it's important that you accurately and succinctly convey important patient information to him during that time. When a doctor is assessing a patient on the unit, you need to relay assessment findings, laboratory data and patient care issues in a concise report.

You'll often collaborate with doctors on patient care decisions; you may even suggest additional treatments or interventions that may benefit the patient. In addition, you need to know when it's important to call the doctor with a change in the patient's condition. Be sure to have important information at hand before you call. (See *Timesaving tip*.)

Working with advanced nurse practitioners

ANPs are increasingly seen working on critical care units. An ANP may be employed to perform roles previously regarded as medical and assist nurses in caring for and monitoring patients. The ANP assists staff nurses in clinical decision-making and enhances the quality of patient care, which improves patient care outcomes.

On a role

An ANP performs roles that may include:
- conducting comprehensive health assessments
- diagnosing
- prescribing pharmacological and nonpharmacological treatments.

An ANP may also conduct research, manage care setting individualised patient care plans and perform advanced procedures, such as removing chest tubes and inserting central lines.

Advice from the experts

Timesaving tip

Make sure that you have everything you need before calling the doctor, including:

- assessment data
- laboratory results
- radiology results.

Be clear about who and where you are and which patient you are calling about. Be ready to report exactly the reason for your call and your level of concern. Having all the necessary information at your fingertips before making the phone call saves time for everyone involved.

Clinical tools

The multidisciplinary team uses various tools to promote safe and comprehensive holistic care. These tools include clinical pathways, practice guidelines and protocols.

Clinical pathways

Clinical pathways (also known as *integrated pathways of care* [*IPOCs*]) are care management plans for patients with a given diagnosis or condition.

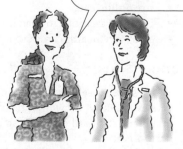

Remember: an ANP works under the supervision of a doctor but has autonomy in making medical decisions.

Follow the path

Clinical pathways are typically generated and used by units that deliver care for similar conditions to many patients. A multidisciplinary group usually develops clinical pathways. The overall goals are to:
- establish a standardised approach to care for all providers in the facility
- establish clear roles for various members of the health care team
- provide a framework for collecting data on patient progress and outcomes.

Tried and true

Pathways are based on evidence from reliable sources, such as benchmarks, research and guidelines. The group gathers and uses information from peer-reviewed literature and experts outside the unit.

Outlines and timelines

Clinical pathways usually outline the duties of all professionals involved with patient care. They follow specific timelines for indicated actions. They also specify expected patient progress and outcomes, which serve as checkpoints for the patient's progress and caregiver's performance.

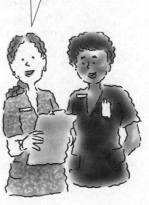

A registered nurse delegates tasks to a health care assistant. Together, they deliver the best possible patient care.

Policies

Policies specify courses of action to be taken in response to a condition or situation. They reflect value judgments about the relative importance of various health and economic outcomes. The policies may come from the Department of Health or be Trust specific.

Policies aid decision making by the health care team. They're multidisciplinary in nature and can be used to coordinate care by multiple providers. Deviation from or disregard for a policy requires careful consideration and discussion with senior staff because adhering to the policy should be the norm.

Let an expert be your guide

Expert health care providers usually write policies. They condense large amounts of information into easily usable formats, combining clinical expertise with the best available clinical evidence. Policies are used to:
- streamline care
- control variations in practice patterns
- distribute health care resources more effectively.

The evidence is in

Policies are valuable sources of information and should be based on up-to-date evidence and reviewed regularly. They also provide a framework for building a standard of care (a statement describing an expected level of care or performance).

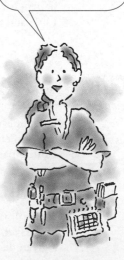

In critical care, we're all packing the most efficient tools to get the job done.

Consider the source

Like research-based information, policies should be evaluated for the quality of their sources. It's a good idea to read the developers' policy statement about how evidence was selected and what values were applied in making recommendations for care.

Protocols

Protocols are unit or Trust-established sets of procedures for a given circumstance. Their purpose is to outline actions that are most likely to produce optimal patient outcomes.

First things first

Protocols describe a sequence of actions a health care professional should take to establish a diagnosis or begin a treatment regimen. For example, a pain management protocol outlines a bedside strategy for managing acute pain.

Protocols facilitate delivery of consistent, cost-effective care. They're also educational resources for clinicians who strive to keep abreast of current best practices. Protocols may be either highly directive or flexible, allowing individuals to use clinical judgment.

Input from experts

Nursing or medical experts write protocols, commonly with input from other health care providers. Hospital committees may approve certain types of protocols for various areas within the Trust.

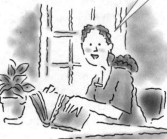

> Oh, my! I must have taken a wrong turn at that last fork. Better march it back to the critical care unit!

> It's the responsibility of every nurse to stay up to date on the latest policies and protocols.

Best practices

As new procedures and medicines become available, nurses committed to excellence regularly update and adapt their practices. An approach known as *best practice* is an important tool for providing high quality care.

Best for all concerned

The term *best practice* refers to clinical practices, treatments and interventions that result in the best possible outcomes for both the patient and your unit.

The best practice approach is generally a team effort that draws on various types of information. Common sources of information used to identify best practices are research data, personal experience and expert opinion. The majority of critical care nurses will not undertake research themselves. More commonly nurses need to be aware of the latest developments and recommendations for practice and be able to review and critique literature, recognising the quality of the findings and the rigour with which the research has been conducted.

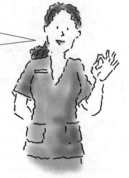

> Simply put, the best practice results in the best possible outcomes for both the patient and your unit—and that's OK with me!

The goal of critical care research is to improve the delivery of care and, thereby, improve patient outcomes. Nursing care is commonly based on evidence that's derived from research. Evidence can be used to support current practices or to change practices.

The most common and best way to get involved in research is to be a good consumer of nursing research. You can do so by reading nursing journals and being aware of the quality of research and reported results.

Share and share alike

Don't be afraid to share research findings with colleagues. Sharing promotes sound clinical care, and everyone involved may learn about easier and more efficient ways to care for patients. This sharing of information might come from unit journal clubs, displaying literature on notice boards, feeding back from critical care courses or study days or just talking to other staff. All critical care nurses have a responsibility to share their knowledge with other staff.

As part of formal critical care education and degree or masters courses you may be involved in undertaking audit or research. Remember that the quality in conducting the research will directly affect the quality of any findings. (See *Research and nursing*.)

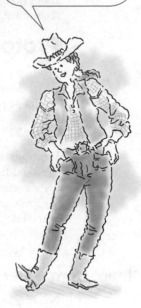

It seems there are more than *two steps* in this research process!

Research and nursing

All scientific research is based on the same basic process.

Research steps

The research process consists of the following steps:

1. **Identify a problem.** Identifying problems in the critical care environment isn't difficult. An example of such a problem is skin breakdown.
2. **Conduct a literature review.** The goal of this step is to see what has been published about the identified problem.
3. **Formulate a research question or hypothesis.** In the case of skin breakdown, one question is, 'Which type of mattress is most protective to the pressure areas of a patient on bed rest?'
4. **Design a study.** The study may be experimental or nonexperimental. The nurse must decide what data are to be collected and how to collect that data.
5. **Obtain consent.** The nurse must obtain consent from the study participants to conduct research. Most hospitals have an internal review board that must approve such permission for studies.
6. **Collect data.** After the study is approved, the nurse can begin conducting the study and collecting the data.
7. **Analyse the data.** The nurse analyses the data and states the conclusions derived from the analysis.
8. **Share the information.** Finally, the researcher shares the collected information with other nurses through publications and presentations.

Evidence-based care

Health care professionals have long recognised the importance of laboratory research and developed ways to make research results more useful in clinical practice. One way is by delivering evidence-based care.

Evidence-based care isn't based on tradition, custom or intuition. It's derived from various concrete sources, such as:

- formal nursing research
- clinical knowledge
- scientific knowledge.

An evidence-based example

Research results may provide insight into the treatment of a patient who, for example, doesn't respond to a medication or treatment that seemed effective for other patients.

In this example, you may believe that a certain drug should be effective for sedation based on previous experience with that drug. The trouble with such an approach is that other factors can contribute to sedative effectiveness, such as pre-admission drug or alcohol use, dosage, organ failure and other concurrent treatments.

First, last and always

Regardless of the value of evidence-based care, you should always use professional clinical judgment when dealing with critically ill patients and their families. Remember that each individual patient's condition ultimately dictates treatment. Critically ill patients have complex conditions and needs and what works with one patient will not necessarily work with another; the skill of critical care nursing is adapting your care to the individual.

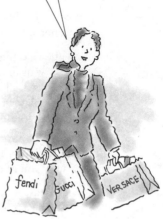

Well, I'm just following the book's advice . . . I read that shopping can be very therapeutic for busy nurses. Isn't this a way of being a good consumer of nursing research?

The goal of delivering evidence-based care is to improve nursing care and patient outcomes.

Quick quiz

1. The most dependent patients in critical care will usually be classified as:
    A. level 0.
    B. level 1.
    C. level 2.
    D. level 3.

Answer: D. Level 3 is intensive care for patients with two or more organ failure/support or requiring mechanical ventilation. Nurse to patient ratios for this level of care have been suggested as one nurse to one patient.

2. Advocacy in critical care nursing focuses on:
    A. the nurse making decisions for the patient.
    B. negotiating on behalf of the patient and their family.

C.   protecting the rights of the health care team.
D.   ensuring the patient survives.

Answer: B. Advocacy focuses on negotiating with other members of the health care team on behalf of the patient and their family.

3.   The purpose of the multidisciplinary team is to:
A.   reduce nursing workload.
B.   replace the concept of primary care in the acute care setting.
C.   minimise costs in critical care.
D.   provide holistic, comprehensive care to the patient.

Answer: D. The purpose of the multidisciplinary team is to provide comprehensive care to the critically ill patient.

4.   When alerting a doctor about a change in a patient's condition, you need to:
A.   wait until he attends the unit.
B.   have all assessment data and laboratory and radiology results available.
C.   ask for treatment ideas.
D.   delegate the phone call to the charge nurse.

Answer: B. Save time by having all assessment data and laboratory and radiology results available when you make the phone call. Let the doctor know why you're calling and what your specific concern is.

5.   The easiest way to participate in research is to:
A.   be a good consumer of research.
B.   collect research data.
C.   conduct a research study.
D.   participate in your hospital's internal research review board.

Answer: A. Being a good consumer of research by reading research articles and judging whether they're applicable to your practice. Research findings aren't useful if they aren't incorporated into practice.

6.   The purpose of evidence-based practice is to:
A.   validate traditional nursing practices.
B.   improve patient outcomes.
C.   remove the need for clinical judgment.
D.   establish a body of knowledge unique to nursing.

Answer: B. Although evidence-based practices may validate or refute traditional practice, the purpose is to improve patient outcomes.

Scoring

☆☆☆   If you answered all six questions correctly, take a bow. You're basically a wiz when it comes to critical care basics.

☆☆   If you answered four or five questions correctly, there's no room for criticism. Your critical thinking skills are basically intact.

☆   If you answered fewer than four questions correctly, the situation is critical. Review the chapter and you'll be on the right pathway.

2 Holistic care issues

Just the facts

In this chapter, you'll learn:

♦ how risk management and safety checks are a vital part of the critical care nurse role

♦ how infection control issues can be managed in critical care

♦ how illness affects family dynamics and family members' ability to cope

♦ about the most common issues that affect critically ill patients and their families

♦ about cognitive issues that affect critically ill patients

♦ how to maintain patient comfort

♦ how to assess and manage pain in critically ill patients

♦ how to assess and manage sedation in critically ill patients

♦ about important questions to consider when faced with decision-making

♦ about concepts related to end-of-life decisions and how they're important to your care.

Here's the whole story about holistic health care.

What is holistic health care?

Holistic health care revolves around a notion of totality. The goal of holistic care is to meet not just the patients' physical needs but also their social and emotional needs.

The whole is the goal

Holistic care addresses all dimensions of a person, including:
• physical
• emotional

- social
- spiritual.

Only by considering all dimensions of a person can the health care team provide high-quality holistic care. You should strive to provide holistic care to all critically ill patients, even though their physical needs may seem more pressing than their other needs.

The issues

The road to the goal of delivering the best holistic care is riddled with various problems or concerns, including:

- risk management and safety issues
- infection control issues
- patient and family issues
- cognitive issues
- patient comfort issues
- pain control issues
- sedation issues
- consent issues
- legal issues
- ethical issues.

Risk management and safety issues

Critical care is a hazardous environment because of the patients' severity of illness and the wide range of complex therapies. The high nurse-to-patient ratios help to reduce risk but you can also practice in a way that helps to keep patients, visitors and staff safe. It is important that patients are not exposed to unnecessary risks in critical care. Both they and their relatives will want assurances of a safe environment.

Be prepared

Critical illness means the patient can deteriorate rapidly so it is important to ensure your patient area or bed-space is prepared for this. Equipment to cope with electricity or medical gas failure should be readily available. Knowing what to do if a patient is accidentally extubated, has a cardiac arrest or develops a tension pneumothorax, and where any necessary equipment is stored should all be part of your preparation. Maintaining a clean and tidy well-stocked bed-space and ensuring infusions and oxygen supplies do not run out are also important.

Extra preparation can be undertaken prior to more hazardous situations like patient admission, transfer, intubation or tracheostomy insertion. Ensuring equipment is to hand will make any procedure easier for all staff and safer for the patient.

Deadly situations—safe systems

Unfortunately human error will always exist so systems should be in place to reduce risk. Education, training and competency assessments all help to make critical care safer. Adhering to set practices and policies is also beneficial. This includes following structured routines at handover periods, such as discussing blood results, providing regular medication and checking ventilator settings and infusions which help to identify and reduce errors. Staffing and skill mix also affect safety. Ensuring that inexperienced staff are supervised by senior staff and the severity of the patient's condition does not exceed staffing competence protects both staff and patients from dangerous situations.

Recognise and report

All staff must be encouraged to undertake risk assessments and act when appropriate to reduce risk or report their concerns to the appropriate person. Examples of risk assessments might include:
- assessment of a delirious patient
- storage of equipment
- manual handling of a patient
- inexperience of a junior nurse.

In accordance with clinical governance guidelines all hospitals have a system of critical incident reporting. These forms are completed whenever an untoward incident occurs, the incident is then investigated and the appropriate follow-up action taken. The incidents are collected centrally and themed allowing recognition of particular hazards. Examples of critical incidents may include:
- equipment unavailability
- equipment failure
- patient/staff falls or other accidents
- delays in treatment
- drug errors.

Safety and risk reduction in critical care is also augmented by the National Patient Safety Agency (NPSA) who inform, support and influence the UK health service by developing guidelines and policies, and the Medicines and Healthcare Products Regulatory Agency (MRHA) who ensure medicines and products work and are safe and if there are any concerns take action to ensure patients and staff are protected.

Infection control issues

The control of infection is important for all nurses but in critical care it is especially important because patients are at increased risk of developing infections and dying from them. Patients should be protected from preventable infections.

Acquiring an infection

Patients in critical care units are often admitted suffering from infections and are also at very high risk of developing infections. The usual host defence mechanisms of skin, mucous membranes and cilia are often disturbed, allowing bacteria to enter. The immune system may be working hard fighting the primary disorder so is unable to carry out its usual detect and destroy functions as effectively. Infections are more common in the elderly, those with underlying chronic conditions, during steroid or immunosuppressive therapies and during prolonged hospital admissions.

Nosocomial or healthcare associated infections (HCAIs) are linked with increased mortality and morbidity and extra health care costs. The most common are urinary tract infections, wound infections and nosocomial pneumonia. Infections associated with vascular access devices, like central lines and arterial lines, are also common.

Recognising infection and screening

An important role of the critical care nurse is to recognise infection and take the appropriate action. Temperature, white blood cell count, respiratory and cardiovascular system changes can all be significant. (See 'Sepsis, severe sepsis and septic shock ', Chapter 10.) Close monitoring and screening of the following are important:
- Sputum—monitor amount, consistency and colour, send sputum sample
- Urine—monitor amount, odour, debris and colour, send urine sample
- Stool—monitor amount, odour and texture, send stool sample
- Invasive line/drain sites—monitor for redness, inflammation and pus, remove if possible and send tip for culture
- Wounds—monitor for redness, inflammation, pus and odour, send wound swab

In addition whenever severe infection or sepsis is suspected, blood cultures must also be sent. (See 'Sepsis, severe sepsis and septic shock ', Chapter 10.)

To find out more information about HCAIs many critical care units are now screening patients on admission particularly for methicillin-resistant *Staphylococcus aureus* (MRSA) and *Clostridium difficile* (C. Diff) if diarrhoea is present. Regular screening may then continue throughout the patients' stay for early identification with the aim of reducing spread to other patients.

Spreading infection

Critical care units are reservoirs of pathogenic organisms. Large numbers of very sick patients, staff transferring organisms between patients and wide use of equipment and antibiotics all contribute to infections. Spread of infection via contamination from hand contact, usually of staff between patients, and endogenous flora on the patient gaining access to sterile areas, e.g. lungs, blood or urine, are the most common causes. In bacterial infections antibiotic resistance reducing eradication increases the number of patients likely to be infected. Following close guidelines for antibiotic prescribing helps limit the incidence and spread of resistance.

Standard precautions

The value of hand washing to reduce HCAIs has been reported for over 100 years. Ensuring that staff and relatives wash their hands before and after patient contact can significantly reduce infection rates. Wearing gloves and aprons when there is a risk of exposure to body fluids reduces risks for patients and staff. A variety of care bundles to reduce HCAIs have been developed as part of a Department of Health campaign (see Chapter 5 for details of the ventilator-associated pneumonia [VAP] care bundle). The care bundles are made up of elements that are known to reduce infection, they provide information, for example, on urinary catheter and central venous catheter insertion and ongoing care. If there is 100% compliance with the elements of these bundles it is suggested that HCAI rates will be virtually nonexistent, so it is probably wise to adopt these care bundles as a standard practice. Keeping the critical care environment clean, decontaminating equipment and bed-spaces and utilising single patient use equipment where possible should also be standard practice.

Special measures

All critical care units will have the support of infection control teams and microbiologists. They will review infection control policies and procedures, monitor and investigate infection outbreaks and antibiotic resistance and have a key role in educating staff. In certain situations or with certain patients special measures need to be taken to prevent infection. Policies and the infection control team provide guidance on the need for isolation nursing and any other specific precautions, e.g. masks and visors. For example, patients with MRSA or C. Diff will be closely monitored and routes of transmission investigated. Any organisms with antibiotic resistance and high risks of transmission will usually require patient isolation. In all these cases isolation aims to prevent other patients from contracting the infection.

Patients with compromised immune systems will require protective isolation to prevent them from becoming infected. Haematological conditions, e.g. leukaemia or following a bone marrow transplant, can result in neutropenia and these patients must be protected.

Certain diseases must legally be notified to a consultant for communicable disease control. Amongst others these include:
- acute encephalitis
- meningitis and Meningococcal sepsis
- dysentery (amoebic and bacillary)
- food poisoning (or suspected)
- malaria

- measles
- mumps
- rubella
- scarlet fever
- smallpox
- tetanus
- tuberculosis
- viral hepatitis A, B, C and other
- hooping cough (Pertussis).

In any situations where advice is required the infection control team will usually be able to provide support and guidance.

Patient and family issues

A family is a group of two or more persons who may live together in the same household, perform certain interrelated social tasks and share an emotional bond. Families can profoundly influence the individuals within them. Some families will already have complex or difficult relationships.

Family ties

A family is a dynamic system. During stress-free times, this system may maintain homeostasis, meaning that it exists in a stable state of harmony and balance. However, when a crisis sends a family member into a critical care environment, family members may feel a tremendous strain and family homeostasis is thrown off. The major effects of such imbalances are:

- increased stress levels for family members
- fear of death for the patient
- reorganisation of family roles
- the need for contact between members who may be estranged.

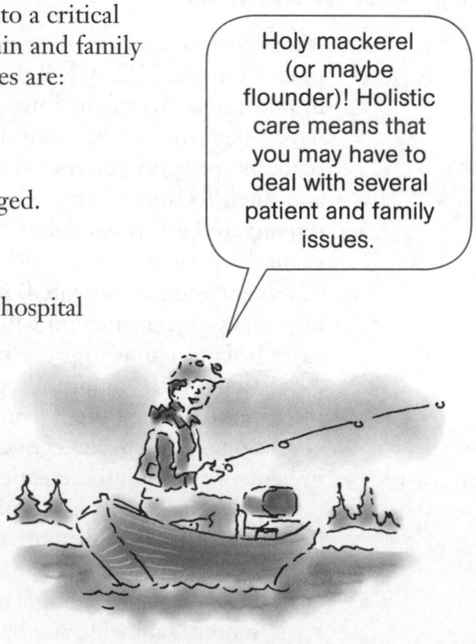

Unprepared for the worst

The family may be caught off-guard by sudden exposure to the hospital environment, causing homeostasis to be disrupted. Family members may worry about the possible death of the ill family member. The ramifications of the patient's illness may cause other family members to feel hopeless and helpless.

Circle out of round

When critical illness or injury disrupts the family circle, the patient can no longer fulfil certain role responsibilities. Such roles are typically:

- financial (if the patient is a major contributor to the family's monetary stability)

> Holy mackerel (or maybe flounder)! Holistic care means that you may have to deal with several patient and family issues.

- social (if the patient fills such roles as spouse, parent)
- emotional (if the patient fills such roles as supporter, mediator or disciplinarian).

One thing leads to another

A sudden shift in the patient's ability to bear family responsibilities can create havoc and a feeling of overwhelming responsibility for other family members. The family members may blame themselves (or the health care team) for the patient being critically ill.

Nursing responsibilities

Because a critical illness or injury greatly affects family members as well, be sure to provide care to the family too. Members of the patient's family need guidance and support during the patient's hospital stay. The critical care nurse's responsibility to family members is to provide information about:
- nursing care
- the patient's prognosis and expected treatments
- ways to communicate with the patient
- what they can do to help the patient
- support services that are available.

Slipping on emotional turmoil

The critically ill patient's condition may change rapidly (within minutes or hours). The result of such physiological instability is emotional turmoil for the family.

The family may use whatever coping mechanisms they have, such as seeking support from friends or clergy. The longer the patient remains in critical care, the more stress for both the patient and their family. The result can be a slow deterioration of the family system.

Step in and lend a helping hand

Because you're regularly exposed to members of the patient's family, you can help them during their time of crisis. For example, you can observe the anxiety level of family members and, if necessary, refer them to another member of the multidisciplinary team, such as a social worker.

You can also help family members solve problems by assisting them to:
- verbalise the immediate problem
- identify support systems
- recall how they handled stress in the past.

Such assistance helps family members to focus on the present issue. It also allows them to solve problems and regain a sense of control over their lives.

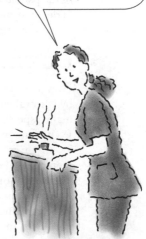

Stand by to answer whatever questions family members have. They may turn to you for guidance and support.

Lean on me

You can also help family members cope with their feelings during this stressful time. Two ways to do this are by encouraging them to express their feelings (such as by crying or discussing the issue) and by providing empathy. You can help them practically by providing them with information about travel to and from the hospital, parking availability and the on-site shops and amenities. You will also need to let them know the location of the nearby waiting and visitor rooms as well as details of hospital accommodation.

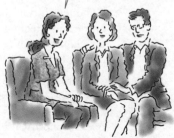

Be prepared to orientate the family to the critical care environment.

Since you asked

During a patient's critical illness, family members come to rely on the opinions of professionals and commonly ask for their input. They need honest information to be given to them in terms they can understand. In many cases, you're the health care team member who provides this information. (See *Tips for helping the family cope*, page 27.)

A dose of reality

The best way to respond to concerned family members is to acknowledge their feelings and ambivalences and to lend reality to their statements, e.g. 'It must be difficult for you having to look after the children and support them as well as visiting the hospital every day'.

Living with the decision

The nurse can provide the facts to the family but then needs to accept that different people will act in different ways. Using such phrases as 'It is entirely up to you whether you decide to stay here or go home tonight, whatever you feel you want to do is okay' means the critical care nurse can reinforce and acknowledge the family's decision and accept their feelings and decisions. But it is important that the nurse is sure that the relatives have grasped the severity of the patient's condition prior to making decisions. Another important issue in decision-making is highlighting to the family the legal responsibilities of the medical staff with regard to treatment limits or withdrawal.

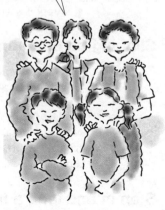

Always honour the cultural beliefs and values of patients and family members.

Cultural considerations

How a family copes with the hospitalisation of a loved one can be influenced by cultural characteristics. A patient's cultural background can also affect many aspects of care, such as:
- patient and family roles during illness
- communication between health care providers and the patient and family members
- feelings of the patient and family members about end-of-life issues
- patient and family views regarding health care practices
- pain management
- nutrition
- spiritual support.

Tips for helping the family cope

A significant role for the nurse is orientating a patient's family to the critical care unit. Here are some useful tips for dealing with family members of critically ill patients.

The environment

If it the first time the relatives have visited it is a good idea to greet the family at the door and explain to them what to expect. Ensure the relatives can see the patient by seating them on the side the patient is lying and lowering the bed if necessary. Make the relatives feel welcome and not a hindrance by introducing yourself and spending time with them. Explain what the equipment is for and what alarms mean. Explain the infection control measures.

Please touch

Let family members know that it's okay to touch the patient. Many are afraid to touch a critically ill loved one for fear of interfering with monitoring equipment or invasive lines. Let them know if there are any special considerations when touching the patient.

How's the weather?

Many family members spend their visitation time looking at equipment in the room and asking the patient questions such as, 'Are you in pain?' Encourage them to focus on the patient, not necessarily their pain or surroundings. You may have to explain on a daily basis how they should behave depending on changes in condition, for example, if the patient is agitated they should be calm and reassuring and if the patient is apathetic they should be upbeat and positive.

Let family members know how to be visitors. The patient wants to hear about the outside world— not reminders that they're ill and hospitalised. They may want to hear about other family members, the family pet and who won the latest football match. It is important to encourage and motivate the patient and remind them about what they have to get better for.

One at a time, please

Ask the family to appoint one spokesperson for the group. This is especially important when families are large. The spokesperson is the person who should call the unit for updates on the patient's condition. The spokesperson can then spread the word to the rest of the family. It may also be helpful to identify a primary nursing contact for the family.

Should they stay or should they go?

Allow family members to stay at the patient's bedside when appropriate. For example, a patient may require constant monitoring to keep them from trying to climb out of bed. If a family member is available to stay with such a patient, the use of sedatives and restraints could be avoided.

On the other hand, some patients appear to be agitated and have adverse changes in their vital signs when certain family members are present. Remember: Your first role is to be a patient advocate and to do what's best for the patient. Ask them whether they want to have visitors and whom they want to visit. If having a family member is best for the patient, then allow the visitor to stay. Many units have open visitation policies but this should also be matched with needs of the relatives who should not be made to feel guilty if they find visiting difficult.

Ensure support

Ensure that support services are available to family members if they need them. If they belong to a particular church, offer to call someone if needed. Most facilities provide spiritual care for families if they request it.

Practical help

Providing information about rest facilities, patient accommodation, parking availability and on-site shops and amenities all help to make the relatives' experience in critical care less distressing.

Culture-clued for care

Because your knowledge about cultural characteristics affects care, you should perform a cultural assessment. (See *Assessing cultural considerations*, page 29.)

Conducting a cultural assessment enables you to:
- recognise a patient's cultural responses to illness and hospitalisation
- determine how the patient and their family define health and illness
- determine the family's beliefs about the cause of the illness.

To provide effective holistic care, you must honour the patient's cultural beliefs and values.

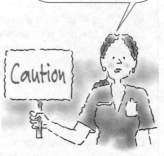

Although it's good to be aware of cultural considerations, make sure that you don't stereotype patients based on their cultural backgrounds.

Cognitive issues

Patients on a critical care unit may feel overwhelmed by the technology around them. Although this equipment is essential for patient care, it can create an environment that's foreign to the patient, which can result in disturbed cognition (thought-related function). In addition, the disease process can affect cognitive function in a critically ill patient. For example, patients with metabolic disturbances or hypoxia can experience confusion and changes in mental clarity.

The way things were

When assessing cognitive function, the first question you should ask is, 'What activities were you able to perform by yourself?' If the patient can't answer this question, ask a family member. If the patient has been transferred to critical care from another ward, ask the nurse who provided care before the transfer.

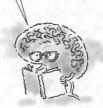

Uh-oh! It says here that the disease process can affect cognitive function.

It's a factor

Many factors affect a patient's cognitive function whilst critically ill, including:
- medications
- sensory input
- invasion of personal space
- emotional status
- medical diagnosis
- spiritual status.

Medications

Some medications that can cause adverse central nervous system reactions and affect cognitive function include:
- inotropes—such as digoxin, which can cause agitation, hallucinations, malaise, dizziness, vertigo and parasthesia
- barbiturates—such as phenobarbital, which can cause drowsiness, lethargy, hangover symptoms, physical and psychological dependence and paradoxical excitement (in elderly patients)

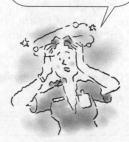

Inotropic medications can cause a patient to become agitated or to hallucinate.

Advice from the experts

Assessing cultural considerations

A cultural assessment yields the information you need to administer high quality nursing care to members of various cultural populations. The goal of the cultural assessment quest is to gain awareness and understanding of cultural variations and their effects on the care you provide. For each patient, you and other members of the multidisciplinary team use the findings of a cultural assessment to develop an individualised care plan.

When performing a cultural assessment, be sure to ask questions that yield information about the patient and their family, including information about:

- cultural health beliefs
- communication methods
- cultural restrictions
- social networks
- nutritional status
- religion
- values and beliefs

Here are examples of the types of questions you should consider for each patient.

Cultural health beliefs

- What does the patient believe caused their illness? A patient may believe that their illness is the result of an imbalance in yin and yang, punishment for a past transgression or the result of divine wrath.
- How does the patient express pain?
- What does the patient believe promotes health? Beliefs can range from eating certain foods to wearing amulets for good luck.
- In what types of healing practices (such as herbal remedies and healing rituals) does the patient engage?
- Who do the patients go to when they're ill? (Some patients may go to a doctor, a medicine man or a holistic practitioner.)

Communication methods

- What language does the patient speak?
- Does the patient require an interpreter?

- How does the patient want to be addressed?
- What are the styles of nonverbal communication (eye contact, touching)?

Cultural restrictions

- How does the patient's cultural group express emotion?
- How are feelings about death, dying and grief expressed?
- How is modesty expressed?
- Does the patient have restrictions related to exposure of any parts of the body?

Social networks

- What are the roles of each family member during health and illness?
- Who makes the decisions?

Nutritional status

- What's the meaning of food and eating to the patient?
- What types of food do they eat?
- Does the patient's food need to be prepared in a certain way?
- Are there dietary restrictions?

Religion

- What's the role of religious beliefs and practices during illness?
- Does the patient believe that special rites or blessings need to be performed?
- Are there healing rituals or practices that must be followed?

Values and beliefs

- What particular values do the patient and their family hold? (For example a wife may wish to provide all physical care)
- Are their any particular beliefs within the culture?

- corticosteroids—such as prednisone, which can cause euphoria, psychotic behaviour, insomnia, vertigo, headache, paraesthesia and seizures
- benzodiazepines—such as lorazepam, which can cause drowsiness, sedation, disorientation, amnesia, unsteadiness and agitation
- opioid analgesics—such as morphine, which can cause sedation, difficulty concentrating or processing information, euphoria, dizziness, light-headedness and somnolence.

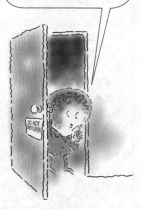

Shhh! Keep it down as much as possible because noise can result in delirium.

Sensory input

Sensory stimulation in any environment may be perceived as pleasant or unpleasant and comfortable or painful. The critical care environment tends to stimulate all five senses:
- auditory
- visual
- taste
- olfactory
- tactile.

Too much or too little

Patients in critical care don't have control over the environmental stimulation around them. They may experience sensory deprivation, sensory overload or both. Sensory deprivation can result from a reduction in the quantity and quality of normal and familiar sensory input, such as the normal sights and sounds encountered at home, especially if the patient is in isolation. Sensory overload results from an increase in the amount of unfamiliar sounds and sights in the critical care environment, such as beeping cardiac monitors, ringing telephones, ventilator and pump alarms, voices and attachment to monitoring and invasive devices.

When environmental stimuli exceed the patient's ability to cope with the stimulation, the patient may experience anxiety, confusion and panic as well as delusions.

A sensitive subject

Sensory deprivation or overload can lead to such problems as sleep disturbances, reality disturbances, delirium and emotional distress.

Sleep disturbances

Because the critical care environment is typically noisy due to staff, other patients and equipment alarms, patients commonly experience sleep disturbances.

Other factors that interfere with sleep include nursing interventions, pain, fear, breathlessness, thirst, hunger, temperature derangements, loss of circadian rhythm, inability to create darkness and restrictions in movement.

Torture chamber

Sleep deprivation can cause anxiety, restlessness, disorientation, depression, irritability, confusion, aggression and hallucinations.

In addition, sleep deprivation can cause further medical problems, such as:

- immunosuppression
- decreased pain tolerance
- decreased muscle strength.

In other words, sleep deprivation can impede the recovery process and contribute to new problems.

Quiet time

To promote rest, the critical care nurse can take steps to provide a quieter environment for patients.

For example, the nurse may reduce light and noise by not having loud conversations near the patient and by closing the door to the patient's room if it's safe to do so. Using eye masks and earplugs may be appropriate for some patients. Creating a pre-sleep routine like bed bathing, providing a warm milky drink and relaxing music or a hand massage may help. Careful positioning and extra blankets in apyrexial patients are useful. It is worth remembering that air flow mattresses are notoriously cool especially at night. Some patients may welcome fans in warm weather. Make sure any concerns the patient has are addressed before they try to sleep and determine whether the patient feels better with you in close proximity or wishes you to retreat to a safe distance.

An average sleep cycle passing through all four stages of sleep and including rapid eye movement (REM) sleep, which is closely linked to psychological wellbeing, lasts around 90 minutes. Therefore every effort should be made to ensure sleeping patients are left undisturbed for this period at the very least.

Opinions differ greatly regarding resumption of circadian rhythms. Preventing patients from sleeping in the day so that they will sleep at night can cause increased agitation and confusion in an already sleep-deprived patient. Sleep requirements increase with illness and it is rare that any patients on a critical care unit achieve an optimal amount of good quality sleep. Performing activities during the day such as sitting out in a chair but also allowing periods of rest and sleep if desired is probably a reasonable option.

Hypnotics and sedatives should be avoided if possible owing to their association with delirium. They should only be considered if the patient normally uses them or all other interventions have failed.

Reality disturbances

Integration of the senses is necessary for a person to process environmental information. Disturbances in reality occur when a patient's ability to interpret the environment is altered. Examples of reality disturbances are:

- disorientation to time
- inability to decipher whether it's night or day
- misinterpretation of environmental stimuli—for example, thinking that alarms and noises from equipment are phones ringing for the patient.

I know how hard it is when I don't get all my sleep. Imagine what it's like for a sleep-deprived patient ... pure torture!

When your reality is altered, it isn't a pretty sight.

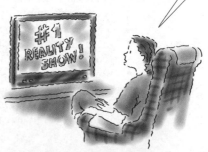

The surreal world

Hearing or vision loss or loss of consciousness (caused, for example, by a head injury) can make a patient especially vulnerable to reality disturbances. Lack of one or more sensory mechanisms that are necessary to function makes it hard for the patient to adapt to the critical care environment.

Delirium

Delirium (acute confusion) is an altered state of consciousness and cognition which cannot be explained by a pre-existing condition. It consists of confusion, distractibility, disorientation, delusional thinking, defective perception and agitation or hypoactivity. It has been referred to by different names over time, e.g. *ICU psychosis*, acute confusional state and ICU syndrome. Delirium has a rapid onset and is generally reversible. It is unrecognised in large numbers of patients and incidence is increasing with a growing elderly population. It is estimated that over 50% of critically ill patients develop delirium.

Common contributors

In addition to sensory deprivation or overload, contributing factors that affect patients in critical care include:
- infection
- poor pain control
- immobility
- drug/alcohol/nicotine withdrawal
- organ failure
- visual, hearing and communication impairment
- malnutrition
- electrolyte derangement
- medications given (opiates, benzodiazepines, drugs with anticholinergic effects, e.g. frusemide and digoxin).

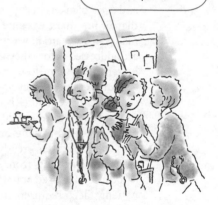

The critical care environment doesn't allow for much personal space—for you or the patient!

Antidelirium

The nurse can assist the patient suffering from delirium by:
- minimising common contributors where possible, e.g. appropriate drug withdrawal regimes, good hydration, nutrition and pain control
- promoting rest and facilitating sleep
- decreasing noise and artificial light in the room at rest times
- encouraging mobility when possible, especially sitting out in a chair as soon as possible
- providing repeated orientation to the patient
- removing monitors, lines and catheters as soon as possible
- providing cognitive stimulation several times per day, e.g. asking about previous employment/hobbies/family, radio, television etc.
- using communication adjuncts
- involving family in care provision.

Antidelirium—pharmacological management

If nonpharmacological measures remain unsuccessful, the nurse can assist the patient suffering from delirium by:
- reviewing current medication
- providing appropriate replacement therapy if the patient is suffering withdrawal symptoms, e.g. nicotine patches for smokers, morphine or methodone for heroin addiction, chlordiazepoxide or lorazepam for alcohol withdrawal and lorazepam or diazepam for benzodiazepine withdrawal
- administering the antipsychotic Haloperidol if the patient is unmanageable
- sedating with Lorazepam for chemical restraint if the patient continues to be a danger to themselves and others and all other therapies have been unsuccessful; however, the risks of causing further delirium must be evaluated.

Antidelirium—physical restraint

Physical restraint is less culturally acceptable in the UK than some other countries but in some situations it may be thought necessary. If nonpharmacological measures remain unsuccessful the nurse can protect the patient suffering from delirium by:
- ensuring a comprehensive multidisciplinary assessment is made and documented (this should focus on whether the patient is a danger to themselves or others)
- applying equipment specifically designed for physical restraint, e.g. padded mits (boxing gloves)
- reassessing the patient on a regular basis (2–4 hourly) to determine whether the physical restraint is still required and removing the restraints as soon as possible
- providing reassurance and explanation to the patient and their relatives regarding the restraints.

Space invasion—respecting privacy and dignity

Personal space is the unmarked boundary or territory around a person; protection of this is usually maintained by respect for individual privacy and dignity. Several factors—such as cultural background and social situation—influence a patient's interpretation of personal space, privacy and dignity. A patient's personal space and privacy is limited in many ways by the critical care environment—for example, due to the confines of bed rest, need to access parts of the body, dependence on others for care and use of invasive equipment. The Department of Health has implemented policies to ensure single-sex accommodation for patients. Although critical care areas are exempt from this it seems important to promote separation whenever possible.

You can try to increase your patient's sense of personal space and respect their privacy and dignity—even within the critical care environment—by simply remembering to show common courtesy, such as:

- asking permission to perform a procedure or look at a wound or dressing
- pulling the curtain or closing the door
- knocking before you enter the patient's room
- nursing same sex patients in adjacent beds or bays
- dressing the patient in a gown or nightwear
- keeping the patient partially covered when bed bathing
- involving the family where appropriate in personal care.

Patient comfort issues

Providing comfort to patients is a vital part of the critical care nurse role. It consists of many elements including aiding, encouraging, reassuring and consoling. To provide comfort you need to be attentive to your individual patient's needs, recognise the problem and be able to modify care. Pain, sleep and rest are specific comfort issues and are covered in separate sections; other comfort issues are:

- providing physical care such as positioning, mouthcare, washing and styling hair
- creating a therapeutic nurse–patient relationship by trust, respect, patience and open communication
- demonstrating your availability for physical and psychological care as well as respecting patient privacy
- minimising the constraints of the technical environment, e.g. ensuring alarm parameters are set appropriately, lowering the bed and cotsides if safe to do so when visitors are present
- allowing the individuals to continue their familiar rituals and routines, e.g. watching soap operas, not eating breakfast.

If comfort issues are respected and prioritised to the same extent as physical and technical elements of care, there is more patient, family and staff satisfaction.

Pain control issues

Because fear of pain is a major concern for many critically ill patients, pain management is an important part of your care.

Critical care patients are exposed to many types of procedures—such as I.V. procedures, cardiac monitoring and intubation—that cause discomfort and pain. Pain is classified as acute or chronic.

Acute pain

Acute pain is caused by tissue damage due to injury or disease. It varies in intensity from mild to severe and usually resolves as the patient recovers from their illness or the injury heals (lasts generally up to 6 months).

Acute pain is considered a protective mechanism because it warns of present or potential tissue damage or organ disease. It may result from a traumatic injury, surgical or diagnostic procedure or medical disorder. Examples of acute pain are:

- pain experienced during a dressing change
- pain related to surgery
- pain of acute myocardial infarction
- pain of immobility
- generalised pain from joints and tissues because of the immune response.

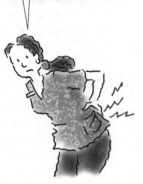

Acute pain can be managed effectively, and it generally subsides when the underlying problem is resolved. That's a relief!

Help is at hand

Acute pain can be managed effectively with analgesics, such as opioids, paracetamol and nonsteroidal antiinflammatory drugs (NSAIDs). It generally subsides when the underlying problem is resolved.

Chronic pain

Chronic pain is pain that has lasted 6 months or longer and is ongoing. It may be as intense as acute pain. It may signify tissue damage, for example, osteo or rheumatoid arthritis, or nerve damage in diabetic neuropathy, or there may be no damage to explain the pain in, for example, long-term low back pain. Some patients in critical care experience chronic as well as acute pain.

Examples of chronic pain include:

- arthritis pain
- back pain
- pain from cancer.

Don't look for the signs

The nervous system adapts to pain. This means that many typical manifestations of pain—such as abnormal vital signs and facial grimacing—reduce but are apparent when pain increases or is new. Therefore, in critical care chronic pain should be assessed as often as acute pain (generally, at least every 2 hours or more often, depending on the patient's condition). Assess pain by questioning the patient.

Pain assessment

When it comes to pain assessment for critical care patients, it's especially important for the nurse to have good assessment skills. Pain assessment is most important as a tool to evaluate the efficacy of treatment and the course of disease. The most valid pain assessment comes from the patient's own reports of pain.

A pain assessment includes questions about:
• location—ask the patient to tell you where the pain is; there may be more than one area of pain
• intensity—ask the patient to rate the pain using a pain scale
• quality—ask how the pain feels: sharp, dull, aching or burning
• onset, duration and frequency—ask when the pain started, how long it lasts and how often it occurs
• alleviating and aggravating factors—ask what makes the pain feel better and what makes it worse
• associated factors—ask whether other problems are associated with the pain, such as nausea and vomiting.

When it comes to pain, the best validation comes from the patient's own reports of pain.

Choose a tool

Many pain assessment tools are available. Whichever you choose, make sure it's used consistently so that everyone on the health care team is speaking the same language when addressing the patient's pain.

The four most common pain assessment tools used by clinicians are verbal pain-rating, behavioural pain-rating, numerical rating and the faces scale. (See *Common pain-rating scales*, page 37.) The tool should be readily available for all to use and pain assessment should be performed regularly (usually when recording observations) and documented. Pain should be assessed at rest and on movement. If the assessment identifies the patient has moderate or severe pain, action must be taken to alleviate the pain then reassessed until mild pain or no pain remains on movement.

Uncontrollable pain

If severe pain persists despite maximum therapy, other contributory factors should be considered:
• equipment or cannula malfunction affecting delivery of the analgesia
• adjuvants like antidepressants, anticonvulsants or nerve blocks
• worsening patient condition like internal infection or ischaemia elevating pain levels
• psychological elements of pain
• preadmission analgesia usage (prescribed and nonprescribed).

Prevention is better than cure

Once a patient is experiencing severe pain, it is more difficult to achieve a pain-free state and the patient will be fearful of the pain returning. Therefore it is important to have a plan for pain management with drugs prescribed before severe pain emerges. This can readily be undertaken with elective patients and should be prioritised with emergency patients. When administering analgesia the aim is to maintain patients as pain-free or with mild pain on movement.

Common pain-rating scales

These scales are examples of the rating systems you can use to help a patient quantify pain levels.

Verbal pain-rating scale

To use the verbal pain-rating scale, ask the patients to categorise their current level of pain. They should be asked, giving the options below, how they feel both at rest and on movement.

No pain **Mild pain** **Moderate pain** **Pain as bad as it can be**

Behavioural pain-rating scale

Sedated or confused patients may not be able to report their level of pain so the nurse has to use other information to determine presence of pain. Objective cues like tachycardia, hypertension, sweating, pupil dilation, fighting the ventilator, grimacing or guarding should all be considered in the assessment.

No pain—patient appears comfortable on interventions like suctioning or moving

Mild pain—patient shows some signs of discomfort on intervention which settle immediately

Moderate pain—patient shows signs of discomfort in the absence of interventions

Severe pain—patient appears distressed and agitated despite adequate sedation and reassurance

Numerical pain-rating scale

To use the numeric rating scale ask the patient to choose a number from 0 (indicating no pain) to 10 (indicating the worst pain imaginable) to describe their current pain level. The patient may circle the number on the scale or verbally state the number that best describes the pain.

No pain 0 1 2 3 4 5 6 7 8 9 10 **Pain as bad as it can be**

Faces scale

A paediatric or adult patient with language difficulty may not be able to describe the current pain level using the visual analogue scale or the numeric rating scale. In that case, use a faces scale like the one below. Ask your patient to choose the face on a scale from 1 to 6 that best represents the severity of current pain.

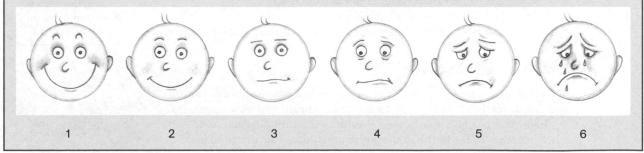

1   2   3   4   5   6

The sounds of silence

Many patients can't verbally express feelings of pain. For example, a patient may be unable to speak due to intubation or have an altered level of consciousness (LOC) ranging from confusion to unresponsiveness. In such cases, it's up to the nurse to ascertain the patient's pain level and this is notoriously difficult.

Body and mind

There are many physiological and psychological responses to pain that the nurse should watch for during a pain assessment. But you must remember that physiological responses are transient and a patient can be in pain without evidence of physiological response.

Some examples of the physiological responses to pain are:
- tachycardia
- tachypnoea
- dilated pupils
- increased or decreased blood pressure
- pallor
- grimacing
- guarding
- ventilator asynchrony
- nausea and vomiting
- loss of appetite.

Psychological responses to pain may manifest as:
- fear
- anxiety
- confusion
- depression
- sleep deprivation.

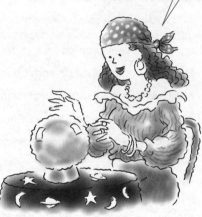

When a patient can't tell you about feelings of pain, it's up to you to see the unspoken signs.

Pain particulars

When communicating aspects of a patient's pain to the doctor or other health care providers, make sure you:
- describe the pain by location, intensity and duration
- indicate possible causes of the pain if known
- describe how the patient is responding to the pain or treatment interventions.

Enjoy the rest, pal. Once we're called up to critical care, there's no break until the end of the first half.

Pain management

Achieving adequate pain control in critical care depends on effective pain assessment and the use of pharmacological and nonpharmacological treatments.

To provide the best holistic care possible, work with the doctor and other members of the health care team to develop an individualised pain management programme for each patient.

Pharmacological pain management

Pharmacological pain management is common in critical care.

The WHO analgesic ladder

The World Health Organisation (WHO) developed a three-step ladder (shown here) to guide pain-relief efforts for patients. Analgesics are selected based on the intensity of the patient's pain. The ladder includes three categories of drugs: nonopioids, opioids and adjuvant drugs. Adjuvant drugs such as antidepressants and anticonvulsants can be used on any step of the ladder.

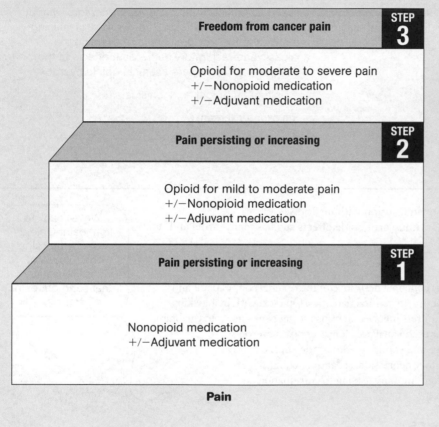

Freedom from cancer pain

STEP 3

Opioid for moderate to severe pain
+/−Nonopioid medication
+/−Adjuvant medication

Pain persisting or increasing

STEP 2

Opioid for mild to moderate pain
+/−Nonopioid medication
+/−Adjuvant medication

Pain persisting or increasing

STEP 1

Nonopioid medication
+/−Adjuvant medication

Pain

When the patient's pain reaches the moderate-to-severe level, administer more potent opioid drugs, including morphine, oxycodone, fentanyl or diamorphine. Nonopioid drugs may be continued.

Add opioid drugs, such as low-dose oral or sub-cut morphine or tramadol, for the patient with mild-to-moderate pain that isn't relieved by a nonopioid. If the patient is already taking NSAIDs, continue to use them as they add to the analgesic effect.

Administer nonopioid analgesics, such as paracetamol, and nonsteroidal antiinflammatory drugs (NSAIDs), to the patient just beginning to experience discomfort and mild pain. Although the patient's pain might not be adequately controlled with nonopioid drugs, their use may reduce the overall amount of opioids needed to achieve pain control.

Take three and call in the morning

Three classes of medications commonly used by the critical care nurse are:
- nonopioids
- opioids
- adjuvant medications. (See *The WHO analgesic ladder*.)

Nonopioids

Nonopioids are the first choice for managing mild pain. They decrease pain by inhibiting inflammation at the injury site. Examples of nonopioids are:
- paracetamol (caution with hepatic impairment)
- NSAIDs, such as ibuprofen and diclofenac (caution with renal failure, asthmatics, ulcer disease and clotting abnormalities)

Opioids

Opioids block the release of neurotransmitters that send pain signals to the brain. The three categories of opioids are opioid agonists (narcotic analgesics), opioid antagonists (narcotic reversal agents) and mixed agonist–antagonists.

Opioid agonists

Opioid agonists relieve pain by binding to pain receptors, which, in effect, produces pain relief Examples of opioid agonists are:

- morphine
- fentanyl
- alfentanil
- pethidine
- tramadol
- codeine
- dihydrocodeine
- oxycodone.

Opioid antagonists

Opioid antagonists attach to opiate receptors without producing agonistic effects. They work by displacing the opioid at the receptor site and reversing the analgesic and respiratory depressant effects of the opioid; therefore, they are useful in opioid overdose.

Example of an opioid antagonist is:

- naloxone (Narcan)

- salicylates such as aspirin (caution with ulcer disease)
- nefopam (may have antimuscarinic side effects such as tachycardia and dry mouth).

Opioids

Opioids are narcotics that contain a derivative of the opium (poppy) plant and other synthetic drugs that imitate natural narcotics. Opioids work by blocking the release of neurotransmitters involved in transmitting pain signals to the brain. Morphine is still the most useful analgesic for severe pain even though it can cause nausea and vomiting. Other side effects of opioids include respiratory depression, sedation, itching, vasodilation and reduced gut motility leading to constipation (See *Opioids*).

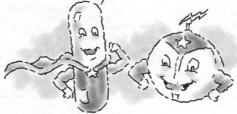

We're ready to fight pain! Opioids work by blocking the release of neurotransmitters that send out pain signals.

Adjuvant analgesics

Adjuvant analgesics are drugs that have other primary indications but are used as analgesics in some circumstances.

Alone or together

Adjuvants may be given in combination with opioids or alone to treat patients with chronic pain and acute pain. Drugs used as adjuvant analgesics include:

- anticonvulsants, such as carbamazepine and gabapentin especially for neuropathic pain
- tricyclic antidepressants, such as amitriptyline
- benzodiazepines, such as diazepam
- corticosteroids, such as dexamethasone and methylprednisolone.

Drug administration

One route of pain medication administration in critical care is I.V. bolus on an as-needed basis. It's the preferred route for opioid therapy, especially when short-term pain relief is needed—for example, during procedures such as wound care. The benefit of this method is rapid pain control. On the downside, with I.V. bolus administration, as well as risks of hypotension, the patient experiences alternating periods of pain control and pain and the analgesia is not given until pain is recognised by the nurse.

Round-the-clock control

Using continuous infusions ensures that steady levels of drugs prevent exacerbations of pain. This type of dosing has many benefits for critically ill patients who have difficulty communicating their pain because of altered LOC or endotracheal intubation. Unfortunately there are risks of overdosage especially in patients with renal or hepatic dysfunction. Therefore pain and sedation assessment must be performed regularly.

Patients overpower pain

Some patients are candidates for patient-controlled analgesia (PCA). PCA provides a supply of pain medication allowing the patient to self-administer as needed. Lock-out controls are set to prevent excessive self-administration. (See *Understanding PCA*.) Because analgesia is not administered unless the patient presses, the control it is important that they are able to operate it properly.

> Round-the-clock dosing controls pain better than as-needed administration.

Understanding PCA

A patient-controlled analgesia (PCA) system can provide an optimal opioid dose administered by the patient, thus maintaining a more stable concentration of the drug.

Pump and port

A PCA system consists of a specialised syringe-type injection pump delivering drugs intravenously, epidurally or subcutaneously.

By pressing a button, the patient receives a preset bolus dose of an opioid, for example, 1 mg morphine. The practitioner orders the bolus dose. The lock-out time between boluses is usually 5 minutes thus reducing the risk of overdose. The device automatically records the number of times the patient presses the button, helping you to determine analgesic requirements.

Patient at the controls

Using a PCA system may reduce a patient's drug dosage need. This may be because the patient using PCA is more in control of pain and typically feels reassured knowing that an analgesic is quickly available.

Patients usually report that they have more control over pain levels when using PCA. In some cases they may require more analgesia than the pump is set to administer and the bolus amount may have to be increased or a background continuous infusion may have to be set. Patients using PCA still require close assessment and evaluation for responses to treatment and amount of drug used. Most PCA pumps record the number of times the patient has tried to administer analgesia. If there is a large number of tries in the lock-out period, the patient may either have severe pain or may not understand fully how the PCA works.

A caveat

Note that PCA may not be appropriate for patients with altered LOC or those with renal or hepatic abnormalities.

Local anaesthesia

Local anaesthesia is an important and common method of analgesia used in critical care units that is not included in the WHO analgesic ladder. Most commonly epidural anaesthesia is used in elective abdominal and orthopaedic surgery. Pleural and sternal blocks may be seen in trauma cases with fractured ribs or sternums, and local anaesthesia with lignocaine may be seen for invasive procedures, e.g. central line and chest drain insertion. For epidurals the local anaesthetic bupivacaine is usually used and fentanyl and bupivacaine pre-prepared infusions are included in many hospital epidural policies.

Local anaesthesia can provide very effective pain relief if coverage of the block is adequate. Assessment of pain, insertion site, motor and sensory block should be routinely performed to ensure adequate analgesia without risks. The complications of epidurals specifically include hypotension, bradycardia, itching, infection, urinary retention (if not catheterised), haemorrhage and autonomic dysreflexia (hypertension secondary to stimuli below the level of block).

Nonpharmacological pain management

Pain control isn't achieved solely with medications. Nonpharmacological means are useful adjuncts in managing pain. Most importantly a therapeutic nurse–patient relationship with good communication and attention to comfort measures will aid pain control. Pain will be increased by fear and anxiety and therefore nursing care should be targeted to alleviate these feelings.

Some other common nonpharmacological pain control methods are:
- distraction—such as television viewing, reading and chatting
- music therapy—a form of sound therapy using rhythmic sound to communicate, relax and encourage healing (this method works for brief periods).

You're getting sleepy

- hypnosis—used to achieve *symptom suppression*, to block awareness of pain, or *symptom substitution*, which allows a positive interpretation of pain
- imagery—in which the patient visualises a soothing image while the nurse describes pleasant sensations (for example, the patient may picture himself at the beach while you describe the sounds of the waves and birds and the feel of the warm sun and a breeze on the patient's skin)
- relaxation therapy—a form of meditation used to focus attention on a single sound or image or on the rhythm of breathing
- heat application (thermotherapy)—application of dry or moist heat to decrease pain (heat enhances blood flow, increases tissue metabolism and decreases vasomotor tone; it may also relieve pain due to muscle aches or spasms, itching or joint pain)
- cold application (cryotherapy)—constricts blood vessels at the injury site, reducing blood flow to the site (cold slows oedema development, prevents further tissue damage and minimises bruising; it may be more effective than heat in relieving such pain as muscle aches or spasms, itching, incision pain, headaches and joint pain)
- transcutaneous electrical nerve stimulator (TENS)—in which electrodes transmit mild electrical impulses to the brain to block pain impulses
- massage therapy—used as an aid to relaxation
- reflexology—used as an aid to relaxation and to reduce pain.

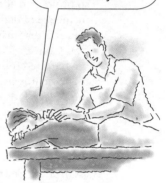

Massage therapy helps to control pain by inducing relaxation. Ahhh! I feel better already.

Sedation issues

A large number of patients will require sedation during their stay in the critical care unit, particularly those requiring mechanical ventilation. (See *Understanding sedatives* in Chapter 5, page 325.) It is important to recognise why the patient requires sedation and remember that sedation is not a replacement for analgesia and nonpharmacological comfort measures.

Need for sedation

Sedation regimes can be very beneficial for critically ill patients and are used for a variety of reasons:
- to facilitate mechanical ventilation
- to prevent awareness especially when administering paralysing agents
- to treat anxiety and agitation
- to provide amnesia
- to reduce the stress response
- to improve tolerance to interventions
- to reduce oxygen consumption and improve oxygenation, e.g. by suppressing laboured breathing in respiratory failure, suppressing cerebral metabolic rate in neurological injury and suppressing basal metabolic rate in sepsis.

Drug choice

The drug choice should be dependent on the reason for sedating the patient and consideration of any acute or chronic conditions that they may have. (See *Understanding sedatives* in Chapter 5, page 325.). Usual continuous regimes include concurrent opioid infusion to enhance sedation.

Problems with sedatives

Like many therapies within critical care the use of sedatives can be detrimental to patients. Boluses of sedatives given to agitated or delirious patients can cause increased confusion. No sedative provides REM sleep, so prolonged administration causes patients to be REM deprived increasing incidence of delirium. There are risks of accumulation with prolonged infusion that may result in prolonged mechanical ventilation and critical care stay. Conversely tolerance may occur during infusion, meaning higher doses are required to produce the same sedative effects. When sedation is stopped the patient may suffer withdrawal symptoms especially if sedatives have been infused for 7 days or longer. Many cause hypotension resulting in increased vasoconstrictor and inotrope requirements. Sedation causing vasodilation in the lungs can have detrimental pulmonary effects with ventilation perfusion (VQ) mismatch and reduced oxygenation. Reduced gastrointestinal motility is another common side effect and can cause problems with enteral feed absorption. Sedatives reduce accuracy of neurological assessment and may mask the presence of fitting. All these problems can be reduced by careful monitoring and administration.

Calm down

If a patient appears agitated it is important to determine and treat any underlying causes prior to assuming they are under sedated and administering sedation. Consideration of pain, fear and anxiety should be at the forefront of a critical care nurse's mind. Remember that sedatives have no analgesic properties therefore should not be used if pain is suspected. Good communication, reassurance and explanation may reduce the amount of sedative required.

You are feeling sleepy

It has been recognised that there is a general tendency to over sedate patients. This increases the problems as detailed earlier as well as increasing incidence of tissue viability problems and constipation by reduced movement and increased sputum retention by suppressing the cough reflex. Unless directed otherwise patients should be rousable but able to sleep when undisturbed. The exception to this will be patients with neurological problems or respiratory failure requiring high ventilatory pressures, who either are paralysed or require deep sedation levels.

What is the score?

To reduce the risk of over and under sedation, a sedation score can be used. If nurses and doctors are using a standardised subjective sedation scale, the doctor can prescribe the level of sedation for an individual patient and the nurse can titrate the sedation to achieve this. Subjective data should be used, e.g. opens eyes to voice and no response to painful stimuli. Whoever is measuring the sedation level should be able to reach the same score if the assessment is repeated.

There are a variety of sedation scales available, most use a numerical scale and are similar in content to the AVPU assessment (see Chapter 3). For scoring to be successful it must be determined what level to aim for in the patient. The nurse must also measure the sedation score on a regular basis (1–2 hourly) and feel confident in adjusting the doses of sedative and, at times, analgesia.

Give us a break

Collation of several elements that have been shown to be beneficial to mechanically ventilated patients has created the VAP care bundle. If all elements of this bundle are consistently undertaken, it is suggested that significant improvements in mortality and morbidity will be seen. As part of reducing VAP and reducing time spent on mechanical ventilation, daily interruption of sedative infusions has been recommended. This 'sedation break' allows 'lightening' of patients' sedation level, reducing risks of accumulation. The sedation can be stopped as long as the patient has no contraindications, e.g. high ventilatory pressures and raised intracranial pressure. When the patient becomes responsive, sedation may be retitrated and usually recommenced at a lower rate than before. Sedation breaks may last between 5 minutes and many hours. The patient must be assessed closely throughout the break to maintain safety and minimise risks of anxiety. Concurrent opioid infusions will normally not be discontinued unless the patient fails to wake after an extended break in sedation.

Consent, legal and ethical issues

Nurses who work in critical care routinely deal with complex decision-making about minor and major issues. Primarily they may be required to make decisions on the patient's behalf because the patient is unable to consent to care. In an emergency situation life saving treatment must be carried out based on a principle of necessity. As soon as time allows information should be obtained from medical records, relatives and health care professionals involved in the patient's care to find out what the patient's wishes are. Life saving technology allows patients, lives to be prolonged, but it is important to look at the quality of life as well. Lots of things should be considered when decisions are made about patient care and clear documentation will assist this.

Consent considerations

As a critical care nurse you should know:
- what to do to help patients make their own decisions
- how to work out whether a patient can make their own decisions
- what to do if a patient can't make a decision about something at a particular time.

Consent in critical care covers a wide range of decisions; from asking a patient if they will get out of bed into a chair, to deciding whether the patient should have renal replacement therapy. The underlying principles of consent include:
- assuming everyone can make their own decisions until proven otherwise
- giving patients support to make decisions, e.g. using communication aids in nonverbal patients and explaining clearly what the implications of the decision may be
- not stopping patients from making their own decision even if you think it is wrong or bad
- making sure that if someone does something or makes a decision on behalf of a patient who hasn't got capacity to consent, it must be in the patient's best interests (to work this out they must listen to what the patient wants and talk to anyone who knows them)
- trying to limit the patient's freedom and rights as little as possible.

Some patients may have appointed a deputy to act in their best interests in the event that they cannot make decisions themselves, this is called *lasting power of attorney* and can relate to decisions around health, welfare, property and money. For patients who have no family or friends an *independent mental capacity advocate* can provide help with decisions.

Legal liabilities

The law underpins many areas of critical care nursing. The four key areas applicable to nurses are:
- criminal law—if a nurse does something illegal and is prosecuted, e.g. stealing and violence to others
- civil law—if a nurse's care causes harm to another, action may be taken by that person or their representative to claim compensation from the nurse or nurse's employer, e.g. failure to report patient's deterioration
- employment law—on commencing employment the nurses sign a contract agreeing to comply with the policies and procedures of the organisation; if they fail to comply they may be disciplined or have their employment terminated, e.g. failing to comply with the roles and responsibilities detailed in their job description
- professional law—qualified nurses practicing in the UK are registered with the Nursing and Midwifery Council (NMC). Requirements to maintain registration are provided and a code of conduct is specified. If these are not adhered to registration may be removed preventing the nurse from practicing, e.g. verbal abuse of patients.

In many cases a nurse will be subject to actions from more than one of the areas if actions or omissions have been detrimental. A good understanding of these legal areas will aid your decision-making.

Ethical evaluations

The need to perform ethical evaluations occur regularly for critical care nurses. They commonly present as ethical dilemmas. You'll recognise a situation as an ethical dilemma if:
- more than one solution exists, i.e. there's no clear 'right' or 'wrong' way to handle a situation
- each solution carries equal weight
- each solution is ethically defensible.
  Examples of ethical dilemmas might include:
- closing the unit for admissions because of staff shortages and fears that care of existing patients may be compromised while recognising that other critically ill patients will then have to be transferred to other hospitals
- administering sedation to patients to prevent them extubating themselves but results in extended mechanical ventilation because the nurses are busy with another patient.

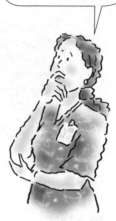

Ethical dilemmas are commonly faced by nurses in critical care. Always remember to respect the patient's personal values.

The value of values

Ethical dilemmas in critical care commonly revolve around quality-of-life issues for the patient, especially if they relate to end-of-life decisions—such as do-not-resuscitate orders, life support and patients' requests for no heroic measures. When considering quality of life, make sure others don't impose their own value system on the patient. Each person has a set of personal values that are influenced by environment and culture. Nurses also have a set of professional values.

End-of-life decisions

The threat of death is common in critical care. Perhaps at no other time is the holistic care of patients and their families as important as it is during this time.

End-of-life decisions are almost always difficult for patients, families and health care professionals to make. Nurses are in a unique position as advocates to assist patients and their families through this process.

Unsolvable mysteries

Your primary role as a patient advocate is to promote the patient's wishes. In many instances, however, a patient's wishes aren't known. That's when ethical decision-making takes priority. Decisions aren't always easy to make and the answers aren't usually clear-cut. At times, such ethical dilemmas may seem insolvable.

A question of quality

It's sometimes difficult to determine what can be done to achieve a good quality of life and what can simply be achieved, technologically speaking. Technological advances sometimes seem to exceed our ability to analyse the ethical dilemmas associated with them.

Years ago, death was considered a natural part of life and most people died at home, surrounded by their families. Today, most people die in hospitals and death is commonly regarded as a medical failure rather than a natural event. Sometimes it's hard for you to know whether you're assisting in extending the patient's life or delaying the patient's death.

Consulting the crowd

Legally if the patients lack the capacity to make their own decisions then the senior doctor in charge of their care can make decisions regarding what is in their best interests. However it is important that all other relevant parties should be consulted, for example, family, friends and general practitioner.

Determining medical futility

Medical futility refers to treatment that's hopeless or interventions that aren't likely to benefit the patient even though they may appear to be effective. For example, a patient with a terminal illness who's expected to die experiences cardiac arrest. Cardiopulmonary resuscitation may be effective in restoring a heartbeat but may still be deemed futile because it doesn't change the patient's outcome.

Withholding or withdrawing treatment

The issue of withholding or withdrawing treatment in critical care presents some ethical dilemmas. When withdrawing treatment from a patient—even at the patient's request—controversy over the principle of nonmaleficence (to prevent harm) may arise.

Harm alarm

Such controversy revolves around the definition of harm. The withdrawal of extraordinary measures that are prolonging the patient's life, like inotropes or mechanical ventilation, can be discontinued if not in the patient's best interests. This withdrawal may involve reducing or discontinuing mechanical ventilation and inotropes but maintaining sedative and analgesia infusions to ensure patient comfort. The monitor alarms will usually be turned off at this stage or the patient disconnected from the monitor. The relatives can be encouraged to have close contact with the patient and privacy to grieve as they desire.

Basic comfort measures like fluids, artificial nutrition and analgesia cannot be withdrawn unless a patient refuses them. The primary principle in these situations is to maintain comfort and promote dignity. (See *Approaching ethical decisions*, page 49.)

Dealing with cardiac arrest

In case of cardiac arrest (sudden stoppage of the heart), a critically ill patient may have a do not attempt resuscitation (DNAR) status. This describes the orders written by the senior doctor caring for the patient, i.e. what resuscitation measures should be carried out by the nurse and whether the patient's wishes regarding resuscitation measures should be considered. When cardiac arrest occurs, you must ensure that resuscitative efforts are initiated or that unwanted resuscitation doesn't occur.

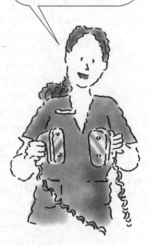

Futile treatment isn't a good use of health care resources and it doesn't change the patient's outcome.

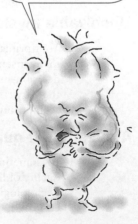

During cardiac arrest, it's typically up to you to ensure that resuscitation is initiated or that unwanted resuscitation doesn't occur.

Approaching ethical decisions

When faced with an ethical dilemma, consider the following questions:

- What health issues are involved?
- What ethical issues are involved?
- What further information is necessary before a judgement can be made?
- Who will be affected by this decision? (Include the decision maker and other caregivers if they'll be affected emotionally or professionally.)
- What are the values and opinions of the people involved?
- What conflicts exist between the values and ethical standards of the people involved?
- Must a decision be made and, if so, who should make it?
- What alternatives are available?
- For each alternative, what are the ethical justifications?
- For each alternative, what are the possible outcomes?

Who decides?

The wishes of a competent, informed patient should always be honoured. However, when a patient can't make decisions, the health care team—consisting of the patient's family, nursing staff and doctors—may have to make end-of-life decisions for the patient.

Advance decisions

Most people prefer to make their own decisions regarding end-of-life care. It's important that patients discuss their wishes with their loved ones; however, many don't. Instead, total strangers may be asked to make important health care decisions when a patient can't do so. That's why it's important for people to make choices ahead of time and to make these choices known by developing advance decisions.

Where there's a will, there's a law

An advance decision states which treatments a patient will accept and which the patient will refuse if they lack capacity in the future. For example, a patient may be willing to accept artificial nutrition but not haemodialysis.

It takes two

If an advance decision to refuse treatment that may keep the patient alive is made, it must be clearly stated and signed by the patient and a witness. All people with capacity are free to make advance decisions but they must understand the consequences. The document can be altered or cancelled at any time.

Organ donation

When asked, most people say that they support organ donation. However, only a small percentage of qualified organs are ever donated. Tens of thousands of names are on waiting lists for organs and the waiting lists are getting longer. The number of organs donated has remained static for several years. Organ transplantation is successful for many patients, giving them additional, high quality years of life.

The Human Tissue Act governs the donation of organs and tissues. In addition the government is actively promoting organ donation with an increase in transplant coordinators and the organ donor register. Become familiar with your local transplant coordinators and local policies.

Don't miss out

Medical criteria for organ donation are specified across the UK. Some transplant coordinators want to be notified of all deaths and imminent deaths so that they, not the medical staff, can determine if the patient is a potential candidate for organ donation. All suitable patients should be considered and transplant coordinators may be utilised to approach the family because of their expert counselling skills.

No, thank you

The following conditions usually preclude any organ or tissue donation:
• advanced age
• metastatic cancer
• history of human immunodeficiency virus or acquired immunodeficiency syndrome
• sepsis.

Donations accepted

Any heart beating patients who donate organs must first be declared brain dead. The exceptions to this are living donors, who most commonly donate a kidney or a segment of the lung, liver, pancreas or intestine. Death used to be defined as the cessation of respiratory and cardiac function. However, with developments in technology, this definition has become obsolete. We now rely on brain stem death criteria in determining death of an individual. This assessment must be performed by two qualified doctors who have determined that there are no pre-existing conditions that may mask brain stem function, e.g. sedatives, paralysing agents, hypothermia, metabolic or electrolyte abnormalities. (See *Assessing brain death*, page 51.)

Complex care

Care of a heart beating patient who's to be an organ donor is very complex. It's imperative that haemodynamic variables and electrolyte values be kept within very tight ranges for successful organ transplantation. You have a vital role in caring for the patient and in supporting the patient's family during this difficult time.

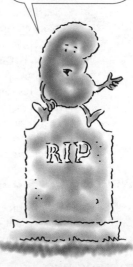

Despite the best intentions, only a small percentage of qualified organs are ever donated. Make sure you know your patient's wishes about organ donation before it's too late.

Assessing brain death

Methods for determining brain death vary, but several of the following criteria are commonly used:

- The patient must be unresponsive to all stimuli.
- Pupillary responses are absent.
- All brain functions cease.
- No eye movements are noted when cold water is instilled into the ears (caloric test). Normally, the eyes move towards the ear irrigated with cold water.
- No corneal reflex is present.
- No gag reflex is present.

- Quick rotation of the patient's head from left to right (doll's eyes test) causes the eyes to remain fixed, suggesting brain death. Normally, the eyes move in the opposite direction of the head movement.
- No response to painful stimuli is present.
- An apnoea test reveals no spontaneous breathing. Usually the carbon dioxide level is allowed to rise, then the patient is removed from the ventilator. Oxygen is entrained into the endotracheal tube and the patient is monitored for evidence of respiration.

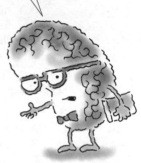

Although the methods for determining brain death vary, the most commonly used criteria are listed here.

When caring for an organ donor, it's essential to:
- maintain haemodynamic stability so that vital organs are perfused adequately
- assess urine output hourly to detect diabetes insipidus
- monitor laboratory results—such as electrolyte levels, complete blood count, liver and renal function tests—to assess organ function.

Non-heart-beating donors

Patients can donate some organs straight after death (lungs and liver less than 1 hour after death and kidneys less than 2 hours and skin, bone, tendons, corneas within 24 hours, and heart valves within 48 hours). However for organ donation, in this case, the patient must have died within a short space of time so that organs are not damaged by underperfusion for prolonged periods. The practice of obtaining organs from non-heart-beating donors increases organ availability and allows more patients to have the opportunity to donate.

After death

Whatever the cause of death or process of dying the nurse's role does not stop until the relatives have left the hospital and the patient has left the unit. Performing last offices will vary according to local hospital policies and religious and cultural beliefs and is an important final stage in caring for a critically ill patient. As well as emotional support the relatives will need information about what to do next. It is useful to provide written information as well as ensuring any questions are answered before the relatives leave.

Quick quiz

1. Which statement regarding a patient's culture and their hospitalisation experience is true?

    A.   Culture affects a patient's experience during hospitalisation because the patient has to adapt to the hospital culture.

    B.   Culture doesn't affect the patient's hospitalisation.

    C.   Cultural factors can affect patient and family roles during illness.

    D.   Culture rarely affects decisions about health.

Answer: C. Cultural factors can have a major impact on patient and family roles during illness. Culture affects the patient's and family members' feelings about illness, pain and end-of-life issues, among other things.

2. Factors that can affect a critically ill patient's cognitive function include:

    A.   medications.

    B.   health condition.

    C.   sleep disturbances.

    D.   all of the above.

Answer: D. All of these factors can affect the patient's cognitive function while in critical care.

3. When dealing with the family of a patient in critical care, the nurse should:

    A.   consider them an integral part of the team.

    B.   allow them to visit only during posted visiting times.

    C.   refer them to the patient's doctor for all information.

    D.   tell them not to touch the patient.

Answer: A. Family members know the patient better than anyone else does and should be considered an important part of the team caring for the patient.

4. Pain assessment in an unconscious patient:

    A.   isn't necessary because unconscious patients don't experience pain.

    B.   requires astute assessment skills by the nurse.

    C.   can be achieved through the use of visual analogue scales.

    D.   will be helped by increasing sedation.

Answer: B. Nurses should be especially vigilant in assessing for nonverbal signs of pain in an unconscious patient.

5. When considering issues of consent you should:

    A.   assume the patients cannot consent.

    B.   give the patients all the support they need to make decisions.

    C.   stop the patients from making decisions that may prevent their recovery.

    D.   try to limit the patients' freedom as much as possible.

Answer: B. The law states that patients should be assumed to have mental capacity until proven otherwise, should be helped to make decisions and not prevented from making decisions and any decisions made by others should aim to limit the patients' freedom as little as possible.

Scoring

☆☆☆ If you answered all five questions correctly, jump for joy. You're well versed in holistic care issues.

☆☆ If you answered four questions correctly, we won't issue a complaint. You're ready to join the team.

☆ If you answered fewer than four questions correctly, don't worry; it isn't an ethical dilemma. Just review the chapter and try again.

Just the facts

In this chapter, you'll learn:

♦ anatomy and physiology of the nervous system

♦ assessment of the nervous system

♦ diagnostic tests and procedures

♦ neurological disorders and treatments.

Understanding the nervous system

The nervous (or neurological) system is the organ system that coordinates all body functions. This complex system allows a person to adapt to changes within their body and in the environment.

Two systems in one

The nervous system consists of:

☝ the central nervous system (CNS), which includes the brain and spinal cord

✌ the peripheral nervous system, which includes the cranial nerves, spinal nerves and autonomic system.

Central nervous system

The organs of the CNS—the brain and spinal cord—collect and interpret motor and sensory stimuli. In the process, voluntary and involuntary sensory impulses travel along neural pathways to the brain. (See *A close look at the CNS*.)

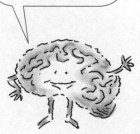

We're both central features of the central nervous system. I'm the smart one!

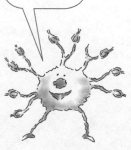

I'm the sensitive one!

A close look at the CNS

This illustration depicts a cross-section of the brain and spinal cord, which together make up the central nervous system (CNS). The brain joins the spinal cord at the base of the skull and ends near the second lumbar vertebrae. Note the butterfly-shaped mass of grey matter in the spinal cord.

Cross-section of the brain

Cerebellum

Cerebrum

Thalamus

Hypothalamus

Midbrain

Pituitary gland

Pons

Medulla

Spinal cord

Cross-section of the spinal cord

Ventral horn
(relays motor impulses)

Dorsal horn
(relays sensory impulses)

White matter
(forms ascending and descending tracts)

Grey matter

Brain

The brain consists of three parts:
- cerebrum
- cerebellum
- brain stem.

Brain work

The brain collects, integrates and interprets all stimuli, and initiates and regulates voluntary and involuntary motor activity. Four major arteries supply the brain with oxygen.

Cerebrum

The cerebrum, or cerebral cortex, is the largest part of the brain.

Nerve Centre

Tissues of the cerebrum make up a nerve centre that controls sensory and motor activities and intelligence. It's encased by the bones of the skull and

The cerebrum contains the nerve centre that controls sensory and motor activities and intelligence.

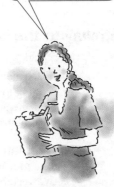

enclosed by three meninges (membrane layers): the dura mater, arachnoid and pia mater.

Relay and regulate

The diencephalons, another part of the cerebrum, contain the thalamus and hypothalamus. The thalamus is a relay station for sensory impulses.

The hypothalamus has many regulatory functions, such as:
- temperature control
- pituitary hormone production
- sleep and wake cycles
- water balance.

Divided in two

The cerebrum is divided into two hemispheres, left and right. The right hemisphere controls the left side of the body. The left hemisphere controls the right side of the body.

The two hemispheres of the brain are composed of four lobes. Each of the four lobes controls different functions. (See *Basic brain functions*.)

Cerebellum
The cerebellum—the brain's second largest region—lies behind and below the cerebrum. Like the cerebrum, it has two hemispheres.

Smooth moves

The cerebellum contains the major motor and sensory pathways. It enables smooth, coordinated muscle movement and helps maintain equilibrium.

Brain stem
The brain stem lies below the diencephalons and includes the:
- midbrain
- pons
- medulla.

Pathway to the brain

The brain stem contains the cranial nerves III to XII. It's a major sensory and motor pathway for impulses running to and from the cerebral cortex. It also regulates automatic body functions, such as heart rate, breathing, swallowing and coughing.

Circulation to the brain
The four major blood vessels of the brain include two vertebral and two carotid arteries.

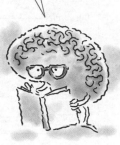

Golly, am I good? I didn't even know I could walk and chew gum at the same time let alone control the right side of the body with my left hemisphere and vice versa.

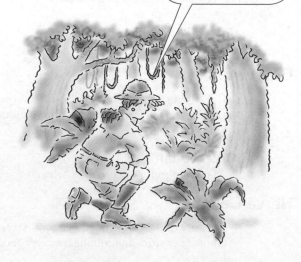

The brain stem is a sensory and motor pathway to and from the cerebral cortex. It also regulates automatic functions.

Basic brain functions

The basic structures and functions of the brain are depicted here. The cerebrum is divided into four lobes, based on location and function. The lobes—parietal, occipital, temporal and frontal—are named for the cranial bones over them.

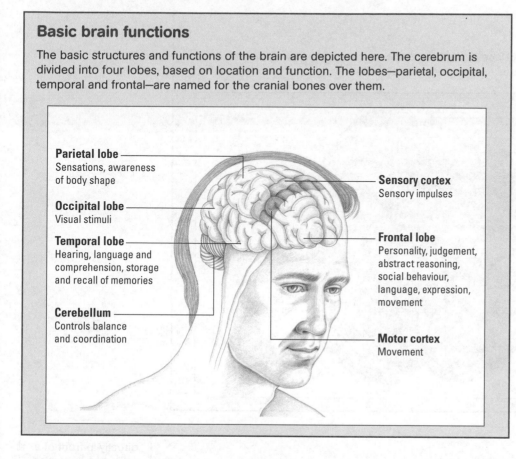

Parietal lobe
Sensations, awareness of body shape

Occipital lobe
Visual stimuli

Temporal lobe
Hearing, language and comprehension, storage and recall of memories

Cerebellum
Controls balance and coordination

Sensory cortex
Sensory impulses

Frontal lobe
Personality, judgement, abstract reasoning, social behaviour, language, expression, movement

Motor cortex
Movement

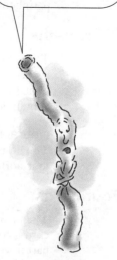

The circle of Willis ensures a constant supply of oxygen to the brain even if a major vessel is interrupted. Whew!

Two arteries converge

The two vertebral arteries converge to become the basilar artery. The basilar artery supplies oxygenated blood to the posterior parts of the brain.

Two arteries diverge

The common carotid arteries branch into the two internal carotids, which further divide to supply oxygenated blood to the anterior and middle areas of the brain. These vessels interconnect and form the circle of Willis at the base of the brain. The circle of Willis ensures that oxygen is continuously circulated to the brain even if any of the brain's major vessels is interrupted. (See *Arteries of the brain*, page 58.)

Spinal cord

The spinal cord extends from the upper border of the first cervical vertebrae to the lower border of the first lumbar vertebrae. It's encased by the same membrane structure as the brain and is protected by the bony vertebrae of the spine.

Arteries of the brain

Here's how the inferior surface of the brain appears. The anterior and posterior arteries join smaller arteries to form the circle of Willis.

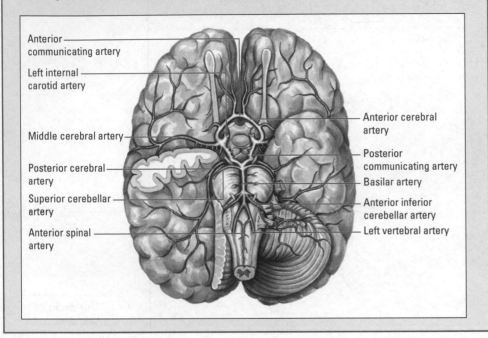

Anterior communicating artery

Left internal carotid artery

Middle cerebral artery

Posterior cerebral artery

Superior cerebellar artery

Anterior spinal artery

Anterior cerebral artery

Posterior communicating artery

Basilar artery

Anterior inferior cerebellar artery

Left vertebral artery

Long paths

The spinal cord is the primary pathway for messages travelling between the peripheral parts of the body and the brain.

Short paths

The spinal cord also mediates the sensory-to-motor transmission path known as the *reflex arc*. Because the reflex arc enters and exits the spinal cord at the same level, reflex pathways don't need to travel up and down the way other stimuli do. (See *Understanding the reflex arc,* page 59.)

Neural horns

The butterfly-shaped mass of grey matter in the spinal cord is divided into four horns, which consist mainly of neurone cell bodies.

Four horns

The main function of cells in the two dorsal (posterior) horns of the spinal cord is to relay sensations; those in the two ventral (anterior) horns play a part in voluntary and reflex motor activity.

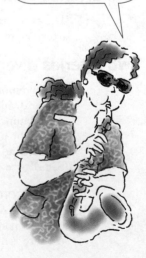

Don't stand directly in front of a patient when testing this reflex!

Understanding the reflex arc

Spinal nerves—which have sensory and motor portions—control deep tendon and superficial reflexes. A simple reflex arc requires a sensory (or afferent) neurone and a motor (or efferent) neurone.

Knee-jerk reaction

The knee-jerk, or patellar, reflex illustrates the sequence of events in a normal reflex arc:

• First, a sensory receptor detects the mechanical stimulus produced by the reflex hammer striking the patellar tendon.

• Then the sensory neuron carries the impulse along its axon by way of the spinal nerve to the dorsal root, where it enters the spinal column.

• Next, in the anterior horn of the spinal cord, shown below, the sensory neuron joins with a motor neurone, which carries the impulse along its axon by way of the spinal nerve to the muscle. The motor neurone transmits the impulse to muscle fibres through stimulation of the motor end plate. This triggers the muscle to contract and the leg to extend.

Patellar reflex arc

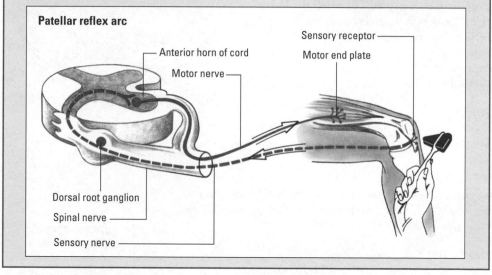

Anterior horn of cord
Motor nerve
Sensory receptor
Motor end plate
Dorsal root ganglion
Spinal nerve
Sensory nerve

White matter matters

White matter surrounds the four horns. This white matter consists of myelinated nerve fibres grouped in vertical columns, or tracts:
• The *dorsal* (posterior) white matter contains the ascending tracts, which carry impulses up the spinal cord to higher sensory centres.
• The *ventral* (anterior) white matter contains the descending tracts, which transmit motor impulses down from higher motor centres to the spinal cord.

Sensory impulse pathways

Sensory impulses travel along the afferent (sensory or ascending) neural pathways to the sensory cortex in the parietal lobe of the brain. There, the impulses are interpreted.

Dorsal horn

Pain and temperature sensations enter the spinal cord through the dorsal horn. After immediately crossing to the opposite side of the cord, these impulses travel to the thalamus by way of the spinothalamic tract.

Ganglia

Sensations such as touch, pressure and vibration enter the cord by way of relay stations, called *ganglia,* which are masses of nerve cell bodies on the dorsal roots of spinal nerves. Impulses travel up the dorsal column to the medulla, cross to the opposite side and enter the thalamus. There, the sensory cortex interprets the impulses.

> Sensations of touch, pressure and vibration enter the spinal cord by way of relay stations called ganglia.

Motor impulse pathways

Motor impulses travel from the brain to muscles by way of the efferent (motor or descending) pathway. Motor impulses begin in the motor cortex of the frontal lobe and travel along the upper motor neurons to reach the lower motor neurones of the peripheral nervous system.

Upper motor neurons originate in the brain and form two major systems:
• the pyramidal system
• the extrapyramidal system.

Pyramidal system

The pyramidal system (corticospinal tract) is responsible for fine and skilled movements of skeletal muscle.

All the right moves

Impulses in this system travel from the motor cortex through the internal capsule to the medulla. At the medulla, they cross to the opposite side and continue down the spinal cord.

Extrapyramidal system

The extrapyramidal system (extracorticospinal tract) controls gross motor movements.

Extra, extra! Read all about it!

Impulses in this system originate in the premotor area of the frontal lobe. They then travel to the pons, where they cross to the opposite side and travel down the spinal cord to the anterior horns. They're then relayed to the lower motor neurons, which carry the impulses to muscles.

> The pyramidal system controls fine and skilled movements of skeletal muscle.

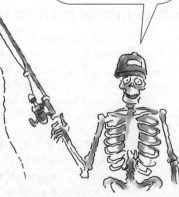

Peripheral nervous system

The peripheral nervous system includes the cranial nerves, spinal nerves and autonomic nervous system.

Identifying cranial nerves

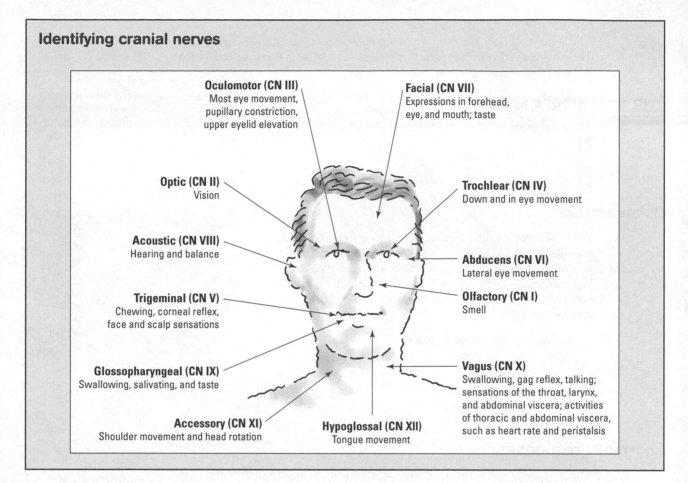

Oculomotor (CN III)
Most eye movement, pupillary constriction, upper eyelid elevation

Facial (CN VII)
Expressions in forehead, eye, and mouth; taste

Optic (CN II)
Vision

Trochlear (CN IV)
Down and in eye movement

Acoustic (CN VIII)
Hearing and balance

Abducens (CN VI)
Lateral eye movement

Trigeminal (CN V)
Chewing, corneal reflex, face and scalp sensations

Olfactory (CN I)
Smell

Glossopharyngeal (CN IX)
Swallowing, salivating, and taste

Vagus (CN X)
Swallowing, gag reflex, talking; sensations of the throat, larynx, and abdominal viscera; activities of thoracic and abdominal viscera, such as heart rate and peristalsis

Accessory (CN XI)
Shoulder movement and head rotation

Hypoglossal (CN XII)
Tongue movement

Cranial nerves

The 12 pairs of cranial nerves are the primary motor and sensory pathways between the brain and the head and neck. All cranial nerves except the olfactory and optic nerves exit from the midbrain, pons or medulla oblongata of the brain stem. (See *Identifying cranial nerves*.)

Spinal nerves

There are 31 pairs of spinal nerves, each named for the vertebra immediately below its exit point from the spinal cord.

The nerve of nerves

Each spinal nerve consists of afferent (sensory) and efferent (motor) neurones, which carry messages to and from specific body regions, called *dermatomes*.

What's in a name?

Well, each pair of spinal nerves is named for the vertebra below its exit point from the spinal cord.

Autonomic nervous system

The large autonomic nervous system supplies nerves to all internal organs. These visceral efferent nerves carry messages to the viscera from the brain stem and neuroendocrine system.

Two sympathetic systems

The autonomic nervous system includes two major parts:

- the sympathetic nervous system
- the parasympathetic nervous system.

Balancing act

When one part of the autonomic nervous system stimulates smooth muscles to contract or a gland to secrete, the other part of the system inhibits that action. Through such dual innervation, the sympathetic and parasympathetic systems counterbalance each other's activities to keep body systems running smoothly.

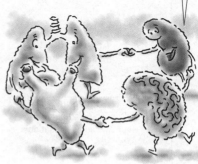

> The autonomic nervous system supplies nerves to all internal organs.

Sympathetic nervous system

Sympathetic nerves, called *preganglionic neurons,* exit the spinal cord between the first thoracic and second lumbar vertebrae and enter relay stations (ganglia) near the cord. These ganglia form the links of a chain that sends impulses to postganglionic neurons, which reach the organs and glands.

Enormous responses

The postganglionic neurons of the sympathetic nervous system produce widespread, generalised responses sometimes called the 'fight or flight' response, including:

- vasoconstriction
- elevated blood pressure
- enhanced blood flow to skeletal muscles
- increased heart rate and contractility
- increased respiratory rate
- smooth-muscle relaxation of the bronchioles, GI tract and urinary tract
- sphincter contraction
- pupillary dilation and ciliary muscle relaxation
- increased sweat gland secretion
- reduced pancreatic secretion.

> The sympathetic and parasympathetic systems counterbalance each other to keep body systems running smoothly.

Parasympathetic nervous system

Fibres of the parasympathetic nervous system leave the CNS by way of the cranial nerves from the midbrain and medulla and the spinal nerves between the second and fourth sacral vertebrae.

After leaving the CNS, the preganglionic fibre of each parasympathetic nerve travels to a ganglion near a specific organ or gland. The postganglionic fibre of the nerve enters that organ or gland.

Subtle responses

The postganglionic fibres of the parasympathetic nervous system produce responses involving one specific organ or gland, and may be deemed as resting or usual responses, such as:
• reductions in heart rate, contractility and conduction velocity
• bronchial smooth-muscle constriction
• increased GI tract tone and peristalsis, with sphincter relaxation
• increased bladder tone and urinary system sphincter relaxation
• vasodilatation of external genitalia, causing erection
• pupil constriction
• increased pancreatic, salivary and lacrimal secretions.

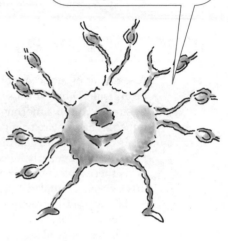

The postganglionic fibres of the parasympathetic nervous system produce responses that involve one specific organ or gland.

Key physiological principles

To understand more about how the nervous system works it is useful to know what circumstances it needs to function best.

What cells need in the brain and spinal cord

To maintain normality the cells need the following balance of things, such as:
• oxygen, a constant supply is required or irreversible damage can occur
• blood flow to maintain oxygen delivery and waste removal
• fluid to ensure the cells are hydrated but not oedematous
• electrolytes to maintain osmolarity, especially sodium
• glucose as the main energy source for the brain
• vitamins and trace elements, especially B vitamins
• removal of wastes and toxins; carbon dioxide, urea and ammonia to name a few.

The Monro–Kellie hypothesis

The intracranium is the brain inside a rigid box (the skull), and is made up of blood, cerebrospinal fluid and brain cells. The hypothesis states that the volume of the intracranium is the sum of the three components. So any situation that increases the volume of one or more of these will increase the pressure within the brain, known as the *intracranial pressure* 'ICP'. The nervous system will try to compensate but when a certain ICP is reached it will no longer be able to cope and rapid deterioration will occur. A normal ICP is around 5–10 mmHg.

Blood supply in the brain

Because a good supply of oxygenated blood is so important to the brain, it tries to keep a constant pressure in the brain and adapt to any changes in blood flow. This *cerebral perfusion pressure* (CPP) is balanced by the patient's *mean arterial pressure* (MAP) and ICP. In other words CPP = MAP − ICP. If CPP stays around 60–90 mmHg, the cerebral circulation will be adequate.

Neurological assessment

Assessment of subtle and elusive changes in the complex nervous system can be difficult. When you assess a patient for possible neurological impairment, be sure to collect a thorough health history and investigate physical signs of impairment. You are trying to answer the following questions:
- Is there an acute neurological problem?
- Is there an underlying chronic neurological condition?
- Is there a potential for neurological deterioration?

To carry out a complete assessment it is useful to adopt a structured approach:
- History of the present complaint
- Health history
- Clinical assessment and monitoring
- Results and significance of diagnostic tests.

Check the records

If you can't interview a critically ill patient due to impairment, you may gather history information from the patient's medical record. In many cases, you will need to ask their family members or the nurse transferring the patient to the critical care unit for information.

History of the present complaint

With a little help from their friends (and family)

A patient with neurological impairment may have trouble remembering. If members of the patient's family or close friends are available, include them in the assessment process. They may be able to corroborate or correct the details of the patient's health history.

Current health
Discover the patient's chief complaint by asking such questions as, 'Why did they come to the hospital?' or 'What has happened over the past 24 hours?'

Common complaints

If your patient is suffering from a neurological disorder, you may hear reports of headaches, motor disturbances (such as weakness, paresis and

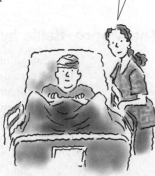

Ask members of the patient's family to fill in details of the health history if the patient can't remember.

paralysis), seizures, sensory deviations, altered level of consciousness (LOC) or a history of trauma or cardiac arrest.

Details, please

Encourage the patient/relatives to describe details of the current condition by asking such questions as:
• Do you have headaches? How often do you have them? What precipitates them?
• Do you feel dizzy from time to time? How often do you feel this way? What seems to precipitate the episodes?
• Do you ever feel a tingling or prickling sensation or numbness? If so, where?
• Have you ever had seizures or tremors? Have you ever had weakness or paralysis in your arms or legs?
• Do you have trouble urinating, walking, speaking, understanding others, reading or writing?
• How is your memory and ability to concentrate?

Health history

To collect a thorough health history, gather details about the patient's previous health status, lifestyle and family health.

Previous health

Many chronic diseases affect the neurological system, so ask questions about the patient's past health and what medications they're taking. Specifically, ask whether the patient has had any:
• major illnesses
• recurrent minor illnesses
• accidents
• injuries
• surgical procedures
• allergies.

Lifestyle

Ask questions about the patient's cultural and social background because these affect care decisions. Note the patient's occupation and hobbies.

Family health

Information about the patient's family may reveal a hereditary disorder. Ask if anyone in the family has had diabetes, cardiac or renal disease, high blood pressure, cancer, a bleeding disorder, a mental disorder or a stroke.

Clinical assessment and monitoring

As in any situation it is useful to begin with an ABCDE assessment. The rapid survey will allow immediate problems to be detected and treated.
A—Is the patient able to maintain their own airway? Patients with a Glasgow coma score of less than 8 usually can't.

B—Is the patient breathing adequately to maintain a good oxygen supply to the brain and eliminate carbon dioxide?

C—Is the circulation perfusing the brain properly?

D—What is the GCS? What are the pupil sixes and reactions? What is the blood sugar?

E—Are there any other features to note on a top-to-toe examination? For example, marked weakness and rashes.

Following this a complete neurological examination can be done. This is often long and detailed and it's unlikely that you would perform one in its entirety. However, if initial screening suggests a neurological problem, it may be necessary for medical staff to conduct a more detailed assessment and you may observe this or be asked to assist.

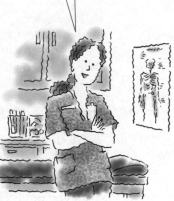

Mental status assessment begins with a health history. Your patient's responses reveal clues about their mental status.

Top-to-bottom examination

The patient's neurological system should be examined in an orderly way. Beginning with the highest levels of neurological function and working down to the lowest:

- mental status
- cranial nerve functions
- sensory function
- motor function
- reflexes.

Mental status

Mental status assessment begins when you talk to the patient during the health history. Responses to your questions reveal clues about the patient's orientation and memory. Use such clues as a guide during the physical assessment.

No easy answers

Make sure that you ask questions that require more than yes-or-no answers. Otherwise, confusion or disorientation might not be apparent. If you have doubts about a patient's mental status, perform a screening examination. (See *Quick check of mental status,* page 67.)

Three-part assessment

Use the mental status examination to check these three parameters:

- LOC
- speech
- cognitive function.

Level of consciousness

Watch for any change in the patient's LOC. It's the earliest and most sensitive indicator that their neurological status has changed.

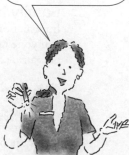

Watch for a change in the patient's GCS—the earliest and most sensitive indicator of neurological status change.

Advice from the experts

Quick check of mental status

To quickly screen your patient for disordered thought processes, ask the questions below. An incorrect answer to any question may indicate the need for a complete mental status examination. Make sure that you know the correct answers before asking the questions.

Question	Function screened
What's your name?	Orientation to person
What's your mother's name?	Orientation to other people
What year is it?	Orientation to time
Where are you now?	Orientation to place
How old are you?	Memory
Where were you born?	Remote memory
What did you have for breakfast?	Recent memory
What is the name of the Queen?	General knowledge
Can you count backwards from 20 to 1?	Attention span and calculation skills

Descriptions and definitions

Many terms are used to describe LOC, and definitions differ slightly among practitioners. To avoid confusion, you can clearly describe the patient's response to various stimuli using the AVPU scale:
- *Alert*—Patient follows commands and responds completely and appropriately to stimuli.
- *Voice*—Patient is drowsy, has delayed responses to verbal stimuli, and may drift off to sleep during the examination.
- *Pain*—Patient requires vigorous stimulation for a response.
- *Unresponsive*—Patient doesn't respond appropriately to verbal or painful stimuli and can't follow commands or communicate verbally.

Looking at LOC

Start by quietly observing the patient's behaviour. If the patient is sleeping, try to rouse them by providing an appropriate stimulus, in this order:

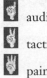 auditory

tactile

painful.

Always start with a minimal stimulus, increasing intensity as necessary. The Glasgow Coma Scale offers a more holistic objective way to assess the patient's LOC. (See *Using the Glasgow Coma Scale*, page 69.)

Speech
Listen to how well the patients express thoughts. Do they choose the correct words or seem to have problems finding or articulating words?

It's hard to say

To assess for dysarthria (difficulty forming words), ask the patient to repeat the phrase, 'No ifs, ands or buts'. Assess speech comprehension by determining the patient's ability to follow instructions and cooperate with your assessment.

Language changes

Keep in mind that language performance tends to fluctuate with the time of day and changes in physical condition. A healthy person may have language difficulty when ill or fatigued. However, increasing speech difficulties may indicate a deteriorating neurological status, which warrants further evaluation.

Cognitive function
You can assess cognitive function by testing the patient's:
- memory
- orientation
- attention span
- calculation ability
- thought content
- abstract thinking
- judgement
- insight
- emotional status.

Thanks for the memories

Short-term memory is commonly affected first in a patient with neurological disease. A patient with intact short-term memory can generally remember and repeat five to seven nonconsecutive numbers right away and again 10 minutes later.

When then who

To quickly test your patient's orientation, memory and attention span, use the mental status screening questions. Orientation to time is usually disrupted first; orientation to person, last.

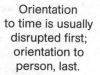

Listen up! Increasing speech difficulties may indicate deteriorating neurological status.

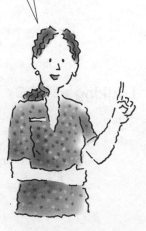

Orientation to time is usually disrupted first; orientation to person, last.

Take charge!

Using the Glasgow Coma Scale

You can use the Glasgow Coma Scale to describe the patient's baseline mental status and detect and interpret changes in the level of consciousness.

To use the scale, test the patient's ability to respond to verbal, motor and sensory stimulation and base your findings on the scale. A patient who's alert, can follow simple commands and is oriented to time, place and person receives a score of 15 points. A lower score in one or more categories may signal an impending neurological crisis. A total score of 8 or less indicates severe neurological damage.

Test	Score	Patient's response
Eye-opening response		
Spontaneously	4	Opens eyes spontaneously
To speech	3	Opens eyes when told to
To pain	2	Opens eyes only on painful stimulus
None	1	Doesn't open eyes in response to stimulus
Motor response		
Obeys	6	Sticks tongue out when asked
Localises	5	Reaches towards painful stimulus and tries to remove it
Withdraws	4	Moves away from painful stimulus
Abnormal flexion	3	Assumes a decorticate posture (shown below)
Abnormal extension	2	Assumes a decerebrate posture (shown below)
None	1	No response, just lies flaccid—an ominous sign
Verbal response		
Oriented	5	Tells current date
Confused	4	Tells incorrect year
Inappropriate words	3	Replies randomly with incorrect word
Incomprehensible	2	Moans or screams
None	1	No response
Total score		

Always consider the patient's environment and physical condition when assessing orientation. For example, a patient admitted to the critical care unit for several days may not be oriented to time because of the constant activity and noise of the monitoring equipment.

Attention and calculation

When testing attention span and calculation skills, keep in mind that lack of mathematical ability and anxiety can affect the patient's performance. If they have difficulty with numerical computation, ask them to spell the word 'world' backwards. While they're performing these functions, note their ability to pay attention.

Thought content

Disordered thought patterns may indicate delirium or psychosis. Assess thought pattern by evaluating the clarity and cohesiveness of the patient's ideas. Is their conversation smooth, with logical transitions between ideas? Do they have hallucinations (sensory perceptions that lack appropriate stimuli) or delusions (beliefs not supported by reality)?

Hypothetically speaking...

Test the patient's judgement by asking them how they would respond to a hypothetical situation. For example, what would they do if they were in a public building and the fire alarm sounded? Evaluate the appropriateness of their answer.

Insight on insight

Test your patient's insight by finding out:
• whether they have a realistic view of themselves
• whether they're aware of their illness and circumstances.
Assess insight by asking, for example, 'What do you think caused your chest pain?' Expect different patients to have different degrees of insight. For instance, a patient may attribute chest discomfort to indigestion rather than acknowledge that they have had a heart attack.

Lost in emotion

Throughout an assessment, consider your patient's emotional status. Note their mood, emotional lability or stability and the appropriateness of their emotional responses. Also, assess the patient's mood by asking how they feel about themselves and their future. Keep in mind that signs and symptoms of depression in an elderly patient may be atypical. (See *Depression and elderly patients*.)

Test your patient's judgment: Ask how they would respond to a hypothetical situation, and then evaluate his answer.

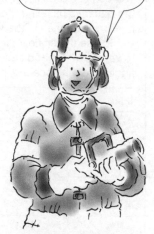

Senior moment

Depression and elderly patients

Symptoms of depression in elderly patients may be different from those found in other patients. For example, rather than the usual sad effects seen in patients with depression, your elderly patient may exhibit such atypical signs as decreased function and increased agitation.

Cranial nerve function

Cranial nerve assessment reveals valuable information about the condition of the CNS, especially the brain stem.

Under pressure

Because of their location, some cranial nerves are more vulnerable to the effects of increasing ICP. Therefore, a neurological screening assessment of the CNS focuses on these key nerves:
- optic (II)
- oculomotor (III)
- trochlear (IV)
- abducens (VI).

Go on

Also evaluate other nerves if the patient's history or symptoms indicate a potential CNS disorder or when performing a complete nervous system assessment. (See *Checking brain stem function,* page 72.)

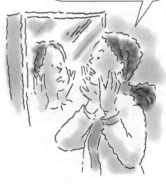

Look for symmetry when you test the motor portion of the facial nerve.

See about sight

- To assess the optic nerve, check visual acuity, visual fields and retinal structures. This may be done by asking the patient to read a newspaper, starting with large headlines and moving to small print.
- To assess the oculomotor nerve, check pupil size, pupil shape and pupillary response to light. When assessing pupil size, look for trends such as a gradual increase in the size of one pupil or appearance of unequal pupils. (See *Recognising pupillary changes,* page 73.)

Check three nerves at once

Assess the coordinated function of the oculomotor (CN III), trochlear (CN IV) and abducens (CN VI) nerves simultaneously. Here's how these nerves normally work:
- The oculomotor nerve (CN III) controls extraocular movement, pupillary constriction and raising of the eyelid.
- The trochlear nerve (CN IV) controls downwards and inwards eye movement.
- The abducens nerve (CN VI) controls lateral eye movement.

Here's how

Make sure that the patient's pupils constrict when exposed to light and that their eyes adapt to seeing objects at various distances. This can be done by asking the patient to follow your finger.

Checking brain stem function

In an unconscious patient, assist the doctor in assessing brain stem function by testing for the oculocephalic (doll's eye) reflex and the oculovestibular reflex. If the patient has a cervical spine injury, expect to use the oculovestibular reflex test as an alternative. The oculovestibular reflex test may also be used to determine the status of the vestibular portion of the acoustic nerve (CN VIII).

Oculocephalic reflex

Before beginning, examine the patient's cervical spine. Don't perform this procedure if you suspect the patient has a cervical spine injury. If the patient has no cervical spine injury, proceed as follows:

- Place both hands on either side of their head and use your thumbs to gently hold their eyelids open.
- While watching the patient's eyes, briskly rotate the head from side to side (as shown at right) or briskly flex and extend the patient's neck.
- Observe how the patient's eyes move in relation to head movement. In a normal response, which indicates an intact brain stem, the eyes appear to move opposite to the movement of the head. For example, if the neck is flexed, the eyes appear to look upwards. If the neck is extended, the eyes gaze downwards.

Abnormal response

With an abnormal (doll's eye) response, the eyes appear to move passively in the same direction as the head, indicating the absence of oculocephalic reflex. Such a response suggests a deep coma or severe brain stem damage at the level of the pons or midbrain.

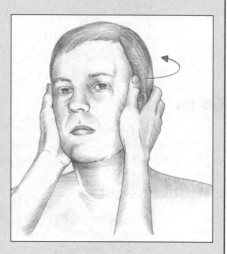

Oculovestibular reflex

To assess the oculovestibular reflex, the doctor first determines that the patient has an intact tympanic membrane and a clear external ear canal. Then follow these steps:

- Elevate the head of the bed 30 degrees.
- Using a large syringe with a small catheter on the tip, slowly irrigate the external auditory canal with 20–200 ml of cold water or ice water (as shown at right).
- During irrigation, watch the patient's eye movements. In a patient with an intact oculovestibular reflex, the eyes deviate towards the side being irrigated with cold water.

Abnormal responses

If the patient is conscious to some degree, there may be nystagmus (involuntary, rapid movement of the eyeball) with rapid jerking of the eyes away from the side being irrigated. In a normal conscious individual, as little as 10 ml of ice water may produce such a response and may also cause nausea. In a comatose patient with an intact brain stem, the eyes tonically deviate towards the stimulated ear. Absence of eye movement suggests a brain stem lesion.

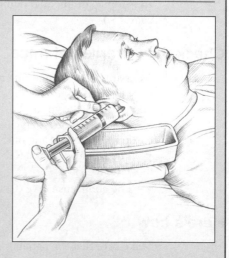

Recognising pupillary changes

Use this table as a guide to recognise pupillary changes and identify possible causes.

Pupillary change	Possible causes
Unilateral, dilated (4 mm) fixed and nonreactive 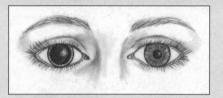	• Uncal herniation with oculomotor nerve damage • Brain stem compression • Increased intracranial pressure • Tentorial herniation • Head trauma with subdural or epidural haematoma • May be normal in some people
Bilateral, dilated (4 mm), fixed and nonreactive 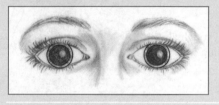	• Severe midbrain damage • Cardiopulmonary arrest (hypoxia) • Anticholinergic poisoning
Bilateral, midsize (2 mm), fixed and nonreactive 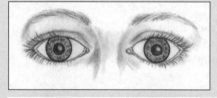	• Midbrain involvement caused by oedema, haemorrhage, infarctions, lacerations or contusions
Bilateral, pinpoint (<1 mm) and usually nonreactive 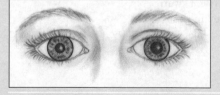	• Lesions of pons, usually after haemorrhage
Unilateral, small (1.5 mm) and nonreactive 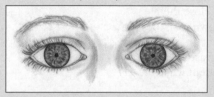	• Disruption of sympathetic nerve supply to the head caused by spinal cord lesion above the first thoracic vertebra

Pause slightly before moving from one position to the next, to assess the patient for nystagmus, or involuntary eye movement, and the ability to hold gaze in that particular position.

Sensory function

Assess the sensory system to evaluate:
- ability of the sensory receptors to detect stimulus
- ability of the afferent nerves to carry sensory nerve impulses to the spinal cord
- ability of the sensory tracts in the spinal cord to carry sensory messages to the brain.

Four sensations

During assessment, four types of sensation may be checked, including pain, light touch, position and discrimination.

This might hurt

To test for pain sensation, have the patient close their eyes; then, touch all the major dermatomes, first with the sharp end of a safety pin and then with the dull end. Proceed in this order:
- fingers
- shoulders
- toes
- thighs
- trunk.

While testing, occasionally alternate sharp and dull ends. Ask the patient to tell you when they feel the sharp stimulus. If the patient have known deficits, start in the area with the least sensation and move towards the area with the most sensation.

Use a light touch

To test for the sense of light touch, follow the instructions for pain sensation, using a wisp of cotton or tissue. Lightly touch the patient's skin; don't swab or sweep the skin. A patient with peripheral neuropathy might retain the sensation for light touch after losing pain sensation.

Where the toes are

To experience position sense, the patient needs intact vestibular and cerebellar function. To assess for position sense, have the patient close their eyes. Then, grasp the sides of their big toe and move it up and down. Ask the patient what position the toe is in.

To perform the same test on the patient's upper extremities, grasp the sides of their index finger and move it back and forth. Ask the patient what position the finger is in.

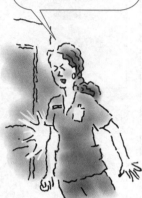

Ouch! To test for pain in a more sensible fashion, touch all the major dermatomes with the sharp end of a safety pin and then with the dull end.

Motor function

Assess motor function to aid evaluation of these structures and functions:
- the cerebral cortex and its initiation of motor activity by way of the pyramidal pathways
- the corticospinal tracts and their capacity to carry motor messages down the spinal cord
- the lower motor neurons and their ability to carry efferent impulses to the muscles
- the muscles and their capacity to carry out motor commands
- the cerebellum and basal ganglia and their capacity to coordinate and fine-tune movement.

> Motor function assessment yields a truckload of information about neurological structures and functions.

Tone test

Muscle tone represents muscular resistance to passive stretching. To test muscle tone of the arm, move the patient's shoulder through its passive range of movement (ROM); you should feel a slight resistance. When you let the patient's arm drop to their side, it should fall easily.

To test leg muscle tone, guide the patient's hip through its passive ROM, and then let their leg fall to the bed. If it falls in an externally rotated position, note this abnormal finding.

Feats of strength

To assess arm muscle strength, ask the patient to push you away as you apply resistance. Then ask the patient to extend both arms, palms up. Have them close their eyes and maintain this position for 20–30 seconds. Observe the arm for downwards drifting and pronation.

Strength of feet

Assess leg movement by first asking the patient to move each leg and foot. If they fail to move the leg on command, watch for spontaneous movement.

Grace and gait

Assess the patient's coordination and balance through cerebellar testing. Note whether the patient can sit and stand without support. While observing the patient, note imbalances and abnormalities. When cerebellar dysfunction is present, the patient has a wide-based, unsteady gait. Deviation to one side may indicate a cerebellar lesion on the side.

Extreme coordination

Test the extremities for coordination by having the patient touch their nose and then your outstretched finger as you move it. Have them do this faster and faster. Their movements should be accurate and smooth.

Test cerebellar function further by assessing rapid alternating movements. Tell the patient to use the thumb of one hand to touch each finger of the same hand in rapid sequence. Repeat with the other hand.

Present and absent actions

Motor responses in an unconscious patient may be appropriate, inappropriate or absent. Appropriate responses, such as localisation or withdrawal, mean that the sensory and corticospinal pathways are functioning. Inappropriate responses, such as decorticate or decerebrate posturing, indicate a dysfunction. (See *Using the Glasgow Coma Scale* for pictures of these positions, page 69.)

It can be challenging to assess motor responses in a patient who can't follow commands or is unresponsive. Make sure that you note whether any stimulus produces a response and what that response is.

Reflexes

Reflexes may be assessed to learn about the integrity of the sensory receptor organ. This can also evaluate how well afferent nerves relay sensory messages to the spinal cord or brain stem segment to mediate reflexes.

How deep is your reflex?

Deep tendon reflexes are tested by checking the responses of the biceps, triceps, brachioradialis, patellar and Achilles tendons:
*   The biceps reflex contracts the biceps muscle and forces flexion of the forearm.
*   The triceps reflex contracts the triceps muscle and forces extension of the forearm.
*   The brachioradialis reflex causes supination of the hand and flexion of the forearm at the elbow.
*   The patellar reflex forces contraction of the quadriceps muscle in the thigh with extension of the leg.
*   The Achilles reflex forces plantar flexion of the foot at the ankle.

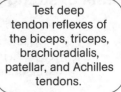

When assessing coordination and balance, note any imbalance or abnormality.

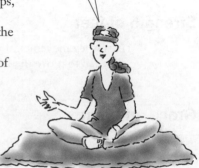

Test deep tendon reflexes of the biceps, triceps, brachioradialis, patellar, and Achilles tendons.

Monitoring plan

Results and significance of diagnostic tests and investigations

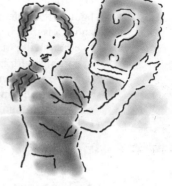

Diagnostic testing can be frightening. Make sure that you prepare the patient and their family members for each test.

Diagnostic testing to evaluate the nervous system typically includes imaging studies, angiography and electrophysiological studies. Other tests, such as lumbar puncture and transcranial Doppler studies, may also be used.

Tell it like it is

Diagnostic testing may be routine for you, but it can be frightening for the patient. Make sure that the patient and their family are prepared for each test and follow-up monitoring procedure. Some tests can be performed at the patient's bedside, but many require transfer to the imaging department.

Imaging studies

The most common imaging studies used to detect neurological disorders include computed tomography (CT) scan, magnetic resonance imaging (MRI), skull and spinal x-rays.

Computed tomography scan

CT scanning of intracranial structures combines radiology and computer analysis of tissue density (determined by contrast dye absorption). CT scanning doesn't show blood vessels as well as an angiogram does; however, it carries less risk of complications and causes less trauma than cerebral angiography.

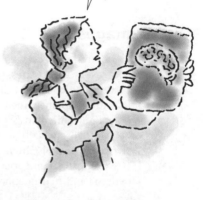

Thanks to CT scanning, you can see much of what may be wrong in the patient's brain.

Spine scanning

CT scanning of the spine is used to assess such disorders as herniated disk, spinal cord tumours and spinal stenosis.

Brain scanning

CT scanning of the brain is used to detect brain contusion, brain calcifications, cerebral atrophy, hydrocephalus, inflammation, space-occupying lesions (tumours, haematomas, oedema and abscesses) and vascular anomalies (arteriovenous malformation [AVM], infarctions, blood clots and haemorrhage). The quality of the information obtained and the minimal risks for the patient mean that CT scanning is performed for a wide range of neurological conditions. It is recommended by the National

Institute for Clinical Excellence (NICE) as part of traumatic head and spinal injury management.

Nursing concerns

- Confirm that the patient isn't allergic to iodine or shellfish to avoid an adverse reaction to the contrast medium.
- If the test calls for a contrast medium, the patient needs dedicated patent large-bore I.V. access.
- Preprocedure testing should include evaluation of renal function (serum creatinine and urea) because the contrast medium can cause acute renal failure. Renal failure is not an absolute contraindication and scans may be performed without contrast if required. Acetylcysteine may be infused prior and post the procedure in patients with impaired renal function to reduce the detrimental effects of the contrast.
- Warn the patient that they may feel flushed or notice a metallic taste in their mouth when the contrast medium is injected.
- Tell them that the CT scanner circles around them for 10–30 minutes, depending on the procedure and type of equipment.
- The patient must lie still during the test. In patients with neurological abnormalities, this can be difficult because of confusion and agitation. The patient may require sedation and intubation in order that an acceptable quality CT scan can be obtained.
- The contrast medium may discolour their urine for 24 hours. Suggest that they drink more fluids to flush the medium out of their body, unless this is contraindicated or they have oral intake restrictions; otherwise, the doctor may prescribe increased I.V. fluids.

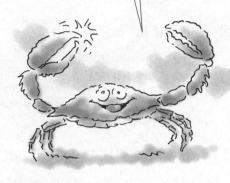

Before CT scanning of the brain, make sure that the patient isn't allergic to iodine or shellfish, which may foretell an adverse reaction to the contrast medium.

Magnetic resonance imaging

MRI generates detailed pictures of body structures. The test may involve the use of a contrast medium such as gandolinium.

Sharper images

Compared with conventional x-rays and CT scans, MRI provides superior contrast of soft tissues, sharply differentiating healthy, benign and cancerous tissue and clearly revealing blood vessels. In addition, MRI permits imaging in multiple planes, including sagittal and coronal views in regions where bones normally hamper visualisation.

MRI is especially useful for studying the CNS because it can reveal structural and biochemical abnormalities associated with such conditions as transient ischaemic attack (TIA), tumours, multiple sclerosis (MS), cerebral oedema and hydrocephalus.

Nursing concerns

• Confirm that the patient isn't allergic to the contrast medium (usually gandolinium).
• If the test calls for a contrast medium, the patient needs dedicated patent large-bore I.V. access.
• Explain that the procedure can take up to 1 hour, and the patient must remain still for intervals of 5–20 minutes.
• All metallic items must be removed, such as hair clips, jewellery (including body-piercing jewellery), watches, eyeglasses, hearing aids and dentures. This often causes problems with ventilated and monitored critically ill patients. Liaising with the scanning department and planning the procedure carefully should ensure that patient safety and therapies are maintained.
• Explain that the test is painless, but that the machinery may seem loud and frightening and the tunnel confining. Tell the patient that they'll receive earplugs to reduce the noise.
• Provide sedation, as ordered, to promote relaxation during the test.
• After the procedure, increase the I.V. fluids as prescribed, or encourage the patient to increase their fluid intake to flush the contrast medium from their system.

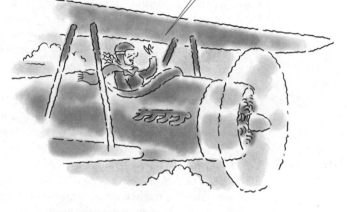

MRI is painless, but the machinery may seem loud, confining and frightening to your patients.

Skull and spinal x-rays

Skull x-rays are typically taken from two angles: anteroposterior and lateral. The doctor may order other angles to examine the frontal and maxillary sinuses, facial bones and eye orbits.

Having one's head examined

Skull x-rays are used to detect fractures; bony tumours or unusual calcifications; pineal displacement, which indicates a space-occupying lesion; skull or sella turcica erosion, which indicates a space-occupying lesion; and vascular abnormalities.

Spinal findings

The doctor may order anteroposterior and lateral spinal x-rays when:
• spinal disease is suspected
• injury to the cervical, thoracic, lumbar or sacral vertebral segments exists.

Depending on the patient's condition, other x-ray images may be taken from special angles, such as the open-mouth view (to confirm odontoid fracture).

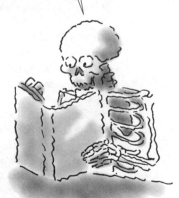

Skull x-rays are typically taken from the anteroposterior and lateral angles.

Spinal x-rays are used to detect spinal fracture; displacement and subluxation due to partial dislocation; destructive lesions, such as primary and metastatic bone tumours; arthritic changes or spondylolisthesis; structural abnormalities, such as kyphosis, scoliosis and lordosis; and congenital abnormalities.

Nursing concerns

• Reassure the patient that x-rays are painless.

• As ordered, administer an analgesic before the procedure if the patient has existing pain, so that they'll be more comfortable.

• A normal x-ray does not rule out spinal cord injury (neurological examination usually confirms this) so do not remove a patient's cervical collar or discontinue log rolling until a doctor permits it.

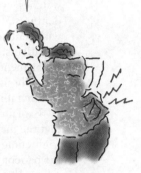

Critical care nursing seems like backbreaking work, but an x-ray is needed to confirm the diagnosis.

Angiography

Angiographic studies include cerebral angiography and digital subtraction angiography (DSA).

Cerebral angiography

During cerebral angiography, the doctor injects a radiopaque contrast medium, into the brachial artery (through retrograde brachial injection) or femoral artery (through catheterisation).

Why it's done

This procedure highlights cerebral vessels, making it easier to:

• detect stenosis or occlusion associated with thrombus or spasm

• identify aneurysms and AVMs

• locate vessel displacement associated with tumours, abscesses, cerebral oedema, haematoma or herniation

• assess collateral circulation.

Cerebral angiography is used to detect and identify problems affecting the cerebral vessels.

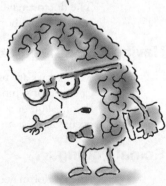

Nursing concerns

• Explain the procedure to the patient, and answer all questions honestly.

• Confirm that the patient isn't allergic to iodine or shellfish because a person with such allergies may have an adverse reaction to the contrast medium.

• Include evaluation of renal function (creatinine and urea levels) and potential risk of bleeding (prothrombin time [PTT] and platelet count) in preprocedure testing. Notify the doctor of abnormal results.

• Encourage the patient to lie still during the procedure.

• Explain that they may feel a flushed sensation as the dye is injected.

• Maintain bed rest, as ordered, and monitor the patient's vital signs.

• Monitor the catheter injection site for signs of bleeding.

• Monitor the patient's peripheral pulse in the arm or leg used for catheter insertion, and mark the site.

• Unless contraindicated, encourage the patient to drink more fluids to flush the dye from the body; alternatively, increase the I.V. fluids as prescribed.
• Monitor the patient for neurological changes and such complications as hemiparesis, hemiplegia, aphasia and impaired LOC. This may be particularly difficult in a sedated patient.
• Monitor for adverse reactions to the contrast medium, which may include restlessness, tachypnoea and respiratory distress, tachycardia, facial flushing, urticaria, and nausea and vomiting.

Digital subtraction angiography

Like cerebral angiography, DSA highlights cerebral blood vessels. DSA is done in the following way:
• Using computerised fluoroscopy, a technician takes an image of the selected area, which is then stored in a computer's memory.
• After administering a contrast medium, the technician takes several more images.
• The computer produces high-resolution images by manipulating the two sets of images.

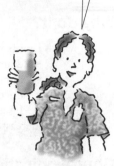

Encourage fluid consumption to flush out the contrast dye after testing, unless it's contraindicated.

Electrophysiological studies

The commonest electrophysiological study is electroencephalography (EEG).

Electroencephalography

During EEG, the brain's continuous electrical activity is recorded. The results are used to identify seizure disorders; head injury; intracranial lesions, such as abscesses and tumours; TIAs; and stroke.

EEG is used to identify problems that affect the brain's electrical activity.

Nursing concerns
• Explain that a technician applies paste and attaches electrodes to areas of skin on the patient's head and neck after these areas have been lightly abraded to ensure good contact.
• Instruct the patient to remain still during the test.
• Discuss what the patient may be asked to do during the test, such as hyperventilating for 3 minutes or sleeping, depending on the purpose of the EEG.
• Use acetone to remove any remaining paste from the patient's skin.

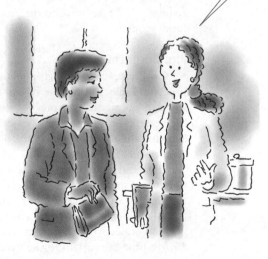

Other Tests

Other neurological tests include lumbar puncture and transcranial Doppler studies.

Lumbar puncture

During lumbar puncture, a sterile needle is inserted into the subarachnoid space of the spinal canal, usually between the third and fourth lumbar vertebrae. A doctor does the lumbar puncture, with a nurse assisting. It requires sterile technique and careful patient positioning. The cerebrospinal fluid should be clear.

Why do it?

Lumbar puncture is used to:
- detect blood in cerebrospinal fluid (CSF)
- obtain CSF specimens for laboratory analysis
- inject dyes or gases for contrast in radiological studies.
  It's also used to administer drugs or anaesthetics and to relieve increased ICP by removing CSF.

Contraindications and cautions

Lumbar puncture is contraindicated in patients with lumbar deformity or infection at the puncture site. It's performed very cautiously in patients with increased ICP because the rapid decrease of pressure that follows withdrawal of CSF can cause herniation of the brain through the foramen magnum ('coning') and medullary compression resulting in brain stem death. Any patient with risk of raised ICP will require a CT scan prior to the procedure or at least an eye examination for fundoscopy.

Nursing concerns
- Calmly describe lumbar puncture to the patient, explaining that the procedure may cause some discomfort and assist them into a curled lateral position pushing out their lower spine to the doctor. This increases space between the vertebrae, allowing the doctor to insert the needle.
- Reassure the patient that a local anaesthetic is administered before the test. Tell them to report any tingling or sharp pain they feel as the anaesthetic is injected.
- To prevent headache after the test, instruct the patient to lie flat or semi-recumbent after the procedure, local hospital policy will provide further guidance.
- Monitor the patient for neurological deficits and complications, such as headache, fever, back spasms or seizures, according to facility policy.

Transcranial Doppler studies

In transcranial Doppler studies, the velocity of blood flow through cerebral arteries is measured. The results

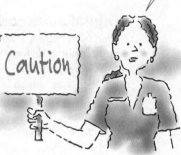

Be careful! If the patient has increased ICP, the rapid drop in ICP after CSF is withdrawn can lead to serious problems.

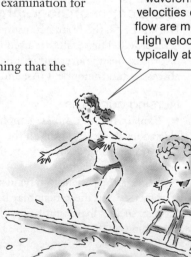

In transcranial Doppler studies, waveforms and velocities of blood flow are measured. High velocities are typically abnormal.

provide information about the presence, quality and changing nature of blood flow to an area of the brain.

What blood flow tells you

The types of waveforms and velocities obtained by testing indicate whether disease exists. Test results commonly aren't definitive, but this is a noninvasive way to obtain diagnostic information.

High velocities are typically abnormal, suggesting that blood flow is too turbulent or the vessel is too narrow. They may also indicate stenosis or vasospasm. High velocities may also indicate AVM due to the extra blood flow associated with stenosis or vasospasm.

Nursing concerns

- Tell the patient that the study usually takes less than 1 hour, depending on the number of vessels examined and any interfering factors.
- Explain that a small amount of gel is applied to the skin and that a probe is then used to transmit a signal to the artery being studied.

Treatments

Initial treatments for all types of acute, chronic and potential neurological dysfunctions should focus on optimising the cells. Going back to what the cells need is the priority:

- Ensure adequate oxygenation is maintained by providing supplemental supply as required and monitoring oxygen saturations and blood gases if required.
- Maintain blood pressure and perfusion, administering fluids and vasoactive drugs as required to maintain CPP.
- Maintain hydration and fluid balance, administering fluids as prescribed.
- Maintain electrolyte balance by taking blood samples for analysis and reviewing fluid therapy with medical staff to ensure large water loads are avoided.
- Maintain the glucose energy source by monitoring blood sugar levels and providing glucose or insulin as prescribed.
- Consider which patients are high risk for vitamin and trace element derangements and administer supplements as prescribed.
- Examine blood results for evidence of waste and toxin build-up and liaise with medical staff regarding treatments.

Sedation and mechanical ventilation might be used to help meet these requirements. Ensure an adequate level of sedation which reduces cerebral metabolic rate. Ventilator settings should be adjusted to maintain good arterial oxygen supply and carbon dioxide levels at the lower range of normal. Additional treatments for patients with neurological dysfunction may include medication therapy, surgery and other forms of treatment.

Medication therapy

For many of your patients with neurological disorders, medication or drug therapy is essential. For example:

- thrombolytics may be used to treat patients with acute ischaemic stroke
- anticonvulsants are used to control seizures
- corticosteroids are used to reduce inflammation.

Types of drugs commonly used to treat patients with neurological disorders include:

- analgesics
- anticonvulsants
- anticoagulants and antiplatelets
- barbiturates
- benzodiazepines
- calcium channel blockers

> Watch for severe adverse reactions and interactions with other drugs.

Common neurological drugs

Use this table to find out about common neurological drugs, their indications and adverse effects, and related monitoring measures.

Drug	Indications	Adverse effects
Nonopioid analgesics		
Paracetamol	• Mild pain, headache	• Severe liver damage, neutropenia, thrombocytopenia
Opioid analgesics		
Morphine	• Severe pain	• Respiratory depression, apnoea, bradycardia, seizures, sedation
Codeine	• Mild to moderate pain	• Respiratory depression, bradycardia, sedation, constipation
Anticonvulsants		
Carbamazepine	• Generalised tonic-clonic seizures, complex partial seizures, mixed seizures	• Heart failure, worsening of seizure, atrioventricular block, hepatitis, thrombocytopenia, Stevens–Johnson syndrome
Fosphenytoin	• Status epilepticus, seizures during neurosurgery	• Increased intracranial pressure, cerebral oedema, somnolence, bradycardia, QT prolongation, heart block
Phenytoin	• Generalised tonic-clonic seizures, status epilepticus, nonepileptic seizures after head trauma	• Agranulocytosis, thrombocytopenia, toxic hepatitis, slurred speech, Stevens–Johnson syndrome
Primidone	• Generalised tonic-clonic seizures, focal seizures and complex partial seizures	• Thrombocytopenia, drowsiness, ataxia

- corticosteroids
- diuretics
- thrombolytics.

Heads up!

When caring for a patient undergoing medication therapy, stay alert for severe adverse reactions and interactions with other drugs. Some drugs such as barbiturates also carry a high risk of toxicity.

Stay the course

Successful therapy hinges on strict adherence to the medication schedule. Compliance is especially critical for drugs that require steady blood levels for therapeutic effectiveness such as anticonvulsants. (See *Common neurological drugs,* pages 84 to 87.)

Practice pointers

- Monitor total daily intake of paracetamol because of risk of liver toxicity. Use with caution in elderly patients and those with liver disease.

- Monitor for respiratory depression. Use with caution in elderly patients and those with head injury, seizures, or increased intracranial pressure (ICP). Contraindicated in patients with acute bronchial asthma.
- Monitor for respiratory depression. Use with caution in elderly patients and those with head injury, seizures or increased ICP.

- Use cautiously in patients with mixed seizure disorders because it can increase the risk of seizure. Use cautiously in patients with hepatic dysfunction. Obtain baseline liver function studies, complete blood count and creatinine and urea levels. Monitor blood levels of the drug; therapeutic level is 4–12 mcg/ml.
- Stop drug with acute hepatotoxicity. May cause hyperglycaemia; monitor blood glucose in diabetic patients. Fosphenytoin should be prescribed and dispensed in PE units. Monitor for cardiac arrhythmias and QT prolongation.

- Abrupt withdrawal can trigger status epilepticus. Contraindicated in patients with heart block. Use cautiously in patients with hepatic disease and myocardial insufficiency. Monitor blood levels of the drug; therapeutic range is 10–20 mcg/ml. If rash appears, stop the drug.

- Abrupt withdrawal can cause status epilepticus. Reduce dosage in elderly patients.

(continued)

Common neurological drugs (Continued)

Drug	Indications	Adverse effects
Sodium valproate	Complex partial seizures, simple and complex absence seizures	Thrombocytopenia, pancreatitis, toxic hepatitis, sedation, ataxia
Anticoagulants		
Heparin/Enoxaparin Sodium	Embolism prophylaxis after cerebral thrombosis in evolving stroke	Haemorrhage, thrombocytopenia
Antiplatelets		
Aspirin	Transient ischaemic attacks, thromboembolic disorders	GI bleeding, acute renal insufficiency, thrombocytopenia, liver dysfunction
Clopidogrel	Thrombotic stroke prophylaxis	GI bleeding, rarely thrombocytopenia
Barbiturates		
Phenobarbitone	All types of seizures except absence seizures and febrile seizures in children; also used for status epilepticus, sedation and drug withdrawal	Respiratory depression, apnoea, bradycardia, angioedema, Stevens–Johnson syndrome
Benzodiazepines		
Clonazepam	Absence and atypical seizures, generalised tonic-clonic seizures, status epilepticus, panic disorders	Respiratory depression, thrombocytopenia, leukopenia, drowsiness, ataxia
Diazepam	Status epilepticus, anxiety, acute alcohol withdrawal, muscle spasm	Respiratory depression, bradycardia, cardiovascular collapse, drowsiness, acute withdrawal syndrome
Lorazepam	Status epilepticus, anxiety, agitation	Drowsiness, acute withdrawal syndrome
Calcium channel blockers		
Nimodipine	Neurological deficits caused by cerebral vasospasm after congenital aneurysm rupture	Decreased blood pressure, tachycardia, oedema
Corticosteroids		
Dexamethasone, methylprednisolone	Cerebral oedema, severe inflammation, especially associated with malignancy	Heart failure, cardiac arrhythmias, oedema, circulatory collapse, thromboembolism, pancreatitis, peptic ulceration
Diuretics		
Furosemide (loop)	Oedema, hypertension	Renal failure, thrombocytopenia, agranulocytosis, volume depletion, dehydration
Mannitol (osmotic)	Cerebral oedema, increased ICP	Heart failure, seizures, fluid and electrolyte imbalance
Thrombolytics		
Alteplase (recombinant tissue plasminogen activator)	Acute ischaemic stroke	Cerebral haemorrhage, spontaneous bleeding, allergic reaction
Streptokinase	Acute ischaemic stroke	Cerebral haemorrhage, spontaneous bleeding, allergic reaction

- Obtain baseline liver function tests. Avoid use in patients at high risk for hepatotoxicity. Abrupt withdrawal may worsen seizures. Monitor blood levels of the drug; therapeutic range is 50–100 mcg/ml.

- Monitor for bleeding. Obtain baseline APTT ratio (APTT/INR) and prothrombin time (PTT). Monitor APTT at regular intervals. Protamine sulphate reverses the effects of heparin. Low molecular weight heparins do not alter clotting times specifically but clotting should still be monitored. They are better for longer term use as the effects take longer to stop on discontinuation of treatment than standard heparin.

- Monitor for bleeding. Avoid use in patients with active peptic ulcer and GI inflammation. Check allergy status.

- Monitor for bleeding. Avoid use in patients with active peptic ulcer and GI inflammation.

- Monitor for respiratory depression and bradycardia. Keep resuscitation equipment on hand when administering I.V. dose; monitor respirations.

- Abrupt withdrawal may precipitate status epilepticus. Elderly patients are at a greater risk for central nervous system (CNS) depression and may require a lower dose.

- Monitor for respiratory depression and cardiac arrhythmia. Don't stop suddenly; can cause acute withdrawal in physically dependent persons.

- Don't stop abruptly; can cause withdrawal. Monitor for CNS depressant effects in elderly patients.

- Use cautiously in hepatic failure. Monitor for hypotension and tachycardia.

- Use cautiously in patients with recent myocardial infarction, hypertension, renal disease and GI ulcer. Monitor blood pressure and blood glucose levels.

- Monitor blood pressure, pulse and intake and output. Monitor serum electrolyte levels, especially potassium levels. Monitor for cardiac arrhythmias.

- Contraindicated in severe pulmonary congestion and heart failure. Monitor blood pressure, heart rate and intake and output. Monitor serum electrolyte levels. Use with caution in patients with renal dysfunction.

- Contraindicated in patients with intracranial or subarachnoid haemorrhage. The patient must meet criteria for thrombolytic therapy before initiation of therapy. Monitor baseline laboratory values: haemoglobin level, haematocrit, APTT, PT/INR. Monitor vital signs. Monitor for signs of bleeding. Monitor puncture sites for bleeding.

- Contraindicated in patients with intracranial or subarachnoid haemorrhage. The patient must meet criteria for thrombolytic therapy before initiation of therapy. Monitor baseline laboratory values: haemoglobin level, haematocrit, APTT, PT/INR. Monitor vital signs. Monitor for signs of bleeding. Monitor puncture sites for bleeding.

Surgery

Life-threatening neurological disorders may call for emergency surgery in a specialist neurosurgical centre.

Opening up

Surgery commonly involves craniotomy, a procedure to open the skull and expose the brain.

Be ready before and after

You may be responsible for the patient's care before and after surgery. Here are some general preoperative and postoperative pointers:
• The prospect of surgery usually causes fear and anxiety, so give ongoing emotional support to the patient and their family. Make sure that you're ready to answer their questions.
• Postoperative care may include teaching about diverse topics, such as ventricular shunt care and tips about cosmetic care after craniotomy. Be ready to give good advice after surgery.

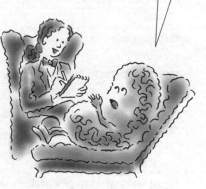

I feel so exposed. Life-threatening neurological disorders may call for emergency surgery, beginning with craniotomy.

Craniotomy

During craniotomy, a surgical opening into the skull exposes the brain. This procedure allows various treatments, such as ventricular shunting, excision of a tumour or abscess, haematoma aspiration and aneurysm clipping (placing one or more surgical clips on the neck of an aneurysm to destroy it). In extreme circumstances a craniotomy is performed to prevent coning in a patient with massive ICP.

Condition and complexity count

The degree of risk depends on your patient's condition and the complexity of the surgery. Craniotomy raises the risk of having various complications, such as:
• infection
• haemorrhage
• respiratory compromise
• increased ICP.

Nursing concerns
• Encourage the patient and family members to ask questions about the procedure. Provide clear, honest answers to reduce their confusion and anxiety and to enhance effective coping.
• Explain that the patient's head will be shaved before surgery and that the skull section may not be replaced immediately.
• Discuss the recovery period so the patient understands what to expect. Explain that they'll awaken with a dressing on their head to protect the incision and may have a surgical drain.
• Tell them to expect a headache and facial swelling for 2–3 days after surgery, and reassure them that they'll receive pain medication.

- Monitor the patient's neurological status and vital signs, and report any acute change immediately. Watch for signs of increased ICP, such as pupil changes, weakness in extremities, headache and change in GCS.
- Monitor the incision site for signs of infection or drainage.
- Provide emotional support to the patient and their family members as they cope with remaining neurological deficits.

Cerebral aneurysm repair

Surgical intervention is the only sure way to prevent rupture or rebleeding of a cerebral aneurysm.

Hats off

In cerebral aneurysm repair, a craniotomy is performed to expose the aneurysm. Depending on the shape and location of the aneurysm, the surgeon then uses one of several corrective techniques, such as:
- clamping the affected artery
- wrapping the aneurysm wall with a biological or synthetic material
- clipping or ligating the aneurysm.

Nursing concerns
- Tell the patient and their family members that monitoring is done in the critical care unit before and after surgery. Explain that several I.V. lines, intubation and mechanical ventilation may be needed.
- Monitor the incision site for signs of infection or drainage.
- Monitor the patient's neurological status and vital signs, and report acute changes immediately. Watch for signs of increased ICP, such as pupil changes, weakness in extremities, headache and a change in LOC.
- Give emotional support to the patient and their family members to help them cope with remaining neurological deficits.

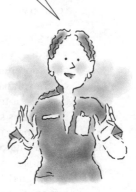

After craniotomy, provide emotional support to the patient and their family members to help them cope with any remaining deficits.

Other treatments

Other treatments include barbiturate coma, CSF drainage, ICP monitoring and plasmapheresis.

Barbiturate coma

Occasionally the doctor may order barbiturate coma when conventional treatments, such as fluid restriction, diuretic or corticosteroid therapy or ventricular shunting, don't correct sustained or acute episodes of increased ICP.

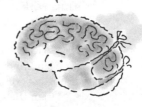

The corrective technique used in cerebral aneurysm repair depends on the shape and location of the aneurysm.

High I.V.

During barbiturate coma, the patient receives high I.V. doses of a short-acting barbiturate to produce a comatose state. The drug reduces the patient's metabolic rate and cerebral blood flow. Once heavy sedation is achieved a paralysing agent may also be added.

Last resort

The goal of barbiturate coma is to relieve increased ICP and protect cerebral tissue. It's a last resort for patients with:
- acute ICP elevation (over 40 mmHg)
- persistent ICP elevation (over 20 mmHg)
- rapidly deteriorating neurological status that's unresponsive to other treatments.

If barbiturate coma doesn't reduce ICP, the patient's prognosis for recovery is poor.

Nursing concerns
- Focus your attention on the patient's family. The patient's condition and apprehension about the treatment is likely to frighten them. Provide clear explanations of the procedure and its effects, and encourage them to ask questions. Convey a sense of optimism but provide no guarantees of the treatment's success.
- Prepare the family for expected changes in the patient during therapy, such as hypotension and loss of muscle tone and reflexes.
- Closely monitor the patient's ICP, electrocardiogram (ECG) and vital signs. Notify the doctor of increased ICP, arrhythmias or hypotension.
- Check serum barbiturate levels frequently as ordered.
- Because the patient is in such deep level drug-induced coma, devote special attention to eye care and preventing pressure ulcers.

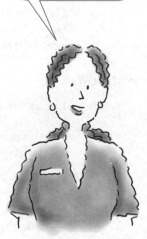

Devote special care to pressure ulcer prevention when your patient is in a drug-induced coma.

Cerebrospinal fluid drainage

The goal of CSF drainage is to reduce ICP to the desired level and keep it at that level. Fluid is withdrawn from the lateral ventricle through ventriculostomy.

To place the ventricular drain a patient will need to be in a neurosurgical centre. A doctor inserts a ventricular catheter through a burr hole in the patient's skull. This is usually done in the operating room. (See *CSF closed drainage system*, page 91.)

Nursing concerns
- Maintain a continuous hourly output of CSF by raising or lowering the drainage system drip chamber.
- Drain the CSF, as ordered, by putting on gloves and turning the main stopcock on to drainage and allowing the CSF to collect in the drip chamber.
- To stop drainage, turn off the stopcock to drainage. Record the time and the amount of collected CSF.
- Check the patient's dressing frequently for drainage.
- Check the tubing for patency by watching the CSF drops in the drip chamber.
- Observe the CSF for colour, clarity, amount, blood and sediment.
- Maintain the patient on bed rest with the head of the bed at 30–45 degrees to promote drainage.

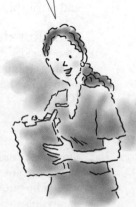

Rapid CSF drainage is an emergency! Watch for signs and symptoms, including headache, tachycardia, diaphoresis and nausea.

CSF closed drainage system

The goal of cerebrospinal fluid (CSF) drainage is to control intracranial pressure (ICP) during treatment for traumatic injury or other conditions that cause increased ICP. Here's one common procedure.

Ventricular drain

For a ventricular drain, the doctor makes a burr hole in the patient's skull and inserts the catheter into the ventricle. The distal end of the catheter is connected to a closed drainage system.

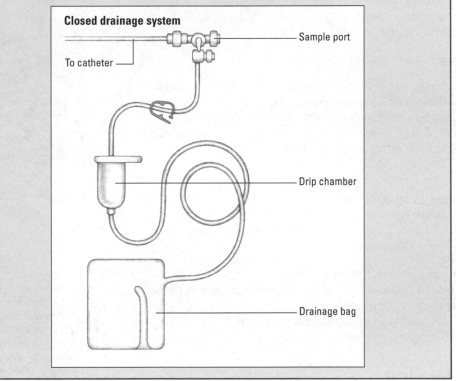

Closed drainage system

To catheter

Sample port

Drip chamber

Drainage bag

• Observe for complications, such as excessive CSF drainage, characterised by headache, tachycardia, diaphoresis and nausea. Overly rapid accumulation of drainage is a neurosurgical emergency. Cessation of drainage may indicate clot formation.

Intracranial pressure monitoring

In ICP monitoring, pressure exerted by the brain, blood and CSF against the inside of the skull is measured. In many hospitals ICP monitoring is rarely performed and assumptions about the ICP are made from clinical signs and CT scan results.

Clinical signs which can show evidence of increasing ICP include:
- changes in GCS and pupillary responses
- increasing blood pressure
- increased urine output from diabetes insipidus because the increased ICP reduces antidiuretic hormone secretion.

Invasive ICP monitoring does provide a specific measurement to inform intervention, which can avert damage caused by cerebral hypoxia and shifts of brain mass.

Indications for ICP monitoring include:
- head trauma with bleeding or oedema
- overproduction or insufficient absorption of CSF
- cerebral haemorrhage
- space-occupying lesions.

Four similar systems

There are four basic types of ICP monitoring systems. (See *Monitoring ICP*, page 93.) Regardless of which system is used, the insertion procedure is usually performed by a neurosurgeon in the operating room or critical care unit. Insertion of an ICP monitoring device requires sterile technique to reduce the risk of CNS infection.

Doctors do this

The doctor inserts a ventricular catheter or subarachnoid screw through a twist-drill hole created in the skull. Devices have built-in transducers that convert ICP into electrical impulses that allow constant monitoring.

Nursing concerns
- Observe digital ICP readings and waveforms.
- Assess the patient's clinical status and monitor routine and neurological vital signs every hour or as ordered.
- Calculate CPP hourly. To calculate CPP, subtract ICP from MAP.
- Inspect the insertion site at least every 24 hours for redness, swelling and drainage.

Nursing ways to reduce ICP

In any patient where raised ICP is confirmed or suspected, the nurse should concentrate on reducing this by ensuring that brain cell requirements are met by aiming to:
- Minimise patient stimulation, create a quiet environment.
- Position the patient 30 degrees head up with head in the midline to promote venous drainage.
- If intubated make sure ties are not too tight restricting venous drainage.

Plasmapheresis
Symptoms of several neurological disorders are reduced through plasma exchange, or plasmapheresis.

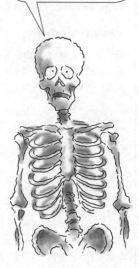

A neurosurgeon always inserts an ICP monitoring device.

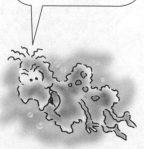

Looks like I'm movin' out! In plasmapheresis, plasma is filtered to remove toxins and disease mediators from the patient's blood.

Monitoring ICP

Intracranial pressure (ICP) can be monitored using one of the following four systems.

Intraventricular catheter monitoring

In intraventricular catheter monitoring, used to monitor ICP directly, the doctor inserts a small polyethylene or silicone rubber catheter into the lateral ventricles through a burr hole.

Although this method is most accurate for measuring ICP, it carries the greatest risk of infection. This is the only type of ICP monitoring that allows evaluation of brain compliance and significant drainage of cerebrospinal fluid (CSF).

Contraindications usually include stenotic cerebral ventricles, cerebral aneurysms in the path of catheter placement and suspected vascular lesions.

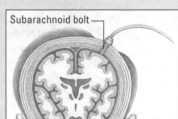
Ventricular catheter

Subarachnoid bolt monitoring

Subarachnoid bolt monitoring involves insertion of a special bolt into the subarachnoid space through a twist-drill burr hole in the front of the skull, behind the hairline.

Placing the bolt is easier than placing an intraventricular catheter, especially if a computed tomography scan reveals that the cerebrum has shifted or the ventricles have collapsed. This type of ICP monitoring also carries less risk of infection and parenchymal damage because the bolt doesn't penetrate the cerebrum.

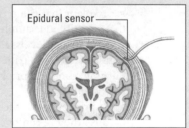
Subarachnoid bolt

Epidural or subdural sensor monitoring

ICP can also be monitored from the epidural or subdural space. For epidural monitoring, a fibre-optic sensor is inserted into the epidural space through a burr hole. This system's main drawback is its questionable accuracy because ICP isn't being measured directly from a CSF-filled space.

For subdural monitoring, a fibre-optic transducer-tipped catheter is tunnelled through a burr hole and is placed on brain tissue under the dura mater. The main drawback of this method is its inability to drain CSF.

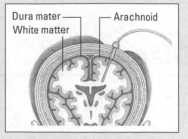
Epidural sensor

Intraparenchymal monitoring

In intraparenchymal monitoring, the doctor inserts a catheter through a small subarachnoid bolt and, after punctuating the dura, advances the catheter a few centimetres into the brain's white matter. There's no need to balance or calibrate the equipment after insertion.

This method doesn't provide direct access to CSF, but measurements are accurate because brain tissue pressure correlates well with ventricular pressures. Intraparenchymal monitoring may be used to obtain ICP measurements in patients with compressed or dislocated ventricles.

Dura mater — Arachnoid
White matter

Out with the bad

In plasmapheresis, blood from the patient flows into a cell separator, which separates plasma from formed elements. The plasma is then filtered to remove toxins and disease mediators, such as immune complexes and autoantibodies, from the patient's blood. The equipment is similar to that used for renal dialysis.

In with the good

The cellular components are then transfused back into the patient using fresh frozen plasma or albumin in place of the plasma removed.

Who benefits?

Plasmapheresis benefits patients with neurological disorders such as Guillain–Barré syndrome and, especially, myasthenia gravis. In myasthenia gravis, plasmapheresis is used to remove circulating antiacetylcholine receptor antibodies.

Plasmapheresis is used most commonly for patients with long-standing neuromuscular disease, but it can also be used to treat patients with acute exacerbations. Some acutely ill patients require treatment up to four times per week; others about once every 2 weeks. When it's successful, treatment may relieve symptoms for months, but results vary.

> Administer prescribed medications after plasmapheresis; otherwise, they're removed from the blood during treatment.

Nursing concerns

• Discuss the treatment and its purpose with the patient and their family members.
• Explain that the procedure can take up to 5 hours. During that time, blood samples are taken frequently to monitor calcium and potassium levels. Blood pressure and heart rate are checked regularly. Tell the patient to report any paraesthesia (numbness, burning, tingling, prickling or increased sensitivity) during treatment.
• If possible, give the patient prescribed medications after treatment because they're removed from the blood during treatment.
• Monitor the patient's observation signs according to your unit's policy.
• Check puncture sites for signs of bleeding or extravasation.

Disorders

In the general critical care unit many patients may have disorders with associated neurological compromise such as reduced LOC secondary to shock states, risk of stroke/bleeding secondary to their primary condition and delirium of unknown cause. Initial management of such patients will usually focus on an ABCDE approach with close monitoring of GCS to detect deterioration early and trying to ensure the cells get what they need so that further damage is minimised. (See *Using the Glasgow Coma Scale,* page 69 and *What cells need in the brain and spinal cord,* page 63.) Management of delirium is discussed in more detail in Chapter 2.

Care of specific disorders you're likely to encounter are acute spinal cord injury, AVM, cerebral aneurysm, encephalitis, Guillain–Barré syndrome, traumatic closed head injury, hypoxic brain damage, meningitis, seizure disorders and stroke. Liver failure encephalopathy may also be encountered and this is discussed in Chapter 6.

Acute spinal cord injury

Spinal injuries include fractures, contusions and compressions of the vertebral column. They usually result from trauma to the head or neck. Fractures of the 5th, 6th or 7th cervical; 12th thoracic; and 1st lumbar vertebrae are most common. In critical care a number of patients may be admitted in an unconscious state with a suspected spinal cord injury but this cannot be confirmed or ruled out until the patient regains consciousness. These patients should be treated as if they have spinal cord injury until proven otherwise.

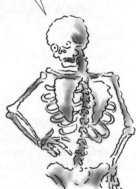

The real danger with spinal injury is spinal cord damage.

Dangerous damage

The real danger with spinal injury is spinal cord damage due to cutting, pulling, twisting and compression. Spinal cord injury can occur at any level, and the damage it causes may be partial or involve the entire cord.

Complications of spinal cord injury include neurogenic shock and spinal shock. (See *Complications of spinal cord injury,* page 96.)

What causes it

The most serious spinal cord trauma typically results from motor vehicle accidents, falls, sports injuries, diving into shallow water and gunshot or stab wounds. Less serious injuries usually occur from lifting heavy objects and minor falls, although elderly patients may get injuries disproportionate to their trauma owing to reduced bone density.

Spinal dysfunction may also result from hyperparathyroidism, neoplastic lesions and abcesses.

Pathophysiology

Spinal cord trauma results from acceleration, deceleration or other deforming forces. Types of trauma include:
• hyperextension due to acceleration–deceleration forces
• hyperflexion from sudden and excessive force
• vertebral compression from downwards force from the top of the cranium, along the vertical axis and through the vertebra
• rotational twisting, which adds shearing forces.

Take charge!

Complications of spinal cord injury

When you assess your patient, watch for these two complications related to spinal cord injuries.

Neurogenic shock

Neurogenic shock is an abnormal vasomotor response that occurs secondary to disruption of sympathetic impulses from the brain stem to the thoracolumbar area. It's most common in patients with cervical cord injury. It causes temporary loss of autonomic function below the level of injury and leads to cardiovascular changes.

Signs of neurogenic shock include:

- orthostatic hypotension
- bradycardia
- inability to sweat below the level of the injury.

Spinal shock

Spinal shock is the loss of autonomic, reflex, motor and sensory activity below the level of the cord lesion. It occurs secondary to damage of the spinal cord usually lasting around 48 hours.

Signs of spinal shock include:

- flaccid paralysis
- loss of deep tendon and perianal reflexes
- loss of motor and sensory function.

Trauma trail

Here's what happens during spinal cord trauma:
- An injury causes microscopic haemorrhages in the grey matter and pia-arachnoid.
- The haemorrhages gradually increase in size until all of the grey matter is filled with blood, which causes necrosis.
- From the grey matter, the blood enters the white matter, where it impedes circulation within the spinal cord.
- Resulting oedema causes compression and decreases the blood supply.
- The spinal cord loses perfusion and becomes ischaemic. The oedema and haemorrhage are usually greatest in the two segments above and below the injury.
- The oedema temporarily adds to the patient's dysfunction by increasing pressure and compressing the nerves. For example, oedema near the 3rd to 5th cervical vertebrae may interfere with respiration.

> Careful! The most serious causes of spinal cord trauma are car collisions and other accidents.

After acute injury

Here's what happens following acute trauma:
• In the white matter, circulation usually returns to normal within 24 hours after injury.
• In the grey matter, an inflammatory reaction prevents restoration of circulation.
• Phagocytes appear at the site within 35–48 hours after injury.
• Macrophages engulf degenerating axons and collagen replaces the normal tissue.
• Scarring and meningeal thickening leaves the nerves in the area blocked or tangled.

What to look for

In your assessment, look for:
• history of trauma, a neoplastic lesion, an infection that could produce a spinal abscess or an endocrine disorder
• muscle spasm and back or neck pain that worsens with movement; in cervical fractures, pain that causes point tenderness; in dorsal and lumbar fractures, pain that may radiate to other areas, such as the legs
• mild paraesthesia to quadriplegia and shock, if the injury damages the spinal cord; in milder injury, symptoms that may be delayed for several days or weeks.

Speaking specifically

Specific signs and symptoms depend on the type and degree of injury. (See *Types of spinal cord injury,* page 98.)

What tests tell you

Diagnoses of acute spinal cord injuries are based on the results of the following diagnostic tests:
• Spinal x-rays (the most important diagnostic measure) reveal fracture.
• Myelography shows the location of fracture and site of compression.
• CT scan and MRI show the location of fracture and the site of compression and reveal spinal cord oedema and a possible spinal cord mass.
• Neurological evaluation is used to locate the level of injury and detect cord damage.
• Lumbar puncture shows increased CSF pressure from a lesion or trauma in spinal compression.

How it's treated

The primary treatment after spinal injury is immediate immobilisation to stabilise the spine and prevent cord damage. Other treatment is supportive.
Cervical injuries require immobilisation, using sandbags on both sides of the patient's head, a hard cervical collar or skeletal traction with skull tongs or a halo device.

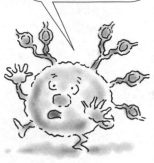

After acute spinal injury, scarring and meningeal thickening leaves the nerves in the area blocked or tangled.

Types of spinal cord injury

Spinal cord injury may be classified as complete or incomplete. Incomplete injury may be an anterior cord syndrome, central cord syndrome or Brown–Séquard's syndrome, depending on which area of the cord is affected. Here are the characteristic signs and symptoms of each.

Type	Description	Signs and symptoms
Complete transection	• All tracts of the spinal cord completely disrupted • All functions involving the spinal cord below the level of transection lost • Complete and permanent loss	• Loss of motor function (quadriplegia) with cervical cord transection; paraplegia with thoracic cord transection • Muscle flaccidity • Loss of all reflexes and sensory function below the level of injury • Bladder and bowel atony • Paralytic ileus • Loss of vasomotor tone in lower body parts with low and unstable blood pressure • Loss of perspiration below level of injury • Dry, pale skin • Respiratory impairment
Incomplete transection: Central cord syndrome	• Centre position of cord affected • Typically from hyperextension injury	• Motor deficits greater in upper than in lower extremities • Variable degree of bladder dysfunction
Incomplete transection: Anterior cord syndrome	• Occlusion of anterior spinal artery • Occlusion from pressure of bone fragments	• Loss of motor function below the level of injury • Loss of pain and temperature sensations below the level of injury • Intact touch, pressure, position and vibration senses
Incomplete transection: Brown–Séquard's syndrome	• Hemisection of cord affected • Most common in stabbing and gunshot wounds • Damage to cord on only one side	• Ipsilateral paralysis or paresis below the level of injury • Ipsilateral loss of touch, pressure, vibration and position sense below the level of injury • Contralateral loss of pain and temperature sensations below the level of injury

What to do

Here's what you should do for patients with spinal cord injuries:
• Refer to specialist spinal injuries unit as soon as possible because patient outcomes are shown to be better if patients are cared for in these specialist areas.
• Ensure ongoing stabilisation of the patient's spine. As with all spinal injuries, suspect cord damage until proven otherwise.

- Perform a neurological assessment to establish a baseline and continually reassess neurological status for changes.
- Assess respiratory status closely at least every hour, initially. Obtain baseline tidal volume, vital capacity, negative inspiratory forces and minute volume.
- Auscultate breath sounds and check secretions as necessary, perform suction as required but monitor closely because of high risks of bradycardia from vagal stimulation.
- Monitor oxygen saturation levels and administer supplemental oxygen as indicated. Aim to optimise respiratory function by adequate humidification, considering additional saline nebulisers if required.
- Remember that if intubation is required it will be relatively difficult because of cervical immobilisation so it should ideally be undertaken by an experienced clinician in an elective manner with difficult intubation equipment available (fibreoptic and McCoy laryngoscopes and bougie).
- Assess cardiac status frequently, at least every hour initially. Begin cardiac monitoring. Monitor blood pressure and hemodynamic status frequently.
- If your patient becomes hypotensive, prepare to administer vasopressors (e.g. noradrenaline) as neurogenic and spinal shock cause vasodilation.
- Prepare the patient for surgical stabilisation, if necessary.
- Assess GI status closely for signs of ulceration or bleeding. Anticipate nasogastric (NG) tube insertion and regular aspiration. Assess the abdomen for distention, auscultate bowel sounds and report any decrease or absence. Be alert for paralytic ileus, which usually occurs 72 hours after injury.
- Monitor intake and output for fluid imbalance.
- Insert an indwelling urinary catheter as ordered to prevent urinary retention. Commence daily PR examination and administration of laxatives and/or enemas according to specialist spinal injury unit policies.
- Begin measures to prevent skin breakdown due to immobilisation, including repositioning, padding and care of equipment such as halo or traction devices.
- Monitor laboratory and diagnostic test results, including urea and creatinine levels, full blood count (FBC) and urine culture (if indicated).
- Be alert to other potentially undiagnosed injuries that have been missed owing to patient paralysis.
- Monitor the patient for deep vein thrombosis and pulmonary embolism. Apply antiembolism stockings or intermittent sequential compression devices as ordered.
- Provide emotional support to the patient and their family members.
- Begin rehabilitation as soon as possible.

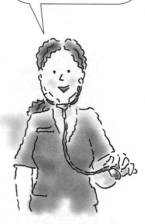

After the spine is immobilised, begin a neurological assessment to establish baselines. Be alert at all times for changes.

Arteriovenous malformation

AVMs are tangled masses of thin-walled, dilated blood vessels between arteries and veins which aren't connected by capillaries. Abnormal channels between the arterial and venous system mix oxygenated and unoxygenated blood. This prevents adequate perfusion of brain tissue.

Looking for AVMs

AVMs are common in the brain, especially in the posterior parts of the cerebral hemispheres. They range in size from a few millimetres to large malformations extending from the cerebral cortex to the ventricles. More than one AVM is commonly found.

Males and females are affected equally, and some evidence exists that AVMs occur in families. Most AVMs are present at birth, but symptoms typically occur later, when the person is 10–20 years old.

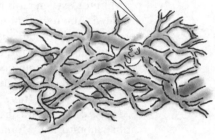

Uh-oh! AVMs are tangled masses of blood vessels that prevent adequate perfusion of brain tissue.

Uh-oh

Complications depend on the severity (location and size) of the AVM and include:
• aneurysm development and subsequent rupture
• haemorrhage (intracerebral, subarachnoid or subdural, depending on the location of the AVM)
• hydrocephalus.

What causes it

Causes of AVMs may be either:
• congenital—due to a hereditary defect
• acquired—due to penetrating injuries such as trauma.

Pathophysiology

AVMs lack the typical structural characteristics of the blood vessels; the vessels of an AVM are very thin.

Blood pressure, aneurysm and haemorrhage

One or more arteries feed into the AVM; the typically high-pressured arterial blood flow moves into the venous system through connecting channels. This increases venous pressure, engorging and dilating the venous structures, which may result in the development of an aneurysm.

If the AVM is large enough, the shunting can deprive the surrounding tissue of adequate blood flow. Additionally, the thin-walled vessels may ooze small amounts of blood or rupture, causing haemorrhage into the brain or subarachnoid space.

Shunting can deprive tissues of adequate blood flow.

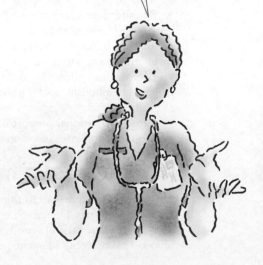

What to look for

Typically, patients exhibit few, if any, signs and symptoms unless the AVM is large or it leaks or ruptures.

Some signs and symptoms

In some patients, signs and symptoms include:
• chronic mild headache and confusion from AVM dilation, vessel engorgement and increased pressure
• seizures secondary to compression of the surrounding tissues by the engorged vessels
• systolic bruit over the carotid artery, mastoid process or orbit, indicating turbulent blood flow
• focal neurological deficits (depending on the location of the AVM) resulting from compression and diminished perfusion
• symptoms of intracranial (intracerebral, subarachnoid or subdural) haemorrhage, including sudden severe headache, seizures, confusion, lethargy and meningeal irritation from bleeding into the brain tissue or subarachnoid space
• hydrocephalus from AVM extension into the ventricular lining.

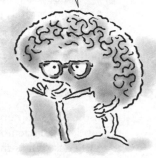

Loss of blood through thin-walled vessels can lead to rupture and hemorrhage.

What tests tell you

The following tests are used to diagnose AVM:
• Cerebral angiography yields the most definitive diagnostic information. It's used to localise the AVM and allow visualisation of large feeding arteries and drainage veins.
• CT scan with a contrast medium is used to differentiate AVM from a clot or tumour.
• MRI is used to determine the location and size of AVM.
• EEG is used to locate AVM.
• Doppler ultrasonography of the cerebrovascular system is used to find abnormal and turbulent blood flow.

How it's treated

The choice of treatment depends on the:
• size and location of the AVM
• feeder vessels supplying it
• age and condition of the patient.

Supportive, corrective or both

Treatment can be supportive, corrective or both, including:
• support measures, such as aneurysm precautions to prevent possible rupture
• surgery—block dissection, laser or ligation—to repair the communicating channels and remove the feeding vessels
• embolisation or radiation therapy if surgery isn't possible, to close the communicating channels and feeder vessels and thus reduce blood flow to the AVM.

What to do

If haemorrhage hasn't occurred in your patient with AVM, focus your efforts on bleeding prevention.

Steps to take

To prevent bleeding, follow these steps to control hypertension and seizure activity:
- Maintain a quiet therapeutic environment.
- Monitor and control associated hypertension with drug therapy as ordered.
- Conduct ongoing neurological assessment.
- Monitor vital signs frequently.
- Assess and monitor characteristics of headache, seizure activity or bruit as needed.
- Provide emotional support.

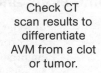

Check CT scan results to differentiate AVM from a clot or tumor.

Rupture measures

If the AVM ruptures, work to control elevated ICP and intracranial haemorrhage. Follow the steps described earlier as well as those listed here:
- refer to neurosurgical centre
- monitor neurological status and vital signs frequently
- maintain sedation and ventilation as required
- monitor arterial blood gases (ABGs), fluid balance and electrolyte levels.

Cerebral aneurysm

In intracranial or cerebral aneurysm, a weakness in the wall of a cerebral artery causes that area of the artery to dilate or bulge. The most common form is the berry aneurysm, a saclike outpouching in a cerebral artery.

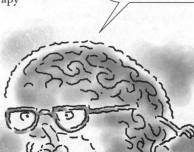

In cerebral aneurysm, blood pressure against a weak arterial wall stretches the vessel like a balloon, making it likely to rupture.

The usual place

Cerebral aneurysms usually arise at an arterial junction in the circle of Willis, the circular anastomosis forming the major cerebral arteries at the base of the brain. Cerebral aneurysms commonly rupture and cause subarachnoid haemorrhage.

The usual patient

The incidence of cerebral aneurysm is slightly higher in women than in men, especially those in their late 40s or early to mid-50s, but a cerebral aneurysm can occur at any age in either sex.

The usual prognosis

The prognosis for any patient with cerebral aneurysm is guarded. About 50% of all patients who suffer a subarachnoid haemorrhage die immediately.

Take charge!

Signs of increased ICP

The earlier you spot signs of increased intracranial pressure (ICP), the quicker you can intervene and the better your patient's chance of recovery. By the time late signs appear, interventions may be useless.

Assessment area	Early signs	Late signs
Level of consciousness	• Requires increased stimulation • Subtle orientation loss • Restlessness and anxiety • Sudden quietness	• Unarousable
Pupils	• Pupil changes on side of lesion • One pupil constricts but then dilates (unilateral hippus) • Sluggish reaction of both pupils • Unequal pupils	• Pupils fixed and dilated or 'blown'
Motor response	• Sudden weakness • Motor changes on side opposite the lesion • Positive pronator drift: With palms up, one hand pronates	• Profound weakness
Vital signs	• Intermittent increases in blood pressure	• Increased systolic pressure with widening pulse pressure, bradycardia and abnormal respirations (Cushing's triad)

Of those who survive untreated, 40% die from the effects of haemorrhage and another 20% die later from recurring haemorrhage. New treatments are improving the prognosis.

The major complications of cerebral aneurysm include death from increased ICP and brain herniation, rebleeding and vasospasm. (See *Signs of increased ICP*.)

What causes it

Causes of cerebral aneurysm include:
• congenital defect
• degenerative process
• combination of congenital defect and degenerative process
• trauma.

Pathophysiology

Blood flow exerts pressure against a weak arterial wall, stretching it like an overblown balloon and making it likely to rupture.

Right after rupture

Rupture is followed by a subarachnoid haemorrhage, in which blood spills into the space normally occupied by CSF. Sometimes, blood also spills into brain tissue, where a clot can cause potentially fatal increased ICP and brain tissue damage.

What to look for

Occasionally, your patient may exhibit signs and symptoms due to blood oozing into the subarachnoid space. The symptoms, which may persist for several days, include:
• headache
• intermittent nausea
• nuchal rigidity
• stiff back and legs.

Rupture without warning

Aneurysm rupture usually occurs abruptly and without warning, causing:
• sudden severe headache caused by increased pressure from bleeding into a closed space, can be described like being hit on the head
• nausea and projectile vomiting related to increased ICP
• altered LOC, possibly including deep coma, depending on the severity and location of bleeding, due to increased pressure caused by increased cerebral blood volume
• meningeal irritation due to bleeding into the meninges and resulting in nuchal rigidity, back and leg pain, fever, restlessness, irritability, occasional seizures, photophobia and blurred vision
• hemiparesis, hemisensory defects, dysphagia and visual defects due to bleeding into the brain tissues
• diplopia, ptosis, dilated pupil and inability to rotate the eye caused by compression on the oculomotor nerve if the aneurysm is near the internal carotid artery.

Grading severity

Typically, the severity of a ruptured intracranial aneurysm is graded according to the patient's signs and symptoms. (See *Grading cerebral aneurysm rupture.*)

What tests tell you

The following tests aid in the diagnosis of cerebral aneurysm:
• Cerebral angiography confirms a cerebral aneurysm that isn't ruptured and reveals altered cerebral blood flow, vessel lumen dilation and differences in arterial filling.
• CT scan reveals evidence of aneurysm and possible haemorrhage.

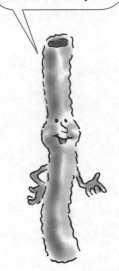

If your patient reports headache, nausea, and back and leg stiffness lasting for several days, suspect cerebral aneurysm.

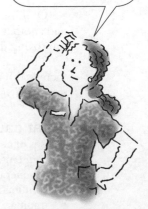

A cerebral aneurysm typically ruptures before symptoms are seen. Signs after rupture are sudden and severe.

Grading cerebral aneurysm rupture

The severity of symptoms varies from patient to patient, depending on the site and amount of bleeding. Five grades characterise ruptured cerebral aneurysm:

- *Grade I: minimal bleeding*—The patient is alert, with no neurological deficit; they may have a slight headache and nuchal rigidity.
- *Grade II: mild bleeding*—The patient is alert, with a mild-to-severe headache and nuchal rigidity; they may have third-nerve palsy.
- *Grade III: moderate bleeding*—The patient is confused or drowsy, with nuchal rigidity and, possibly, a mild focal deficit.
- *Grade IV: severe bleeding*—The patient is stuporous, with nuchal rigidity and, possibly, mild-to-severe hemiparesis.
- *Grade V: moribund (usually fatal)*—If the rupture is nonfatal, the patient is in a deep coma or decerebrate.

- MRI is used to detect vasospasm and locate the bleeding.
- PET scan shows the chemical activity of the brain and extent of tissue damage.

How it's treated

Emergency treatment begins with oxygenation and ventilation and then emergency referral to a neurosurgical centre, where to reduce the risk of rebleeding, the doctor may attempt to repair the aneurysm. Surgical repair usually includes clipping, ligating or wrapping the aneurysm neck with muscle.

New and improved

Newer techniques for surgery include interventional radiology in conjunction with endovascular balloon therapy. This technique occludes the aneurysm or vessel and uses cerebral angiography to treat arterial vasospasm.

In some cases, a type of nonsurgical repair called electrothrombosis is used. (See *Endovascular aneurysm repair*, page 106.)

Conservative whys

The patient may receive conservative treatment when surgical correction poses too much risk, such as when:
- the patient is elderly
- the patient has heart, lung or other serious disease
- the aneurysm is in a dangerous location
- vasospasm necessitates a delay in surgery.

Conservative ways

Conservative treatment methods include:
- bed rest in a quiet, darkened room with the head of bed flat or raised less than 30 degrees, which may continue for 4–6 weeks

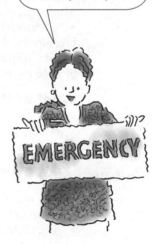

Think fast! Emergency treatment begins with oxygenation and ventilation before the doctor attempts aneurysm repair.

Endovascular aneurysm repair

When surgery isn't appropriate for intracranial aneurysm repair, a recently developed endovascular treatment method called electrothrombosis may be used. Electrothrombosis is most successful in aneurysms with small necks and those without significant intrafundal thrombus.

Electrothrombosis

Here's what happens in electrothrombosis:

- Soft platinum coils soldered to a stainless steel delivery wire are positioned in the aneurysm.
- After the coil is positioned within the fundus of the aneurysm, a 1-mA current is applied to the delivery wire.
- The delivery wire is removed, leaving the platinum coil in place and another coil is introduced into the fundus.

- The process is continued until the aneurysm is densely packed with platinum and no longer opacifies during diagnostic contrast injections.

How it works

The positively charged platinum left in the aneurysm theoretically attracts negatively charged blood elements, such as white and red blood cells, platelets and fibrinogen. This induces intra-aneurysmal thrombosis.

The coils provide immediate protection against further haemorrhage by reducing blood pulsations in the fundus and sealing the hole or weak portion of the artery wall. Eventually, clots form and the aneurysm is separated from the parent vessel by the formation of new connective tissue.

- avoidance of coffee, other stimulants and aspirin to reduce the risk of rupture and elevation of blood pressure
- possible administration of codeine or other analgesics
- administration of antihypertensives, if the patient is hypertensive
- administration of corticosteroids to reduce oedema
- cautious administration of a sedative but recognising that this may affect neurological assessment
- administration of a vasoconstrictor to maintain an optimum blood pressure level (20–40 mmHg above normal), if necessary
- administration of a fibrinolysis inhibitor, to minimise the risk of rebleeding by delaying blood clot lysis (the effectiveness of these drugs is under dispute).

What to do

When caring for a patient with an intact cerebral aneurysm, an accurate neurological assessment, good patient care, patient and family teaching and psychological support can speed recovery and reduce complications.

Your next step

During the initial treatment after haemorrhage use an ABCDE approach with particular attention to the following:
- Establish and maintain a patent airway and anticipate the need for supplementary oxygen or mechanical ventilatory support. Monitor ABG levels.
- Position the patient to promote pulmonary drainage and prevent upper airway obstruction. If intubated, preoxygenate with 100% oxygen before suctioning.
- Impose aneurysm precautions (such as bed rest, limited visitors and avoidance of coffee and physical activity) to minimise the risk of rebleeding and avoid increased ICP.

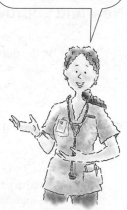

When surgical correction is too risky for your patient, implement these conservative treatment methods.

- Administer a stool softener, as ordered, to prevent straining.
- Monitor LOC and vital signs frequently.
- Accurately measure intake and output.
- Be alert for danger signs that may indicate an enlarging aneurysm, rebleeding, intracranial clot, increased ICP or vasospasm, including decreased LOC, unilateral enlarged pupil, onset or worsening of hemiparesis or motor deficit, increased blood pressure, slowed pulse rate, worsening of headache or sudden onset of a headache, renewed or worsened nuchal rigidity and renewed or persistent vomiting.
- If the patient develops vasospasm—evidenced by focal motor deficits, increasing confusion and worsening headache—the doctor may initiate hypervolaemic–haemodilution therapy, such as the administration of normal saline, whole blood, packed red cells, human albumin solution and crystalloid solution. The calcium channel blocker, nimodipine, may reduce smooth-muscle spasm and maximise perfusion during spasm. During therapy, assess the patient for fluid overload.
- Turn the patient often, apply antiembolism stockings or intermittent sequential compression devices to the patient's legs and begin measures to prevent skin breakdown.
- If the patient has facial weakness, assist during meals. If they can't swallow, insert an NG tube feeding over 24 hours.
- If mannitol is used, administer as prescribed. Be alert for subsequent rebound of increased ICP, which may occur 8–12 hours after administration.
- Prepare the patient for surgery, as appropriate.
- Inform the patient and their family members about the condition.

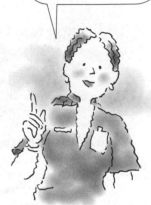

Aneurysm precautions may minimize your patient's risk of rebleeding and prevent increased ICP.

Encephalitis

Encephalitis is severe inflammation of the brain, it can be caused by a variety of viruses transmitted by accidental injection or inhalation.

What causes it
Causes include herpes virus, mumps virus, human immunodeficiency virus, adenoviruses and demyelinating diseases following measles, chicken pox, rubella or vaccination.

Pathophysiology
With encephalitis, intense lymphocytic infiltration of brain tissues and the leptomeninges causes cerebral oedema, degeneration of the brain's ganglion cells and diffuse nerve cell destruction.

What to look for
Watch for the signs and symptoms that signal the beginning of acute illness, including:
- hyperpyrexia (38.9–40.6°C)
- headache
- vomiting.

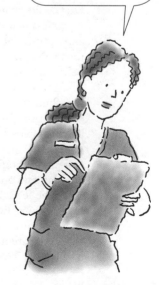

When a patient presents with fever, headache, vomiting and stiff neck and back, suspect encephalitis.

Negative progression

The illness can progress to include signs and symptoms of meningeal irritation, such as stiff neck and back. Be alert for signs of neurone damage, such as:

- drowsiness
- coma
- paralysis
- seizures
- ataxia
- organic psychoses.

Stay alert for changes! Symptoms can escalate to include drowsiness, coma, paralysis, and other signs of neurone damage.

What tests tell you

The following diagnostic tests are used in the diagnosis of encephalitis:

- CSF or blood analysis used to identify the causative virus confirms the diagnosis.
- CT scan may disclose localised abnormalities.

How it's treated

Most of the treatments for patients with encephalitis are entirely supportive:

- The antiviral agent, acyclovir, is effective in treatment for herpes encephalitis.
- Anticonvulsants and corticosteroids reduce cerebral inflammation and oedema.
- Mannitol can reduce cerebral swelling.
- Sedatives may be given to alleviate restlessness.
- Paracetamol relieves headache and reduces fever.
- Fluids and electrolytes prevent dehydration and electrolyte imbalance.
- Antibiotics are used to fight an associated infection such as pneumonia.

What to do

During the acute phase of the illness, follow these guidelines:

- Assess neurological function frequently. Check for changes in GCS and signs of increased ICP. Watch for signs and symptoms of cranial nerve involvement, such asptosis, strabismus, diplopia, abnormal sleep patterns and behaviour changes.
- Monitor intake and output carefully to maintain fluid balance. Be aware that fluid overload can increase cerebral oedema.
- Position and move the patient carefully to prevent joint stiffness and neck pain.
- Provide analgesia and a quiet, darkened room to ease headache and photophobia.
- Maintain adequate nutrition by giving small, frequent meals or NG tube feedings as prescribed.
- Reassure the patient and their family members that behaviour changes caused by encephalitis usually disappear.
- If the patient is disoriented or confused, attempt to reorient them frequently. Place a calendar or clock in the patient's room to aid in orientation.

If your patient with encephalitis is disoriented, place a calendar or clock in the room.

Guillain–Barré syndrome

Guillain–Barré syndrome, or acute idiopathic polyneuritis, is also known as *infectious polyneuritis*. It's an acute, rapidly progressive and potentially fatal form of polyneuritis that causes muscle weakness and mild distal sensory loss.

Equal opportunity syndrome

This syndrome can occur at any age but is most common in people between ages 30 and 50. It affects both sexes equally.

Recovery is spontaneous and complete in about 95% of patients; however, mild motor or reflex deficits may persist in the feet and legs. The prognosis is best when symptoms resolve sooner than 15–20 days after onset.

Three-phase syndrome

Guillain–Barré syndrome occurs in three phases:

 The acute phase begins with the onset of the first definitive symptom and ends 1–3 weeks later. Further deterioration doesn't occur after the acute phase.

The plateau phase lasts several days to 2 weeks.

The recovery phase coincides with remyelinisation and regrowth of axonal processes. Recovery commonly takes 4–6 months, but may take as long as 2–3 years in severe cases.

Commonly complicated syndrome

Common complications include thrombophlebitis, pressure ulcers, muscle wasting, sepsis, joint contractures, respiratory tract infections, respiratory failure and loss of bladder and bowel control.

What causes it

The precise cause of Guillain–Barré syndrome isn't known, but it may be a cell-mediated immune response to a virus. About 50% of patients with Guillain–Barré syndrome have a recent history of minor febrile illness, usually an upper respiratory tract infection or, less commonly, gastroenteritis. When infection precedes the onset of Guillain–Barré syndrome, signs of infection subside before neurological features appear.

Possible precipitators

Other possible precipitating factors include:
- surgery
- Hodgkin's or other malignant disease
- systemic lupus erythematosus.

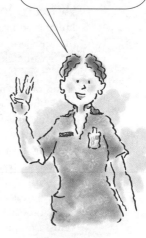

In a severe case, your patient with Guillain-Barré syndrome may take 2–3 years to recover.

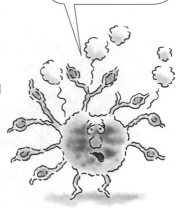

Guillain–Barré syndrome causes sensory and motor losses at the same time...

Pathophysiology

The major pathological feature of Guillain–Barré syndrome is segmental demyelination of the peripheral nerves, which prevents the normal transmission of electrical impulses along the sensorimotor nerve roots.

Double trouble

Guillain–Barré syndrome causes inflammation and degenerative changes in both the posterior (sensory) and the anterior (motor) nerve roots. That's why signs of sensory and motor losses occur simultaneously. Additionally, autonomic nerve transmission may be impaired.

What to look for

During your assessment, look for symptoms that are progressive and include:
• Symmetrical muscle weakness (the major neurological sign), appearing first in the legs (in the ascending type of the syndrome, which is the most common form) and then extending to the arms and facial nerves within 24–72 hours, due to impaired anterior nerve root transmission.
• Muscle weakness developing in the brainstem, in the cranial nerves and progressing downwards in the arms first (in the descending type of the syndrome) or in the arms and legs simultaneously, due to impaired anterior nerve root transmission.
• Normal muscle strength (in mild forms of the syndrome) or weakness affecting only the cranial nerves.
• Paraesthesia, sometimes preceding muscle weakness but vanishing quickly, due to impairment of the dorsal nerve root transmission.
• Diplegia, possibly with ophthalmoplegia (ocular paralysis), from impaired motor nerve root transmission and involvement of cranial nerves III, IV and VI.
• Dysphagia or dysarthria and, less commonly, weakness of the muscles supplied by CN XI (the spinal accessory nerve).
• Hypotonia and areflexia from interruption of the reflex arc.

...thanks to changes in both the sensory and motor nerve roots. Thanks, but no thanks!

What tests tell you

The following diagnostic tests aid in the diagnosis of Guillain–Barré syndrome:
• CSF analysis reveals protein levels that begin to increase several days after the onset of symptoms and peak in 4–6 weeks.
• FBC early in illness shows leukocytosis and immature forms of white blood cells (immature neutrophils, called *bands*).
• Electromyography may show repeated firing of the same motor unit instead of widespread sectional stimulation.
• Nerve conduction velocities slow soon after paralysis develops.
• Serum immunoglobulin levels are elevated due to an inflammatory response.

How it's treated
- Treatments are primarily supportive and include endotracheal (ET) intubation or tracheostomy if respiratory muscle involvement causes difficulty in clearing secretions.
- A trial dose of steroids may be given to reduce inflammatory response if the disease is relentlessly progressive; if there is no noticeable improvement after 7 days, the drug is discontinued.
- High dose I.V. immunoglobulins may be infused as some evidence shows demyelination is due to postinfectious autoimmunity.
- Plasmapheresis is useful during the initial phase, but of no benefit if started 2 weeks after onset.
- Continuous ECG is used to monitor for possible arrhythmias due to autonomic dysfunction. Beta-blockers are used to reduce tachycardia and hypertension. Atropine is given for bradycardia. Volume replacement is used in treating patients with severe hypotension.

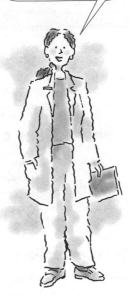

Stand by to provide supportive treatments, such as ET intubation or tracheostomy.

What to do
When caring for a patient with Guillain–Barré syndrome:
- Watch for ascending sensory loss, which precedes motor loss.
- Monitor vital signs and GCS.
- Assess and treat patients with respiratory dysfunction, monitoring vital capacity.
- Auscultate breath sounds, turn and position patient, and encourage coughing and deep breathing. Begin respiratory support at the first sign of respiratory failure, which may include ET intubation and mechanical ventilation.
- Provide meticulous skin care to prevent skin breakdown.
- Perform passive ROM exercises within the patient's pain limits.
- Administer analgesia as prescribed, pain is usually neuropathic in nature so gabapentin and amitriptyline may be used.
- To prevent aspiration, test the gag reflex and elevate the head of the bed before the patient eats. If the gag reflex is absent, give NG tube feedings until the gag reflex returns.
- As the patient regains strength and can tolerate a vertical position, be alert for hypotension. Change the patient's position slowly.
- Apply antiembolism stockings and a sequential compression device to the legs.
- If the patient has facial paralysis, provide eye and mouth care every 4 hours.
- Watch for urine retention. Use an indwelling urinary catheter if necessary.
- To prevent constipation, provide a high-fibre diet. Administer laxatives asprescribed and monitor bowels closely.
- liaise closely with physiotherapists.

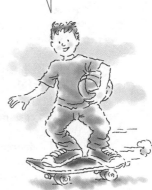

Ahh! It's no surprise that most patients with head injuries are toddlers, young adults, or elderly people.

Head injury

Head injury is any insult to the brain that can cause physical, intellectual, emotional, social or vocational changes. Children aged 6 months to 2 years, adults aged 15 to 24 and elderly adults are most at risk for head injury.

To put it bluntly

Head injury is generally categorised as closed or open. Closed (or blunt) trauma is more common. It typically occurs when the head strikes a hard surface or a rapidly moving object strikes the head. The dura is intact, and no brain tissue is exposed to the external environment. A closed head injury may also result from hypoxic brain damage when oxygen has not been supplied to the brain for a period of time, hypoglycaemia when glucose has not been supplied or hyponatraemia when the sodium level has been very low, less than 120 mmol/L.

In open head injury, as the name suggests, an opening in the scalp, skull, meninges or brain tissue (the dura) exposes the cranial contents to the environment. The risk of infection is high.

Complications are possible

Possible complications include:
- increased ICP
- infection (in open trauma)
- respiratory depression and failure
- brain herniation resulting in brain stem death.

On the decline

Mortality from head injury has declined as a result of:
- advances in preventive measures, such as air bags and seat belts
- quicker emergency response and transport times
- improved treatment measures.

What causes it

Head injury commonly results from:
- motor vehicle collisions (the number one cause)
- falls
- sports-related accidents
- assaults and other crimes
- respiratory and cardiac arrests
- insulin overdose
- water intoxication, incorrect I.V. fluid administration.

How it happens

In trauma the patient's brain is shielded by the cranial vault (comprised of skin, bone, meninges and CSF), which intercepts the force of a physical blow. Below a certain level of force, the cranial vault prevents energy from affecting the brain.

The degree of traumatic head injury usually is proportional to the amount of force reaching the cranial tissues. In addition, unless it's ruled out, you may presume that neck injuries are present in patients with traumatic head injuries.

In hypoxic and hypoglycaemic head injury diffuse cell damage can occur from ischaemia or lack of glucose resulting in necrosis of brain cells. In hyponatraemia the myelin sheath covering the nerves is damaged often irreversibly.

Case closed

Closed trauma is typically a sudden acceleration–deceleration or coup–contrecoup injury. In coup–contrecoup injury, the head hits a more stationary object, injuring cranial tissues near the point of impact (coup); the remaining force then pushes the brain against the opposite side of the skull, causing a second impact and injury (contrecoup).

Contusions and lacerations may also occur during contrecoup as the brain's soft tissues slide over the rough bone of the cranial cavity. The cerebrum may endure rotational shear, damaging the upper midbrain and areas of the frontal, temporal and occipital lobes.

What to look for

Types of head trauma include:
- concussion
- contusion
- epidural haematoma
- subdural haematoma
- intracerebral haematoma
- skull fractures.

Each type is associated with specific signs and symptoms. (See *Types of head injury*, pages 114 to 117.) Signs and symptoms of head trauma in elderly patients may not be readily apparent. (See *Hidden haematoma*.)

What tests tell you

These diagnostic tests are used in diagnosing head injury:
- Skull x-rays show the location of the fracture, unless the cranial vault is fractured. (A CT scan will show a fracture of the cranial vault.)
- Cerebral angiography shows the location of vascular disruption due to internal pressure or injuries that result from cerebral contusion or skull fracture.
- CT scan shows intracranial haemorrhage from ruptured blood vessels, ischaemic or necrotic tissue, cerebral oedema, a shift in brain tissue and subdural, epidural and intracerebral haematomas.
- MRI may show intracranial haemorrhage from ruptured blood vessels in a patient with a skull fracture.

How it's treated

Treatment may be surgical or supportive.

It's surgical

Surgical treatment includes:
- evacuation of a haematoma
- craniotomy.

Senior moment

Hidden haematoma

An older person with cerebral atrophy can tolerate a larger subdural haematoma for a longer time than a younger person can before the haematoma causes neurological changes. That's why a haematoma in an older patient can become rather large before you see any symptoms, even in an acute condition.

Check skull x-rays for the location of a fracture.

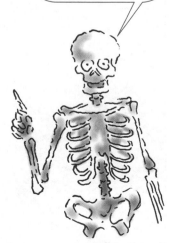

Types of head injury

Here's a summary of the signs and symptoms and diagnostic test findings for different types of head injury.

Type	Description
Concussion (closed head injury)	• A blow to the head hard enough to make the brain hit the skull, but not hard enough to cause a cerebral contusion; causes temporary neural dysfunction. • Recovery is usually complete within 24–48 hours. • Repeated injuries have a cumulative effect on the brain.
Contusion (bruising of brain tissue; more serious than concussion)	• Most common in 20–40-year-olds. • Most result from arterial bleeding. • Blood commonly accumulates between skull and dura. Injury to middle meningeal artery in parietotemporal area is most common and is typically accompanied by linear skull fractures in temporal region over middle meningeal artery. • Less commonly arises from dural venous sinuses.
Epidural haematoma	• Acceleration—deceleration or coup—contrecoup injuries disrupt normal nerve functions in bruised area. • Injury is directly beneath the site of impact when the brain rebounds against the skull from the force of a blow (a beating with a blunt instrument, for example), when the force of the blow drives the brain against the opposite side of the skull or when the head is hurled forward and stopped abruptly (as in an automobile crash when a driver's head strikes the windshield). • Brain continues moving and slaps against the skull (acceleration), then rebounds (deceleration). Brain may strike bony prominences inside the skull (especially the sphenoidal ridges), causing intracranial haemorrhage or haematoma that may result in tentorial herniation.
Subdural haematoma	• Meningeal haemorrhages, resulting from accumulation of blood in subdural space (between dura mater and arachnoid). • May be acute, subacute and chronic: unilateral or bilateral. • Usually associated with torn connecting veins in cerebral cortex; rarely from arteries. • Acute haematomas are a surgical emergency.

Signs and symptoms	Diagnostic test findings
• Short-term loss of consciousness secondary to disruption of reticular activating system, possibly due to abrupt pressure changes in the areas responsible for consciousness, changes in polarity of the neurones, ischaemia or structural distortion of neurones • Vomiting from localised injury and compression • Anterograde and retrograde amnesia (patient can't recall events immediately after the injury or events that led up to the traumatic incident) correlating with severity of injury; all related to disruption of reticular activating system • Irritability or lethargy from localised injury and compression • Behaviour out of character due to focal injury • Complaints of dizziness, nausea or severe headache due to focal injury and compression	• Computed tomography (CT) scan reveals no sign of fracture, bleeding or other nervous system lesion.
• Severe scalp wounds from direct injury • Laboured respiration and loss of consciousness secondary to increased pressure from bruising • Drowsiness, confusion, disorientation, agitation or violence from increased intracranial pressure (ICP) associated with trauma • Hemiparesis related to interrupted blood flow to the site of injury • Decorticate or decerebrate posturing from cortical damage or hemispheric dysfunction • Unequal pupillary response from brain stem involvement	• CT scan shows changes in tissue density, possible displacement of the surrounding structures and evidence of ischaemic tissue, haematomas and fractures. • Lumbar puncture with cerebrospinal fluid (CSF) analysis reveals increased pressure and blood (not performed if haemorrhage is suspected). • EEG recordings directly over the area of contusion reveal progressive abnormalities by appearance of high-amplitude theta and delta waves.
• Brief period of unconsciousness after injury reflects the concussive effects of head trauma, followed by a lucid interval varying from 10–15 minutes to hours or, rarely, days • Severe headache	• CT scan or magnetic resonance imaging (MRI) identifies abnormal masses or structural shifts within the cranium.
• Progressive loss of consciousness and deterioration in neurological signs result from expanding lesion and extrusion of medial portion of temporal lobe through tentorial opening • Compression of brain stem by temporal lobe causes clinical manifestations of intracranial hypertension • Deterioration in level of consciousness results from compression of brain stem reticular formation as temporal lobe herniates on its upper portion	

(continued)

Types of head injury (Continued)

Type	Description
Subdural haematoma (*continued*)	
Intracerebral haematoma	• Subacute haematomas have better prognosis because venous bleeding tends to be slower. • Traumatic or spontaneous disruption of cerebral vessels in brain parenchyma cause neurological deficits, depending on site and amount of bleeding. • Shear forces from brain movement frequently cause vessel laceration and haemorrhage into the parenchyma. • Frontal and temporal lobes are common sites. Trauma is associated with few intracerebral haematomas; most are caused by hypertension.
Skull fracture	• There are four types: linear, comminuted, depressed and basilar. • Fractures of anterior and middlefossae are associated with severe head trauma and are more common than those of posterior fossa. • Blow to the head causes one or more of the types. May not be problematic unless the brain is exposed or bone fragments are driven into neural tissue.

Signs and symptoms	Diagnostic test findings
• Respirations, initially deep and laboured, become shallow and irregular as brain stem is impacted • Contralateral motor deficits reflect compression of corticospinal tracts that pass through the brain stem • Ipsilateral (same side) pupillary dilation due to compression of third cranial nerve • Seizures possible from high ICP • Continued bleeding leads to progressive neurological degeneration, evidenced by bilateral pupillary dilation, bilateral decerebrate response, increased systemic blood pressure, decreased pulse and profound coma with irregular respiratory patterns	
• Similar to epidural haematoma but significantly slower in onset because bleeding is typically of venous origin • Unresponsive immediately or experiencing a lucid period before lapsing into a coma from increasing ICP and mass effect of haemorrhage • Possible motor deficits and decorticate or decerebrate responses from compression of corticospinal tracts and brain stem	• CT scan, x-rays and arteriography reveal mass and altered blood flow in the area, confirming a haematoma. • CT scan or MRI reveals evidence of masses and tissue shifting. • The CSF is yellow and has relatively low protein (chronic subdural haematoma). • CT scan or cerebral arteriography identifies the bleeding site. CSF pressure is elevated, and the fluid may appear bloody or xanthochromic (yellow or straw-coloured) from haemoglobin breakdown.
• May not produce symptoms, depending on underlying brain trauma • Discontinuity and displacement of bone structure with severe fracture • Motor sensory and cranial nerve dysfunction with associated facial fractures • Persons with anterior fossa basilar skull fractures may have periorbital ecchymosis (raccoon eyes), anosmia (loss of smell due to first cranial nerve involvement) and pupil abnormalities (second and third cranial nerve involvement) • CSF rhinorrhoea (leakage through nose), CSF otorrhoea (leakage from the ear), hemotympanum (blood accumulation at the tympanic membrane), ecchymosis over the mastoid bone (Battle's sign) and facial paralysis (seventh cranial nerve injury) accompany middle fossabasilar skull fractures • Signs of medullary dysfunction such as cardiovascular and respiratory failure accompany posterior fossa basilar skull fracture	• CT scan and MRI reveal swelling and intracranial haemorrhage from ruptured blood vessels. • Skull x-ray may reveal a fracture. • A lumbar puncture is contraindicated by expanding lesions.

The goal of surgery is to remove fragments driven into the brain and to extract foreign bodies and necrotic tissue. Such measures reduce the risk of infection and further brain damage due to fractures.

It's supportive

Provide supportive treatment, which includes:
- close observation of GCS to detect changes in neurological status suggesting further damage or expanding haematoma
- cleaning and debridement of any wounds associated with skull fractures
- diuretics such as mannitol to reduce cerebral oedema
- analgesics such as codeine or paracetamol to relieve complaints of headache
- anticonvulsants such as phenytoin to prevent seizures
- respiratory support, including elective sedation, mechanical ventilation and ET intubation for patients with raised ICP or respiratory failure from brain stem involvement
- control of oxygen and carbon dioxide levels within normal ranges
- fluid therapy to maintain adequate hydration without overload and osmolarity, usually with normal saline I.V.
- use of vasopressors (noradrenaline) to maintain blood pressure within normal range
- active cooling in postarrest patients for 12–24 hours down to 32–34°C
- prophylactic antibiotics to prevent the onset of meningitis from CSF leakage associated with skull fractures.

What to do

- Initially assess using ABCDE, monitor vital signs continuously and check for additional injuries.
- Continue to check vital signs and neurological status, including GCS and pupil size, every 15–60 minutes.
- Maintain a patent airway. Monitor oxygen saturation levels through pulse oximetry and ABG analysis as ordered.
- Assess hemodynamic parameters to aid in evaluating CPP.
- Administer medications as ordered. If necessary, use continuous infusions of such agents as midazolam, morphine or propofol and alfentanil to reduce metabolic demand and the risk of increased ICP.
- Observe the patient closely for signs of hypoxia or increased ICP, such as headache, dizziness, irritability, anxiety and changes in behaviour such as agitation.
- Monitor elderly patients especially closely because they may have brain atrophy and, therefore, more space for cerebral oedema. This means ICP may increase without showing signs until later.
- If an ICP monitoring system is inserted, continuously monitor ICP waveforms and pressure.
- Carefully observe the patient for CSF leakage. Check the bed sheets for a blood-tinged spot surrounded by a lighter ring (halo sign). If the patient

has CSF leakage or is unconscious, elevate the head of the bed 30 degrees or leave it flat. Such a patient is at risk for jugular compression that leads to increased ICP when not positioned on their back.

• Position the patient so that secretions drain properly. If you detect CSF leakage from the nose, place a gauze pad under the nostrils. Don't suction through the nose, but use the mouth. If CSF leaks from the ear, position the patient so their ear drains naturally.

• Monitor intake and output frequently to maintain fluid balance.

• Institute seizure precautions as necessary. Use safety precautions to minimise the risk of injury.

• Cluster nursing activities to provide rest periods, thus reducing metabolic demands and reducing the risk of sustained increases in ICP.

• Prepare the patient for craniotomy as indicated.

• After the patient is stabilised, clean and dress superficial scalp wounds using strict sterile technique. Monitor wounds for signs and symptoms of infection.

• Explain all procedures and treatments to the patient and their family members to reduce anxiety.

• Aim to reduce activity which may increase ICP.

Surgical intervention may be needed to reduce your patient's risk of infection and further brain damage due to fractures.

Meningitis

In meningitis, the brain and the spinal cord meninges become inflamed, usually because of bacterial infection. Such inflammation may involve all three meningeal membranes—the dura mater, arachnoid and pia mater.

Promptness improves the prognosis

If meningitis is recognised early and the infecting organism responds to treatment, the prognosis is good. Complications are rare and may include increased ICP, hydrocephalus, cerebral infarction, cranial nerve deficits causing optic neuritis and deafness, brain abscess, seizures or coma.

Time matters. Prompt recognition and treatment improves the meningitis patient's prognosis.

What causes it

Meningitis is usually a complication of bacteraemia, especially from pneumonia, empyema, osteomyelitis or endocarditis. Aseptic meningitis may result from a virus or other organism. Sometimes no causative organism can be found.

Uh-oh, other infections

Other infections associated with meningitis include:
• sinusitis
• otitis media
• encephalitis

- myelitis
- brain abscess, usually caused by *Neisseria meningitidis, Haemophilus influenzae, Streptococcus pneumoniae* and *Escherichia coli*.

Any opening

Meningitis may follow trauma or invasive procedures, including skull fracture, penetrating head wound, lumbar puncture and ventricular shunting.

Pathophysiology

Meningitis commonly begins as inflammation of the pia-arachnoid tissue. It may progress to congestion of adjacent tissues and destroy some nerve cells.

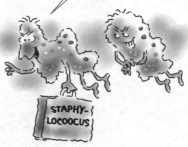

> Your patient with meningitis may play host to a whole host of infective organisms.

It enters here...

The causative organism typically enters the CNS by one of four routes:

 the blood (most common)

a direct opening between the CSF and the environment as a result of trauma

 along the cranial and peripheral nerves

through the mouth or nose.

...and triggers a response...

The invading organism triggers an inflammatory response in the meninges. To ward off the invasion, neutrophils gather in the area and produce an exudate in the subarachnoid space, causing the CSF to thicken. The thickened CSF flows less readily around the brain and spinal cord. This can block the arachnoid villi, further obstructing CSF flow and causing hydrocephalus.

> Meningitis that begins as inflammation may progress to congestion of adjacent tissues and destroy some nerve cells.

...and yet more responses

The exudate also:
- exacerbates the inflammatory response, increasing the pressure in the brain
- can extend to the cranial and peripheral nerves, triggering additional inflammation
- irritates the meninges, disrupting their cell membranes and causing oedema.

Truth or consequences

The consequences of meningitis are:
- elevated ICP
- engorged blood vessels

- disrupted cerebral blood supply
- possible thrombosis or rupture
- cerebral infarction if ICP isn't reduced
- possible encephalitis (a secondary infection of the brain tissue).

In aseptic meningitis, lymphocytes infiltrate the pia-arachnoid layers, but usually not as severely as in bacterial meningitis; no exudate is formed. Thus, this type of meningitis is self-limiting.

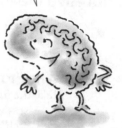

Thickened CSF flows slowly around the brain and spinal cord, sometimes causing hydrocephalus.

What to look for

Look for the signs of meningitis, which typically include:
- fever, chills and malaise resulting from infection and inflammation
- headache, vomiting and, rarely, papilloedema (inflammation and oedema of the optic nerve) from increased ICP.

Signs of irritation

Signs of meningeal irritation include:
- nuchal rigidity
- positive Brudzinski's (flexion of the neck causing flexion of the hips and knees) and Kernig's (inability to straighten leg) signs
- exaggerated and symmetrical deep tendon reflexes
- opisthotonos (a spasm more common in infants and children in which the back and extremities arch backwards so that the body rests on the head and heels).

Further features

Other features of meningitis may include:
- sinus arrhythmias due to irritation of autonomic nerves
- irritability due to increasing ICP
- photophobia, diplopia and other visual problems due to cranial nerve irritation
- delirium and coma due to increased ICP and cerebral oedema.

What tests tell you
- Lumbar puncture shows elevated CSF pressure (from obstructed CSF outflow at the arachnoid villi), cloudy or milky-white CSF, high protein levels, positive Gram stain and culture (unless a virus is responsible) and decreased glucose concentration.
- Positive Brudzinski's and Kernig's signs indicate meningeal irritation.
- Cultures of blood, urine and nose and throat secretions reveal the offending organism.
- Chest x-ray may reveal pneumonitis or lung abscess, tubercular lesions or granulomas secondary to a fungal infection.
- Sinus and skull x-rays may identify paranasal sinusitis as the underlying infectious process or a skull fracture as the mechanism for entrance of microorganisms.
- White blood cell count reveals leukocytosis.

How it's treated
Treatment includes administration of:
- antibiotic therapy, usually for 2 weeks
- mannitol to decrease cerebral oedema
- sedative to reduce restlessness
- paracetamol to relieve headache and fever.

Supportive measures

Supportive measures include bed rest; fever reduction, which may include tepid baths or cooling blankets; and isolation, if necessary.

What to do
Take the following steps when caring for a patient with meningitis:
- Assess neurological function 1–2 hourly.
- Watch for deterioration, especially temperature increase, deteriorating GCS, onset of seizures and altered respirations.
- Monitor fluid balance. Maintain adequate fluid intake to avoid dehydration, but avoid fluid overload because of the danger of cerebral oedema.
- Position the patient to prevent joint stiffness and neck pain.
- Maintain adequate nutrition and elimination.
- Maintain a quiet environment.
- Follow strict sterile technique when treating patients with head wounds or skull fractures.
- Provide emotional support.

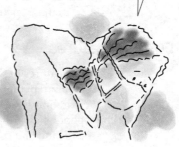

Remember: Meningitis is usually due to infection, so use sterile technique for patients with a head or skull injury.

Seizure disorder

Seizure disorder, or epilepsy, is a condition of the brain characterised by recurrent seizures (paroxysmal events associated with abnormal electrical discharges of neurons in the brain).

Primary and secondary

Primary seizure disorder or epilepsy is idiopathic without apparent structural changes in the brain.

Secondary epilepsy, characterised by structural changes or metabolic alterations of the neuronal membranes, causes increased automaticity.

Who's affected...

Epilepsy affects 1–2% of the population; approximately 1 million people live with epilepsy. The incidence is highest in childhood and old age. The prognosis is good if the patient adheres strictly to the prescribed treatment.

...and how

Complications of epilepsy may include hypoxia or anoxia due to airway occlusion, traumatic injury, brain damage and depression and anxiety.

What causes it

In about one-half of seizure disorder cases, the cause is unknown. Some possible causes are:
- birth trauma (such as inadequate oxygen supply to the brain, blood incompatibility or haemorrhage)
- perinatal infection
- anoxia
- infectious diseases (meningitis, encephalitis or brain abscess)
- head injury or trauma.

Pathophysiology

Some neurons in the brain may depolarise easily or be hyperexcitable, firing more readily than normal when stimulated. On stimulation, the electrical current spreads to surrounding cells, which fire in turn. The impulse thus cascades to:
- one side of the brain (a partial seizure)
- both sides of the brain (a generalised seizure)
- cortical, subcortical and brain stem areas.

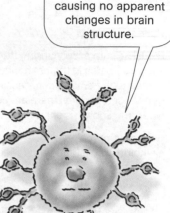

I'm clueless. Primary epilepsy is idiopathic, causing no apparent changes in brain structure.

Increase O₂, or else

The brain's metabolic demand for oxygen increases dramatically during a seizure. If this demand isn't met, hypoxia and brain damage result.

Firing of inhibitory neurons causes the excited neurons to slow their firing and eventually stop. Without this inhibitory action, the result is status epilepticus (seizures occurring one right after another). Without treatment, resulting anoxia is fatal.

What to look for

The hallmarks of seizure disorders are recurring seizures, which can be classified as partial or generalised. Some patients are affected by more than one type. (See *Types of seizures,* page 124.)

What tests tell you

The results of primary diagnostic tests for seizure disorders may include the following:
- CT scan to show density readings of the brain may indicate abnormalities in internal structures.
- MRI may indicate abnormalities in internal brain structures.
- EEG is used to confirm the diagnosis of epilepsy by providing evidence of the continuing tendency to have seizures.

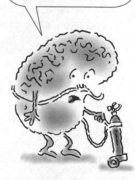

In epilepsy, some neurones in the brain fire more readily than normal when stimulated.

Types of seizures

Use the guidelines below to understand different seizure types. Keep in mind that some patients may be affected by more than one type.

Partial seizures

Partial seizure activity arising from a localised area in the brain may spread to the entire brain, causing a generalised seizure. There are several types and subtypes of partial seizures:

- simple partial seizures, which include jacksonian and sensory seizures
- complex partial seizures
- secondarily generalised partial seizures (partial onset leading to generalised tonic–clonic seizure).

Jacksonian seizures

A jacksonian seizure begins as a localised motor seizure, characterised by a spread of abnormal activity to adjacent areas of the brain.

The patient experiences stiffening or jerking in one extremity, with a tingling sensation in the same area. The patient seldom loses consciousness, but the seizure may progress to a generalised tonic–clonic seizure.

Sensory seizure

Symptoms of a sensory seizure include hallucinations, flashing lights, tingling sensations, vertigo, déjà vu and smelling a foul odour.

Complex partial seizure

Signs and symptoms of a complex partial seizure are variable but usually include purposeless behaviour, including a glassy stare, picking at clothes, aimless wandering, lip-smacking or chewing motions and unintelligible speech.

An aura may occur first, and seizures may last a few seconds to 20 minutes. Afterwards, mental confusion may last for several minutes and may be mistaken for alcohol or drug intoxication or psychosis. The patient has no memory of their actions during the seizure.

Secondarily generalised partial seizure

A secondarily generalised partial seizure can be simple or complex and can progress to a generalised seizure. An aura may occur first, with loss of concentration immediately or 1–2 minutes later.

Generalised seizure

Generalised seizures cause a generalised electrical abnormality in the brain. Types include absence, myoclonic, clonic, tonic, generalised tonic–clonic and atonic.

Absence seizure

Absence seizure, also known as petit mal seizure, is most common in children. It usually begins with a brief change in the level of consciousness, signalled by blinking or rolling of the eyes, a blank stare and slight mouth movements. The patient retains their posture and continues preseizure activity without difficulty.

Such seizures last 1–10 seconds and impairment is so brief that the patient may be unaware of it. If not properly treated, seizures can recur up to 100 times a day and progress to a generalised tonic–clonic seizure.

Myoclonic seizure

Myoclonic seizure is marked by brief, involuntary muscle jerks of the body or extremities and typically occurs in early morning.

Clonic seizure

Clonic seizure is characterised by bilateral rhythmic movements.

Tonic seizure

Tonic seizure is characterised by a sudden stiffening of muscle tone, usually of the arms but may also include the legs.

Generalised tonic–clonic seizure

Typically, a generalised tonic–clonic seizure begins with a loud cry, caused by air rushing from the lungs and through the vocal cords. The patient falls to the ground, losing consciousness. The body stiffens (tonic phase) and then alternates between episodes of muscle spasm and relaxation (clonic phase). Tongue biting, incontinence, laboured breathing, apnoea and cyanosis may also occur.

The seizure stops in 2–5 minutes, when abnormal electrical conduction of the neurones is completed. Afterwards, the patient regains consciousness but is somewhat confused. They may have difficulty talking and may have drowsiness, fatigue, headache, muscle soreness and arm or leg weakness. They may fall into a deep sleep afterwards.

Atonic seizure

Atonic seizure is characterised by a general loss of postural tone and temporary loss of consciousness. It occurs in children and is sometimes called a 'drop attack' because the child falls.

How it's treated

Generally, treatment consists of drug therapy specific to the type of seizures. The goal is to reduce seizures using a combination of the fewest drugs.

For tonic–clonic seizures

The most commonly prescribed drugs for generalised tonic–clonic seizures (alternating episodes of muscle spasm and relaxation) include carbamazepine, lamotrigine, sodium valproate and topiramate.

For absence seizures

Drugs commonly prescribed for absence seizures (brief changes in LOC) include sodium valproate and clonazepam.

For myoclonic seizures

Response to treatment varies considerably, sodium valproate, clonazepam and levetiracetam may be used.

Surgery and new approaches

If drug therapy fails, treatment may include surgical removal of a focal lesion in an attempt to stop seizures. A new approach for managing seizures is the vagus nerve stimulation device which acts on the brain the way a pacemaker acts on the heart. It sends electrical signals to the brain to inhibit seizure activity.

Because the device is implanted in the chest and neck, adverse effects include voice changes, throat discomfort and shortness of breath, all of which usually occur when the device is turned on.

Emergency management of status epilepticus

Repeated uncontrolled fitting requires emergency treatment (see *Understanding status epilepticus*, page 126):
• I.V. administration of diazepam emulsion, lorazepam, phenytoin or fosphenytoin with recognition of potential airway management requirements
• if fitting subsides perform ABCDE assessment, administer oxygen and consider the causes of the status epilepticus (poor compliance with medication regime, infections, head injury, hypoglycaemia, alcohol withdrawal)
• if seizures recur or fail to respond within 60 minutes anaesthesia with thiopentone, midazolam or propofol should be instituted with full anaesthetic support
• 50% dextrose I.V. (when seizures are secondary to hypoglycaemia)
• thiamine I.V. (in chronic alcoholism or withdrawal)
• antibiotics I.V. (in infections)
• CT scan (in suspected head injury).

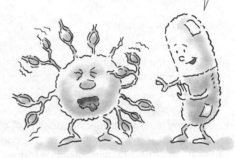

Treatment for a patient with a seizure disorder generally consists of drug therapy specific to the type of seizure.

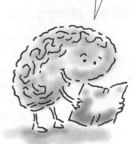

The vagus nerve stimulation device is like a pacemaker for the brain. It sends electrical signals to me to inhibit seizure activity.

Take charge!

Understanding status epilepticus

Status epilepticus is a continuous seizure state that must be interrupted by emergency measures. It can occur during all types of seizures. For example, generalised tonic–clonic status epilepticus is a continuous generalised tonic–clonic seizure without an intervening return of consciousness.

Always an emergency

Status epilepticus is accompanied by respiratory distress. It can result from withdrawal of antiepileptic medications, hypoxic or metabolic encephalopathy, acute head trauma or septicaemia secondary to encephalitis or meningitis.

Act fast

Emergency treatment usually consists of diazepam, phenytoin or phenobarbitone; I.V. dextrose 50% when seizures are secondary to hypoglycaemia; and I.V. thiamine in patients with chronic alcoholism or those who are undergoing withdrawal.

What to do
- Monitor a patient taking anticonvulsants constantly for signs of toxicity, such as nystagmus, ataxia, lethargy, dizziness, drowsiness, slurred speech, irritability, nausea and vomiting.
- When administering phenytoin I.V. use a large vein, administer according to guidelines (not more than 50 mg/minute) and monitor vital signs often.
- Encourage the patient's family to express their feelings about the patient's condition.
- Stress the need for compliance with the prescribed drug schedule.
- Emphasise the importance of having blood levels of anticonvulsants checked at regular intervals.

Tonic–clonic interventions

Generalised tonic–clonic seizures may necessitate the following interventions:
- Avoid restraining the patient during a seizure.
- Help the patient to a lying position, loosen any tight clothing and place something flat and soft, such as a pillow, under their head.
- Clear the area of hard objects.
- Don't force anything into the patient's mouth if their teeth are clenched.

> When caring for seizure patients, stress the need to have blood levels of anticonvulsants checked regularly.

- Turn the patient's head or turn them on their side to provide an open airway
- After the seizure, reassure the patient that they're all right, orient them to time and place and tell them that they had a seizure.

Stroke

Stroke, also known as a *cerebrovascular accident* (CVA), is a sudden impairment of cerebral circulation in one or more blood vessels. A stroke interrupts or diminishes oxygen supply and commonly causes serious damage or necrosis in the brain tissues.

The sooner, the better

The sooner circulation returns to normal after a stroke, the better your patient's chances are for a complete recovery. However, about one-half of the patients who survive a stroke remain permanently disabled and experience a recurrence within weeks, months or years. It's the leading cause of admission to long-term care.

Numbers and odds

Stroke is the third most common cause of death in the UK and the most common cause of neurological disability. It affects more than 150,000 people each year and is fatal in about one-half of these cases.

What causes it

Stroke typically results from one of three causes:

thrombosis of the cerebral arteries supplying the brain or of the intracranial vessels occluding blood flow.

embolism from thrombus outside the brain, such as in the heart, aorta or common carotid artery.

haemorrhage from an intracranial artery or vein, such as from hypertension, ruptured aneurysm, AVM, trauma, haemorrhagic disorder or septic embolism.

Risk factor facts

Risk factors that predispose patients to stroke include:
- hypertension
- family history of stroke
- history of TIA (see *TIA and elderly patients*.)
- cardiac disease, including arrhythmias, coronary artery disease, acute myocardial infarction, dilated cardiomyopathy and valvular disease
- diabetes
- familial hyperlipidaemia
- cigarette smoking
- increased alcohol intake

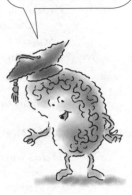

The sooner circulation in the brain returns to normal, the better your patient's chances are for a complete recovery after a stroke.

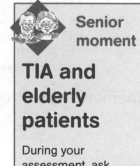

Senior moment

TIA and elderly patients

During your assessment, ask an elderly patient about recent falls—especially frequent falls. This is important because an older patient is less likely to forget about or minimise frequent falls than they are to report other signs of a transient ischaemic attack (TIA).

- obesity, sedentary lifestyle
- use of hormonal contraceptives.

Pathophysiology

Regardless of the cause, the underlying event leading to stroke is oxygen and nutrient deprivation. Here's what happens:

- Normally, if the arteries become blocked, autoregulatory mechanisms maintain cerebral circulation until collateral circulation develops to deliver blood to the affected area.
- If the compensatory mechanisms become overworked or cerebral blood flow remains impaired for more than a few minutes, oxygen deprivation leads to infarction of brain tissue.
- The brain cells cease to function because they can't engage in anaerobic metabolism or store glucose or glycogen for later use.

> Regardless of the cause, the underlying event leading to stroke is oxygen and nutrient deprivation.

Ischaemic stroke

Here's what happens when a thrombotic or embolic stroke causes ischaemia:

- Some of the neurones served by the occluded vessel die from lack of oxygen and nutrients.
- The result is cerebral infarction, in which tissue injury triggers an inflammatory response that in turn increases ICP.
- Injury to the surrounding cells disrupts metabolism and leads to changes in ionic transport, localised acidosis and free radical formation.
- Calcium, sodium and water accumulate in the injured cells, and excitatory neurotransmitters are released.
- Consequent continued cellular injury and swelling set up a vicious cycle of further damage.

Haemorrhagic stroke

Here's what happens when a haemorrhage causes a stroke:

- Impaired cerebral perfusion causes infarction, and the blood acts as a space-occupying mass, exerting pressure on the brain tissues.
- The brain's regulatory mechanisms attempt to maintain equilibrium by increasing blood pressure to maintain CPP. Remember CPP = MAP − ICP. The increased ICP forces CSF out, thus restoring equilibrium.
- If the haemorrhage is small, the patient may have minimal neurological deficits. If the bleeding is heavy, ICP increases rapidly and perfusion stops. Even if the pressure returns to normal, many brain cells die.
- Initially, the ruptured cerebral blood vessels may constrict to limit the blood loss. This vasospasm further compromises blood flow, leading to more ischaemia and cellular damage.
- If a clot forms in the vessel, decreased blood flow also promotes ischaemia. If the blood enters the subarachnoid space, meningeal irritation occurs.
- Blood cells that pass through the vessel wall into the surrounding tissue may break down and block the arachnoid villi, causing hydrocephalus.

> Stroke on the left causes symptoms on the right…

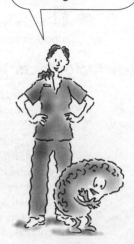

What to look for

Clinical features of stroke vary, depending on the artery affected (and, consequently, the portion of the brain it supplies), the severity of the damage and the extent of collateral circulation that develops to help the brain compensate for decreased blood supply. (See *Stroke signs and symptoms*.)

Stroke signs and symptoms

With stroke, functional loss reflects damage to the area of the brain that's normally perfused by the occluded or ruptured artery. Although one patient may experience only mild hand weakness, another may develop unilateral paralysis.

Hypoxia and ischaemia may produce oedema that affects distal parts of the brain, causing further neurological deficits. Here are the signs and symptoms that accompany stroke at different sites.

Site	Signs and symptoms	Site	Signs and symptoms
Middle cerebral artery	• Aphasia • Dysphasia • Dyslexia (reading problems) • Dysgraphia (inability to write) • Visual field cuts • Hemiparesis on the affected side, which is more severe in the face and arm than in the leg	Anterior cerebral artery	• Confusion • Weakness • Numbness on the affected side (especially in the arm) • Paralysis of the contralateral foot and leg • Incontinence • Poor coordination
Internal carotid artery	• Headaches • Weakness • Paralysis • Numbness • Sensory changes • Visual disturbances such as blurring on the affected side • Altered level of consciousness • Bruits over the carotid artery • Aphasia • Dysphagia • Ptosis	Vertebral or basilar artery	• Impaired motor and sensory functions • Personality changes, such as flat affect and distractibility • Mouth and lip numbness • Dizziness • Weakness on the affected side • Visual deficits, such as colour blindness, lack of depth perception and diplopia • Poor coordination • Dysphagia • Slurred speech • Amnesia • Ataxia
		Posterior cerebral artery	• Visual field cuts • Sensory impairment • Dyslexia • Coma • Blindness from ischaemia in the occipital area

Left is right and right is left

A stroke in the left hemisphere produces symptoms on the right side of the body; in the right hemisphere, symptoms on the left side.

Common signs and symptoms of stroke include sudden onset of:
- hemiparesis on the affected side (may be more severe in the face and arm than in the leg)
- unilateral sensory defect (such as numbness or tingling) generally on the same side as the hemiparesis
- slurred or indistinct speech or the inability to understand speech
- blurred or indistinct vision, double vision or vision loss in one eye (usually described as a curtain coming down or grey-out of vision)
- mental status changes or loss of consciousness (particularly if associated with one of the above symptoms)
- very severe headache (with haemorrhagic stroke).

What tests tell you

Here are some test findings that can help you diagnose a stroke:
- CT scan discloses structural abnormalities, oedema and lesions, such as nonhaemorrhagic infarction and aneurysms. Results are used to differentiate a stroke from other disorders, such as a tumour or haematoma. Patients with TIA generally have a normal CT scan. CT scan shows evidence of haemorrhagic stroke immediately and of ischaemic (thrombotic or embolic) stroke within 72 hours after onset of symptoms. CT scan should be obtained immediately after the patient arrives in the emergency department, and results should be immediately available to determine whether haemorrhage is present. If haemorrhagic stroke is present, thrombolytic therapy is contraindicated.
- MRI is used to identify areas of ischaemia and infarction and cerebral swelling.
- Cerebral angiography shows details of disruption or displacement of the cerebral circulation by occlusion or haemorrhage.
- DSA is used to evaluate patency of the cerebral vessels and shows evidence of occlusion of the cerebral vessels, a lesion or vascular abnormalities.
- Carotid duplex scan is a high-frequency ultrasound that shows blood flow through the carotid arteries and reveals stenosis due to atherosclerotic plaque and blood clots.
- Transcranial Doppler studies are used to evaluate the velocity of blood flow through major intracranial vessels, which can indicate vessel diameter.
- Brain scan shows ischaemic areas but may not be conclusive for up to 2 weeks after stroke.

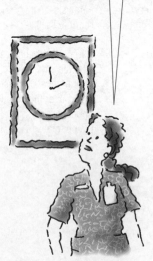

...stroke on the right causes symptoms on the left.

- Single photon emission CT scanning and PET scan show areas of altered metabolism surrounding lesions that aren't revealed by other diagnostic tests.
- Lumbar puncture reveals bloody CSF when stroke is haemorrhagic.
- EEG is used to identify damaged areas of the brain and to differentiate seizure activity from stroke.
- No laboratory tests confirm the diagnosis of stroke, but some tests aid diagnosis and some are used to establish a baseline for thrombolytic treatment. A blood glucose test shows whether the patient's symptoms are related to hypoglycaemia. Haemoglobin level and haematocrit may be elevated in severe occlusion. Baselines obtained before thrombolytic therapy begins include FBC, platelet count, partial thromboplastin time, PTT, fibrinogen level and urea and electrolytes.

How it's treated
The goal is to begin treatment as soon as possible after your patient presents.

Drugs of choice

Thrombolytics (also called fibrinolytics) are being introduced as the drugs of choice in treating a stroke patient. The patient must first meet certain criteria to be considered for this type of treatment.

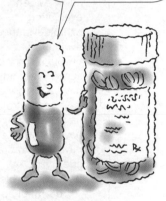

Antihypertensives and antiarrhythmics are given to patients with risk factors for recurrent stroke.

Drugs of choice for management

Drug therapy for the management of stroke includes:
- thrombolytics for emergency treatment of ischaemic stroke
- aspirin or clopidogrel as an antiplatelet agent to prevent recurrent stroke
- benzodiazepines to treat patients with seizure activity
- anticonvulsants to treat patients with seizures or to prevent them after the patient's condition has stabilised
- stool softeners to avoid straining, which increases ICP
- antihypertensives and antiarrhythmics to treat patients with risk factors for recurrent stroke.
- analgesics to relieve the headaches that may follow a haemorrhagic stroke.

Medical management

Medical management of stroke commonly includes physical rehabilitation, dietary and drug regimens to reduce risk factors, surgery and care measures to help the patient adapt to deficits, such as motor impairment and paralysis.

Who's suited for thrombolytic therapy?

Not every stroke patient is a candidate for thrombolytic therapy. Each is evaluated to see whether established criteria are met.

Criteria that must be present

Criteria that must be present for a patient to be considered for thrombolytic therapy include:

- acute ischemic stroke associated with significant neurologic deficit
- onset of symptoms less than 3 hours before treatment begins.

Criteria that must *not* be present

In addition to meeting the above criteria, the patient must not:

- show evidence of intracranial hemorrhage during pretreatment evaluation
- exhibit evidence of subarachnoid hemorrhage during pretreatment evaluation
- have a history of recent (within 3 months) intracranial or intraspinal surgery, serious head trauma, or previous stroke
- have a history of intracranial hemorrhage
- have uncontrolled hypertension at the time of treatment
- have experienced a seizure at the onset of stroke
- have active internal bleeding
- have an intracranial neoplasm, arteriovenous malformation, or aneurysm
- have known bleeding diathesis involving, but not limited to:
  - current use of oral anticoagulants such as warfarin, international normalized ratio greater than 1.7, or prothrombin time greater than 15 seconds
  - receipt of heparin within 48 hours before the onset of stroke and having an elevated partial thromboplastin time
  - platelet count less than 100,000 per µL.

Under the knife

Depending on the cause and extent of the stroke, the patient may undergo:
- a craniotomy to remove a haematoma
- a carotid endarterectomy to remove atherosclerotic plaques from the inner arterial wall
- an extracranial bypass to circumvent an artery that's blocked by occlusion or stenosis.

Cut it out! Surgical intervention after stroke is called for in some cases.

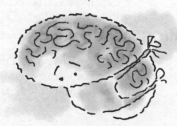

Call for help

Your hospital may have a stroke protocol and stroke team composed of specially trained nurses who respond to potential stroke patients. When a patient shows signs and symptoms of a stroke, first assess the patient using an ABCDE approach.

After your initial assessment, call for senior medical help, who will evaluate the patient, complete a neurological assessment, report findings to the doctor and facilitate rapid and appropriate care of the patient, including emergency interventions, diagnostic tests and transfer if required to a neurosurgical unit.

What to do

• Secure and maintain the patient's airway and anticipate the need for ET intubation and mechanical ventilation.
• Monitor oxygen saturation levels via pulse oximetry and ABG levels as indicated. Administer supplemental oxygen as prescribed to maintain oxygen saturation greater than 95%.
• Place the patient on a cardiac monitor, and monitor for cardiac arrhythmias.
• Assess the patient's neurological status frequently, at least every 15–30 minutes, initially, then hourly as indicated. Observe for signs of increased ICP.
• Elevate the head of the bed to 30 degrees to aid ICP reduction.
• Assess hemodynamic status frequently. Give fluids as ordered and monitor I.V. infusions to avoid overhydration, which may increase ICP.
• For a patient receiving thrombolytic therapy, assess the patient for signs and symptoms of bleeding every 15–30 minutes and institute bleeding precautions. Monitor results of coagulation tests.
• Monitor the patient for seizures and administer anticonvulsants as prescribed. Institute safety precautions to prevent injury.
• If the patient had a TIA, administer antiplatelet agents. Administer anticoagulants such as heparin if they show signs of stroke progression, unstable signs of stroke (such as TIA) or evidence of embolic stroke. Monitor coagulation tests closely.
• Turn the patient often and position them using careful body alignment. Apply antiembolism stockings or intermittent sequential compression devices.
• Take steps to prevent skin breakdown.
• Begin exercises as soon as possible. Perform passive ROM exercises for both the affected and unaffected sides. Teach and encourage the patient to use their unaffected side to exercise their affected side.

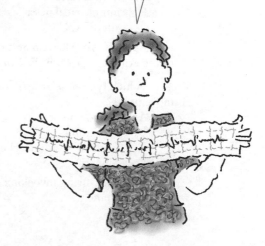

Come back soon! For your patient is on thrombolytic therapy, check for signs of bleeding every 15–30 minutes.

• Manage GI problems. Be alert for signs of straining at stool as it increases ICP. Assess swallowing ability.
• Modify and supplement the patient's diet, as appropriate. Aim to maintain adequate hydration without overload avoiding hypotonic solutions.
• Provide meticulous eye and mouth care.
• Maintain communication with the patient. If they're aphasic, set up a simple method of communicating.
• Provide psychological support.

Quick quiz

1. The most sensitive indicator of neurological status change is:
   A. GCS.
   B. speech.
   C. behaviour.
   D. cognitive function.

Answer: A. Change in GCS is the earliest and most sensitive indicator of neurological status change.

2. Signs of an adverse reaction to contrast medium include all of the following except:
   A. restlessness.
   B. bradycardia.
   C. urticaria.
   D. facial flushing.

Answer: B. A sign of adverse reaction to the contrast medium is tachycardia.

3. The major neurological symptom of Guillain–Barré syndrome is:
   A. headache.
   B. nuchal rigidity.
   C. muscle weakness.
   D. altered GCS.

Answer: C. Muscle weakness usually appears in the legs first, then extends to the arms and face within 2 weeks or less.

4. Which type of seizure is characterised by brief, involuntary muscle movements?
   A. Jacksonian
   B. Myoclonic
   C. Generalised tonic–clonic
   D. Akinetic

Answer: B. During myoclonic seizures, the patient has brief, involuntary muscle movements.

Scoring

☆☆☆ If you answered all four questions correctly, you may already know this: You're a brainiac!

☆☆ If you answered three questions correctly, don't feel sad. You have all the brainpower you need to succeed.

☆ If you answered fewer than three questions correctly, don't be nervous. Review the chapter and then take the test again.

4 Cardiovascular system

Just the facts

In this chapter, you'll learn:

♦ structure and function of the cardiovascular system

♦ assessment of the cardiovascular system

♦ diagnostic tests and procedures for the cardiovascular system

♦ cardiovascular disorders and treatments.

Understanding the cardiovascular system

The cardiovascular system consists of the heart and the blood vessels.

Bring it on...and take it away

This complex system functions to:
- carry life-sustaining oxygen and nutrients in the blood to all cells of the body
- remove metabolic waste products from the cells
- move hormones from one part of the body to another.

Heart

The heart is about the size of a closed fist. It lies beneath the sternum in the mediastinum (the cavity between the lungs), between the second and sixth ribs.

The right border of the heart aligns with the right border of the sternum. The left border aligns with the midclavicular line. The exact position of the heart varies slightly in each patient.

> You might say the cardiovascular system is a mover and remover!

Pericardium

The pericardium is a sac that surrounds the heart. It's composed of an outer (fibrous) layer and inner (serous) layer. The serous layer of the pericardium is composed of a visceral (inner) layer and parietal (outer) layer.

Liquid cushion

The pericardial space separates the visceral and parietal layers of the serous pericardium. This space contains 10–30 ml of thin, clear pericardial fluid, which lubricates the two surfaces of the serous pericardium and cushions the heart.

Heart wall

The heart's wall is composed of three layers:

Epicardium includes the outer layer of the heart wall and the visceral layer of the serous pericardium. It's made up of squamous epithelial cells overlying connective tissue.

Myocardium is the middle and largest portion of the heart wall. This layer of muscle tissue contracts with each heartbeat.

Endocardium is the innermost layer of the heart wall. It contains endothelial tissue made up of small blood vessels and bundles of smooth muscle.

Four chambers

The heart has four chambers:
* right atrium
* left atrium
* right ventricle
* left ventricle. (See *A close look at the heart*, on page 138.)

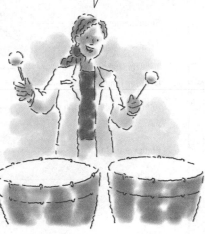

The myocardium is composed of muscle tissue that contracts with each heartbeat.

Thanks for giving blood today!

The right and left atria serve as reservoirs for blood. The right atrium receives deoxygenated blood returning from the body. The left atrium receives oxygenated blood from the lungs. Contraction of the atria forces blood into the ventricles below.

Powerful pumps

The right and left ventricles are the pumping chambers of the heart. The ventricles—which have thicker walls and are larger than the atria—are composed of highly developed muscles.

The right ventricle receives blood from the right atrium and pumps it through the pulmonary arteries to the lungs, where it picks up oxygen and drops off carbon dioxide. The left ventricle receives oxygenated blood from the

A close look at the heart

This illustration provides a detailed look at the internal structures of the heart.

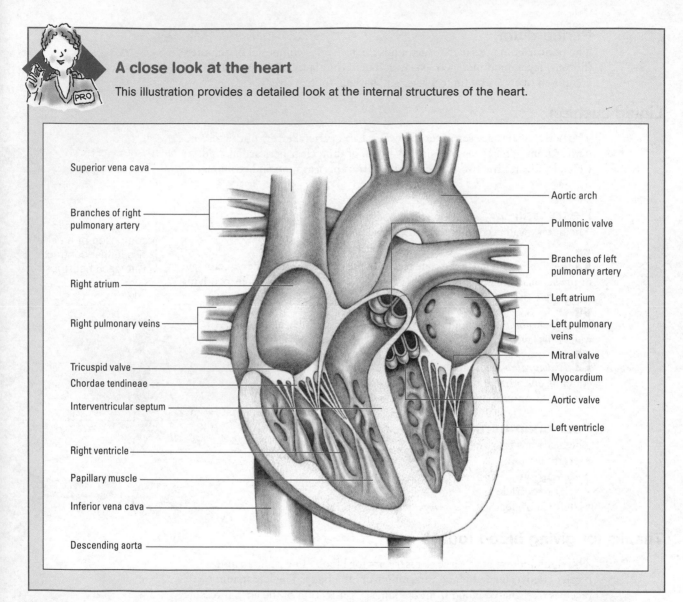

Superior vena cava

Branches of right pulmonary artery

Right atrium

Right pulmonary veins

Tricuspid valve

Chordae tendineae

Interventricular septum

Right ventricle

Papillary muscle

Inferior vena cava

Descending aorta

Aortic arch

Pulmonic valve

Branches of left pulmonary artery

Left atrium

Left pulmonary veins

Mitral valve

Myocardium

Aortic valve

Left ventricle

left atrium and pumps it through the aorta and then out to the rest of the body. The interventricular septum separates the ventricles and helps them to pump.

Heart valves

Valves in the heart keep blood flowing in one direction.

One way

Healthy valves open and close passively as a result of pressure changes in the four heart chambers. The valves prevent blood from travelling the wrong way.

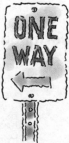

Where the valves are

Valves between the atria and ventricles are called *atrioventricular* (AV) *valves* and include the tricuspid valve on the right side of the heart and the mitral valve on the left side. Valves between the ventricles and the pulmonary artery and the aorta are called *semilunar valves* and include the pulmonary valve on the right (between the right ventricle and the pulmonary artery) and the aortic valve on the left (between the left ventricle and the aorta).

On the cusp

The leaflets, or cusps, of each valve keep the valves tightly closed. The tricuspid valve has three cusps. The mitral valve has two.

The cusps are anchored to the heart wall by cords of fibrous tissue called *chordae tendineae*, which are controlled by papillary muscles.

Great vessels

Leading into and out of the heart are the great vessels:
- The aorta, which carries blood away from the left ventricle, is the main trunk of the systemic artery system.
- The inferior and superior vena cavae carry deoxygenated blood from the body into the right atrium.
- The pulmonary artery is a large artery that carries blood away from the right ventricle. Above the heart, it splits to form the right and left pulmonary arteries, which carry blood to the right and left lungs.
- The four pulmonary veins—two on the left and two on the right—carry oxygenated blood from the left and right lungs to the left atrium.

Coronary arteries

Like all other organs, the heart needs an adequate blood supply to survive. The coronary arteries, which lie on the surface of the heart, supply the heart muscle with blood and oxygen. (See *Heart vessels*, on page 140.)

Coronary ostium

The coronary ostium is an opening in the aorta near the aortic valve. It feeds blood to the coronary arteries.

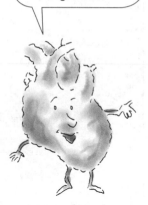

The great vessels carry blood into and out of the heart. Aren't they great?

Ostium action

When the left ventricle is pumping blood through the aorta, the aortic valve is open and the coronary ostium is partly covered. When the left ventricle is filling with blood, the aortic valve is closed and the coronary ostium is open, enabling blood to fill the coronary arteries. Thus the heart muscle is perfused in diastole; that is, the faster the heartbeats the less time there is for perfusion of cardiac muscle.

Right coronary artery

The right coronary artery supplies blood to the right atrium, the right ventricle and part of the left ventricle. It also supplies blood to the bundle of His (muscles that connect the atria with the ventricles) and the AV node

Heart vessels

These two views of the heart depict the great vessels and some of the major coronary vessels.

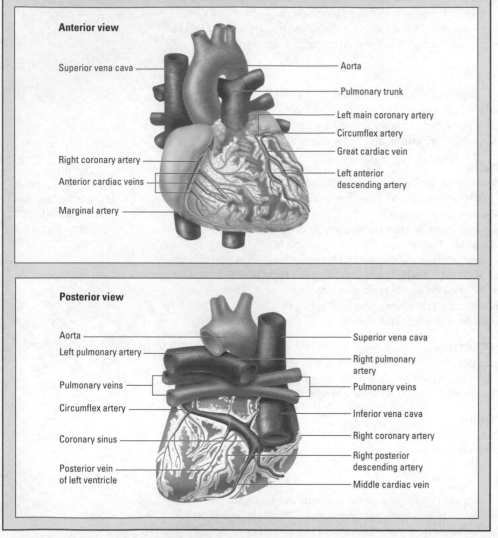

Anterior view

Superior vena cava

Aorta

Pulmonary trunk

Left main coronary artery

Circumflex artery

Great cardiac vein

Right coronary artery

Left anterior descending artery

Anterior cardiac veins

Marginal artery

Posterior view

Aorta

Superior vena cava

Left pulmonary artery

Right pulmonary artery

Pulmonary veins

Pulmonary veins

Circumflex artery

Inferior vena cava

Coronary sinus

Right coronary artery

Right posterior descending artery

Posterior vein of left ventricle

Middle cardiac vein

(fibres at the base of the interatrial septum that transmit the cardiac impulses from the sinoatrial [SA] node).

What do you SA about that?

In about half the population, the right coronary artery also supplies blood to the SA node of the right atrium. The SA node consists of a typical muscle fibres that establish the rhythm of cardiac contractions.

Left coronary artery

The left coronary artery runs along the surface of the left atrium, where it splits into two major branches: the left anterior descending artery and the left circumflex artery.

Left out

The left anterior descending artery supplies blood to the:
- anterior wall of the left ventricle
- interventricular septum
- right bundle branch (a branch of the bundle of His)
- left anterior fasciculus (small cluster) of the left bundle branch.

The branches of the left anterior descending artery—the septal perforators and the diagonal arteries—supply blood to the walls of both ventricles.

Circumflex-ability

The circumflex artery supplies oxygenated blood to the lateral walls of the left ventricle, the left atrium and, in about 50% of the population, the SA node.

Circle left

In addition, the circumflex artery supplies blood to the left posterior fasciculus of the left bundle branch. This artery circles around the left ventricle and provides blood to the ventricle's posterior portion.

Veins

Like other parts of the body, the heart has veins, called *cardiac veins*, that collect deoxygenated blood from the capillaries of the myocardium. These cardiac veins join together to form an enlarged vessel called the *coronary sinus*. The right atrium receives deoxygenated blood from the heart through the coronary sinus.

Pulmonary circulation

During pulmonary circulation, blood travels to the lungs to pick up oxygen in exchange for carbon dioxide.

Heart to lungs to heart

Here's what happens during pulmonary circulation:
- Deoxygenated blood travels from the right ventricle through the pulmonary semilunar valve into the pulmonary arteries.
- Blood passes through smaller arteries and arterioles into the capillaries of the lungs.
- Blood reaches the alveoli and exchanges carbon dioxide for oxygen.
- Oxygenated blood returns through the venules and veins to the pulmonary veins.
- The pulmonary veins carry the oxygenated blood back to the left atrium of the heart.

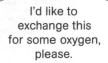

The left coronary artery splits into two major branches that supply blood to the rest of the heart.

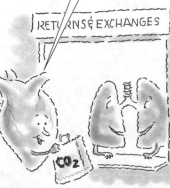

I'd like to exchange this for some oxygen, please.

RETURNS & EXCHANGES

CO2

Cardiac rhythm

Contractions of the heart occur in a rhythm that's regulated by impulses normally initiated at the SA node—thus we call this normal rhythm 'Sinus rhythm'.

Nature's pacemaker

The SA node is the heart's pacemaker. Impulses initiated at the SA node are conducted from there throughout the heart. Impulses from the autonomic nervous system affect the SA node and alter its firing rate to meet the body's needs.

The cardiac cycle

The cardiac cycle consists of two phases: systole and diastole.

Out with systole, in with diastole

During systole, the heart contracts and sends blood on its outward journey. During diastole, the heart relaxes and fills with blood; the mitral and tricuspid valves are open, and the aortic and pulmonary valves are closed.

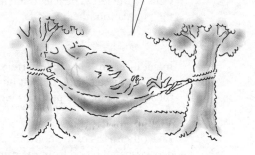

During diastole, the heart relaxes and fills with blood.

Filling and more filling

Diastole consists of ventricular filling and atrial contraction. During ventricular filling, 70% of the blood in the atria drains into the ventricles passively, by gravity. The active period of diastole, atrial contraction (also called *atrial kick*), accounts for the remaining 30% of blood that passes into the ventricles.

The pressure's on

Systole is when the atria and ventricles contract. With contraction comes an increase in pressure in the chambers. When the pressure in the ventricles is greater than the pressure in the aorta and pulmonary artery, the aortic and pulmonary valves open. Blood then flows from the ventricles into the pulmonary artery, then to the lungs and into the aorta, and then to the rest of the body.

The pressure's off

At the end of ventricular contraction, pressure in the ventricles drops below the pressure in the aorta and pulmonary artery. The difference in pressure forces blood back up towards the ventricles and causes the aortic and pulmonary valves to snap shut.

As the valves shut, the atria fill with blood in preparation for the next period of diastolic filling, and the cycle begins again.

Out in a minute

Cardiac output (CO) is the amount of blood the heart pumps in 1 minute. It's equal to the heart rate multiplied by the stroke volume (the amount of blood ejected with each heartbeat).

Stroke volume depends on three major factors:

☝ preload

✌ afterload

✌ contractility. (See *Understanding preload, afterload and contractility*.)

Blood vessels

The vascular system is the complex network of blood vessels throughout the body that conducts systemic circulation. Blood carries oxygen and other nutrients to body cells and transports waste products for excretion.

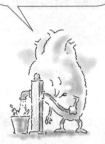

Cardiac output is the amount of blood the heart pumps in 1 minute.

Understanding preload, afterload and contractility

If you think of the heart as a balloon, it will help you understand preload, afterload and contractility.

Blowing up the balloon

Preload is the stretching of muscle fibres in the ventricles. This stretching results from blood volume in the ventricles at end-diastole. According to Starling's law, the more the heart muscles stretch during diastole, the more forcefully they contract during systole. Think of preload as the balloon stretches as air is blown into it. The more air the greater the stretch.

The balloon's stretch

Contractility refers to the inherent ability of the myocardium to contract normally. Contractility is influenced by preload. The greater the stretch the more forceful the contraction—or, the more air in the balloon, the greater the stretch, and the farther the balloon will fly when air is allowed to expel.

The narrow neck of the balloon

Afterload refers to the pressure that the ventricular muscles must generate to overcome the higher pressure in the aorta to get the blood out of the heart. *Resistance* is the narrow neck of the end of the balloon, which the balloon has to work against to get the air out.

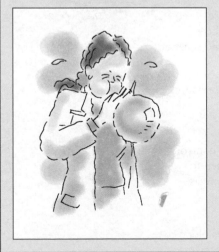

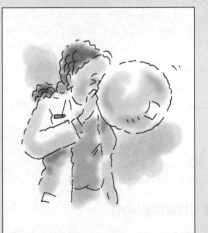

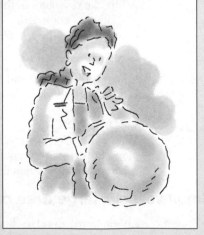

Arteries

The major artery—the aorta—branches into vessels that supply blood to specific organs and areas of the body.

Upper blood suppliers

Three arteries arise from the arch of the aorta and supply blood to the brain, arms and upper chest. These are the:
- left common carotid artery
- left subclavian artery
- innominate artery.

Descending distribution

As the aorta descends through the thorax and abdomen, its branches supply blood to the GI and genitourinary organs, spinal column and lower chest and abdominal muscles. Then the aorta divides into the iliac arteries, which further divide into the femoral arteries—ultimately supplying blood to the legs and feet.

Arterioles

As the arteries divide into smaller units, the number of vessels increases, thereby increasing the area of perfusion. These smaller units are known as *arterioles*. Arterioles can dilate or constrict because of their muscular structure. The greater the constriction the greater the resistance to the blood being pumped by the heart, thus elevating the blood pressure. With greater dilation comes lower resistance to blood flow and thus lower blood pressure.

> Dilated arterioles decrease blood pressure. Constricted arterioles increase blood pressure.

A principle of pressure

The relationship between blood flow out of the heart (cardiac output [CO]), the resistance of the blood vessels to the flow of blood because of dilation of constriction (systemic vascular resistance [SVR]) and the pressure within the arteries (blood pressure) can be summarised in the equation:

Blood pressure = Cardiac output × systemic vascular resistance

Thus higher CO and higher resistance result in higher blood pressure. Lower CO and lower resistance result in lower blood pressure.

Capillaries

Where the arterioles end, the capillaries begin. Strong sphincters control blood flow from the capillaries into the tissues. The sphincters open to permit more flow when needed and close to shunt blood to other areas.

Small vessels, large area of distribution

Although the capillary bed contains the smallest vessels, it supplies blood to the largest area. Capillary pressure is extremely low to allow for exchange of nutrients, oxygen and carbon dioxide with body cells. However, this low pressure means that it is relatively easy for pressures applied to the capillary to prevent blood supply getting to the tissues.

Venules and veins

From the capillaries, returning blood flows into venules and, eventually, into veins. Valves in the veins prevent blood backflow, and the pumping action of skeletal muscles assists venous return.

Branching back to the right atrium

The veins merge until they form branches that return blood to the right atrium. The two main branches include the superior vena cava (coming from above the heart) and the inferior vena cava (coming from below the heart).

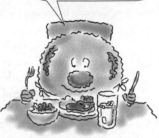

Low capillary pressure allows for the exchange of nutrients, oxygen and carbon dioxide with body cells.

Summary of key physiological concepts related to critical illness

• The cardiovascular system is in essence a pump (the heart) and a network of tubes (blood vessels).
• The key function of this system is to deliver oxygen (mainly bound to haemoglobin) and nutrients (e.g. glucose) to the cells of the body in order that they can perform their vital and specific functions. Waste products from cell metabolism are also transported away from cells to be broken down and eliminated.
• The ideal system has adequate pressure within it (blood pressure) and it has an adequate amount of blood being pumped around the body (CO).
• The basic concepts to remember are about blood pressure, flow and resistance in the vascular system.
• BP (blood pressure) is produced by pumping blood from the heart, so-called CO, into a system of narrowing blood vessels which offer resistance to the flow of blood. SVR is the total resistance offered throughout all the blood vessels (in summary: BP is a product of CO and SVR).
• If the blood vessels offer little resistance (↓SVR—e.g. as in anaphylaxis or sepsis) CO will increase to compensate but there will not be enough pressure (BP) in the vascular system to push blood into the organs and perfuse them.
• Alternatively, if the CO falls (e.g. after a myocardial infarction or because of inadequate blood volume in the system) the SVR will rise to compensate—perhaps maintaining a normal BP. But there will not be an adequate volume of blood ejected from the heart (CO) and delivered to the organs.
• Thus there is a balance to be struck in order to achieve an adequate pressure and flow of blood for oxygen and nutrient delivery to cells.
• Cardiovascular failure means that there is inadequate circulation of blood to meet cellular metabolic needs. (Remember—respiratory failure will also result in inadequate oxygen deliver to cells caused by inadequate oxygenation of the blood.)

- This inadequate oxygen and nutrient delivery to the tissues results in cell and organ dysfunction and an increase in circulating lactic acid (Lactic acidosis) as a by-product of this anaerobic (without oxygen) metabolism.
- The cells of the body don't function well in an acid environment so the cells of the heart are less able to contract delivering oxygen and glucose to other cells. The less oxygen and glucose they receive the more acid they produce.
- Without oxygen and glucose the cells enter a downward spiral of dysfunction causing cardiovascular failure and then death.
- When there is sustained inadequate oxygen delivery due to cardiovascular dysfunction it is described as 'shock'. 'shock' is a state of low tissue perfusion.
- Shock is a common and serious manifestation of critical illness which ultimately leads to death if there is no intervention to support cardiovascular functioning and restore adequate oxygen and nutrient delivery to cells.
- These are important concepts to bear in mind when assessing and monitoring the cardiovascular system of critically ill individuals.

Cardiovascular assessment

An important domain of the registered nurse's role is the assessment and monitoring of important physiological systems. However, this is usually a collaborative process reflected in the multidisciplinary approach which is a salient feature of critical care. When assessing and monitoring the cardiovascular system it is important to focus on the key physiological concepts outlined earlier.

This domain of practice involves thinking critically about how the system is functioning, what is 'normal' for the patient and how chronic or acute health problems might be affecting important functions.

It is perhaps best to think of assessment as a single episode of information gathering and critical thinking about the information in order to form a judgement about the patient. Monitoring, on the other hand, is a process of considering assessment findings over a period of time.

Cardiovascular monitoring is a major part of critical care nursing and will usually take place continually with parameters recorded on charts every 1 to 2 hours, though it could be more frequent in extreme situations where things are changing very quickly or life is in acute danger. The types of monitoring and their clinical use will be discussed later. First it is important to think about a framework for assessment.

Being systematic

Assessment of the cardiovascular system includes knowing the following:
- History of the present complaint
- Health history
- Clinical assessment and monitoring
- Results and significance of diagnostic tests and investigations

History of the present complaint

In essence you need to know why the patient has come into hospital and into critical care, as well as any timescales and key events. In particular, find out any symptoms and how these relate to cardiovascular function.

Health history

Aim to discover the following:
- Current symptoms and complaints—for example, chest pain, dizziness, nausea and dyspnoea.
- Any chronic illnesses—including the severity and treatment.
- Any previous surgery—including reasons for the surgery and outcome.
- Current medication—including the reason for taking these.
- Any behaviours or addictions that might adversely affect health—for example, smoking, alcohol and elicit drug use. Quantify these if possible—for example, pack years (packs per day × years smoked), units of alcohol per week.
- Any allergies.
- Ability to perform activities of daily living.

If your patient has chest pain...

Advice from the experts
Cardiac questions

To thoroughly assess your patient's cardiac function, be sure to ask the following questions:

- Are you in pain?
- Where is the pain located?
- Does the pain feel like a burning, tight or squeezing sensation?
- Does the pain radiate to your arm, neck, back or jaw?

- When did the pain begin?
- What relieves or aggravates it?
- Are you experiencing nausea, dizziness or sweating?
- Do you feel short of breath? Has breathing trouble ever awakened you from sleep?
- Does your heart ever pound or skip a beat? When?

- Do you ever get dizzy or faint? When?
- Do you experience swelling in your ankles or feet? When? Does anything relieve the swelling?
- Do you urinate frequently at night?
- Have you had to limit your activities?

Understanding chest pain

Use this table to help you more accurately assess chest pain.

What it feels like	Where it's located	What makes it worse	What causes it	What makes it better
Aching, squeezing, pressure, heaviness, burning pain; usually subsides within 10 minutes	Substernal; may radiate to jaw, neck, arms and back	Eating, physical effort, smoking, cold weather, stress, anger, hunger, lying down	Angina pectoris	Rest, nitroglycerin (*Note:* Unstable angina appears even at rest)
Tightness or pressure; burning, aching pain, possibly accompanied by shortness of breath, diaphoresis, weakness, anxiety or nausea; sudden onset; lasts 1/2 hour to 2 hours	Typically across chest but may radiate to jaw, neck, arms or back	Exertion, anxiety	Acute myocardial infarction	Opioid analgesics such as morphine, nitroglycerin
Sharp and continuous; may be accompanied by friction rub; sudden onset	Substernal; may radiate to neck or left arm	Deep breathing, supine position	Pericarditis	Sitting up, leaning forward, antiinflammatory drugs
Excruciating, tearing pain; may be accompanied by blood pressure difference between right and left arm; sudden onset	Retrosternal, upper abdominal or epigastric; may radiate to back, neck or shoulders	Not applicable	Dissecting aortic aneurysm	Analgesics, surgery
Sudden, stabbing pain; may be accompanied by cyanosis, dyspnoea or cough with haemoptysis	Over lung area	Inspiration	Pulmonary embolus	Analgesics
Sudden and severe pain; sometimes accompanied by dyspnoea, increased pulse rate, decreased breath sounds or deviated trachea	Lateral thorax	Normal respiration	Pneumothorax	Analgesics, chest tube insertion

Clinical assessment and monitoring

There are many cardiovascular problems that can be present when someone is critically ill. The key questions you should ask yourself when assessing and monitoring a critically ill patient are:
- Is there evidence of inadequate perfusion?
- Are there signs or symptoms of heart failure?
- Is there potential for impaired perfusion or acute heart failure because of current or expected health problems?

Just a minute . . . I'm trying to think of the exact word to describe the pain.

Remember adequate perfusion is a balance of pressure and flow of blood to the tissues. Consider the following as a guide to what clinical assessment information will help in answering these questions:

- Skin—colour, temperature, capillary refill time, diaphoresis/clammy skin
- Pulses—presence at peripheries, volume, rate, visible pulsation in the neck veins
- Blood pressure—systolic, diastolic, mean, pulse pressure
- Heart rate and rhythm
- Respiratory rate and pattern, presence of dyspnoea, crackles or wheeze on auscultation
- Renal function—urine output
- Gastrointestinal function—presence of bowel sounds/gut function
- Central nervous system—conscious level/acute confusion or agitation
- Peripheral 'pitting' oedema
- General inspection from head to toe for any other obvious abnormalities

> Oedema is a telltale sign of possible heart failure, venous insufficiency, varicosities or thrombophlebitis.

Assessing arterial and venous insufficiency

You should be aware of how assessment findings differ between healthy patients and those with arterial insufficiency or chronic venous insufficiency.

Arterial insufficiency

In a patient with arterial insufficiency, pulses may be decreased or absent. The skin is cool, pale and shiny, and the patient may have pain in their legs and feet. Ulcerations typically occur in the area around the toes, and the foot usually turns deep red when dependent. Nails may be thick and ridged.

Chronic venous insufficiency

In a patient with chronic venous insufficiency, check for ulcerations around their ankle. Pulses are present but may be difficult to find because of pitting oedema. The foot may become cyanotic when dependent, and you may see a brown pigmentation and thickening of the skin around the ankle.

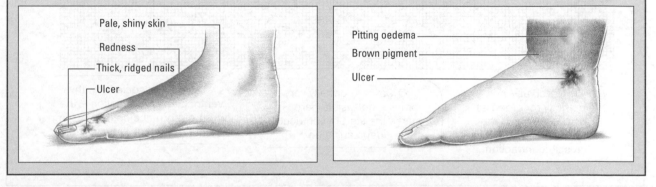

Pale, shiny skin

Redness

Thick, ridged nails

Ulcer

Pitting oedema

Brown pigment

Ulcer

Heart rhythm

Heart rhythm will determine the speed and regularity of cardiac pumping. Abnormalities of rhythm (arrhythmias) are quite common in the critically ill. It is important for the critically ill to have their heart rhythm monitored and for the critical care nurse to be able to identify a normal rhythm (sinus rhythm) as well as common arrhythmias.

Electrocardiogram (ECG)

This can be divided into two related but quite different areas. Firstly, there is bedside cardiac monitoring—the main purpose of which is to establish and monitor the cardiac rhythm. Secondly, there is the 12-lead ECG which allows much more detailed assessment of the electrophysiology of the heart and cardiac rhythm.

It is important to know the normal electrophysiology of the heart and the appearance of the ECG before you can recognise abnormalities. Abnormalities are many, and they are a large topic on their own. Here we'll look at basic principles before moving on later to look at the abnormalities that you'll see in the critically ill.

ECG basics

The normal rhythm of the heart is called 'sinus rhythm'—so-called because the pacemaker that initiates each electrical impulse originates in the sinus node. It

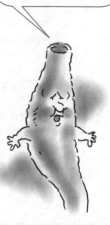

If you detect pulsations too far above the sternal notch, it's due to elevated CVP and jugular vein distention.

Sinus rhythm and the PQRST

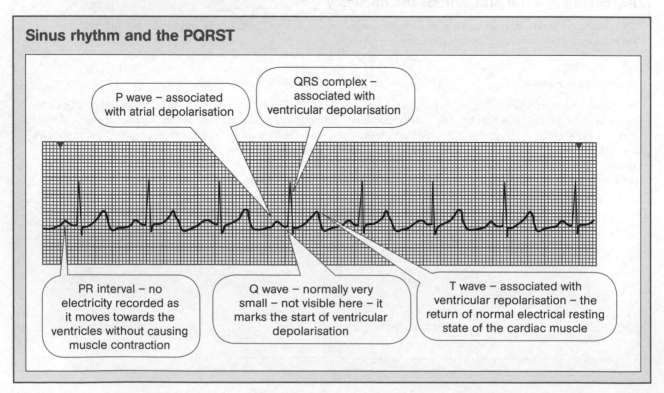

P wave – associated with atrial depolarisation

QRS complex – associated with ventricular depolarisation

PR interval – no electricity recorded as it moves towards the ventricles without causing muscle contraction

Q wave – normally very small – not visible here – it marks the start of ventricular depolarisation

T wave – associated with ventricular repolarisation – the return of normal electrical resting state of the cardiac muscle

then progresses through the conduction system including the AV node, at the junction of the atria and ventricles, and then through the bundle of His where it separates off into the right and left bundle branches and finally into the peripheral conduction pathways—the Purkinje fibres embedded in the cardiac muscle. On its way through the conduction system this wave of electricity causes the cardiac muscle, firstly in the atria, then, the ventricles to contract. The electrical phenomenon that coincides with muscular contraction is called depolarisation—where the electrical charge of cells is momentarily changed as the impulse passes along muscle fibres. The ECG measures this electricity and produces a graph of its amplitude over time. When electricity is moving towards the lead (attached to the patient's skin) there is an upward wave on the

Where the leads of the ECG are placed

As well as a lead on each limb (always labelled to tell you where to put them) the chest leads are placed as shown over heart (the precordium)

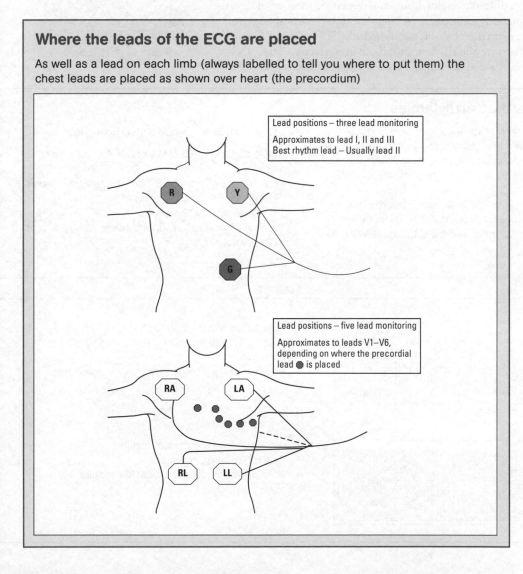

Lead positions – three lead monitoring

Approximates to lead I, II and III
Best rhythm lead – Usually lead II

Lead positions – five lead monitoring

Approximates to leads V1–V6, depending on where the precordial lead ● is placed

graph and a downward one when moving away. There is a characteristic set of waves on the graph recorded either on the 12-lead paper or on the screen of the bedside monitor. The PQRST are the normal waves of each heartbeat (and associated electrical impulse). Knowing the normal appearance of these is the first step to recognising when there are abnormalities.

Cardiac monitoring

Traditionally a cardiac monitor would be capable of viewing the heart from three different angles (leads) but only displaying one of these at a time on the bedside monitor. More modern monitoring systems found in critical care units may be capable of viewing the heart from between five and twelve different angles (leads) and displaying most or all of these simultaneously if necessary (see also '12-lead electrocardiogram'). However, the main use of a continuous bedside ECG monitor is to view the cardiac rate and rhythm since these may adversely affect CO and blood pressure if abnormal and are common in the critically ill.

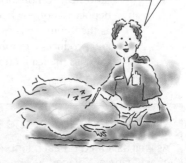

Arrhythmias are generally classified according to whether their origin is ventricular or supraventricular.

Understanding cardiac arrhythmias

Here's an outline of many common cardiac arrhythmias and their features, causes and treatments. Use a normal electrocardiogram strip, if available, to compare normal cardiac rhythm configurations with the rhythm strips shown here.

When caring for any patient with an abnormal rhythm who is causing concern be sure to support ABCs, monitor the patient closely, get medical help, record a 12-lead ECG and look for causes.

Characteristics of normal sinus rhythm include:

- ventricular and atrial rates of 60–100 beats per minute
- regular and uniform QRS complexes and P waves
- PR interval of 0.12–0.20 second
- QRS duration < 0.12 second
- identical atrial and ventricular rates, with constant PR intervals.

Arrhythmia	Features
Sinus tachycardia 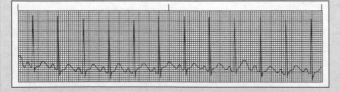	• Atrial and ventricular rhythms regular • Rate > 100 beats per minute; rarely > 160 beats per minute • Normal P waves preceding each QRS complex
Sinus bradycardia 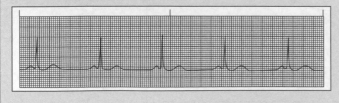	• Atrial and ventricular rhythms regular • Rate < 60 beats per minute • Normal P waves preceding each QRS complex

Cardiac arrhythmias

In cardiac arrhythmia, abnormal electrical conduction or automaticity changes heart rate and rhythm. An overview of the arrhythmias you should become familiar with and look out for are presented in *Understanding cardiac arrhythmias*, on page 152.

12-Lead electrocardiogram

The 12-lead electrocardiogram (ECG) measures the heart's electrical activity and records it as waveforms. It's one of the most valuable and commonly used diagnostic tools as well as being noninvasive and without risk to the patient.

A test with 12 views

The standard 12-lead ECG uses a series of electrodes placed on the patient's extremities and chest wall to assess the heart from 12 different views (leads).

Causes	Treatment
• Normal physiological response to fever, exercise, anxiety, pain, dehydration; may also accompany shock, left-sided heart failure, hyperthyroidism, anaemia, hypovolaemia, pulmonary embolism and anterior wall myocardial infarction (MI) • May also occur with atropine, adrenaline, aminophylline, caffeine, alcohol, cocaine, amphetamine and nicotine use	• Correction of underlying cause
• Normal, in well-conditioned heart, as in an athlete, or during sleep • Increased intracranial pressure; vagal stimulation; vomiting, sick sinus syndrome; hypothyroidism; inferior wall MI; and hypothermia	• Correction of underlying cause • Assess for adverse signs: HR < 40 per minute, heart failure, systolic BP < 90 mmHg • If adverse signs are present give atropine 500 mcgs I.V.

(continued)

Understanding cardiac arrhythmias (continued)

Arrhythmia	Features

Sinus bradycardia (continued)

Paroxysmal supraventricular tachycardia

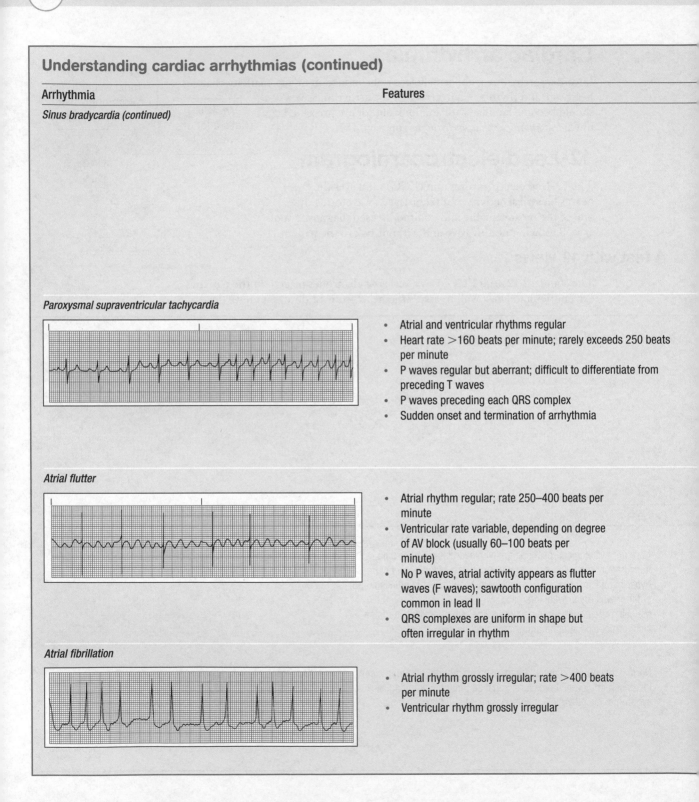

- Atrial and ventricular rhythms regular
- Heart rate >160 beats per minute; rarely exceeds 250 beats per minute
- P waves regular but aberrant; difficult to differentiate from preceding T waves
- P waves preceding each QRS complex
- Sudden onset and termination of arrhythmia

Atrial flutter

- Atrial rhythm regular; rate 250–400 beats per minute
- Ventricular rate variable, depending on degree of AV block (usually 60–100 beats per minute)
- No P waves, atrial activity appears as flutter waves (F waves); sawtooth configuration common in lead II
- QRS complexes are uniform in shape but often irregular in rhythm

Atrial fibrillation

- Atrial rhythm grossly irregular; rate >400 beats per minute
- Ventricular rhythm grossly irregular

Causes	Treatment
• May also occur with calcium channel blockers, beta-adrenergic blocker, digoxin and morphine use	• If response to atropine is not satisfactory assist with preparation for transvenous pacing and interim measures such as repeated atropine or adrenaline infusion • Assess for risk of asystole: recent asystole, complete heart block, Mobitz II, >3 s ventricular pauses; if there is a risk monitor closely and assist with preparation for transvenous pacing and interim measures such as repeated atropine or adrenaline infusion • In the absence of adverse signs and risk of asystole monitor closely
• Stress, hypoxia, hypokalaemia, cardiomyopathy, MI, valvular disease, Wolff–Parkinson–White syndrome, cor pulmonale, hyperthyroidism, anxiety, hypoxia, rheumatic heart disease • May also occur with digoxin toxicity; use of caffeine, marijuana, central nervous system stimulants, nicotine or alcohol	• If patient is unstable (hypotension, chest pain, heart failure, reduced LOC) prepare for immediate electrical cardioversion (up to three attempts) followed by amiodarone 30 mg over 20 minutes, if unsuccessful, prior to further cardioversion attempts • If patient is stable begin with vagal stimulation, e.g. Valsalva's manoeuvre, and carotid sinus massage proceeding to adenosine and amiodarone for chemical cardioversion or rate control with beta blocker
• Heart failure, tricuspid or mitral valve disease, pulmonary embolism, cor pulmonale, pericarditis and hyperthyroidism • May also occur with digoxin toxicity or alcohol use	• If patient is unstable (hypotension, chest pain, heart failure, reduced LOC) prepare for immediate electrical cardioversion (up to three attempts) followed by amiodarone 30 mg over 20 minutes, if unsuccessful, prior to further cardioversion attempts. • If patient is stable begin with vagal stimulation, e.g. Valsalva's manoeuvre, and carotid sinus massage proceeding to adenosine and amiodarone for chemical cardioversion or rate control with beta blocker
• Heart failure, chronic obstructive pulmonary disease, thyrotoxicosis, pericarditis, ischaemic heart disease, pulmonary embolus, hypertension, mitral stenosis, atrial irritation or complication of coronary bypass or valve replacement surgery	• If patient is unstable (hypotension, chest pain, heart failure, reduced LOC) prepare for immediate electrical cardioversion (up to three attempts) followed by amiodarone 30 mg over 20 minutes, if unsuccessful, prior to further cardioversion attempts.

(continued)

Understanding cardiac arrhythmias (continued)

Arrhythmia	Features

Atrial fibrillation (continued)

- QRS complexes of uniform configuration and duration
- PR interval indiscernible
- No P waves, atrial activity appears as erratic, irregular, baseline fibrillatory waves (f waves)

Junctional rhythm

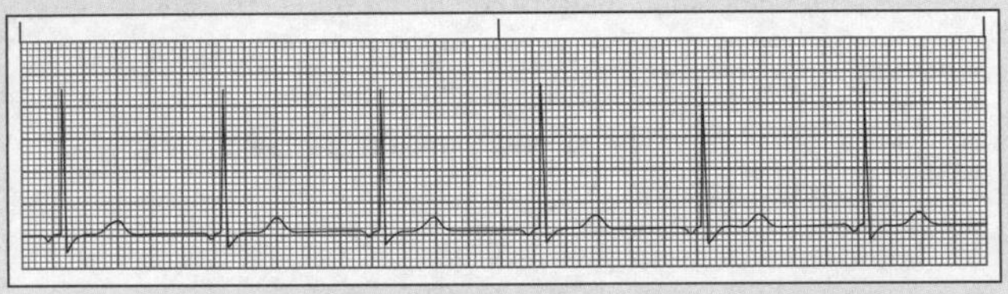

- Atrial and ventricular rhythms regular; atrial rate 40–60 beats per minute; ventricular rate usually 40–60 beats per minute (60–100 beats per minute is accelerated junctional rhythm)
- P waves preceding, hidden within (absent), or after QRS complex; usually inverted if visible
- PR interval (when present) < 0.12 second
- QRS complex configuration and duration normal, except in aberrant conduction

First-degree AV block

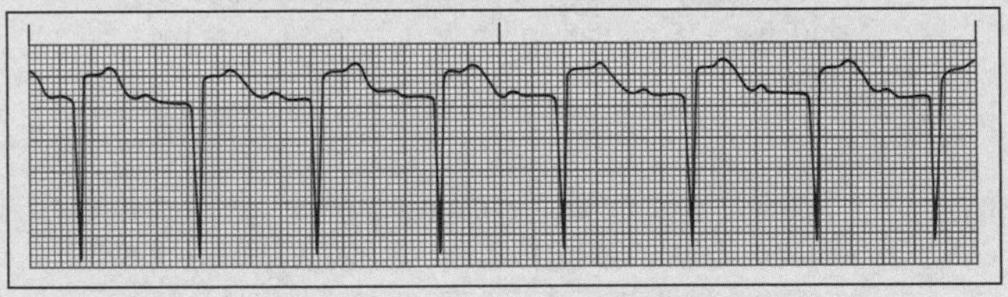

- Atrial and ventricular rhythms regular
- PR interval >0.20 second
- P wave precedes QRS complex
- QRS complex normal

Second-degree AV block

Mobitz I (Wenckebach)

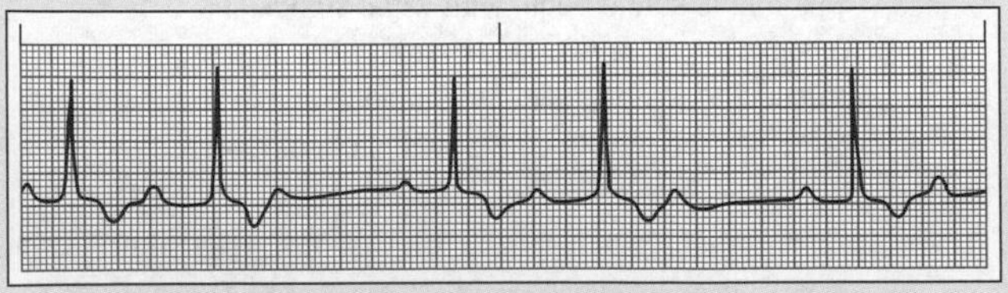

- Atrial rhythm regular
- Ventricular rhythm irregular
- Atrial rate exceeds ventricular rate
- PR interval progressively longer with each cycle until QRS complex disappears (dropped beat); PR interval shorter after dropped beat

Causes	Treatment
• May also occur with nifedipine, digoxin or alcohol use	• If patient is stable: Rate control with digoxin or beta blocker if onset >48 hours or amiodarone 300 mg I.V. over 20–60 minutes then 900 mg over 24 hours to chemically cardiovert if onset <48 hours.
• MI or ischaemia, hypoxia, vagal stimulation and sick sinus syndrome • Valve surgery • May also occur with digoxin toxicity	• Correction of underlying cause. • Discontinuation of digoxin if appropriate. • Assess for adverse signs: HR <40 per minute, heart failure, systolic BP <90 mmHg. • If adverse signs are present give atropine 500 mcgs I.V. • If response to atropine is not satisfactory assist with preparation for transvenous pacing and interim measures such as repeated atropine or adrenaline infusion. • In the absence of adverse signs monitor closely.
• May be seen in healthy persons • MI or ischaemia, hyperkalaemia, complication of coronary bypass or valve surgery • May also occur with digoxin toxicity; use of beta-adrenergic blockers, calcium channel blockers or amiodarone	• Correction of underlying cause. • Possibly atropine if severe symptomatic bradycardia develops. • Cautious use of digoxin, calcium channel blockers and beta-adrenergic blockers.
• Inferior wall MI, cardiac surgery, conduction system defects and vagal stimulation • May also occur with digoxin toxicity; use of beta-adrenergic blockers or calcium channel blockers	• Treatment of underlying cause. • Temporary pacemaker for symptomatic bradycardia (atropine usually not helpful). • Discontinuation of digoxin if appropriate.

(continued)

Understanding cardiac arrhythmias (continued)

Arrhythmia	Features

Second-degree AV block

Mobitz II

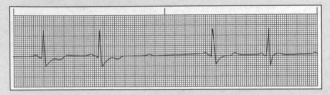

- Atrial rhythm regular
- Ventricular rhythm regular or irregular, with varying degree of block
- PR interval constant for conducted beats
- P waves normal size and shape, but some aren't followed by a QRS complex

Third-degree AV block

(*complete heart block*)

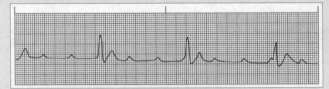

- Atrial rhythm regular
- Ventricular rhythm regular and rate slower than atrial rate
- No relation between P waves and QRS complexes
- No constant PR interval
- QRS duration normal (junctional pacemaker) or wide and bizarre (ventricular pacemaker)

Premature ventricular contraction (PVC)

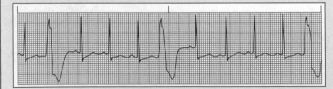

- Atrial rhythm regular
- Ventricular rhythm may be regular except for aberrant beats
- QRS complex premature, usually followed by a complete compensatory pause
- QRS complex wide and distorted, usually >0.12 second; conducted in opposite direction
- Premature QRS complexes occurring alone, in pairs, or in threes, alternating with normal beats; focus from one or more sites
- Ominous when clustered, multifocal, with R wave on T pattern

Causes	Treatment
• Severe coronary artery disease, anterior wall MI, acute myocarditis, hypertension, conduction system defects and complication of cardiac surgery	• Temporary or permanent pacemaker • Adrenaline for symptomatic bradycardia (atropine usually not helpful)
• Inferior or anterior wall MI, hypoxia, postoperative complication of cardiac surgery, postprocedure complication of radiofrequency ablation in or near AV nodal tissue and potassium imbalance • May also occur with digoxin toxicity	• Correction of underlying cause. • Assess for adverse signs: HR <40 per minute, heart failure, systolic BP <90 mmHg. • If adverse signs are present give atropine 500 mcgs I.V. • If response to atropine is not satisfactory assist with preparation for transvenous pacing and interim measures such as repeated atropine or adrenaline infusion. • Assess for risk of asystole: recent asystole, complete heart block, Mobitz II, >3 s ventricular pauses. If there is a risk monitor closely and assist with preparation for transvenous pacing and interim measures such as repeated atropine or adrenaline infusion. • In the absence of adverse signs and risk of asystole monitor closely.
• Heart failure; old or acute MI, ischaemia or contusion; myocardial irritation by ventricular catheter or a pacemaker; hypokalaemia; hypocalcaemia; hypomagnesaemia; cardiomyopathy; hypoxia; and acidosis • May also occur with drug toxicity (digoxin, aminophylline, epinephrine or noradrenaline) • Caffeine, tobacco or alcohol use • Psychological stress, anxiety, pain or exercise	• Treatment of underlying cause. • Discontinuation of drug causing toxicity. • Potassium chloride I.V. if PVC is induced by hypokalaemia. • Magnesium sulphate I.V. if PVC is induced by hypomagnesaemia.

(continued)

Understanding cardiac arrhythmias (continued)

Arrhythmia	Features

Ventricular tachycardia

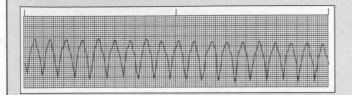

- Ventricular rate 100–250 beats per minute, rhythm usually regular
- QRS complexes wide, bizarre
- P waves not discernible
- May start and stop suddenly

Ventricular fibrillation

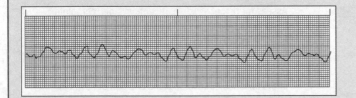

- Ventricular rhythm and rate chaotic and rapid
- QRS complexes wide and irregular; no visible P waves

Asystole

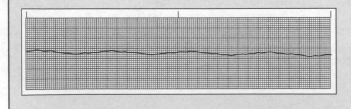

- No atrial or ventricular rate or rhythm
- No discernible P waves, QRS complexes or T waves

Causes	Treatment
• Myocardial ischaemia, MI or aneurysm; coronary artery disease; mitral valve prolapse; cardiomyopathy; ventricular catheters; hypokalaemia; hypocalcaemia; hypomagnesaemia; myocardial reperfusion; acidosis; and hypoxia • May also occur with drug toxicity	• If patient is unstable (hypotension, chest pain, heart failure, reduced LOC) prepare for immediate electrical cardioversion (up to three attempts) followed by amiodarone 30 mg over 20 minutes, if unsuccessful, prior to further cardioversion attempts. • Stable VT—should be treated with amiodarone loading (300 mg per 20 minutes I.V.) followed by maintenance (900 mg per 24 hours I.V.). • If irregular QRS rhythm (polymorphic) and QT interval is prolonged, stop medications that may prolong QT interval; correct electrolyte imbalance; administer magnesium; if ineffective, cardioversion. • If pulseless, initiate CPR; follow ALS protocol for defibrillation, endotracheal intubation and administration of adrenaline, followed by amiodarone and treatment of reversible causes.
• Myocardial ischaemia, MI, untreated ventricular tachycardia, R-on-T phenomenon, hypokalaemia, hypomagnesaemia, hypoxaemia, alkalosis, electric shock and hypothermia • May also occur with digoxin or tricyclic antidepressant toxicity	• Initiate CPR; follow ALS protocol for defibrillation, endotracheal intubation and administration of adrenaline, followed by amiodarone and treatment of reversible causes.
• Myocardial ischaemia, MI, heart failure, hypoxia, hypokalaemia, severe acidosis, shock, ventricular arrhythmia, AV block, pulmonary embolism, heart rupture, hyperkalaemia • May also occur with cocaine overdose	• Initiate CPR; follow ALS protocol for endotracheal intubation and administration of adrenaline and atropine and treatment of reversible causes.

The 12 leads include three bipolar limb leads (I, II and III), three unipolar augmented limb leads (aVR, aVL and aVF) and six unipolar precordial limb leads (V1 to V6). The limb leads and augmented leads show the heart in the frontal or vertical plane. The precordial leads show the heart in the horizontal plane.

The ECG can be used to identify myocardial ischaemia and infarction, rhythm and conduction disturbances, chamber enlargement, electrolyte imbalances and drug toxicity. However much of this is quite complex stuff. It is best to start by understanding the basics:

- Where the heart is being viewed from (each lead)
- What the waves are and how they should normally look
- What the waves might look like when abnormal

This information will then allow you to identify abnormal waves (for example, ST elevation—associated with myocardial damage in MI) and use

Normal ECG waveforms

Each of the 12 standard leads of an electrocardiogram (ECG) takes a different view of heart activity, and each generates its own characteristic tracing. The tracings shown here represent a normal heart rhythm viewed from each of the 12 leads. Keep in mind:

- An upwards (positive) deflection indicates that the wave of depolarisation flows towards the positive electrode.
- A downwards (negative) deflection indicates that the wave of depolarisation flows away from the positive electrode.
- An equally positive and negative (biphasic) deflection indicates that the wave of depolarisation flows perpendicularly to the positive electrode.

Each lead represents a picture of a different anatomic area; when you find abnormal tracings, compare information from the different leads to pinpoint areas of cardiac damage.

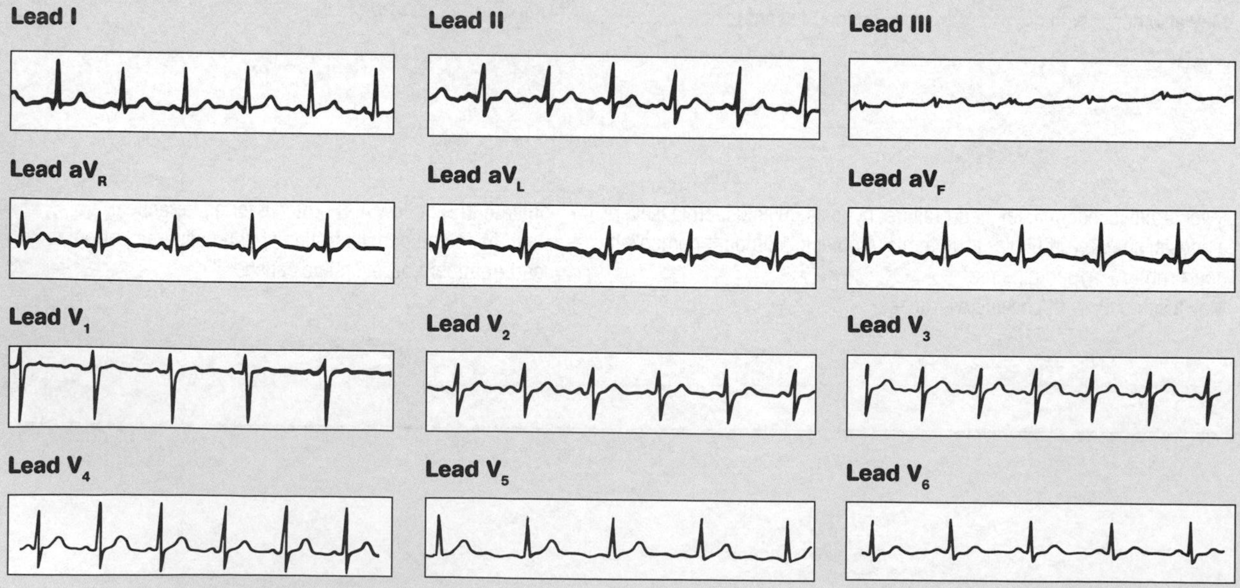

Lead I

Lead II

Lead III

Lead aV$_R$

Lead aV$_L$

Lead aV$_F$

Lead V$_1$

Lead V$_2$

Lead V$_3$

Lead V$_4$

Lead V$_5$

Lead V$_6$

your knowledge of the views of the heart to decide where the abnormality is. Use a systematic approach to interpret the ECG recording. Compare the patient's previous ECG with the current one, if available. This will help you identify changes.

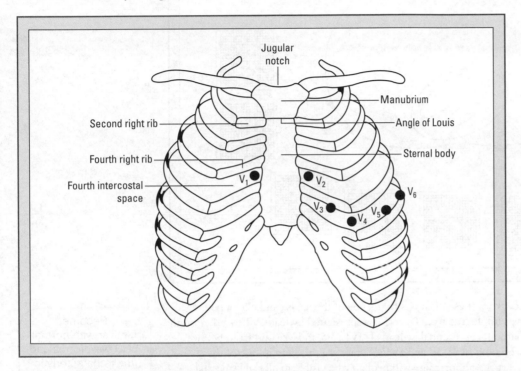

Jugular notch

Manubrium

Second right rib — Angle of Louis

Sternal body

Fourth right rib —

Fourth intercostal space

V₁ V₂ V₆ V₃ V₄ V₅

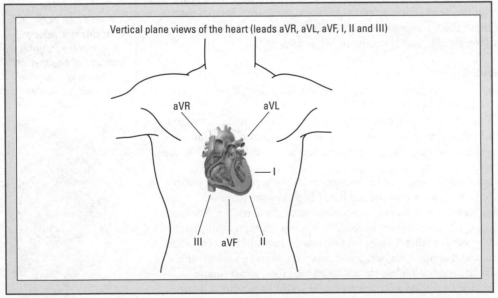

Vertical plane views of the heart (leads aVR, aVL, aVF, I, II and III)

aVR aVL

I

III aVF II

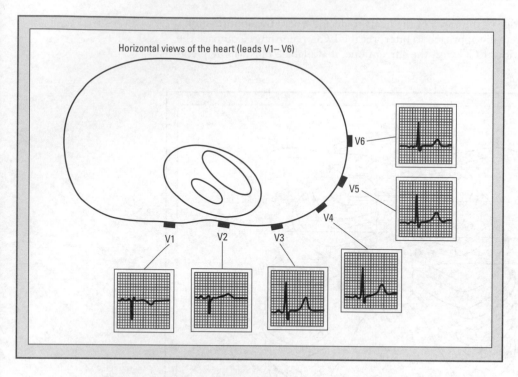

Horizontal views of the heart (leads V1– V6)

You can see from these diagrams that some of the leads can be grouped together. For example, the front (anterior) represented by leads V1 to V4; around the left side (lateral) represented by leads I, aVL, V5 and V6; and from below (inferior) represented by II, III and aVF. If there is a problem in one of these areas of the heart the abnormality will probably be visible in all the leads that look at that area of the heart. For example, significant myocardial infarctions may generate elevation of the ST segment on the ECG—ST elevation in inferior, anterior and/or lateral leads usually means an MI in these areas.

Normal waves

• P waves should be upright except in aVR where they should be inverted (they may also be inverted or biphasic III, aV$_L$ and V$_1$).
• PR intervals should always be constant, just like QRS-complex durations. If they are prolonged there may be conduction disturbance such as heart block. PR interval should be no longer than 0.2 seconds—or five small squares on the graph paper.
• QRS—complex deflections vary in different leads. When they are positive (upright) electricity is flowing towards the lead (thus they are generally upside down in aVR as conduction is downwards and towards the left). A QRS should be no longer than 0.12 seconds—or three small squares on the graph paper. Q waves should be very small. Observe for large pathological Q waves—these mean cardiac muscle damage. (See *Abnormal waves*, on page 165.) A normal Q wave generally has a duration less than 0.04 second (one small square). An abnormal Q wave has either a duration of 0.04 second or more, a depth greater than 4 mm or a height one-fourth of the R wave. Remember

Become familiar with normal ECG waveforms and their characteristic patterns. Then you can spot abnormal waves and configurations indicating a possible problem or disease. It's elementary.

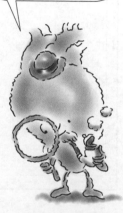

Abnormal waves

Normal PQRST (upright T waves and normal isoelectric line between S wave and T wave)

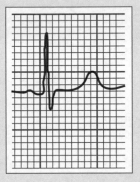

T wave inversion (may be myocardial ischaemia or non-ST-elevation myocardial infarction)

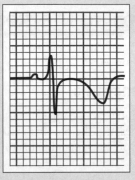

ST depression (signifies myocardial ischaemia or damage in a non-STEMI (ST-elevation myocardial infarction)

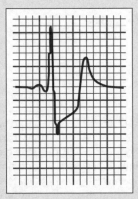

ST elevation (as with STEMI) and large deep pathological Q waves signifying myocardial damage through the full thickness of the myocardium

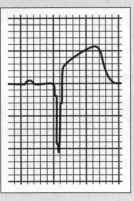

that aVR normally has a large Q wave, so disregard this lead when searching for abnormal Q waves.

• ST segments should be on the baseline as when there is no electrical wave, or have minimal deviation from the isoelectric line (baseline). ST-segment elevation greater than 1 mm above the baseline and ST-segment depression greater than 0.5 mm below the baseline are considered abnormal. ST elevation means damage to heart muscle as in myocardial infarction; ST depression often means ischaemia—a prelude to damage if left untreated.

• The T wave normally deflects upwards in leads I, II and V_3 through V_6. It's inverted in aV_R and variable in the other leads. T-wave changes have many causes and aren't always a reason for alarm. Excessively tall, flat or inverted T waves occurring with symptoms, such as chest pain, may indicate ischaemia.

A fuller discussion of the acute coronary syndromes is included in the section 'Disorders.'

There's a lot more to it

We've covered some ECG basics here. There is much more to the ECG and if you are working in a cardiac unit or want to develop more advanced knowledge on the ECG you'll need to read and study much more.

Cardiac marker studies

Analysis of cardiac markers aids diagnosis of acute coronary syndromes, including MI.

Release the enzymes!

After infarction, damaged cardiac tissue releases significant amounts of enzymes into the blood. Serial measurement of enzyme levels reveals the extent of damage and helps to monitor the progress of healing.

Heart-zymes

The cardiac enzymes include creatine kinase (CK) and its isoenzyme MB (found specifically in heart muscle) and lactate dehydrogenase (LD) and its isoenzymes LD1 and LD2 that occur in heart muscle.

Tests for troponin T and I and myoglobin are more specific to cardiac muscle and can be used to detect damage more quickly, allowing faster and more effective treatment.

Meaning in markers

Here's what the results of cardiac marker studies mean:
• CK-MB levels increase 4–8 hours after the onset of acute MI, peak after 20 hours and may remain elevated for up to 72 hours.
• Troponin levels increase within 3–6 hours after myocardial damage. Troponin I peaks in 14–20 hours, with a return to baseline in 5–7 days. Troponin T peaks in 12–24 hours, with a return to baseline in 10–15 days. Because troponin levels stay elevated for a long time, they can be used to detect an infarction that occurred several days earlier. However, in the context of critical illness, renal dysfunction and poor tissue perfusion, troponin may be elevated even if there has not been an acute myocardial event.
• Myoglobin levels may increase within 30 minutes to 4 hours after myocardial damage, peak within 6–7 hours and return to baseline after 24 hours. However, because skeletal muscle damage may cause myoglobin levels to increase, it isn't specific to myocardial injury.

Did you know that troponin levels stay elevated for long time and can indicate an infarction occurred several days earlier.

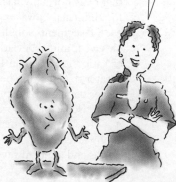

Echocardiography

Echocardiography is used to examine the size, shape and motion of cardiac structures. It's done using a transducer placed at an acoustic window (an area where bone and lung tissue are absent) on the patient's chest. The transducer directs sound waves towards cardiac structures, which reflect these waves.

Echo, echo

The transducer picks up the echoes, converts them into electrical impulses and relays them to an echocardiography machine for display on a screen and for recording on a strip chart or videotape. The most commonly used echocardiographic techniques are M-mode and two-dimensional.

Motion mode

In M-mode (motion mode) echocardiography, a single, pencil-like ultrasound beam strikes the heart, producing an 'ice pick', or vertical, view of cardiac structures. This mode is especially useful for precisely viewing cardiac structures.

Echo in 2-D

In two-dimensional echocardiography, the ultrasound beam rapidly sweeps through an arc, producing a cross-sectional, or fan-shaped, view of cardiac structures; this technique is useful for recording lateral motion and providing the correct spatial relationship between cardiac structures. In many cases, both techniques are performed to complement each other.

TOE combination

In transoesophageal echocardiography (TOE), ultrasonography is combined with endoscopy to provide a better view of the heart's structures. (See *A closer look at TOE*.)

Echo abnormalities

The echocardiogram may detect mitral stenosis, mitral valve prolapse, aortic insufficiency, wall motion abnormalities and pericardial effusion (excess pericardial fluid).

Nursing considerations
• Explain the procedure to the patient and advise them to remain still during the test because movement can distort results. Tell them that conductive gel is applied to the chest and a small transducer is placed directly over it. Because pressure is exerted to keep the transducer in contact with the skin, warn the patient that they may feel minor discomfort.
• After the procedure, remove the conductive gel from the skin.
• Ensure that the patient is informed of the results and significance of the test.

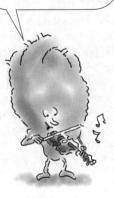

Echocardiography reflects the size, shape and motion of cardiac structures using sound waves.

A closer look at toe

In transoesophageal echocardiography (TOE), ultrasonography is combined with endoscopy to provide a better view of the heart's structures.

How it's done

A small transducer is attached to the end of a gastroscope and inserted into the oesophagus so that images of the heart's structure can be taken from the posterior of the heart. This test causes less tissue penetration and interference from chest wall structures and produces high quality images of the thoracic aorta (except for the superior ascending aorta, which is shadowed by the trachea).

And why

TOE is used to diagnose:
• thoracic and aortic disorders
• endocarditis
• congenital heart disease
• intracardiac thrombi
• tumours.

It's also used to evaluate valvular disease or repairs.

Haemodynamic monitoring

Haemodynamic monitoring is used to assess circulatory function and determine the effectiveness of therapy. This is a major part of the critical care nurse's role. In this section you'll learn about haemodynamic therapies, revise key concepts and become aware of the range of established and more contemporary haemodynamic monitoring available and how to use it in practice.

Fundamentals of the circulatory system and haemodynamics

The ideal cardiovascular system has adequate pressure within it (blood pressure) and it has an adequate volume of blood being pumped around the body (CO), delivering oxygen and nutrients to cells. The three factors that affect CO are preload, afterload and contractility. (See *Understanding preload, afterload and contractility*, page 143.) Blood pressure is a product of CO and SVR.

Therapies directed at optimising the cardiovascular system often rely on accurate haemodynamic measurements. For an overview of how the values you'll see match physiological parameters as outcomes of therapies see *Matching haemodynamic monitoring to therapies*.

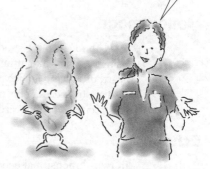

Haemodynamic monitoring is a way of tracking and recording pressures and flow within the circulatory system that allow evaluation of problems and responses to treatment.

Matching haemodynamic monitoring to therapies

Therapies	Physiological parameters affected	Haemodynamic parameters of use in evaluation
Intravenous fluid boluses—increasing circulating volume	Increased 'preload'. As a result will increase contractility and cardiac output within myocardial capabilities. Blood pressure will often increase as well.	Blood pressure Central venous pressure Pulmonary artery wedge pressure Cardiac output
Diuretics or renal replacement therapy—reducing circulating volume; 'offloading'	Reduced 'preload'. In the case of an overfilled (overstretched) heart this may improve contractility, cardiac output and blood pressure.	Blood pressure Central venous pressure Pulmonary artery wedge pressure Cardiac output
Positive inotropic drugs	Increased 'contractility'. Often blood pressure will increase as a result. May also affect 'afterload' (e.g. dobutamine is a vasodilator).	Blood pressure Cardiac output Systemic vascular resistance
Vasopressors	Increase 'afterload'. This will often result in an improvement in blood pressure but will usually reduce cardiac output as well.	Blood pressure Cardiac output Systemic vascular resistance
Vasodilators	Reduce 'afterload'. This will often result in an increased cardiac output. It may, however, reduce blood pressure.	Blood pressure Cardiac output Systemic vascular resistance

Understanding pressures

The pulmonary artery catheter (Swan-Ganz Catheter) provides information on intracardiac pressures, arterial pressure and cardiac output. The CVC measures right atrial pressures. To understand intracardiac pressures, picture the heart and vascular system as a continuous loop with constantly changing pressure gradients that keep the blood moving. Haemodynamic monitoring records the gradients within the vessels and heart chambers. Cardiac output indicates the amount of blood ejected by the heart each minute.

Pressure and description	Normal values	Causes of increased pressure	Causes of decreased pressure
Central venous pressure or right atrial pressure	Normal mean pressure ranges from 1 to 6 mmHg (1.34–8 cmH$_2$0)	• Right-sided heart failure	• Reduced circulating blood volume
The central venous pressure (CVP) or right atrial pressure (RAP) shows right ventricular function and end-diastolic pressure		• Volume overload • Tricuspid valve stenosis or insufficiency • Constrictive pericarditis • Pulmonary hypertension • Cardiac tamponade • Right ventricular infarction	
Right ventricular pressure	Normal systolic pressure ranges from 20 to 30 mmHg; normal diastolic pressure from 0 to 5 mmHg.	• Mitral stenosis or insufficiency	• Reduced circulating blood volume
Typically, the doctor measures right ventricular pressure only when initially inserting a pulmonary artery catheter; right ventricular systolic pressure normally equals pulmonary artery systolic pressure; right ventricular end-diastolic pressure, which reflects right ventricular function, equals RAP		• Pulmonary disease • Hypoxaemia • Constrictive pericarditis • Chronic heart failure • Atrial and ventricular septal defects • Patent ductus arteriosus	
Pulmonary artery pressure	Systolic pressure normally ranges from 20 to 30 mmHg; the mean pressure usually ranges from 10 to 15 mmHg	• Left-sided heart failure	• Reduced circulating blood volume
Pulmonary artery systolic pressure shows right ventricular function and pulmonary circulation pressures; pulmonary artery diastolic pressure		• Increased pulmonary blood flow (left or right shunting, as in atrial or ventricular septal defects)	

(continued)

Understanding pressures (continued)

Pressure and description	Normal values	Causes of increased pressure	Causes of decreased pressure
Pulmonary artery pressure (continued) reflects left ventricular pressures, specifically left ventricular end-diastolic pressure, in a patient without significant pulmonary disease		• Any condition causing increased pulmonary arteriolar resistance (such as pulmonary hypertension, volume overload, mitral stenosis or hypoxia)	
Pulmonary artery wedge pressure	The mean pressure normally ranges from 6 to 12 mmHg	• Left-sided heart failure	• Reduced circulating blood volume
Pulmonary artery wedge pressure (PAWP) reflects left atrial and left ventricular pressures, unless the patient has mitral stenosis; changes in PAWP reflect changes in left ventricular filling pressure		• Mitral stenosis or insufficiency • Pericardial tamponade	

These are the fundamental concepts and relationships that you need to know before you move on to understand and use haemodynamic monitoring. Whether it be an accurate blood pressure measured from an arterial catheter (arterial line), the measurement of central venous pressure (CVP) or pulmonary artery wedge pressure (PAWP) as representations of 'preload' or measurement of CO and calculation of SVR from a pulmonary artery catheter, the clinical agenda is always the same—evaluating the effectiveness of circulation, the nature of problems and the evaluation of responses to treatment.

More on the fundamentals. . .

Accuracy is important in monitoring. The information will often be used to titrate some pretty powerful drugs—so you should follow your organisation's policy or guidelines for setting up, zero referencing, calibrating, maintaining and troubleshooting equipment. Risks to patients exist with all forms of haemodynamic monitoring so you should be aware of the associated complications and how to prevent and monitor these.

Invasive arterial pressure monitoring

In arterial blood pressure monitoring, a catheter (an 'arterial line') is inserted into a distal artery—usually radial (in the wrist) or dorsalis pedis (in the foot). When there are problems, such as shock, that reduce peripheral pulses a more central artery may be used (e.g. brachial or femoral)— however, these are avoided when possible since vessel damage or a clot at this level carries the risk of a loss of circulation to a limb rather than just fingers or toes. The catheter is connected to a bedside monitor with pressure monitoring capabilities and a transducer transforms the pressure into a waveform that appears on the monitor. The catheter also allows access for samples of arterial blood for diagnostic tests such as arterial blood gas (ABG) studies.

'Arterial lines' are usually inserted for reasons such as:
- Unstable blood pressure
- The need to monitor the effects of vasoactive drugs
- Respiratory failure and/or ventilatory support requiring frequent ABGs
- Tissue, limb or anatomical states where use of a cuff and sphygmomanometer is not possible

Nursing considerations
- Explain the procedure to the patient and their family, including the purpose of arterial pressure monitoring.
- After catheter insertion, observe the pressure waveform to assess arterial pressure.
- Document the date and time of catheter insertion and catheter insertion site.
- Follow local policy and guidelines for the prevention of infection and complications.
- Explain the procedure to the patient and their family, including the purpose of CVP monitoring.
- Maintain 300 mmHg pressure in the pressure bag to permit a flush flow of 3–6 ml/hour.
- If fever develops when the catheter is in place, inform the doctor; they may wish to take blood cultures from the line or remove the catheter and send its tip to the laboratory for culture.
- Make sure stopcocks are properly positioned and connections are secure. Loose connections may introduce air into the system or cause leakage of blood or inaccurate pressure readings.

You'll need to monitor for these complications
- Haemorrhage—from the insertion site or from inadvertent disconnection
- Infection—sometimes noticeable at the insertion site or as a fever with bloodstream infection
- Clot formation or air embolus—leading to a dampened waveform on the monitor and ischaemia in distal tissues if released into the artery
- Vessel damage—caused at the time of insertion could result in a swelling at the insertion site
- Injection of drugs into an artery by mistake—may cause tissue ischaemia which can be prevented by clearly labelling the line as ARTERIAL! and following local policy for avoiding intra-arterial administration of drugs.

Central venous pressure monitoring
In CVP monitoring, a catheter (CVC—central venous catheter—or 'central line') is inserted into a central vein (usually internal jugular or subclavian veins). The catheter is advanced until it is in or near the right atrium. The pressure at end-diastole reflects the 'filling pressure' in the right side of the heart—what we've described above as 'preload'. Lots of factors affect this pressure including positive pressure in the thorax, as in mechanical ventilation,

body position (supine increases the venous return and thus CVP) and, importantly, valvular heart disease. You'll need to know if these are present so that you can interpret the measurements in the context of these factors.

The catheter is connected to a bedside monitor with pressure monitoring capabilities and a transducer transforms the pressure into a waveform that appears on the monitor. The catheter also allows access for samples of venous blood and for the administration of drugs and fluids that might inflame or damage peripheral veins.

CVCs are usually inserted for reasons such as:
• The need to monitor CVP to assist in evaluating fluid volume status (and 'preload')
• Difficulty in gaining peripheral venous access
• The need to monitor the effects of vasoactive drugs
• The need to administer drugs or solutions that cannot be administered via peripheral veins

Nursing considerations
• Explain the procedure to the patient and their family, including the purpose of CVP monitoring.
• After catheter insertion, observe the pressure waveform to assess CVP.
• Document the date and time of catheter insertion and catheter insertion site.
• Follow local policy and guidelines for the prevention of infection and complications.
• Maintain 300 mmHg pressure in the pressure bag to permit a flush flow of 3–6 ml/hour.
• If fever develops when the catheter is in place, inform the doctor; they may wish to take blood cultures from the line or remove the catheter and send its tip to the laboratory for culture.
• Make sure stopcocks are properly positioned and connections are secure. Loose connections may introduce air into the system or cause leakage of blood or inaccurate pressure readings.

You'll need to monitor for these complications
• Pneumothorax or haemothorax following insertion via the subclavian route—so a postinsertion chest x-ray is essential
• Haemorrhage—from the insertion site
• Infection—sometimes noticeable at the insertion site or as a fever with bloodstream infection
• Clot formation or air embolus—observe for sudden onset of respiratory compromise and chest pain
• Catheter tip migration—into the right ventricle manifested by ventricular arrhythmias.

Pulmonary artery pressure monitoring (using a Swan-Ganz catheter)
Continuous PAP and intermittent PAWP measurements provide important information about left ventricular function and preload. In addition,

pulmonary artery catheters allow measurement of CO and calculation of SVR. When interpreted in the context of the information available from the other forms of invasive haemodynamic monitoring, discussed above, PAP catheters allow for a comprehensive assessment of the haemodynamic status of the patient and their responses to therapy.

PAP purposes

PAP monitoring is indicated for patients who:
* are haemodynamically unstable
* have complex fluid management issues
* need continuous cardiopulmonary assessment
* are receiving multiple or frequently administered cardioactive drugs.

PAP monitoring can also be very valuable for patients experiencing shock, trauma, severe pulmonary or cardiac disease or multiple organ dysfunction syndrome.

PAP's parts

A pulmonary artery (PA) catheter has up to six lumens that gather haemodynamic information. In addition to distal and proximal lumens used to measure pressures, a PA catheter has a balloon inflation lumen that inflates the balloon for PAWP measurement and a thermistor connector lumen that allows CO measurement.

Some catheters also have a pacemaker wire lumen that provides a port for pacemaker electrodes and measures continuous mixed venous oxygen saturation. (See *PA catheter ports*, on page 174.)

PAP and PAWP procedures

The doctor inserts the balloon-tipped, multilumen catheter into the patient's internal jugular or subclavian vein. When the catheter reaches the right atrium, the balloon is inflated to float the catheter through the right ventricle into the pulmonary artery. This permits PAWP measurement through an opening at the catheter's tip.

The deflated catheter rests in the pulmonary artery, allowing diastolic and systolic PAP readings. The balloon should be totally deflated except when taking a PAWP reading because prolonged wedging can cause pulmonary infarction. (See *Normal PA waveforms*, page C2, C3.)

Nursing considerations
* After catheter insertion, you may inflate the balloon with a syringe to take PAWP readings. Be careful not to inflate the balloon with more than 1.5 cc of air. Overinflation could distend the pulmonary artery causing vessel rupture. Don't leave the balloon wedged for a prolonged period (longer than three respiratory cycles) because this could lead to a pulmonary infarction.
* After each PAWP reading, flush the line; if you encounter difficulty, notify the doctor.
* Maintain 300 mmHg pressure in the pressure bag to permit a flush flow of 3–6 ml/hour.

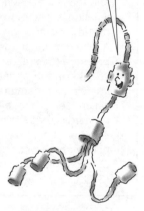

PA catheters have up to six lumens, so various haemodynamic information can be gathered.

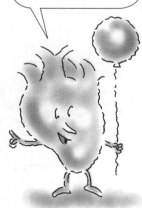

Remember don't leave the balloon wedged for a prolonged period because this could lead to pulmonary infarction.

PA catheter ports

A pulmonary artery (PA) catheter contains several lumen ports to allow various catheter functions:

- The balloon inflation lumen inflates the balloon at the distal tip of the catheter for pulmonary artery wedge pressure (PAWP) measurement.
- A distal lumen measures PA pressure when connected to a transducer and measures PAWP during balloon inflation. It also permits drawing of mixed venous blood samples.
- A proximal lumen measures right atrial pressure (central venous pressure).
- The thermistor connector lumen contains temperature-sensitive wires, which feed information into a computer for cardiac output calculation.
- Another lumen may provide a port for pacemaker electrodes or measurement of mixed venous oxygen saturation ($S\bar{v}O_2$).

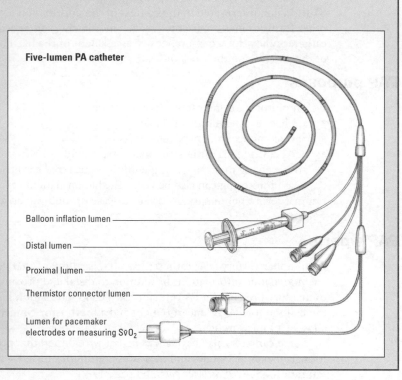

Five-lumen PA catheter

Balloon inflation lumen
Distal lumen
Proximal lumen
Thermistor connector lumen
Lumen for pacemaker electrodes or measuring $S\bar{v}O_2$

- Follow local policy and guidelines for the prevention of infection and complications.
- If fever develops when the catheter is in place, inform the doctor; they may wish to take blood cultures from the line or remove the catheter and send its tip to the laboratory for culture.
- Make sure stopcocks are properly positioned and connections are secure. Loose connections may introduce air into the system or cause leakage of blood or inaccurate pressure readings. Also make sure the lumen hubs are properly identified to serve the appropriate catheter ports.
- Because the catheter can slip back into the right ventricle and irritate it, check the monitor for a right ventricular waveform to detect this problem promptly.
- To minimise valvular trauma, make sure the balloon is deflated whenever the catheter is withdrawn from the pulmonary artery to the right ventricle or from the right ventricle to the right atrium.
- Document the date and time of catheter insertion, the doctor who performed the procedure, the catheter insertion site, pressure waveforms and values for the various heart chambers, balloon inflation volume required to obtain a wedge tracing, arrhythmias that occurred during or after the procedure, type of dressing applied and the patient's tolerance of the procedure.

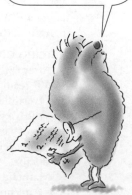

Don't worry I'm just making sure you remember to document everything.

Cardiac output monitoring

CO—the amount of blood ejected by the heart in 1 minute—is monitored to evaluate cardiac function. The normal range for CO is 4–8 L/minute.

When using a pulmonary artery catheter the most widely used method for monitoring CO is the bolus thermodilution technique.

On the rocks or room temperature

To measure CO, a solution is injected into the right atrium through a port on a PA catheter. Iced or room temperature injectate may be used depending on your unit's policy.

This indicator solution mixes with the blood as it travels through the right ventricle into the pulmonary artery, and a thermistor on the catheter registers the change in temperature of the flowing blood. A computer then plots the temperature change over time as a curve and calculates flow based on the area under the curve.

To be continued

Some PA catheters contain a filament that permits continuous CO monitoring. Using such a device, an average CO value is determined over a 3-minute span; the value is updated every 30–60 seconds. This type of monitoring allows close scrutiny of the patient's haemodynamic status and prompt intervention in case problems arise.

Better assessor

CO is better assessed by calculating cardiac index (CI), which takes body size into account. To calculate the patient's CI, divide their CO by their body surface area (BSA), a product of height and weight. The normal CI for adults ranges from 2.5 to 4.2 L/minute/m^2 (3.5–6.5 L/minute/m^2 for pregnant women).

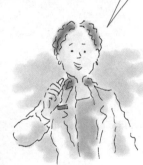

Continuous cardiac output monitoring allows close scrutiny of the patient's haemodynamic status.

Nursing considerations
• Make sure your patient doesn't move during the procedure because movement can cause an error in measurement.
• Perform CO measurements and monitoring at least every 2–4 hours, especially if the patient is receiving vasoactive or inotropic agents or if fluids are being added or restricted.
• Discontinue CO measurements when the patient is haemodynamically stable and weaned from their vasoactive and inotropic medications.
• Monitor the patient for signs and symptoms of inadequate perfusion, including restlessness, fatigue, changes in level of consciousness (LOC), decreased capillary refill time, diminished peripheral pulses, oliguria and pale, cool skin, increasing lactate.
• Record the patient's CO, CI and other haemodynamic values and vital signs at the time of measurement. Note the patient's position during measurement.

More than one way . . .

Along with other measured values such as blood pressure, CVP and arterial oxygen levels the bedside monitor, or other clinical computer, can calculate a range of other values allowing a very comprehensive understanding of a patient's haemodynamic status and responses to therapy. The one pivotal measurement that is essential in calculating values such as SVR and oxygen delivery is CO.

Pulmonary artery catheters have for some time been the most widely used method of measuring CO. However, the technical difficulties of floating the catheter through the heart and the potential for valve damage and other complications has driven the development of other methods and technologies to measure CO. Newer methods of haemodynamic monitoring are less invasive and carry lower risks than PA catheters.

Haemodynamic monitoring methods

Method of monitoring	How it works
Oesophageal Doppler	An ultrasound probe is passed into the oesophagus with the tip adjacent to and facing the ascending aorta. From this position, using the Doppler principle, the probe can monitor cardiac output as blood is ejected from the heart into the aorta. CI and SVR are then calculated and additional parameters are also measured to help evaluation of contractility, preload and afterload. Additional parameters include 'flow time' (the duration of blood ejection) and peak velocity of ejected blood. Frequent adjustment of the probe is often required to refocus the pulse waveform and maintain accurate measurement. The probe can't be used after oesophageal surgery or in conscious patients. The advantage is that it is not an intravascular method and thus there is no associated risk of infection.
Pulse-induced contour cardiac output (PiCCO)	A thermistor tipped arterial catheter is passed into a brachial or femoral artery (in addition to any existing 'arterial line'). The pulse waveform generated is used, in conjunction with thermodilution (via a central venous catheter), to calculate cardiac output. CI and SVR are then calculated and additional parameters are also measured to help haemodynamic evaluation of contractility, preload and afterload. Additional parameters include: stroke volume (SV), stroke volume variation (SVV), global end-diastolic volume (GEDV), intrathoracic blood volume (ITBV), extravascular lung water (EVLW), cardiac function index (CFI). This system requires both central venous and arterial access. All the risks associated with these exist in this system (see also 'Invasive arterial pressure monitoring' and 'Central venous pressure monitoring').
LiDCO	A standard arterial catheter can be used with this system to generate a pulse waveform. The pulse waveform generated is used in conjunction with lithium dilution (via a central venous catheter) to calculate cardiac output. CI and SVR are then calculated and additional parameters are also measured to help haemodynamic evaluation of contractility, preload and afterload. Additional parameters include: systolic pressure variation (SPV), pulse pressure variation (PPV) and stroke volume variation (SVV). This system requires both central venous and arterial access. All the risks associated with these exist in this system (see also 'Invasive arterial pressure monitoring' and 'Central venous pressure monitoring'). The system requires calibration with lithium which may not be accurate if given in the presence of existing lithium therapy or muscle relaxants. Other factors affecting accuracy include: aortic valve regurgitation, patients on an intra-Aortic balloon pump, arterial line damping and pronounced peripheral arterial vasoconstriction.

Understanding the relevance of laboratory tests in cardiovascular assessment

Test	Relevance to cardiovascular assessment
Arterial blood gas analysis PaO_2 9.5–12 kPa $PaCO_2$ 4.6–6 kPa pH 7.36–7.44 HCO_3 22–26 mmol/L Base excess/deficit +/− 2 mmol/L	PaO_2 and $PaCO_2$ are the gold standard measurements of how well gas is exchanging in the lungs. Inadequate oxygen levels in the blood can lead to poor oxygenation of the myocardium and affect the strength of cardiac contraction and pumping. In addition low blood oxygen levels can lead to poor oxygenation of vital organs—even if cardiovascular function (pressure and flow of blood) is adequate.
Lactate 0.63–2.44 mmol/L	Rising lactate means that significant tissue mass is lacking in oxygen—this may be due to cardiovascular and/or respiratory failure.
Creatinine 45–120 µmol/L	Overall a useful and representative marker of renal function—rising levels indicate renal failure. Since kidneys are particularly sensitive to inadequate perfusion this may be a consequence of cardiovascular failure. Underperfusion of the kidneys leads to rising creatinine because filtration pressure is inadequate. Toxic, infective or ischaemic damage to the kidney tubules causes blockage and a resultant back pressure into the glomerular filter. So creatinine also rises in other systemic conditions.
Urea 2–6.5 mmol/L	Urea becomes elevated like creatinine when cardiovascular failure leads to inadequate kidney perfusion. However, it also become elevated in dehydration—an important cause of inadequate circulating volume of blood in the cardiovascular system.
Electrolytes Potassium 3.5–5 mmol/L Sodium 135–145 mmol/L Chloride 100–108 mmol/L Magnesium 0.7–1.0 mmol/L Total calcium 2.2–2.6 mmol/L	Electrolytes are important in normal muscle and nerve function. They facilitate the conduction of impulses through the cardiac conduction system as well as cardiac muscle contraction. Abnormal levels may worsen cardiac failure or cause conduction and rhythm abnormalities.
Haemoglobin Male 13.5–18 g/dl Female 11.5–16 g/dl	Haemoglobin is the carrier of oxygen (and carbon dioxide in the blood). Low levels mean greater work by the lungs and heart to deliver adequate oxygen to cells. Low levels may also mean that the patient is bleeding.
White blood cell count 4–11x10^9 per litre	Elevated levels indicate infection—if severe this can cause sepsis which is a major cause of circulatory failure and shock
Liver function tests (LFT) Total protein 60–80 g/L Albumin 35–50 g/L Globulin 25–34 g/L GGT Males 5–72 U/L Females 5–45 U/L Total bilirubin 0–17 µmol/L	The liver is susceptible to dysfunction if there is poor perfusion—since 75% of the blood it receives is already deoxygenated (from the gut). It is often difficult to interpret LFTs as many of the parameters measured are not specific to the liver and are affected by many factors—commonly drugs. If there is a rise in bilirubin and transaminases such as AST, ALT and GGT there may be cellular damage in the liver. A rise in prothrombin time (part of the coagulation/clotting screen) suggests the synthetic function of the liver is inadequate (also elevated by warfarin therapy).

(continued)

Understanding the relevance of laboratory tests in cardiovascular assessment (continued)

Test	Relevance to cardiovascular assessment
Conjugated bilirubin 0–5 µmol/L *AST 5–55 U/L* *ALT 4–45 U/L* *Alk phosphatase 30–120 U/L*	
Coagulation/clotting tests *PT 10–14 seconds* *INR 1.0* *APTT 35–45 seconds* *Platelet count 150–400x10⁹ per litre*	Elevated clotting times and low platelets may be contributory factors in patients who are bleeding. (Clotting times are also elevated by drugs such as heparin and warfarin.) It is also important to know if there is a coagulation problem prior to the insertion of invasive lines for haemodynamic monitoring and therapy (e.g. central venous catheters)

Results and significance of diagnostic tests and investigations

The value of laboratory and other physiological tests is that they can enhance or help confirm and quantify what might be suspected from clinical assessment. However, it is important to be suspicious of results that seem to contradict the clinical picture built up through assessment.

Laboratory tests

Examples of laboratory tests that might help in the process of cardiovascular assessment are included in *Understanding the relevance of laboratory tests in cardiovascular assessment*, on page 177.

Treatments

Many treatments are available for the critically ill patients with cardiovascular disease. These include:
• Fluid management—including volume replacement for hypovolaemia and dehydration, and fluid restriction or 'offloading' for fluid overload.
• Drug therapy—for prevention of angina and heart failure or continuous infusions aimed at modifying vascular tone and force of cardiac contraction
• Surgery—for vascular aneurysms, heart valve problems, occluded coronary vessels or heart transplantation

- Electrical interventions—such as defibrillation or synchronised cardioversion for arrhythmias and pacemakers for heart block and slow heart rates affecting CO.

It is important for the critical care nurse to have an understanding of the clinical implication of these interventions in order that patients can be prepared for, evaluated during, and helped to recover from common interventions.

Fluid management

Basic fluid physiology

Adequate intravascular volume of blood is essential to ensure adequate preload, CO and oxygen delivery to tissues. Most people can compensate when haemoglobin levels drop to half the normal level by increasing CO. This is not the case when the intravascular volume of blood falls. Profound shock ensues when more than 1.5–2 L (30–40%) of circulating volume is lost. As intravascular volume is depleted CO falls. (For more on hypovolaemic shock, see Chapter 10.)

Ensuring adequate circulating volume is extremely important in the critically ill. However, it can also be complex. In health fluid intake is predominantly through oral fluids—mainly regulated by thirst. Fluid loss is predominantly through urine output—mainly regulated by antidiuretic hormone secretion and renal response to this. In critical illness patients are often unable to regulate their fluid intake and are hydrated by intravenous infusions. If there is renal dysfunction, gastrointestinal dysfunction or other abnormalities of fluid loss, a balance between intake and fluid loss may lead to dehydration or fluid overload.

Understanding the basics of body fluid volumes, fluid volume status assessment and fluid replacement is fundamental to good fluid management in the critically ill. (See *Volumes of water in body compartments*.) The assessment and haemodynamic monitoring described above provide a useful framework for assessing fluid volume status.

Volumes of water in body compartments

	Percentage of body weight	Volume (ml/kg)
• Intracellular	35	350
• Extracellular	25	250
Interstitial	20	200
Plasma	4.5	45
Blood	7.5	75
• Total body water	60	600

Dehydration and rehydration

Dehydration literally means depleted of water. When a person loses fluid through illness (e.g. vomit, diarrhoea, wound drainage, excess urine and sweat) water is lost as well as other constituents of the body fluid (e.g. sodium, potassium and protein). Clinically, rehydration involves calculating or estimating the volume of fluid lost and replacing with an appropriate fluid type. (See *Fluid replacement therapy*.) Rehydration is generally a process undertaken over hours to days.

Hypovolaemia and fluid resuscitation

Hypovolaemia is where there is a low volume of blood in the circulation (intravascular compartment). Replacing intravascular volume rapidly and accurately is important when restoring circulating volume. Estimating the volume lost is critical to this process. (See *Classification of hypovolaemia*, on page 181.) The type of fluid used to replace volume should be guided by the nature of fluid losses.

Drug therapy

Types of drugs used to improve cardiovascular function include cardiac glycosides and phosphodiesterase (PDE) inhibitors, antiarrhythmic drugs, antianginal drugs, antihypertensive drugs, diuretic drugs, adrenergic drugs and beta-adrenergic blockers.

Critical care context

The critical care nurse should understand these drugs and their use in two key ways. Firstly, many patients will be admitted with a history of drug therapies for cardiovascular disease. It is not uncommon for all usual drugs to be stopped during critical illness and phased back in during recovery. Also, some of the drugs described here are used to optimise cardiovascular function in critically ill patients. Their effects in achieving physiological goals and side effects should be a key concern of the critical care nurse.

Fluid replacement therapy

Loss	Comparison with blood	Replacement fluids
Excess urine	Lower sodium	Dextrose saline 0.45% Saline
Sweat	Lower sodium	Dextrose saline 0.45% Saline
GI tract losses	Normal sodium Normal potassium	Hartmann's normal saline + potassium
Serous fluid	Normal sodium Protein loss	Hartmann's consider albumin
Blood	Same	Colloids initially the blood (packed red cells)

Classification of hypovolaemia (estimates based on a 70 kg person)

	Class I	Class II	Class III	Class IV
Blood loss (% of blood)	<15%	15–30%	30–40%	>40%
Blood loss (ml)	<750	750–1500	1500–2000	>2000
Heart rate	<100	>100	>120	>140
SBP	Unchanged	Normal	↓	↓↓
DBP	Unchanged	↑	↓	↓↓
Pulse pressure	Normal	↓	↓	↓↓
Capillary refill	Normal	>2 seconds	>2 seconds	Undetectable
Respiratory rate	14–20	20–30	30–40	>35
Urine output	>30 ml/hour	20–30	5–15	Negligible
CNS/mental status	Alert	Anxious	Anxious and confused	Confused and lethargic/unconscious

Source. Adapted from American College of Surgeons (1997). Reproduced with permission.

Top tip for practice

No one can remember all the drugs used, how they work and how to monitor them. It is therefore important to develop a habit of looking up any drug that you aren't sure about. It takes less time than you think and will save time if it prevents a mistake, an inappropriate drug use or a missed complication.

Cardiac glycosides and PDE inhibitors

Cardiac glycosides and PDE inhibitors increase the force of the heart's contractions.

Cardiac glycosides and PDE inhibitors increase the force of the heart's contractions.

More force

Increasing the force of contractions is known as a *positive inotropic effect*, so these drugs are also called *inotropic agents* (effecting the force or energy of muscular contractions). (See *Understanding cardiac glycosides and PDE inhibitors*, on page 182.)

Slower rate

Cardiac glycosides, such as digoxin, also slow the heart rate (called a negative chronotropic effect) and slow electrical impulse conduction through the AV node (called a negative dromotropic effect).

Understanding cardiac glycosides and PDE inhibitors

Cardiac glycosides and phosphodiesterase (PDE) inhibitors have a positive inotropic effect on the heart, meaning they increase the force of contraction. Use this table to learn about the indications, adverse reactions and practice pointers associated with these drugs.

Drugs	Indications	Adverse reactions	Practice pointers
Digoxin	Heart failure, supraventricular arrhythmias	• Digoxin toxicity (nausea, abdominal pain, headache, irritability, depression, insomnia, vision disturbances, arrhythmias)	• If immediate effects are required (as with a supraventricular arrhythmia), a loading dose of digoxin is required. • Check apical pulse for 1 minute before administration; report pulse less than 60 beats per minute. • Check with your hospital's laboratory to find out the therapeutic range for digoxin where you work.
PDE inhibitors			
Enoximone, milrinone	Heart failure refractory to digoxin, diuretics and vasodilators	• Arrhythmias • Nausea • Vomiting • Headache • Fever • Chest pain • Hypokalaemia • Thrombocytopaenia • Mild increase in heart rate	• These drugs are contraindicated in patients in the acute phase of myocardial infarction (MI) and after an MI. • Serum potassium levels should be within normal limits before and during therapy.

The short and long of it

PDE inhibitors, such as enoximone and milrinone, are typically used for short-term management of heart failure or long-term management in patients awaiting heart transplant surgery.

Boosting output

PDE inhibitors improve CO by strengthening contractions. These drugs are thought to help move calcium into the myocardial cell or to increase calcium storage in the sarcoplasmic reticulum. By directly relaxing vascular smooth muscle, they also decrease peripheral vascular resistance (afterload) and the amount of blood returning to the heart (preload).

Critical care context

In the context of critical illness and inadequate CO these drugs may not be potent enough to boost a failing heart with increased metabolic demands. If that is the case adrenergic drugs such as dobutamine or adrenaline may be used. (See *Understanding cardiac glycosides and PDE inhibitors*.)

Antiarrhythmics

Antiarrhythmic drugs are used to treat arrhythmias, which are disturbances of the normal heart rhythm. (See *Understanding antihypertensives*, on page 185)

Benefits vs. risks

Unfortunately, many antiarrhythmic drugs can worsen or cause arrhythmias, too. In any case, the benefits of antiarrhythmic therapy need to be weighed against its risks.

Four classes plus . . .

Antiarrhythmics are categorised into four major classes according to the Vaughan Williams' classification system: I (which includes IA, IB and IC), II, III and IV. The mechanisms of action of antiarrhythmic drugs vary widely, and a few drugs exhibit properties common to more than one class. One drug, adenosine, doesn't fall into any of these classes.

Class I antiarrhythmics

Class I antiarrhythmics are sodium channel blockers. This is the largest group of antiarrhythmic drugs. Class I agents are commonly subdivided into classes IA, IB and IC.

Class IA antiarrhythmics

Class IA antiarrhythmics control arrhythmias by altering the myocardial cell membrane and interfering with autonomic nervous system control of pacemaker cells. Class IA antiarrhythmics include: disopyramide and procainamide.

> Class IA antiarrhythmics block parasympathetic stimulation and increase the conduction rate of the AV node.

No (para)sympathy

Class IA antiarrhythmics also block parasympathetic stimulation of the SA and AV nodes. Because stimulation of the parasympathetic nervous system causes the heart rate to slow down, drugs that block the parasympathetic nervous system increase the conduction rate of the AV node.

Rhythmic risks

This increase in the conduction rate can produce dangerous increases in the ventricular heart rate if rapid atrial activity is present, as in a patient with atrial fibrillation. In turn, the increased ventricular heart rate can offset the ability of the antiarrhythmics to convert atrial arrhythmias into a regular rhythm.

Class IB antiarrhythmics

Lidocaine, a class IB antiarrhythmic, is one of the antiarrhythmics used in treating patients with acute ventricular arrhythmias.

Class IB drugs work by blocking the rapid influx of sodium ions during the depolarisation phase of the heart's depolarisation—repolarisation cycle, resulting in a decreased refractory period, which reduces the risk of arrhythmia.

Make a IB line for the ventricle

Because class IB antiarrhythmics especially affect the Purkinje fibres (fibres in the conducting system of the heart) and myocardial cells in the ventricles, they're used only in treating patients with ventricular arrhythmias.

Class IC antiarrhythmics

Class IC antiarrhythmics are used to treat patients with certain severe, refractory (resistant) ventricular arrhythmias. Class IC antiarrhythmics include flecainide. Class IC antiarrhythmics primarily slow down conduction along the heart's conduction system. This decreases the fast inward current of sodium ions of the action potential and depresses the depolarisation rate and effective refractory period.

Class II antiarrhythmics

Class II antiarrhythmics include the beta-adrenergic antagonists, also known as beta-adrenergic blockers. Beta-adrenergic blockers used as antiarrhythmics include:

- atenolol
- metoprolol
- esmolol
- propranolol.

Receptor blockers

Class II antiarrhythmics block beta-adrenergic receptor sites in the conduction system of the heart. As a result, the ability of the SA node to fire spontaneously (automaticity) is slowed. The ability of the AV node and other cells to receive and conduct an electrical impulse to nearby cells (conductivity) is also reduced.

Strength reducers

Class II antiarrhythmics also reduce the strength of the heart's contractions (so they are negative inotropes). When the heart beats less forcefully, it doesn't require as much oxygen to do its work.

Class III antiarrhythmics

Class III antiarrhythmics are used to treat patients with ventricular arrhythmias. Amiodarone is the most widely used class III antiarrhythmic.

(Text continues on page 185)

Pulmonary artery catheterisation

Pulmonary artery catheterisation can give you information about a patient's cardiovascular and pulmonary status. With a basic pulmonary artery catheter, you can measure intracardiac pressure, pulmonary artery wedge pressure (PAWP) and cardiac output.

    When your patient requires a pulmonary artery catheter, your responsibilities include assisting with insertion, caring for the insertion site and catheter, and haemodynamic monitoring. Before you care for a patient who requires pulmonary artery catheterisation, familiarise yourself with a basic catheter.

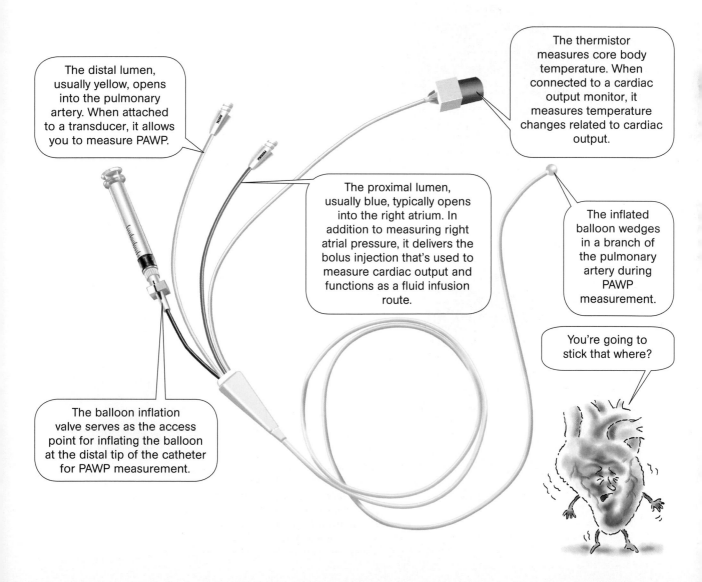

The distal lumen, usually yellow, opens into the pulmonary artery. When attached to a transducer, it allows you to measure PAWP.

The thermistor measures core body temperature. When connected to a cardiac output monitor, it measures temperature changes related to cardiac output.

The proximal lumen, usually blue, typically opens into the right atrium. In addition to measuring right atrial pressure, it delivers the bolus injection that's used to measure cardiac output and functions as a fluid infusion route.

The inflated balloon wedges in a branch of the pulmonary artery during PAWP measurement.

The balloon inflation valve serves as the access point for inflating the balloon at the distal tip of the catheter for PAWP measurement.

You're going to stick that where?

Normal pulmonary artery waveforms

After insertion into a large vein (usually the subclavian, jugular or femoral vein), a pulmonary artery catheter is advanced through the vena cava into the right atrium, through the right ventricle and into a branch of the pulmonary artery. During insertion, the monitor shows various waveforms as the catheter advances through the heart chambers.

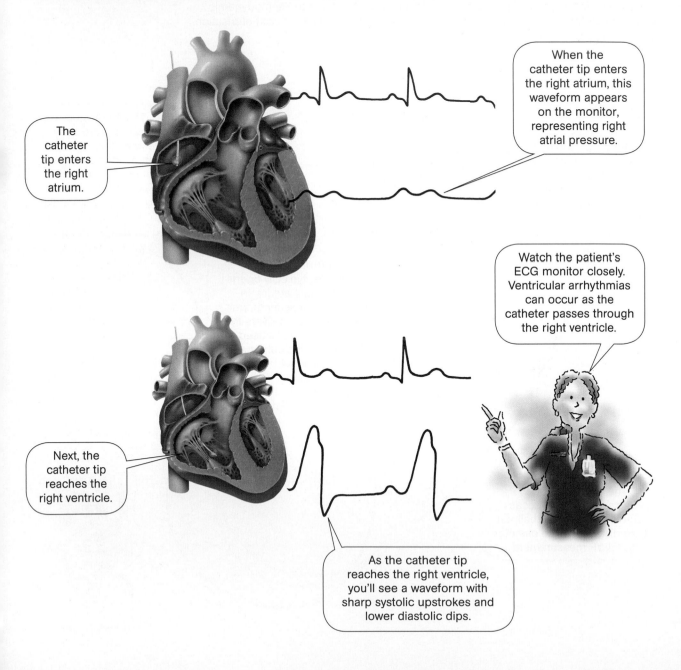

The catheter tip enters the right atrium.

When the catheter tip enters the right atrium, this waveform appears on the monitor, representing right atrial pressure.

Watch the patient's ECG monitor closely. Ventricular arrhythmias can occur as the catheter passes through the right ventricle.

Next, the catheter tip reaches the right ventricle.

As the catheter tip reaches the right ventricle, you'll see a waveform with sharp systolic upstrokes and lower diastolic dips.

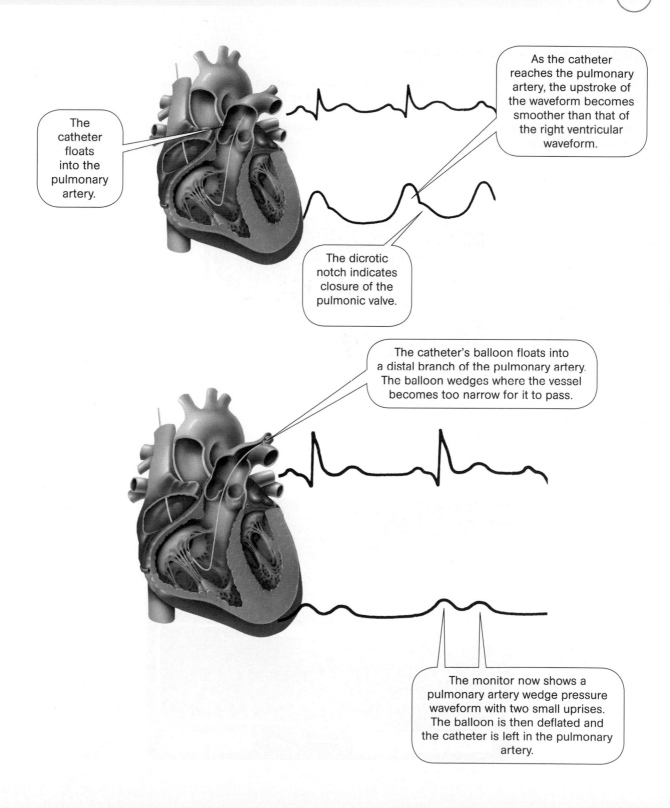

Measuring cardiac output

Measuring cardiac output—the volume of blood ejected from the heart in 1 minute—helps evaluate cardiac function. Normally, cardiac output ranges from 4 to 8 L/minute. To measure cardiac output at the bedside, a pulmonary artery catheter containing a thermistor is inserted. The thermistor detects blood temperature changes and transmits information to a monitoring computer, which calculates and displays cardiac output.

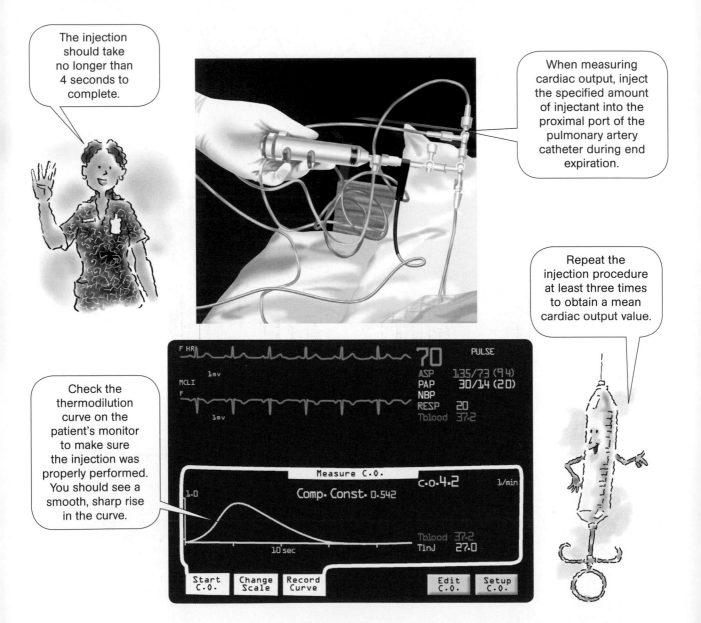

The injection should take no longer than 4 seconds to complete.

When measuring cardiac output, inject the specified amount of injectant into the proximal port of the pulmonary artery catheter during end expiration.

Repeat the injection procedure at least three times to obtain a mean cardiac output value.

Check the thermodilution curve on the patient's monitor to make sure the injection was properly performed. You should see a smooth, sharp rise in the curve.

Understanding antiarrhythmics

Antiarrhythmics are used to restore normal heart rhythm in patients with arrhythmias. Check this table for information about the indications, adverse reactions and practice pointers associated with these drugs.

Drugs	Indications	Adverse reactions	Practice pointers
Disopyramide, procainamide	• Ventricular tachycardia • Atrial fibrillation • Atrial flutter • Paroxysmal atrial tachycardia	• Dry mouth • Blurred vision • Myocardial depression • Hypotension • Arrhythmias • ECG changes (QT, QRS prolongation) • Urinary retention	• Check apical pulse rate before therapy. If you note extremes in pulse rate, hold the dose and notify the doctor. • Use cautiously in patients with asthma.
Lidocaine	• Ventricular tachycardia, ventricular fibrillation	• Drowsiness • Light-headedness • Drowsiness • Confusion • Convulsions • Hypotension • Bradycardia	• IB antiarrhythmics may potentiate the effects of other antiarrhythmics. • Administer I.V. infusions using an infusion pump.
Flecainide	• Ventricular tachycardia, ventricular fibrillation, supraventricular arrhythmias	• Nausea • Vomiting • New arrhythmias • Visual disturbances	• Correct electrolyte imbalances before administration. • Monitor the patient's electrocardiogram before and after dosage adjustments.
Atenolol, esmolol, metoprolol, propranolol	• Atrial flutter, atrial fibrillation, paroxysmal atrial tachycardia	• Arrhythmias • Bradycardia • Heart failure • Hypotension • Nausea and vomiting • Diarrhoea • Bronchospasm	• Monitor apical heart rate and blood pressure. • Abruptly stopping these drugs can exacerbate angina and precipitate myocardial infarction.
Amiodarone	• Life-threatening ventricular arrhythmias (VF/VT), supraventricular/atrial arrhythmias, adjunct to treating arrhythmias resistant to electrical cardioversion	• Nausea • Vomiting • Hypotension • Conduction disturbance and arrhythmias • Hyperthyroidism • Liver enzyme disturbance • Severe pulmonary toxicity/fibrosis • Visual disturbances/corneal deposits	• Amiodarone increases the risk of digoxin toxicity in patients also taking digoxin. • Monitor blood pressure, heart rate and rhythm for changes. • Monitor for signs of pulmonary toxicity (dyspnoea, nonproductive cough and pleuritic chest pain).

(continued)

Understanding antiarrhythmics (continued)

Drugs	Indications	Adverse reactions	Practice pointers
Diltiazem, verapamil	• Supraventricular arrhythmias	• Hypotension • Bradycardia • AV block • Flushing • Heart failure	• Monitor heart rate and rhythm and blood pressure carefully when initiating therapy or increasing dose. • Calcium supplements may reduce effectiveness.
Adenosine	• Paroxysmal supraventricular tachycardia	• Facial flushing • Shortness of breath • Dyspnoea • Chest discomfort	• Adenosine must be administered over 1–2 seconds, followed by a 20 ml flush of normal saline solution. • Record rhythm strip during administration.
Magnesium	• Known hypomagnesaemia, shock refractory VF or VT when hypomagnesaemia is suspected, atrial fibrillation, digoxin toxicity	• Tissue damage associated with extravasation • Muscle weakness • Loss of tendon reflexes • Lethargy, drowsiness • Bradycardia • Hypotension	• Ensure administration into largest vein possible. • Large doses (significantly above those given for arrhythmia treatment) are required to cause hypermagnesaemia—but clinically you should monitor consciousness, muscle tone and strength and deep tendon reflexes and check magnesium and potassium levels after administration.

One-way to two-way

Although the exact mechanism of action isn't known, class III antiarrhythmics are thought to suppress arrhythmias by converting a unidirectional block into a bidirectional block. They have little or no effect on depolarisation.

Class IV antiarrhythmics

The class IV antiarrhythmics include the calcium channel blockers. These drugs block the movement of calcium during phase 2 of the action potential and slow conduction and the refractory period of calcium-dependent tissues, including the AV node. The calcium channel blockers used to treat patients with arrhythmias are verapamil and diltiazem.

Adenosine

Adenosine is an injectable antiarrhythmic drug indicated for acute treatment for paroxysmal supraventricular tachycardia.

Depressing the pacemaker

Adenosine depresses the pacemaker activity of the SA node, reducing the heart rate and the ability of the AV node to conduct impulses from the atria to the ventricles. Because it blocks AV conduction (for a few seconds) it is sometimes used to reveal underlying atrial activity when obscured by a ventricular activity in a tachycardia.

Magnesium

Magnesium is an electrolyte usually present in low concentrations in the plasma (0.8–1.0 mmol/L). It is essential in many enzyme systems and in neurochemical transmission. Magnesium is a membrane stabiliser and a smooth muscle relaxant when levels are above normal plasma. It can be effective in terminating ventricular tachyarrhythmias and ventricular fibrillation. Magnesium has effects similar to potassium in that hypomagnesaemia potentiates the action of digoxin. Low magnesium is not uncommon in hospitalised acutely ill patients and low magnesium potentiates arrhythmias. Magnesium and potassium tend to rise and fall together.

Antianginal drugs

When the oxygen demands of the heart exceed the amount of oxygen being supplied, areas of heart muscle become ischaemic (not receiving enough oxygen). When the heart muscle is ischaemic, a person experiences chest pain. This condition is known as angina or angina pectoris.

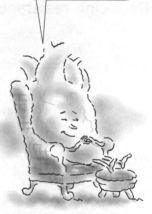

Antianginal drugs take away the pain of angina by reducing myocardial oxygen demand or increasing the supply of oxygen to the heart. Either way, I have more time to relax and just feel good!

Reduce demand, increase supply

Although angina's cardinal symptom is chest pain, the drugs used to treat angina aren't typically analgesics. Instead, antianginal drugs correct angina by reducing myocardial oxygen demand (the amount of oxygen the heart needs to do its work), increasing the supply of oxygen to the heart, or both.

The top three plus two more

Traditionally three classes of commonly used antianginal drugs have been used to improve the balance of myocardial oxygen demand and supply. They include:
- nitrates (for acute angina)
- beta-adrenergic blockers (for long-term prevention of angina)
- calcium channel blockers (used when other drugs fail to prevent angina).
  More recently two more classes of drugs have been used to reduce the risk of myocardial infarction in those with angina and coronary artery disease. These are:
- antiplatelet drugs
- angiotensin converting enzyme inhibitors (ACE inhibitors).

Nitrates
Nitrates are the drug of choice for relieving acute angina. Nitrates commonly prescribed to correct angina include:
- isosorbide dinitrate
- isosorbide mononitrate
- glyceryl trinitrate.

Anti-angina effect

Nitrates cause the smooth muscle of the veins and, to a lesser extent, the arteries to relax and dilate. This is what happens:
• When the veins dilate, less blood returns to the heart.
• This, in turn, reduces the amount of blood in the ventricles at the end of diastole, when the ventricles are full. (This blood volume in the ventricles just before contraction is called preload.)
• By reducing preload, nitrates reduce ventricular size and ventricular wall tension so the left ventricle doesn't have to stretch as much to pump blood. This, in turn, reduces the oxygen requirements of the heart.
• As the coronary arteries dilate, more blood is delivered to the myocardium, improving oxygenation of the ischaemic tissue.

> Nitrates cause veins and arteries to relax and dilate, so more blood is delivered to the myocardium. Gotta go . . . I'm on a tight schedule!

Reducing resistance

The arterioles provide the most resistance to the blood pumped by the left ventricle (called *peripheral vascular resistance*). Nitrates decrease afterload by dilating the arterioles, reducing resistance, easing the heart's workload and easing oxygen demand.

Beta-adrenergic blockers

Beta-adrenergic blockers are used for long-term prevention of angina, and are one of the main types of drugs used to treat hypertension. Beta-adrenergic blockers include:
• atenolol
• metoprolol
• nadolol
• propranolol.

Down with everything

Beta-adrenergic blockers decrease blood pressure and block beta-adrenergic receptor sites in the heart muscle and conduction system, decreasing heart rate and reducing the force of the heart's contractions, resulting in lower demand for oxygen.

> I should have listened to those calcium channel blocker border guards . . . milk overboard!

Calcium channel blockers

Calcium channel blockers are commonly used to prevent angina that doesn't respond to drugs in either of the other antianginal classes. However, beta blockers and calcium channel blockers are both negative inotropes and may cause heart failure if used in combination.

Calcium channel blockers include:
• amlodipine
• diltiazem
• nicardipine
• nifedipine
• verapamil.

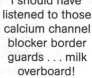

Preventing passage

Calcium channel blockers prevent the passage of calcium ions across the myocardial cell membrane and vascular smooth muscle cells. This causes dilation of the coronary and peripheral arteries, which decreases the force of the heart's contractions and reduces the workload of the heart.

Rate reduction

By preventing arterioles from constricting, calcium channel blockers also reduce afterload. In addition, decreasing afterload decreases oxygen demands of the heart.

Calcium channel blockers also reduce the heart rate by slowing conduction through the SA and AV nodes. A slower heart rate reduces the heart's need for oxygen.

Sticky stuff

Antiplatelet drugs

Antiplatelet drugs prevent clumping of platelets and blood clot formation which reduces the risk of myocardial infarction in patients with atheromatous plaques in their coronary arteries. These drugs include:
- aspirin
- clopidogrel
- dipyridamole.

Angiotensin-converting enzyme inhibitors

These drugs reduce the risk of heart attack in patients with angina. They reduce blood pressure and treat heart failure which may accompany angina. Research also shows that those individuals who have had a myocardial infarction, have high blood pressure or heart failure and who take ACE inhibitors live longer than those who do not. ACE inhibitors include:
- ramipril
- enalapril
- captopril.

Critical care context

Angina experienced in the context of critical illness may require a continuous infusion of nitrates to dilate coronary arteries. In addition, it is important to return to the basic physiological principles of delivering oxygen to tissues (especially the myocardium). This means maximising oxygenation of the blood; thus, supplemental oxygen may be critical in this context.

Antihypertensive drugs

Antihypertensive drugs, which act to reduce blood pressure, are used to treat patients with hypertension, a disorder characterised by high systolic blood pressure, diastolic blood pressure or both.

Understanding antianginal drugs

Antianginal drugs are effective in treating patients with angina because they reduce myocardial oxygen demand, increase the supply of oxygen to the heart or both. Use this table to learn about the indications, adverse reactions and practice pointers associated with these drugs.

Drugs	Indications	Adverse reactions	Practice pointers
Nitrates			
Isosorbide dinitrate, isosorbide mononitrate, glyceryl trinitrate	• Relief and prevention of angina	• Headache • Hypotension • Dizziness • Increased heart rate	• Only sublingual and translingual forms should be used to treat an acute angina attack. • Monitor the patient's blood pressure before and after administration.
Beta-adrenergic blockers			
Atenolol, metoprolol tartrate, nadolol, propranolol	• Long-term prevention of angina • First-line therapy for hypertension	• Bradycardia • Fainting • Fluid retention • Shock • Heart failure • Arrhythmias • Angina • Nausea • Vomiting • Diarrhoea • Bronchial constriction	• Monitor apical pulse rate before administration. Monitor blood pressure, electrocardiogram and heart rate and rhythm frequently. • Signs of hypoglycaemic shock may be masked; watch diabetic patients for sweating, fatigue and hunger.
Calcium channel blockers			
Amlodipine, diltiazem, nicardipine, nifedipine, verapamil	• Long-term prevention of angina (especially Prinzmetal's angina)	• Orthostatic hypotension • Heart failure • Hypotension • Arrhythmias • Dizziness • Headache • Flushing • Weakness • Persistent peripheral oedema	• Monitor cardiac rate and rhythm and blood pressure carefully when initiating therapy or increasing the dose. • Calcium supplementation may decrease the effects of calcium channel blockers.
Antiplatelet drugs			
Aspirin, clopidogrel, dipyridamole	• Prevention of clot formation leading to MI in those with coronary vessel disease	• Bronchospasm in asthmatics (Aspirin) • Dyspepsia and GI disturbances • Gastrointestinal haemorrhage • Hypersensitivity reactions	• Hypertension should be controlled prior to administering antiplatelet drugs because of the increased risk of intracranial haemorrhage. • Monitor for bleeding and GI disturbances.

(continued)

Understanding antianginal drugs (continued)

Drugs	Indications	Adverse reactions	Practice pointers
ACE inhibitors			
Ramipril, enalipril, captopril	• Reduce the risk of MI in those with angina • Heart failure and hypertension accompanying angina	• Hypotension • Renal impairment • Dry cough	• Monitor renal function. • Monitor blood pressure.

Know the programme

Treatment for hypertension begins with a single drug and progresses with the addition of other drugs depending on factors such as age and the presence of other medical problems such as angina or heart failure.

The most commonly used and safest drugs include:
- Diuretics
- Sympatholytics
- Vasodilators
- ACE inhibitors
- Angiotensin II receptor antagonists.

Antihypertensives act to reduce blood pressure. Treatment for hypertension begins with a single drug and progresses with the addition of other drugs depending on factors such as age and the presence of other medical problems such as angina or heart failure.

Diuretics

Diuretics are used to promote the excretion of water and electrolytes by the kidneys. By doing so, diuretics play a major role in treating hypertension and other cardiovascular conditions. (See *Understanding diuretics*, page 192.)

The major diuretics used as cardiovascular drugs include:
- thiazide and thiazide-like diuretics
- loop diuretics
- potassium-sparing diuretics.

Thiazide and thiazide-like diuretics

Thiazide and thiazide-like diuretics are sulphonamide derivatives. Thiazide diuretics include bendroflumethiazide (Bendrofluazide) and metolazone. Thiazide-like diuretics include chlorthalidone and indapamide.

Thiazide and thiazide-like diuretics work by preventing sodium reabsorption in the kidney.

Sodium stoppers

Thiazide and thiazide-like diuretics work by preventing sodium from being reabsorbed in the kidney. As sodium is excreted, it pulls water

Understanding diuretics

Diuretics are used to treat patients with various cardiovascular conditions. They work by promoting the excretion of water and electrolytes by the kidneys. Use this table to learn about the indications, adverse reactions and practice pointers associated with these drugs.

Drugs	Indications	Adverse reactions	Practice pointers
Thiazide and thiazide-like diuretics			
Bendroflumethiazide, benzthiazide, chlorthalidone, hydrochlorothiazide, hydroflumethiazide, indapamide, methyclothiazide, polythiazide, trichlormethiazide	• Hypertension • Oedema	• Hypokalaemia • Orthostatic hypotension • Hyponatraemia	• Monitor serum potassium levels. • Monitor intake and output. • Monitor blood glucose values in diabetic patients. Thiazide diuretics can cause hyperglycaemia.
Loop diuretics			
Bumetanide, ethacrynate sodium, ethacrynic acid, furosemide	• Hypertension • Heart failure • Oedema	• Dehydration • Orthostatic hypotension • Hyperuricaemia • Hypokalaemia • Hypochloraemia • Hyponatraemia • Hypocalcaemia • Hypomagnesaemia	• Monitor for signs of excess diuresis (hypotension, tachycardia, poor skin turgor and excessive thirst). • Monitor blood pressure, heart rate and intake and output. • Monitor serum electrolyte levels.
Potassium-sparing diuretics			
Amiloride, spironolactone, triamterene	• Oedema	• Hyperkalaemia • Diuretic-induced hypokalaemia in patients with heart failure • Cirrhosis • Nephrotic syndrome • Hypertension	• Monitor electrocardiogram for arrhythmias. • Monitor serum potassium levels. • Monitor intake and output.

along with it. Thiazide and thiazide-like diuretics also increase the excretion of chloride, potassium and bicarbonate, which can result in electrolyte imbalances.

Stability with time

Initially, these drugs decrease circulating blood volume, leading to a reduced CO. However, if the therapy is maintained, CO stabilises, but plasma fluid volume decreases.

Loop diuretics

Loop (high-ceiling) diuretics are highly potent drugs. They include:
- bumetanide
- furosemide.

High potency, big risk

The loop diuretics are the most potent diuretics available, producing the greatest volume of diuresis (urine production). They also have a high potential for causing severe adverse reactions.

Bumetanide is the shortest-acting diuretic. It's 40 times more potent than furosemide.

Locating the loop

Loop diuretics receive their name because they act primarily on the thick ascending loop of Henle (the part of the nephron responsible for concentrating urine) to increase the secretion of sodium, chloride and water. These drugs may also inhibit sodium, chloride and water reabsorption.

Potassium-sparing diuretics

Potassium-sparing diuretics have weaker diuretic and antihypertensive effects than other diuretics, but they have the advantage of conserving potassium.

The potassium-sparing diuretics include:
- amiloride
- triamterene
- spironolactone.

Potassium-sparing effects

The direct action of the potassium-sparing diuretics on the distal tubule of the kidneys produces:
- increased urinary excretion of sodium and water
- increased excretion of chloride and calcium ions
- decreased excretion of potassium and hydrogen ions.

These effects lead to reduced blood pressure and increased serum potassiun levels.

Aping aldosterone

Spironolactone, one of the main potassium-sparing diuretics, is structurally similar to aldosterone and acts as an aldosterone antagonist. Aldosterone promotes the retention of sodium and water and loss of potassium; spironolactone counteracts these effects by competing with aldosterone for receptor sites. As a result, sodium, chloride and water are excreted and potassium is retained.

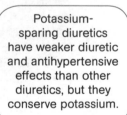

Loop diuretics are the most potent diuretics, producing the most amount of urine. But they also carry the greatest risk of side effects.

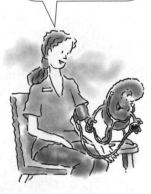

Potassium-sparing diuretics have weaker diuretic and antihypertensive effects than other diuretics, but they conserve potassium.

Sympatholytic drugs

The sympatholytic drugs include several different types of drugs, but work by inhibiting or blocking the sympathetic nervous system, which causes dilation of the peripheral blood vessels or decreases CO, thereby reducing blood pressure.

The sympatholytic drugs are classified by their site or mechanism of action and include:

- central-acting sympathetic nervous system inhibitors, such as clonidine (which may be administered by continuous intravenous infusion to patients (hypertensive and/or agitated) waking from sedation in critical care)
- alpha blockers, such as doxazosin, phentolamine, prazosin, terazosin and indoramin.

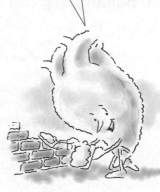

Sympatholytic drugs reduce blood pressure by blocking the sympathetic nervous system.

Vasodilating drugs

The two types of vasodilating drugs include calcium channel blockers and direct vasodilators. These drugs decrease systolic and diastolic blood pressure.

Calcium stoppers

Calcium channel blockers produce arteriolar relaxation by preventing the entry of calcium into the cells. This prevents the contraction of vascular smooth muscle.

Direct dilators

Direct vasodilators act on arteries, veins or both. They work by relaxing peripheral vascular smooth muscles, causing the blood vessels to dilate. This decreases blood pressure by increasing the diameter of the blood vessels, reducing total peripheral resistance.

The direct vasodilators include:

- hydralazine
- minoxidil
- diazoxide
- nitroprusside.

Hydralazine and minoxidil are usually used to treat patients with resistant or refractory hypertension. Diazoxide and nitroprusside are reserved for use in hypertensive crisis.

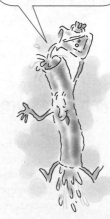

Vasodilators cause the blood vessels to dilate, which decreases blood pressure.

ACE inhibitors

ACE inhibitors reduce blood pressure by interrupting the renin–angiotensin–aldosterone system. Commonly prescribed ACE inhibitors include:

- captopril
- enalapril
- lisinopril
- imidapril
- ramipril.

Without ACE interference

Here's how the renin—angiotensin—aldosterone system works:
- Normally, the kidneys maintain blood pressure by releasing the hormone renin.
- Renin acts on the plasma protein angiotensinogen to form angiotensin I.
- Angiotensin I is then converted into angiotensin II.
- Angiotensin II, a potent vasoconstrictor, increases peripheral resistance and promotes the excretion of aldosterone.
- Aldosterone, in turn, promotes the retention of sodium and water, increasing the volume of blood the heart needs to pump.

With ACE interference

ACE inhibitors work by preventing the conversion of angiotensin I into angiotensin II. As angiotensin II is reduced, arterioles dilate, reducing peripheral vascular resistance.

Less water, less work

By reducing aldosterone secretion, ACE inhibitors promote the excretion of sodium and water, reducing the amount of blood the heart needs to pump, resulting in a lowered blood pressure.

> ACE inhibitors reduce blood pressure by interrupting the rennin–angiotensin–aldosterone system.

Angiotensin II receptor antagonists

Unlike ACE inhibitors, which prevent production of angiotensin, angiotensin II receptor antagonists block the action of angiotensin II by attaching to tissue-binding receptor sites.

Commonly prescribed angiotensin II inhibitors include:
- losartan
- valsartan.

Anticoagulants

Anticoagulants are used to reduce the ability of the blood to clot. (See *Understanding anticoagulants*, on page 197.) Major categories of anticoagulants include heparin, oral anticoagulants and antiplatelet drugs.

Heparin

Heparin, prepared commercially from animal tissue, is used to prevent clot formation. Low-molecular-weight heparin, such as dalteparin and enoxaparin, prevents deep vein thrombosis (a blood clot in the deep veins, usually of the legs) in patients at risk due to factors such as immobility, sepsis, indwelling CVCs and major surgery (this means practically all critically ill patients are at high risk!).

Understanding antihypertensives

Antihypertensives are prescribed to reduce blood pressure in patients with hypertension. Use this table to learn about the indications, adverse reactions and practice pointers associated with these drugs.

Drugs	Indications	Adverse reactions	Practice pointers
Sympatholytic drugs			
• *Central-acting sympathetic nervous system inhibitors* (such as clonidine) • *Alpha blockers* (such as doxazosin, phentolamine, prazosin, terazosin and indoramin)	• Hypertension	• Hypotension (alpha blockers) • Depression • Drowsiness • Oedema • Vertigo (central-acting drugs) • Rebound hypertension (clonidine with rapid withdrawal)	• Monitor blood pressure before and after administration. • Clonidine infusions should be weaned slowly to prevent rebound hypertension.
Vasodilators			
• Diazoxide, hydralazine, minoxidil, nitroprusside	• Used in combination with other drugs to treat moderate-to-severe hypertension	• Tachycardia • Palpitations • Angina • Fatigue • Headache • Severe pericardial effusion • Hepatotoxicity • Nausea • Stevens–Johnson syndrome	• Monitor blood pressure before and after administration.
ACE inhibitors			
• Benazepril, captopril, enalapril, fosinopril, lisinopril, quinapril, ramipril	• Hypertension • Heart failure	• Angioedema • Increased serum potassium concentrations • Persistent cough • Renal insufficiency	• Monitor blood pressure before and after administration. • Monitor renal function.
Angiotensin II receptor blockers			
• Losartan • Valsartan	• Hypertension • Heart failure resistant to ACE inhibitors	• Fatigue • Abdominal pain • Rash • Hypotension	• Monitor blood pressure before and after administration.

No new clots

Because it doesn't affect the synthesis of clotting factors, heparin can't dissolve already formed clots. It does prevent the formation of new thrombi, though. Here's how it works:
• Heparin inhibits the formation of thrombin and fibrin by activating antithrombin III.

Understanding anticoagulants

Anticoagulants reduce the blood's ability to clot and are included in the treatment plans for many patients with cardiovascular disorders. Use this table to learn about the indications, adverse reactions and practice pointers associated with these drugs.

Drugs	Indications	Adverse reactions	Practice pointers
Heparins			
Heparin and low-molecular-weight heparins, such as dalteparin and enoxaparin	• Deep vein thrombosis • Embolism prophylaxis • Prevention of complications after myocardial infarction (MI) • Anticoagulation during renal replacement therapy	• Bleeding • Thrombocytopaenia	• Monitor APTT time; the therapeutic range is 1 1/2 to 2 1/2 times the control. • Monitor the patient for signs of bleeding. • Concomitant administration with nonsteroidal antiinflammatory drugs, or an antiplatelet drug increases the risk of bleeding. • Protamine sulphate reverses the effects of heparin.
Oral anticoagulants			
Warfarin	• Deep vein thrombosis prophylaxis • Prevention of complications of prosthetic heart valves or diseased mitral valves • Atrial arrhythmias	• Bleeding (may be severe) • Hepatitis • Diarrhoea	• Monitor prothrombin time and International Normalised Ratio in patients receiving Warfarin. • Monitor the patient for signs of bleeding. • The effects of oral anticoagulants can be reversed with phytomenadione (vitamin K).
Antiplatelet drugs			
Aspirin, clopidogrel, dipyridamole	• Decreases the risk of death post-MI • Prevention of complications of prosthetic heart valves • Reduction of risk of MI	• GI irritation • Bleeding • Thrombocytopaenia • Angioedema	• Monitor the patient for signs of bleeding. • Aspirin, should be taken with meals to prevent GI irritation. • Dipyridamole should be taken with a full glass of fluid at least 1 hour before meals.

- Antithrombin III then inactivates factors IXa, Xa, XIa and XIIa in the intrinsic and common pathways. The end result is prevention of a stable fibrin clot.
- In low doses, heparin increases the activity of antithrombin III against factor Xa and thrombin and inhibits clot formation. Much larger doses are necessary to inhibit fibrin formation after a clot has formed. This relationship between dose and effect is the rationale for using low-dose heparin to prevent clotting.
- Whole blood clotting time, thrombin time and partial thromboplastin time are prolonged during heparin therapy. However, these times may be only slightly prolonged with low or ultra-low preventive doses.

Circulate freely

Heparin can be used to prevent clotting when a patient's blood must circulate outside the body through a machine, such as a haemofiltration machine, haemodialysis machine or cardiopulmonary bypass machine.

Oral anticoagulants

Oral anticoagulants alter the ability of the liver to synthesise vitamin K–dependent clotting factors, including prothrombin and factors VII, IX and X. Clotting factors already in the bloodstream continue to coagulate blood until they become depleted, so anticoagulation doesn't begin immediately.

Warfarin vs. coagulation

The major oral anticoagulant used is warfarin.

Antiplatelet drugs

Examples of antiplatelet drugs include:
- aspirin
- clopidogrel
- dipyridamole

Thromboembolism prevention

Antiplatelet drugs are used to prevent arterial thromboembolism, especially in patients at risk for MI, stroke and arteriosclerosis (hardening of the arteries). They interfere with platelet activity in different drug-specific and dose-related ways.

Low dose

Low dosages of aspirin (75 mg/day) inhibit clot formation by blocking the synthesis of prostaglandin, which in turn prevents formation of the platelet-aggregating substance thromboxane A_2. Dipyridamole may inhibit platelet aggregation.

While we're on the subject . . .

Aside from cardiovascular disorders the main use of anticoagulants is to prevent clotting within extracorporeal circuits such as in continuous renal replacement therapy. The two most commonly used drugs are heparin (discussed above) and epoprostenol.

Epoprostenol is a prostaglandin derivative which acts as to inhibit platelet aggregation. It is often used to prevent clotting in extracorporeal circuits as in renal replacement therapy. It is generally used when patients suffer complications from heparin, such as bleeding or heparin-induced thrombocytopaenia (HIT). It has a very short half-life—around 3 minutes so needs to be given via intravenous infusion. It is also a potent systemic vasodilator and hence can result in hypotension and sudden hypoxia from increased intrapulmonary shunting. However, because it has such a short half-life the side effects wear off very quickly when an infusion is stopped or reduced.

Oral anticoagulants alter my ability to synthesise vitamin K–dependent clotting factors.

Low doses of aspirin help inhibit clot formation by blocking the synthesis of prostaglandin and the formation of thromboxane A_2.

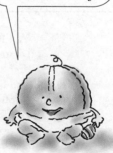

Thrombolytic drugs

Thrombolytic drugs are used to dissolve a pre-existing clot or thrombus, and are commonly used in an acute or emergency situation—most commonly in acute myocardial infarction or large pulmonary embolism. They work by converting plasminogen into plasmin, which lyse (dissolves) thrombi, fibrinogen and other plasma proteins. (See *Understanding thrombolytics*.)

Some commonly used thrombolytic drugs include:

- alteplase
- tenecteplase
- reteplase
- streptokinase.

Adrenergic drugs

Adrenergic drugs are also called *sympathomimetic* drugs because they produce effects similar to those produced by the sympathetic nervous system (in the fight or flight response).

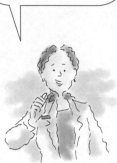

Most adrenergic drugs mimic the action of noradrenaline or adrenaline.

Classified by chemical

Adrenergic drugs are classified into two groups based on their chemical structure—catecholamines (both naturally occurring and synthetic) and noncatecholamines. (See *Understanding adrenergics*, on page 200.)

Understanding thrombolytics

Sometimes called *clot busters*, thrombolytic drugs are prescribed to dissolve a pre-existing clot or thrombus. These drugs are typically used in acute or emergency situations. Use this table to learn about the indications, adverse reactions and practice pointers associated with these drugs.

Drugs	Indications	Adverse reactions	Practice pointers
Thrombolytics			
Alteplase, tenecteplase, reteplase, streptokinase	• Acute myocardial infarction • Acute ischaemic stroke (alteplase) • Pulmonary embolus • Arterial thrombosis/deep vein thrombosis	• Bleeding • Allergic reaction	• Monitor partial thromboplastin time, prothrombin time, International Normalised Ratio, haemoglobin and haematocrit before, during and after administration. • Monitor vital signs frequently during and immediately after administration. Don't use an automatic blood pressure cuff to monitor blood pressure. • Monitor puncture sites for bleeding. Don't use a tourniquet when obtaining blood specimens. • Monitor for signs of bleeding.

Understanding adrenergics

Adrenergic drugs produce effects similar to those produced by the sympathetic nervous system. Adrenergic drugs can affect alpha-adrenergic receptors, beta-adrenergic receptors, or dopamine receptors. However, most of the drugs stimulate the alpha- and beta-receptors, mimicking the effects of noradrenaline and adrenaline. Dopaminergic drugs act on receptors typically stimulated by dopamine.

Use this table to learn about the indications, adverse reactions, and practice pointers associated with these drugs.

Drugs	Indications	Adverse reactions	Practice pointers
Catecholamines			
Dobutamine	• Increase cardiac output in short-term treatment of cardiac decompensation from depressed contractility	Headache, paraesthesia, tingling sensation, bronchospasm, palpitations, tachycardia, cardiac arrhythmias (PVCs), hypotension, hypertension and hypertensive crisis, angina, skin rash, fever, nausea, vomiting, tissue necrosis and sloughing (if catecholamine given I.V. leaks into surrounding tissue)	• Correct hypovolaemia before administering drug. • Incompatible with alkaline solution (sodium bicarbonate); don't mix or give through same line; don't mix with other drugs. • Administer continuous drip on infusion pump. • Give drug into a large vein to prevent irritation or extravasation at site. • Monitor cardiac rate and rhythm and blood pressure carefully when initiating therapy or increasing the dose.
Dopamine	• Adjunct in shock to increase cardiac output and blood pressure, Hypotension	Anxiety, headache, paraesthesia, tingling sensation, dyspnoea, bradycardia, palpitations, tachycardia, conduction disturbance, cardiac arrhythmias (ventricular), hypotension, hypertension and hypertensive crisis, azotaemia, angina, skin rash, fever, nausea, vomiting, may elevate serum glucose, gangrene of extremities in high dose, tissue necrosis and sloughing (if catecholamine given I.V. leaks into surrounding tissue)	• Correct hypovolaemia before administering drug. • Incompatible with alkaline solution (sodium bicarbonate); don't mix or give through same line; don't mix with other drugs. • Administer continuous drip on infusion pump. • Give drug into a large vein to prevent extravasation, if extravasation occurs, stop infusion and treat site with phentolamine infiltrate to prevent tissue necrosis. • Monitor cardiac rate and rhythm and blood pressure carefully when initiating therapy or increasing the dose.
Adrenaline	• Bronchospasm • Hypersensitivity reactions • Anaphylaxis • Circulatory support and restoration of cardiac rhythm in cardiac arrest	Restlessness, anxiety, dizziness, headache, tachycardia, palpitations, cardiac arrhythmias (ventricular fibrillation), hypotension, hypertension and hypertensive crisis, stroke, cerebral haemorrhage, angina, increased blood glucose levels, tissue necrosis and sloughing (if catecholamine given I.V. leaks into surrounding tissue)	• Correct hypovolaemia before administering drug. • Incompatible with alkaline solution (sodium bicarbonate); don't mix or give through same line; don't mix with other drugs. • Administer continuous drip on infusion pump. • Give drug into a large vein to prevent irritation or extravasation at site. • Monitor cardiac rate and rhythm and blood pressure carefully when initiating therapy or increasing the dose.

(continued)

Understanding adrenergics (continued)

Drugs	Indications	Adverse reactions	Practice pointers
Catecholamines (*continued*)			
Noradrenaline	• Maintain blood pressure in acute hypotensive states • Hypotension in septic shock	Restlessness, anxiety, dizziness, headache, bradycardia, tachycardia, palpitations, cardiac arrhythmias (ventricular tachycardia and fibrillation), hypotension, hypertension and hypertensive crisis, stroke, cerebral haemorrhage, angina, gangrene of extremities in high doses, tissue necrosis and sloughing (if catecholamine given I.V. leaks into surrounding tissue)	• Correct hypovolaemia before administering drug. • Incompatible with alkaline solution (sodium bicarbonate); don't mix or give through same line; don't mix with other drugs. • Administer continuous drip on infusion pump. • Give drug into a large vein to prevent extravasation; if extravasation occurs, stop infusion and treat site with phentolamine infiltrate to prevent tissue necrosis. • Monitor cardiac rate and rhythm and blood pressure carefully when initiating therapy or increasing the dose.
Noncatecholamines			
Ephedrine	• Maintain blood pressure in acute hypotensive states, especially with spinal anaesthesia • Treatment of orthostatic hypotension and bronchospasm	Restlessness, anxiety, dizziness, headache, palpitations, cardiac arrhythmias (ventricular fibrillation), hypotension, hypertension, nausea, vomiting	• Correct hypovolaemia before administering drug. • Give drug into a large vein to prevent irritation or extravasation at site. • Monitor cardiac rate and rhythm and blood pressure carefully when initiating therapy or increasing the dose.
Phenylephrine	• Maintain blood pressure in hypotensive states, especially hypotensive emergencies with spinal anaesthesia	Restlessness, anxiety, dizziness, headache, palpitations, cardiac arrhythmias, hypertension, tissue necrosis and sloughing (if noncatecholamine given I.V. leaks into surrounding tissue)	• Correct hypovolaemia before administering drug. • Don't mix with other drugs. • Administer continuous drip on infusion pump. • Give drug into a large vein to prevent extravasation; if extravasation occurs, stop infusion and treat site with phentolamine infiltrate to prevent tissue necrosis. • Monitor cardiac rate and rhythm and blood pressure carefully when initiating therapy or increasing the dose.

Which receptor?

Therapeutic use of adrenergic drugs depends on which receptors they stimulate and to what degree. Adrenergic drugs can affect:
• alpha-adrenergic receptors
• beta-adrenergic receptors
• dopamine receptors.

Mimicking noradrenaline (norepinephrine) and adrenaline (epinephrine)

Most of the adrenergic drugs produce their effects by stimulating alpha- and beta-adrenergic receptors. These drugs mimic the action of norepinephrine or epinephrine.

Doing it like dopamine

Dopaminergic drugs act primarily on receptors in the sympathetic nervous system that are stimulated by dopamine.

Catecholamines

Because of their common basic chemical structure, catecholamines share certain properties. They stimulate the nervous system, dilate or constrict peripheral blood vessels, increase heart rate and dilate the bronchi. They can be manufactured in the body or in a laboratory. Common catecholamines include:

- dobutamine (synthetic)
- dopamine (made by the body)
- adrenaline (made by the body)
- noradrenaline (made by the body).

Direct-acting and excitatory or inhibitory

Catecholamines are primarily direct-acting. When catecholamines combine with alpha- or beta-receptors, they cause either an excitatory or inhibitory effect. Typically, activation of alpha-receptors generates an excitatory response except for intestinal relaxation. Activation of the beta-receptors mostly produces an inhibitory response except in the cells of the heart, where noradrenaline produces excitatory effects.

How heartening

The clinical effects of catecholamines depend on the dosage and the route of administration. Catecholamines are potent inotropes, meaning they make the heart contract more forcefully. As a result, the ventricles empty more completely with each heartbeat, increasing the CO, workload of the heart and the amount of oxygen it needs to do this harder work.

Rapid rates

Catecholamines also produce a positive chronotropic effect, which means they cause the heart to beat faster. That's because the pacemaker cells in the SA node of the heart depolarise at a faster rate. As catecholamines cause

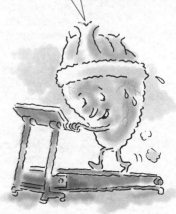

Catecholamines make the heart contract more forcefully so the ventricles empty more completely with each heartbeat, allowing me to do more work.

blood vessels to constrict and blood pressure to increase, the heart rate decreases as the body tries to prevent an excessive increase in blood pressure.

Fascinating rhythm

Catecholamines can cause the Purkinje fibres (an intricate web of fibres that carry electrical impulses into the ventricles of the heart) to fire spontaneously, possibly producing abnormal heart rhythms, such as premature ventricular contractions and fibrillation. Adrenaline is likelier than noradrenaline to produce this spontaneous firing.

Noncatecholamines
Noncatecholamine adrenergic drugs have a variety of therapeutic uses because of the many effects these drugs can have on the body, such as the local or systemic constriction of blood vessels by phenylephrine.

Alpha active

Direct-acting noncatecholamines that stimulate alpha activity include phenylephrine.

Ephedrine is considered a dual-acting noncatecholamine. It combines both beta and alpha actions.

Adrenergic blocking drugs
Adrenergic blocking drugs, also called *sympatholytic drugs*, are used to disrupt sympathetic nervous system function. (See *Understanding adrenergic blockers*, on page 204.)

Impeding impulses

These drugs work by blocking impulse transmission (and thus sympathetic nervous system stimulation) at adrenergic neurons or adrenergic receptor sites. The action of the drugs at these sites can be exerted by:
• interrupting the action of sympathomimetic (adrenergic) drugs
• reducing available noradrenaline
• preventing the action of cholinergic drugs.

Classified information

Adrenergic blocking drugs are classified according to their site of action as alpha-adrenergic blockers or beta-adrenergic blockers.

Alpha-adrenergic blocking drugs
Alpha-adrenergic blocking drugs work by interrupting the actions of sympathomimetic drugs at alpha-adrenergic receptors. This results in:
• relaxation of the smooth muscle in the blood vessels
• increased dilation of blood vessels
• decreased blood pressure.
Drugs in this class include phentolamine and prazosin.

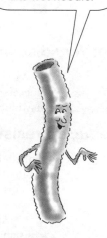

Alpha-adrenergic blocking drugs help to relax smooth muscle in blood vessels, increase dilation of blood vessels and decrease blood pressure. I tell you, I'm so relaxed, I feel like wet noodle.

Understanding adrenergic blockers

Adrenergic blockers block impulse transmission at adrenergic receptor sites by interrupting the action of adrenergic drugs, reducing the amount of norepinephrine available and blocking the action of cholinergics.

Use this table to learn the indications, adverse reactions and practice pointers needed to safely administer these drugs.

Drugs	Indications	Adverse reactions	Practice pointers
Alpha-adrenergic blockers			
Phentolamine, prazosin	• Hypertension • Peripheral vascular disorders • Pheochromocytoma	Orthostatic hypotension, severe hypertension, bradycardia, tachycardia, oedema, difficulty breathing, light-headedness, flushing, arrhythmias, angina, heart attack, shock	• Monitor vital signs and heart rhythm before, during and after administration. • Instruct the patient to rise slowly to a standing position to avoid orthostatic hypotension.
Beta-adrenergic blockers			
Nonselective Labetalol, propranolol, sotalol *Selective* Atenolol, esmolol, metoprolol	• Prevention of complications after myocardial infarction, angina, hypertension, supraventricular arrhythmias, anxiety, essential tremor, cardiovascular symptoms associated with thyrotoxicosis, migraine headaches, pheochromocytoma	Hypotension, bradycardia, peripheral vascular insufficiency, heart failure, bronchospasm, sore throat, atrioventricular block	• Monitor vital signs and heart rhythm frequently. • Beta-adrenergic blockers can alter the requirements for insulin and oral antidiabetic agents.

Alpha-adrenergic blockers work in one of two ways:

Firstly, they interfere with or block the synthesis, storage, release and reuptake of noradrenaline by neurons.

Secondly, they antagonise adrenaline, noradrenaline or adrenergic (sympathomimetic) drugs at alpha-receptor sites.

Not very discriminating

Alpha-receptor sites are either alpha1 or alpha2 receptors. Alpha-adrenergic blockers include drugs that block stimulation of alpha1 receptors and that may block alpha2 stimulation.

Reducing resistance

Alpha-adrenergic blockers occupy alpha-receptor sites on the smooth muscle of blood vessels.

This prevents catecholamines from occupying and stimulating the receptor sites. As a result, blood vessels dilate, increasing local blood flow to the skin and other organs. The decreased peripheral vascular resistance (resistance to blood flow) helps to decrease blood pressure.

Beta-adrenergic blockers

Beta-adrenergic blockers, the most widely used adrenergic blockers, prevent stimulation of the sympathetic nervous system by inhibiting the action of catecholamines and other sympathomimetic drugs at beta-adrenergic receptors.

Selective (or not)

Beta-adrenergic drugs are selective or nonselective. Nonselective beta-adrenergic drugs affect:
- beta1-receptor sites (located mainly in the heart)
- beta2-receptor sites (located in the bronchi, blood vessels and the uterus).

Nonselective beta-adrenergic drugs include labetalol, propranolol and sotalol.

Highly discriminating

Selective beta-adrenergic drugs primarily affect the beta1-adrenergic sites. They include atenolol, esmolol and metoprolol tartrate.

Intrinsically sympathetic

Some beta-adrenergic blockers, such as pindolol and acebutolol, have intrinsic sympathetic activity. This means that instead of attaching to beta-receptors and blocking them, these beta-adrenergic blockers attach to beta-receptors and stimulate them. These drugs are sometimes classified as partial agonists.

Widely effective

Beta-adrenergic blockers have widespread effects in the body because they produce their blocking action not only at the adrenergic nerve endings but also in the adrenal medulla. Effects on the heart include:
- increased peripheral vascular resistance
- decreased blood pressure
- decreased force of contractions of the heart
- decreased oxygen consumption by the heart
- slowed conduction of impulses between the atria and ventricles
- decreased CO.

Selective or nonselective

Some of the effects of beta-adrenergic blocking drugs depend on whether the drug is classified as selective or nonselective. Selective beta-adrenergic blockers, which preferentially block beta1 receptor sites, reduce stimulation of the heart. They're commonly called *cardioselective beta-adrenergic blockers*.

Nonselective beta-adrenergic blockers, which block both beta1 and beta2 receptor sites, reduce stimulation of the heart and cause the bronchioles of the lungs to constrict. This can cause bronchospasm in patients with chronic obstructive lung disorders.

Nonselective beta-adrenergic drugs affect the heart and other sites.

Selective beta-adrenergic drugs primarily affect the heart only.

Nonselective beta-adrenergic blockers can cause bronchospasm in a patient with a chronic obstructive lung disorder.

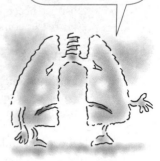

Surgery

Surgeries for treatment of cardiovascular system disorders include coronary artery bypass graft (CABG), heart transplantation, valve surgery, vascular repair and insertion of a ventricular assist device (VAD).

Coronary artery bypass graft

CABG circumvents an occluded coronary artery with an autogenous graft (usually a segment of the saphenous vein from the leg or internal mammary artery), thereby restoring blood flow to the myocardium.

CABG is one of the most commonly performed surgeries because it's done to prevent MI in a patient with acute or chronic myocardial ischaemia. The need for CABG is determined from the results of cardiac catheterisation and patient symptoms. (See *Bypassing coronary occlusions*, on page 207.)

Why bypass?

If successful, CABG can relieve anginal pain, improve cardiac function and possibly enhance the patient's quality of life.

CABG varieties

CABG techniques vary according to the patient's condition and the number of arteries being bypassed.

Newer surgical techniques, such as the mini-CABG and direct coronary artery bypass, can reduce the risk for cerebral complications and accelerate recovery for patients requiring grafts of only one or two arteries.

In some patients it's possible to perform the CABG procedure without using a heart—lung bypass machine. This increases recovery time and decreases complications.

Short and sweet

Some patients may also be candidatures for minimally invasive direct coronary artery bypass (MIDCAB). A MIDCAB is also performed on a beating heart, but instead of the traditional midsternal incision, the surgeon uses a small thoracotomy incision. MIDCAB procedures usually result in shorter hospital stays and fewer complications than traditional CABG.

Nursing considerations

When caring for a CABG patient, your major roles include patient instruction and caring for the patient's changing cardiovascular needs.

Before surgery
• Reinforce the doctor's explanation of the surgery.
• Explain the complex equipment and procedures used in the critical care unit or postanaesthesia care unit (PACU).

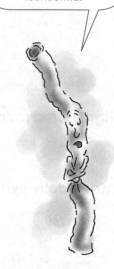

CABG surgery—circumventing an occluded artery with an autogenous graft—may be a viable option for your patient with acute or chronic myocardial ischaemia.

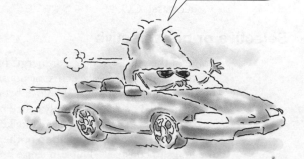

A MIDCAB procedure will have your patient back home much quicker. It usually results in a shorter hospital stay and fewer complications than traditional CABG surgery.

Bypassing coronary occlusions

After the patient receives general anaesthesia, surgery begins with graft harvesting. The surgeon makes a series of incisions in the patient's thigh or calf and removes a saphenous vein segment for grafting. Most surgeons prefer to use a segment of the internal mammarian artery.

Exposing the heart

Once the autografts are obtained, the surgeon performs a medial sternotomy to expose the heart, and then initiates cardiopulmonary bypass.

To reduce myocardial oxygen demands during surgery and to protect the heart, the surgeon induces cardiac hypothermia and standstill by injecting a cold cardioplegic solution (potassium-enriched saline solution) into the aortic root.

One fine sewing lesson

After the patient is prepared, the surgeon sutures one end of the venous graft to the ascending aorta and the other end to a patent coronary artery that's distal to the occlusion. The graft is sutured in a reversed position to promote proper blood flow. The surgeon repeats this procedure for each occlusion to be bypassed.

In the example depicted below, saphenous vein segments bypass occlusions in three sections of the coronary artery.

Finishing up

Once the grafts are in place, the surgeon flushes the cardioplegic solution from the heart and discontinues cardiopulmonary bypass. They then implant epicardial pacing electrodes, insert a chest tube, close the incision and apply a sterile dressing.

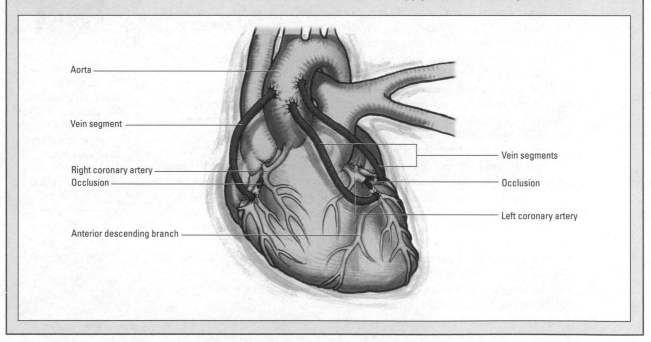

- Explain that the patient awakens from surgery with an endotracheal (ET) tube in place and connected to a mechanical ventilator. They'll also be connected to a cardiac monitor and have in place a nasogastric (NG) tube, a chest tube, an indwelling urinary catheter, arterial lines, epicardial pacing

wires and, possibly, a PA catheter. Tell them that discomfort is minimal and that the equipment is removed as soon as possible.
• Encourage incentive spirometry techniques and limb exercises with the patient.
• Make sure that the patient has signed a consent form.
• Before surgery, prepare the patient's skin as ordered.

After surgery
• Look for signs of haemodynamic compromise, such as severe hypotension, decreased CO and shock.
• Begin warming procedures according to your local policy or guidelines.
• Check and record vital signs and haemodynamic parameters regularly—as per local policy until the patient's condition stabilises. Administer medications and titrate according to the patient's response, as prescribed.
• Monitor ECGs continuously for disturbances in heart rate and rhythm. If you detect serious abnormalities, notify the doctor and be prepared to assist with epicardial pacing or, if necessary, cardioversion or defibrillation.
• To ensure adequate myocardial perfusion, keep arterial pressure within the limits set by the doctor. Usually, mean arterial pressure (MAP) less than 70 mmHg results in inadequate tissue perfusion; pressure greater than 110 mmHg can cause haemorrhage and graft rupture. Monitor PAP, CVP, left atrial pressure and CO according to local policy or guidelines.
• Frequently evaluate the patient's peripheral pulses, capillary refill time, and skin temperature and colour and report abnormalities.
• Evaluate tissue oxygenation by assessing breath sounds, chest excursion and symmetry of chest expansion. Check ABG results every 2–4 hours, and collaborate with medical staff to allow adjustment of ventilator settings to keep ABG values within prescribed limits.
• Maintain chest tube drainage at the ordered negative pressure (usually −10 to −40 cmH$_2$O), and assess regularly for haemorrhage, excessive drainage (greater than 200 ml/hour), and sudden decrease or cessation of drainage.
• Monitor the patient's intake and output, and assess for electrolyte imbalance, especially hypokalaemia and hypomagnesaemia. Assess urine output at least hourly during the immediate postoperative period and then less frequently as the patient's condition stabilises.
• As the patient's incisional pain increases, give an analgesic as prescribed. Give other drugs as prescribed.
• Throughout the recovery period, assess for symptoms of stroke, pulmonary embolism and impaired renal perfusion.
• After weaning the patient from the ventilator and removing the ET tube, assist with chest physiotherapy. Start with incentive spirometry, and encourage the patient to cough, turn frequently and deep-breathe. Assist with limb exercises to enhance peripheral circulation and prevent thrombus formation.
• Explain that postpericardiotomy syndrome commonly develops after open-heart surgery. Instruct the patient about signs and symptoms, such as fever, muscle and joint pain, weakness and chest discomfort.

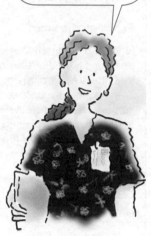

After CABG, look out for signs of haemodynamic compromise, and be ready to assist with epicardial pacing, cardioversion or defibrillation.

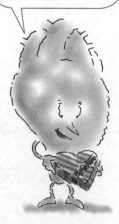

Don't be fooled by the fact that CABG is a fairly common procedure. Remember my heart is in your hands — right up to the time I am discharged home.

• Prepare the patient for the possibility of postoperative depression, which may not develop until weeks after discharge. Reassure them that this depression is normal and should pass quickly.

• Maintain nil-by-mouth status until bowel sounds return. Then begin clear liquids and advance diet as tolerated and as directed by medical staff. Expect sodium and cholesterol restrictions. Explain that this diet can help reduce the risk of recurrent arterial occlusion.

Heart transplantation

Heart transplantation involves the replacement of a person's heart with a donor heart. It's the treatment of choice for patients with end-stage cardiac disease who have a poor prognosis, estimated survival of 6–12 months and poor quality of life. A heart transplant candidate typically has uncontrolled symptoms and no other surgical options.

No guarantee

Transplantation doesn't guarantee a cure. Serious postoperative complications include infection and tissue rejection. Most patients experience one or both of these complications postoperatively.

Rejection and infection

Rejection typically occurs in the first 6 weeks after surgery. The patient is treated with monoclonal antibodies and potent immunosuppressants. The resulting immunosuppression places the patient at risk for life-threatening infection.

Valve surgery

To prevent heart failure, a patient with valvular stenosis or insufficiency accompanied by severe, unmanageable symptoms may require valve replacement (with a mechanical or prosthetic valve), valvular repair or commissurotomy. (See *Types of valve surgery*, on page 210.)

Why valve surgery?

Because of the high pressure generated by the left ventricle during contraction, stenosis and insufficiency most commonly affect the mitral and aortic valves.

Other indications for valve surgery depend on the patient's symptoms and affected valve:

• In aortic insufficiency, the patient undergoes valve replacement after symptoms—palpitations, dizziness, dyspnoea on exertion, angina and murmurs—have developed or if the chest x-ray and ECG reveal left ventricular hypertrophy.

• In aortic stenosis, which may be asymptomatic, the doctor may recommend valve replacement if cardiac catheterisation reveals significant stenosis.

• In mitral stenosis, surgery is indicated if the patient develops fatigue, dyspnoea, haemoptysis, arrhythmias, pulmonary hypertension or right ventricular hypertrophy.

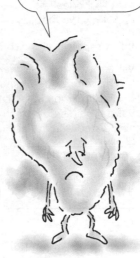

A heart transplant is the treatment of choice for those with end-stage cardiac disease, a poor prognosis, 6–12 months survival and a poor quality of life.

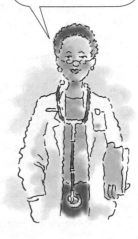

To prevent heart failure, a patient may need valve replacement or other type of surgical repair.

Types of valve surgery

When a patient with valve disease develops severe symptoms, surgery may be necessary. Several surgical procedures are available.

Commissurotomy

During commissurotomy, the surgeon incises fused mitral valve leaflets and removes calcium deposits to improve valve mobility.

Valve repair

Valve repair includes resecting or patching of valve leaflets, stretching or shortening of chordae tendineae or placing a ring in a dilated annulus (annuloplasty). Valve repair is done to avoid the complications associated with the use of prosthetic valves.

Valve replacement

Valvular replacement involves replacement of the patient's diseased valve with a mechanical or biological valve.

In the Ross procedure, the patient's own pulmonic valve is excised and used to replace the diseased aortic valve. An allograft from a human cadaver is then used to replace the pulmonic valve. Advantages of this procedure include the potential for the pulmonary autograft to grow when used in children, anticoagulation isn't necessary and increased durability.

Minimally invasive valve surgery

Minimally invasive valve surgery can be performed without a large median sternotomy incision to repair or replace aortic and mitral valves. Port access techniques may also be used for mitral valve surgery using endovascular cardiopulmonary bypass. Advantages of these types of surgery include a less invasive procedure, shorter hospital stays, fewer postoperative complications, reduced costs and smaller incisions.

• In mitral insufficiency, surgery is usually done when the patient's symptoms—dyspnoea, fatigue and palpitations—interfere with activities of daily living or if insufficiency is acute, as in papillary muscle rupture.

Nursing considerations

Provide the following care measures after valve surgery:
• Closely monitor the patient's haemodynamic status for signs of compromise. Watch especially for severe hypotension, decreased CO and shock. Check and record vital signs regularly until their condition stabilises.
• Monitor the ECG continuously for disturbances in heart rate and rhythm, such as bradycardia, ventricular tachycardia and heart block. Such disturbances may signal injury of the conduction system, which may occur during valve replacement from proximity of the atrial and mitral valves to the AV node. Arrhythmias may also result from myocardial irritability or ischaemia, fluid and electrolyte imbalance, hypoxaemia or hypothermia. If you detect serious abnormalities, notify the doctor and be prepared to assist with temporary epicardial pacing.
• Take steps to maintain the patient's MAP between 70 and 100 mmHg. Also, monitor PAP and left atrial pressure as ordered.
• Frequently assess the patient's peripheral pulses, capillary refill time and skin temperature and colour. Evaluate tissue oxygenation by assessing breath sounds, chest excursion and symmetry of chest expansion. Report any abnormalities.

- Check ABG results every 2–4 hours, and collaborate with medical staff to allow adjustment of ventilator settings to keep ABG values within prescribed limits.
- Maintain chest drainage at the prescribed negative pressure (usually 10–40 cmH$_2$O for adults). Assess chest drains frequently for signs of haemorrhage, excessive drainage (>200 ml/hour) and a sudden decrease or cessation of drainage.
- Administer analgesic, anticoagulant, antibiotic, antiarrhythmic, inotropic and vasopressor medications as well as I.V. fluids and blood products as prescribed. Monitor intake and output and assess for electrolyte imbalances, especially hypokalaemia. When anticoagulant therapy begins, evaluate its effectiveness by monitoring daily coagulation screen.
- Throughout the patient's recovery period, observe carefully for complications.
- After weaning from the ventilator and removing the ET tube, promote chest physiotherapy. Start the patient on incentive spirometry and encourage them to cough, turn frequently and deep-breathe.

Vascular repair

Vascular repair may be needed to treat patients with:
- vessels damaged by arteriosclerotic or thromboembolic disorders, trauma, infections or congenital defects
- vascular obstructions that severely compromise circulation
- vascular disease that doesn't respond to drug therapy or nonsurgical treatments such as balloon catheterisation
- life-threatening dissecting or ruptured aortic aneurysms
- limb-threatening acute arterial occlusion.

Repair review

Vascular repair methods include aneurysm resection, grafting, embolectomy, vena caval filtering and endarterectomy. The surgery used depends on the type, location and extent of vascular occlusion or damage. (See *Types of vascular repair*, on page 212.)

Nursing considerations

Provide care measures before and after vascular repair surgery.

Before surgery
- Make sure the patient and their family understand the explanation of the surgery and possible complications.
- Tell the patient that they'll receive a general anaesthetic and will awaken from the anaesthetic in the critical care unit or postanaesthetic care. Explain that they'll have I.V. hydration, ECG electrodes for continuous cardiac monitoring and possibly an arterial line and central venous catheter to provide continuous pressure monitoring. They may also have a urinary catheter in place to allow accurate output measurement. If appropriate, explain that they'll be intubated and placed on mechanical ventilation.

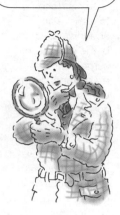

If you detect serious abnormalities in the patient's heart rate and rhythm, be ready to assist with temporary epicardial pacing.

Types of vascular repair

There are several surgical options to repair damaged or diseased vessels. Some of these options are aortic aneurysm repair, vena caval filter insertion, embolectomy and bypass grafting.

Aortic aneurysm repair

Aortic aneurysm repair is done to remove an aneurysmal segment of the aorta. The surgeon first makes an incision to expose the aneurysm site. The patient is placed on a cardiopulmonary bypass machine, if necessary. The surgeon then clamps the aorta. The aneurysm is resected and the damaged portion of the aorta is repaired.

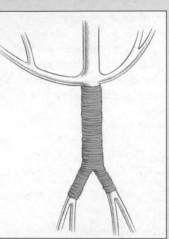

Vena caval filter insertion

A vena caval filter is inserted to trap emboli in the vena cava, preventing them from reaching the pulmonary vessels. A vena caval filter or umbrella is inserted transvenously by catheter. Once in place in the vena cava, the umbrella or filter traps emboli but allows venous blood flow.

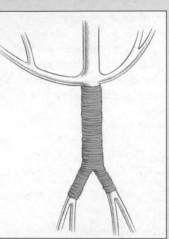

Umbrella

Direction of blood flow

Embolectomy

An embolectomy is done to remove an embolism from an artery. During this procedure, the surgeon inserts a balloon-tipped indwelling catheter into the artery and passes it through the thrombus (top). They then inflate the balloon and withdraw the catheter to remove the thrombus (bottom).

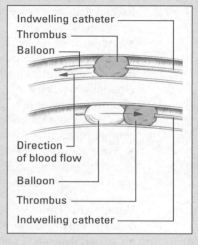

Indwelling catheter
Thrombus
Balloon

Direction of blood flow

Balloon
Thrombus
Indwelling catheter

Bypass grafting

Bypass grafting is used to bypass an arterial obstruction resulting from arteriosclerosis. After exposing the affected artery, the surgeon anastomoses a synthetic or autogenous graft to divert blood flow around the occluded arterial segment. The autogenous graft may be a vein or artery harvested from elsewhere in the patient's body. A femoropopliteal bypass is depicted.

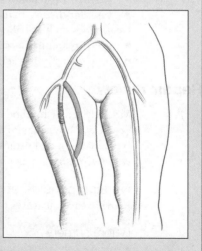

After surgery
• Check and record the patient's vital signs regularly. Report hypotension and hypertension immediately.
• Assess for respiratory and circulatory, gastrointestinal, renal and neurological problems and report concerns to medical staff.
• Assess for complications, and immediately report relevant signs and symptoms. (See *Vascular repair complications*.)
• Check the patient's dressing regularly for excessive bleeding.
• Provide analgesics, as prescribed, for incisional pain.

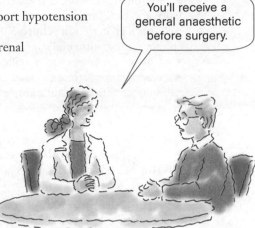

You'll receive a general anaesthetic before surgery.

Vascular repair complications

After a patient has undergone vascular repair surgery, monitor for these potential complications.

Complication	Signs and symptoms
Pulmonary infection	• Fever • Cough • Congestion • Dyspnoea
Infection	• Redness • Warmth • Drainage • Pain • Fever
Renal dysfunction	• Low urine output • Elevated blood urea nitrogen and serum creatinine levels
Occlusion	• Reduced or absent peripheral pulses • Paraesthesia • Severe pain • Cyanosis
Haemorrhage	• Hypotension • Tachycardia • Restlessness and confusion • Shallow respirations • Abdominal pain • Increased abdominal girth

- Frequently assess peripheral pulses, using Doppler ultrasonography if palpation is difficult.
- Check all extremities bilaterally for muscle strength and movement, colour, temperature and capillary refill time.
- Change dressings and provide incision care as per local policy.
- Position the patient to avoid pressure on grafts and to reduce oedema. Administer anticoagulants, as prescribed, and monitor appropriate laboratory values to evaluate effectiveness.
- To prevent atelectasis and respiratory infections encourage the patient to cough, turn and deep-breathe frequently.
- Assist the patient with limb exercises to prevent thrombus formation. Assist with early ambulation to prevent complications of immobility.

Balloon catheter treatments

Balloon catheter treatments of cardiovascular system disorders include intra-aortic balloon pump (IABP) counterpulsation, balloon valvuloplasty and percutaneous transluminal coronary angioplasty (PTCA).

IABP counterpulsation

IABP counterpulsation temporarily reduces left ventricular workload and improves coronary perfusion.

What for?

IABP counterpulsation may benefit patients with:
- cardiogenic shock
- septic shock
- intractable angina before surgery
- intractable ventricular arrhythmias
- ventricular septal or papillary muscle ruptures
- acute MI with left ventricular failure.

It's also used for patients who suffer pump failure before, during or after cardiac surgery and serves as a bridge to other treatments, such as VAD, CABG or heart transplant.

How so?

The doctor may perform balloon catheter insertion at the patient's bedside as an emergency procedure or in the operating room. (See *Understanding a balloon pump*, on page 215.)

Nursing considerations
- Explain to the patient that the doctor is going to place a catheter in the aorta to help their heart pump more easily. Tell them that, while the catheter is in place, they can't sit up, bend their knee or flex their hip more than 45 degrees.

IABP counterpulsation temporarily reduces left ventricular workload and improves coronary perfusion.

Understanding a balloon pump

An intra-aortic balloon pump consists of a polyurethane balloon attached to an external pump console by means of a large-lumen catheter. It's inserted percutaneously through the femoral artery and positioned in the descending aorta just distal to the left subclavian artery and above the renal arteries.

This external pump works in precise counterpoint to the left ventricle, inflating the balloon with helium early in diastole and deflating it just before systole. As the balloon inflates, it forces blood towards the aortic valve, thereby raising pressure in the aortic root and augmenting diastolic pressure to improve coronary perfusion. It also improves peripheral circulation by forcing blood through the brachiocephalic, common carotid and subclavian arteries arising from the aortic trunk.

The balloon deflates rapidly at the end of diastole, creating a vacuum in the aorta. This reduces aortic volume and pressure, thereby decreasing the resistance to left ventricular ejection (afterload). This decreased workload, in turn, reduces the heart's oxygen requirements and, combined with the improved myocardial perfusion, helps prevent or diminish myocardial ischaemia.

Diastole

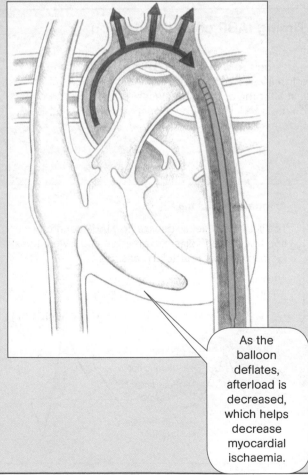

As the balloon inflates, it improves peripheral circulation.

Systole

As the balloon deflates, afterload is decreased, which helps decrease myocardial ischaemia.

- Attach the patient to a continuous ECG monitor and make sure they have an arterial line, a PA catheter and a peripheral I.V. line in place.
- Gather a surgical tray for percutaneous catheter insertion, heparin, normal saline solution, the IABP catheter and the pump console. Connect the ECG monitor to the pump console. Then prepare the femoral site.
- After the IABP catheter is inserted, select either the ECG or arterial waveform to regulate inflation and deflation of the balloon. With the ECG waveform, the pump inflates the balloon in the middle of the T wave (diastole) and deflates with the R wave (before systole). With the arterial waveform, the upstroke of the arterial wave triggers balloon inflation. (See *Timing IABP counterpulsation.*)
- Frequently assess the insertion site. Don't elevate the head of the bed more than 45 degrees, to prevent upward migration of the catheter and occlusion of the left subclavian artery. If the balloon occludes the artery, you may see a diminished left radial pulse, and the patient may report dizziness. Incorrect balloon placement may also cause flank pain or a sudden decrease in urine output.

Timing IABP counterpulsation

Intra-aortic balloon pump (IABP) counterpulsation is synchronised with either the electrocardiogram or arterial waveform. Ideally, balloon inflation should begin just after the aortic valve closes—at the dicrotic notch on the arterial waveform. Deflation should occur just before systole.

Proper timing is crucial

Early inflation can damage the aortic valve by forcing it closed, whereas late inflation permits most of the blood emerging from the ventricle to flow past the balloon, reducing pump effectiveness.

Late deflation increases the resistance against which the left ventricle must pump, possibly causing cardiac arrest.

Arterial waveforms

The illustration below depicts how IABP counterpulsation boosts peak diastolic pressure and lowers peak systolic and end-diastolic pressures.

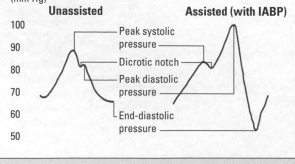

How timing affects waveforms

The arterial waveforms below show correctly and incorrectly timed balloon inflation and deflation.

Inflation

Early   Normal   Late

Deflation

Early   Normal   Late

• Assess distal pulses, colour, temperature and capillary refill of the patient's extremities every 15 minutes for the first 4 hours after insertion. After 4 hours, assess hourly for the duration of IABP therapy.
• Watch for signs of thrombus formation, such as a sudden weakening of pedal pulses, pain and motor or sensory loss.
• If indicated, apply antiembolism stockings.
• Encourage active limb exercises every 2 hours for the arms, the unaffected leg and the affected ankle.
• Maintain adequate hydration to help prevent thrombus formation.
• If bleeding occurs, apply direct pressure and notify the doctor.
• Assess the catheter insertion site every 2 hours.
• Assess the patient's cardiovascular and respiratory status at least every 4 hours
• Administer anticoagulants as ordered to help prevent thrombus formation.

Warning!

• An alarm on the console may indicate a gas leak from a damaged catheter or ruptured balloon. If the alarm sounds or you see blood in the catheter, shut down the pump console and immediately place the patient in Trendelenburg's position (feet higher than the head) to prevent an embolus from reaching the brain. Then notify the doctor.

Ready to wean

• After the signs and symptoms of left-sided heart failure diminish and the patient requires only minimal drug support, the doctor begins weaning them from IABP counterpulsation. This may be accomplished by reducing the frequency of pumping or decreasing the balloon volume; a minimum volume or pumping ratio must be maintained to prevent thrombus formation. Most consoles have a flutter function that moves the balloon to prevent clot formation. Use the flutter function when the patient has been weaned from counterpulsation but the catheter hasn't yet been removed.
• To discontinue the IABP, the doctor deflates the balloon, clips the sutures, removes the catheter and allows the site to bleed for 5 seconds to expel clots.
• After the doctor discontinues the IABP, apply direct pressure for 30 minutes and then apply a pressure dressing. Evaluate the site for bleeding and haematoma formation hourly for the next 4 hours.

Percutaneous balloon valvuloplasty

Performed in the cardiac catheterisation lab, this procedure aims to improve valvular function by enlarging the orifice of a stenotic heart valve caused by a congenital defect, calcification, rheumatic fever or aging. It involves introducing a small balloon valvuloplasty catheter through the skin at the femoral vein. (See *Percutaneous balloon valvuloplasty*, on page 218.)

When surgery isn't the answer

While the treatment of choice for valvular heart disease remains surgery, percutaneous balloon valvuloplasty offers an alternative for individuals considered

Percutaneous balloon valvuloplasty

During valvuloplasty, a surgeon inserts a small balloon catheter through the skin at the femoral vein and advances it until it reaches the affected valve. The balloon is then inflated, forcing the valve opening to widen.

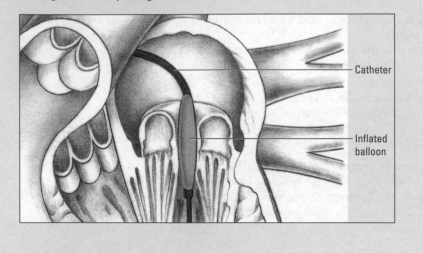

Catheter

Inflated balloon

poor surgical candidates. Unfortunately, elderly patients with aortic disease commonly experience restenosis 1–2 years after undergoing valvuloplasty.

Those complicit complications

Despite the decreased risks as compared with some more invasive procedures, balloon valvuloplasty can lead to complications, including:
• worsening valvular insufficiency as a result of misshaping the valve so that it doesn't close completely
• pieces of the calcified valve breaking off, which may travel to the brain or lungs and cause an embolism
• severe damage to the delicate valve leaflets, requiring immediate surgery to replace the valve (rare)
• bleeding and haematoma formation at the arterial puncture site.

Nursing considerations
Provide these care measures before and after percutaneous balloon valvuloplasty.

Before the procedure
• Explain that a catheter will be inserted into an artery in the patient's groin.
• Reassure the patient that, even though they'll be awake during the procedure, they will receive sedation.

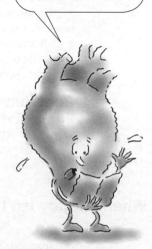

Woah! '…Misshapen valves, pieces of calcified valves breaking off, severe damage to valve leaflets…' And these are the decreased risks compared with more invasive procedures?

Check 'em all off

- Check the patient's history for allergies; if they have had allergic reactions to shellfish, iodine or contrast media, notify the doctor.
- Make sure that the results of coagulation studies, full blood count, serum electrolyte studies, blood typing and cross-matching, blood urea and creatinine are available.
- Obtain baseline vital signs, and assess peripheral pulses.
- Ensure ECG electrodes are applied and I.V. access is present.
- Perform skin preparation according to local policy.
- Give the patient a sedative as ordered.

After the procedure
Check and record the patient's vital signs regularly. Report abnormalities and concerns immediately.

- Monitor their ECG rhythm continuously and assess haemodynamic parameters closely for changes. Be alert for the development of any new cardiac arrhythmias.
- Assess patient's haemodynamic status and notify the doctor of any signs of valve failure.
- Assess peripheral pulses distal to the catheter insertion site as well as the colour, sensation, temperature and capillary refill time of the affected extremity.

Black and blue or bleeding

- Assess the catheter insertion site for haematoma, echymosis and haemorrhage. If bleeding occurs, locate the artery and apply manual pressure, then notify the doctor.
- Monitor the patient's neurological status for any changes and report them to the doctor immediately.

PTCA
PTCA is a nonsurgical way to open coronary vessels narrowed by arteriosclerosis. It's usually used with cardiac catheterisation to assess the stenosis and efficacy of angioplasty. It can also be used as a visual tool to direct the balloon-tipped catheter through a vessel's area of stenosis.

PTCA for pain

In PTCA, a balloon-tipped catheter is inserted into a narrowed coronary artery. This procedure, performed in the cardiac catheterisation laboratory under local anaesthesia, relieves pain due to angina and myocardial ischaemia.

Through one artery and into another

After coronary angiography confirms the presence and location of the occlusion, the doctor threads a guide catheter through the patient's femoral artery and into the coronary artery under fluoroscopic guidance.

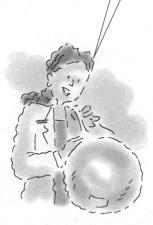

When the balloon is inflated, the plaque is compressed against the vessel wall, allowing coronary blood to flow more freely.

Understanding angioplasty

Percutaneous transluminal coronary angioplasty is used to open an occluded coronary artery without opening the chest. This illustration shows what happens during the procedure.

First, the doctor threads the catheter. When angiography shows the guide catheter positioned at the occlusion site, the doctor carefully inserts a smaller double-lumen balloon catheter through the guide catheter and directs the balloon through the occlusion.

After the balloon is directed through the occlusion, the balloon is inflated, resulting in arterial stretching and plaque fracture. The balloon may need to be inflated and deflated several times until successful dilation occurs.

Plaque, meet Balloon

When the guide catheter's position at the occlusion site is confirmed by angiography, the doctor carefully introduces a double-lumen balloon into the catheter and through the lesion, where a marked pressure gradient is obvious. The doctor alternately inflates and deflates the balloon until arteriography verifies successful arterial dilation and decrease in the pressure gradient. With balloon inflation, the plaque is compressed against the vessel wall, allowing coronary blood to flow more freely.

Placement of a coronary stent may also be done at the same time as an angioplasty. (See *Coronary artery stents*, on page 221.)

Nursing considerations

Provide these care measures before and after cardiac catheterisation.

Before the procedure
• Describe the procedure to the patient and their family and tell them it takes 1–4 hours to complete.
• Explain that a catheter will be inserted into an artery or a vein in the patient's groin and that they may feel pressure as the catheter moves along the vessel.
• Reassure the patient that although they'll be awake during the procedure, they'll be given a sedative. Instruct them to report any angina during the procedure.
• Explain that the doctor injects a contrast medium to outline the lesion's location. Warn the patient that they may feel a hot, flushing sensation or transient nausea during the injection.
• Check the patient's history for allergies; if they have had allergic reactions to shellfish, iodine or contrast media, notify the doctor.
• Give prescribed antiplatelet drugs the evening before the procedure, as ordered, to prevent platelet aggregation.
• Make sure the patient signs a consent form.
• Restrict food and fluids for at least 6 hours before the procedure.
• Make sure that the results of coagulation studies, full blood count, serum electrolytes, blood typing and cross-matching, blood urea and creatinine are available.
• Obtain baseline vital signs and assess peripheral pulses.
• Ensure ECG electrodes are applied and that I.V. access is in place.

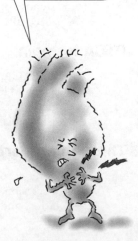

Instruct the patient to report any angina felt during cardiac catheterisation.

Coronary artery stents

An intravascular stent may be used to hold the walls of a vessel open. Some stents are coated with a drug that's slowly released to inhibit further aggregation of fibrin or clots.

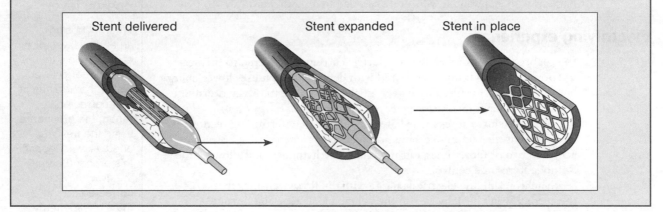

Stent delivered   Stent expanded   Stent in place

- Administer oxygen as prescribed.
- Perform skin preparation according to your facility's policy.
- Give the patient a sedative as ordered.

After the procedure
- Check and record the patient's vital signs regularly. Report abnormalities and concerns immediately.
- Assess peripheral pulses distal to the catheter insertion site as well as the colour, sensation, temperature and capillary refill time of the affected extremity.
- Monitor ECG rhythm continuously, and assess haemodynamic parameters closely for changes.
- Instruct the patient to remain in bed for 8 hours and to keep the affected extremity straight. Elevate the head of the bed 15–30 degrees. If a haemostatic device was used to close the catheter insertion site, anticipate that the patient may be allowed out of bed in only a few hours.
- Assess the catheter site for haematoma, echymosis and haemorrhage. If bleeding occurs, locate the artery and apply manual pressure, then notify the doctor.
- Administer I.V. fluids as prescribed (usually 100 ml/hour) to promote excretion of the contrast medium. Be sure to assess for signs of fluid overload.
- After the catheter is removed, apply direct pressure for at least 10 minutes and monitor the site regularly.
- Document the patient's tolerance of the procedure and status after it, including vital signs, haemodynamic parameters, appearance of catheter site, ECG findings, condition of the extremity distal to the insertion site, complications and necessary interventions.

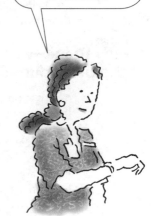

After the catheter is removed, apply direct pressure for at least 10 minutes.

Other therapy

Other treatments for cardiovascular disorders include synchronised cardioversion, defibrillation and pacemaker insertion.

Synchronised cardioversion

Cardioversion is an elective or emergency procedure used to correct tachyarrhythmias (such as atrial tachycardia, atrial flutter, atrial fibrillation and symptomatic ventricular tachycardia). It's also the treatment of choice for patients with arrhythmias who don't respond to drug therapy.

Electrifying experience

In synchronised cardioversion, an electric current is delivered to the heart to correct an arrhythmia. Compared with defibrillation, it uses lower energy levels and is synchronised to deliver an electric charge to the myocardium at the peak R wave. (See *Choosing the correct cardioversion energy level*.)

The procedure causes immediate depolarisation, interrupting reentry circuits (abnormal impulse conduction that occurs when cardiac tissue is activated two or more times, causing reentry arrhythmias) and allowing the SA node to resume control.

Synchronising the electrical charge with the R wave ensures that the current won't be delivered on the vulnerable T wave and disrupt repolarisation. Thus, it reduces the risk that the current will strike during the relative refractory period of a cardiac cycle and induce ventricular fibrillation.

Nursing considerations
- Describe the procedure to the patient and make sure an informed consent is obtained.
- Withhold all food and fluids for 6–12 hours before the procedure. If cardioversion is urgent, withhold food beginning as soon as possible.
- Obtain a baseline 12-lead ECG.
- Connect the patient to a pulse oximeter and blood pressure cuff.
- If the patient is awake, administer a sedative as ordered.
- Place the leads on the patient's chest and assess their cardiac rhythm.
- Apply conductive gel to the paddles or attach defibrillation pads to the chest wall; position the pads so that one pad is to the right of the sternum, just below the clavicle, and the other is at the fifth or sixth intercostal space in the left anterior axillary line.

Ready to jolt—whoever is taking the lead in the procedure should:

- Turn on the defibrillator and select the ordered energy level, usually between 100 and 200 joules initially.
- Activate the synchronised mode by depressing the synchroniser switch.
- Check that the machine is sensing the R wave correctly.
- Place the paddles on the chest, and apply firm pressure.
- Charge the paddles.
- Instruct other personnel to stand clear of the patient and the bed to avoid the risk of an electric shock.

Choosing the correct cardioversion energy level

When choosing an energy level for cardioversion, try the lowest energy level first. If the arrhythmia isn't corrected, repeat the procedure using the next energy level. Repeat this procedure until the arrhythmia is corrected or until the highest energy level is reached. The monophasic energy dose (or clinically equivalent biphasic energy dose) used for cardioversion are:

- 200, 360, 360 joules for unstable regular ventricular tachycardia with a pulse
- 100, 200, 360 joules for unstable paroxysmal supraventricular tachycardia
- 200, 360. 360 joules for unstable atrial fibrillation with a rapid ventricular response
- 100, 200, 360 joules for unstable atrial flutter with a rapid ventricular response.

Letting the sparks fly

• Discharge the current by pushing both paddles' DISCHARGE buttons simultaneously.

• If cardioversion is unsuccessful, repeat the procedure two or three times, as ordered, gradually increasing the energy with each additional shock.

• If normal rhythm is restored, continue to monitor the patient and provide supplemental ventilation as long as needed.

• If the patient's cardiac rhythm changes to ventricular fibrillation, switch the mode from synchronised to defibrillate and defibrillate the patient immediately after charging the machine.

• When using handheld paddles, continue to hold the paddles on the patient's chest until the energy is delivered.

• Remember to reset the SYNC MODE on the defibrillator after each synchronised cardioversion. Resetting this switch is necessary because most defibrillators automatically reset to an unsynchronised mode.

• Document the use of synchronised cardioversion, the rhythm before and after cardioversion, medication given, amperage used and how the patient tolerated the procedure.

Defibrillation

In defibrillation, electrode paddles are used to direct an electric current through the patient's heart. The current causes the myocardium to depolarise, which in turn encourages the SA node to resume control of the heart's electrical activity. (See *Biphasic defibrillators.*)

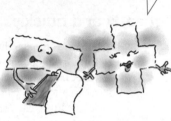

Biphasic defibrillation . . . sounds like one activity that will stimulate both of us, honey.

Biphasic defibrillators

Older defibrillators are monophasic, delivering a single current of electricity that travels in one direction between the two pads or paddles on the patient's chest. A large amount of electrical current is required for effective monophasic defibrillation.

Current flows to and fro

All new defibrillators are biphasic. Pad or paddle placement is the same as with the monophasic defibrillator. The difference is that during biphasic defibrillation, the electrical current discharged from the pads or paddles travels in a positive direction for a specified duration and then reverses and flows in a negative direction for the remaining time of the electrical discharge.

Energy efficient

The biphasic defibrillator delivers two currents of electricity and lowers the defibrillation threshold of the heart muscle, making it possible to successfully defibrillate ventricular fibrillation with smaller amounts of energy.

Adjustable

The biphasic defibrillator is able to adjust for differences in impedance or the resistance of the current through the chest. This reduces the number of shocks needed to terminate ventricular fibrillation.

Less myocardial damage

Because the biphasic defibrillator requires lower energy levels and fewer shocks, damage to the myocardial muscle is reduced. Biphasic defibrillators used at the clinically appropriate energy level may be used for defibrillation and, in the synchronised mode, for synchronised cardioversion.

Automated external defibrillator

An automated external defibrillator (AED) has a cardiac rhythm analysis system. The AED interprets the patient's cardiac rhythm and gives the operator step-by-step directions on how to proceed if defibrillation is indicated. Most AEDs have a 'quick-look' feature that allows visualisation of the rhythm with the paddles before electrodes are connected.

Computer-assisted system

The AED is equipped with a microcomputer that senses and analyses a patient's heart rhythm at the push of a button. It then audibly or visually prompts you to deliver a shock.

All models have the same basic functions but offer different operating options. For example, all AEDs communicate directions by displaying messages on a screen, giving voice commands or both. Some AEDs simultaneously display a patient's heart rhythm.

All devices record your interactions with the patient during defibrillation in a solid-state memory module. Some AEDs have an integral printer for immediate event documentation.

The electrode paddles delivering the current may be placed on the patient's chest or, during cardiac surgery, directly on the myocardium.

Act early and quickly

Because some arrhythmias, such as ventricular fibrillation, can cause death if not corrected, the success of defibrillation depends on early recognition and quick treatment.

In addition to treating ventricular fibrillation, defibrillation may also be used to treat ventricular tachycardia that doesn't produce a pulse, or polymorphic ventricular tachycardia with a pulse.

Nursing considerations

- Assess the patient to determine if they lack a pulse. Call for help and perform cardiopulmonary resuscitation (CPR) until the defibrillator and other emergency equipment arrive. (See *Automated external defibrillator*.)
- Connect the monitoring leads of the defibrillator to the patient and assess their cardiac rhythm.
- Expose the patient's chest and apply conductive pads at the paddle placement positions. (See *Defibrillator paddle placement*, on page 225.)
- Turn on the defibrillator and, if performing external defibrillation, set the energy level at the initial energy level according to current advanced life support guidelines for adult patients.

Charging and shocking—whoever is taking the lead should:

- Place the paddles over the conductive pads and press firmly against the patient's chest, using 25 lb (11.3 kg) of pressure.
- Charge the paddles by pressing the CHARGE buttons, which are located either on the machine or paddles.
- Reassess the patient's cardiac rhythm.
- If the patient remains in a shockable rhythm instruct all personnel to stand clear of the patient and the bed. Also make a visual check to make sure everyone is clear of the patient and the bed.

Defibrillator paddle placement

Here's a guide to correct paddle placement for defibrillation.

Anterolateral placement

For anterolateral placement, place one paddle to the right of the upper sternum, just below the right clavicle, and the other over the fifth or sixth intercostal space at the left anterior axillary line.

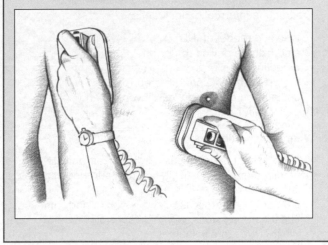

Anteroposterior placement

For anteroposterior placement, place the anterior paddle directly over the heart at the precordium, to the left of the lower sternal border. Place the flat posterior paddle under the patient's body beneath the heart and immediately below the scapulae (but not under the vertebral column).

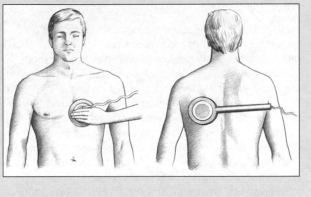

• Discharge the current by pressing both paddle DISCHARGE buttons simultaneously.
• Continue CPR for a further cycle before reassessing cardiac rhythm after defibrillating a pulseless patient.

...then again

• If necessary, prepare to defibrillate a second time. Announce that you're preparing to defibrillate and follow the procedure described previously.
• Reassess the patient and continue CPR.
• Continue according to the current advanced life support guidelines.
• If defibrillation restores a normal rhythm, assess the patient. Obtain baseline ABG levels and a 12-lead ECG. Provide supplemental oxygen, ventilation and medications as needed. Prepare the defibrillator for immediate reuse.

Document everything

• Document the procedure, including the patient's ECG rhythms before and after defibrillation; the number of times defibrillation was performed; the voltage used during each attempt; whether a pulse returned; the dosage, route and time of any drugs administered; whether CPR was used; how the airway was maintained; and the patient's outcome.

Implantable cardioverter-defibrillator

An implantable cardioverter-defibrillator (ICD) is implanted to continually monitor a patient's heart for bradycardia, ventricular tachycardia and ventricular fibrillation. The device also administers either shocks or paced beats. Some ICDs can provide biventricular pacing or administer therapy for atrial fibrillation.

ICDs are generally indicated when drug therapy, surgery or catheter ablation fails to prevent the patient's dangerous arrhythmia.

What it is

An ICD system consists of a programmable pulse generator and one or more leadwires. The pulse generator is a small battery–powered computer that monitors the heart's electrical signals and delivers electrical therapy when an abnormal rhythm is identified.

It also stores information on the heart's activity before, during and after an arrhythmia, along with tracking which treatment was delivered and the outcome of that treatment. Many devices also store electrograms (electrical tracings similar to electrocardiograms). With an interrogation device, a practitioner can retrieve this information to evaluate ICD function and battery status and to adjust ICD system settings.

How it's programmed

When caring for a patient with an ICD, it's important to know how the device is programmed. This information is available through a status report that can be obtained and printed when the practitioner or specially trained technician interrogates the device. This involves placing a specialised piece of equipment over the implanted pulse generator to retrieve pacing function.

If the patient experiences an arrhythmia or if the device delivers a therapy, the programme information is used to evaluate the functioning of the device. Programme information includes:

- type and model of ICD
- status of the device (on or off)
- detection rates
- therapies that will be delivered (pacing, antitachycardia pacing, cardioversion and defibrillation).

What you should know

- If the patient experiences cardiac arrest, initiate cardiopulmonary resuscitation and advanced cardiac life support.
- If the ICD delivers a shock while you're performing chest compressions, you may feel a slight shock. Wear gloves to eliminate this.
- It's safe to also externally defibrillate a patient with an ICD as long as the paddles aren't placed directly over the pulse generator. The anteroposterior paddle position is preferred.

If there are long-term arrhythmias . . .

- Some patients will develop long-term arrhythmias requiring defibrillation to resolve them—because of this they may require an implantable cardioverter-defibrillator. (See *Implantable cardioverter-defibrillator*.)

Permanent pacemaker insertion

A permanent pacemaker is a self-contained device surgically implanted in a pocket under the patient's skin. This is usually done in an operating room or cardiac catheterisation laboratory.

Permanent pacemakers function in the demand mode, allowing the patient's heart to beat on its own but preventing it from falling below a preset rate.

And the nominees for insertion are. . .

Permanent pacemakers are indicated for patients with:
- persistent bradycardia
- complete heart block

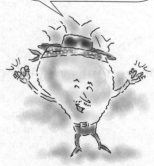

A permanent pacemaker prevents my rate from falling below a preset level so I can keep on dancing.

- congenital or degenerative heart disease
- Stokes–Adams syndrome
- Wolff–Parkinson–White syndrome
- sick sinus syndrome.

Setting the pace

Pacing electrodes can be placed in the atria, ventricles or both chambers (AV sequential or dual chamber). Biventricular pacemakers are also available for cardiac resynchronisation therapy in some patients with heart failure.

To keep the patient healthy and active, some pacemakers are designed to increase the heart rate with exercise.

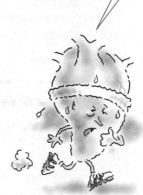

Good news for active patients! Some pacemakers are designed to increase the heart rate with exercise.

Nursing considerations

Provide care measures before and after pacemaker placement. Nursing responsibilities during surgical placement involve monitoring ECG and maintaining sterile technique.

Before surgery
- Explain the procedure to the patient.
- Before pacemaker insertion, clip the hair on the patient's chest from the axilla to the midline and from the clavicle to the nipple line on the side selected by the doctor.
- Ensure that the patient has I.V. access.
- Obtain baseline vital signs and a baseline ECG.
- Provide sedation as ordered.

After surgery
- Monitor the patient's ECG to check for arrhythmias and to ensure correct pacemaker functioning.
- Check the dressing for signs of bleeding and infection.
- Change the dressing according to facility policy.
- Check vital signs and LOC every 15 minutes for the first hour, every hour for the next 4 hours then every 4 hours.
- Provide the patient with an identification card that lists the pacemaker type and manufacturer, serial number, pacemaker rate setting, date implanted and the doctor's name.

Temporary pacemaker insertion

A temporary pacemaker is usually inserted in an emergency. The device consists of an external, battery-powered pulse generator and a lead or electrode system.

Temporary pacemakers typically come in three types, including:

 transcutaneous

transvenous

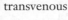 epicardial.

Dire straits

In a life-threatening situation, a transcutaneous pacemaker is the best choice. This device works by sending an electrical impulse from the pulse generator to the patient's heart by way of two electrodes, which are placed on the front and back of the patient's chest.

Transcutaneous pacing is quick and effective, but it's used only until the doctor can institute transvenous pacing.

More comfortable and more reliable

Besides being more comfortable for the patient, a transvenous pacemaker is more reliable than a transcutaneous pacemaker.

Transvenous pacing involves threading an electrode catheter through a vein into the patient's right atrium or right ventricle. The electrode is attached to an external pulse generator that can provide an electrical stimulus directly to the endocardium. (See *Temporary transvenous pacemaker*.)

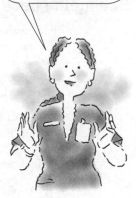

Transcutaneous pacing is used only until transvenous pacing is established.

Temporary transvenous pacemaker

Transvenous pacing provides a more reliable pacing beat. This type of pacing is more comfortable for the patient because the pacing wire is inserted in the heart via a major vein.

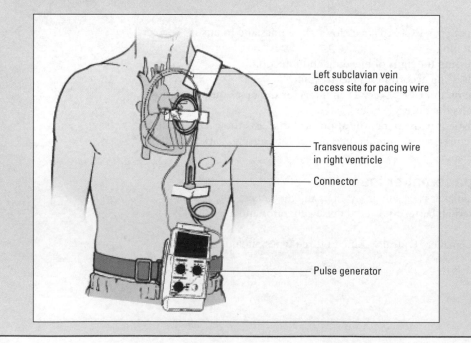

Left subclavian vein access site for pacing wire

Transvenous pacing wire in right ventricle

Connector

Pulse generator

Transvenous pacemaker basics

Indications for a temporary transvenous pacemaker include:
- management of bradycardia
- presence of tachyarrhythmias
- other conduction system disturbances.
    The purpose of temporary transvenous pacemaker insertion is:
- to maintain circulatory integrity by providing for standby pacing in case of sudden complete heart block
- to increase heart rate during periods of symptomatic bradycardia
- occasionally, to control sustained supraventricular or ventricular tachycardia.

Epicardial option

During cardiac surgery, the surgeon may insert electrodes through the epicardium of the right ventricle and, if they want to institute AV sequential pacing, the right atrium. From there, the electrodes pass through the chest wall, where they remain available if temporary pacing becomes necessary. This is called *epicardial pacing*. It uses the same equipment as temporary or transvenous pacers; it is done only after surgery.

Pacemaker no-no's

Among the contraindications to pacemaker therapy are pulseless electrical activity and ventricular fibrillation.

Nursing considerations
- Teach measures to prevent microshock; warn the patient not to use any electrical equipment that isn't grounded.
- Use other safety measures such as placing a plastic cover (supplied by the manufacturer) over the pacemaker controls to avoid an accidental setting change. If the patient needs emergency defibrillation, make sure the pacemaker can withstand the procedure. If you're unsure, disconnect the pulse generator to avoid damage.
- When using a transcutaneous pacemaker, don't place the electrodes over a bony area because bone conducts current poorly. With a female patient, place the anterior electrode under the patient's breast but not over her diaphragm.
- If the doctor inserts the transvenous pacer wire through the brachial or femoral vein, immobilise the patient's arm or leg to avoid putting stress on the pacing wires.
- After insertion of any temporary pacemaker, assess the patient's vital signs, skin colour, LOC and peripheral pulses to determine the effectiveness of the paced rhythm. Perform a 12-lead ECG to serve as a baseline, and then perform additional ECGs daily or with clinical changes. Also, if possible, obtain a rhythm strip before, during and after pacemaker placement; any time the pacemaker settings are changed; and whenever the patient receives treatment because of a complication due to the pacemaker.

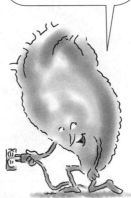

Teach measures to prevent microshock such as using only electrical equipment that's grounded.

- Continuously monitor the ECG reading, noting capture, sensing, rate, intrinsic beats and competition of paced and intrinsic rhythms. If the pacemaker is sensing correctly, the sense indicator on the pulse generator should flash with each beat.
- Record the date and time of pacemaker insertion, the type of pacemaker, the reason for insertion and the patient's response. Note the pacemaker settings. Document any complications and the interventions taken.
- If the patient has epicardial pacing wires in place, clean the insertion site and change the dressing daily. At the same time, monitor the site for signs of infection. Always keep the pulse generator nearby in case pacing becomes necessary.

Disorders

Common cardiovascular disorders include acute coronary syndromes, aneurysms, cardiac arrhythmias, cardiac tamponade, cardiogenic shock, cardiomyopathy, heart failure, hypertensive crisis, pericarditis and valvular heart disease.

Acute coronary syndromes

Patients with acute coronary syndromes have some degree of coronary artery occlusion. The degree of occlusion defines whether the acute coronary syndrome is:
- unstable angina
- non-ST-segment elevated MI (NSTEMI)
- ST segment elevated MI (STEMI).

Plaque's place

The development of any acute coronary syndrome begins with a rupture or erosion of plaque—an unstable and lipid-rich substance. The rupture results in platelet adhesions, fibrin clot formation and activation of thrombin.

What causes it

Patients with certain risk factors appear to face a greater likelihood of developing an acute coronary syndrome. These factors include:
- family history of heart disease
- obesity
- smoking
- high-fat, high-carbohydrate diet
- sedentary lifestyle
- menopause
- stress
- diabetes
- hypertension
- hyperlipidaemia.

How it happens

An acute coronary syndrome most commonly results when a thrombus progresses and occludes blood flow (an early thrombus doesn't necessarily block blood flow). The effect is an imbalance in myocardial oxygen supply and demand.

Degree and duration

The degree and duration of blockage dictate the type of infarct that occurs:
• If the patient has unstable angina, a thrombus partially occludes a coronary vessel. This thrombus is full of platelets. The partially occluded vessel may have distal microthrombi that cause necrosis in some myocytes.
• If smaller vessels infarct, the patient is at higher risk for MI, which may progress to NSTEMI. Usually, only the innermost layer of the heart is damaged.
• STEMI results when reduced blood flow through one of the coronary arteries causes myocardial ischaemia, injury and necrosis. The damage extends through all myocardial layers.

What to look for

A patient with angina typically experiences:
• burning
• squeezing
• crushing tightness in the substernal or precordial chest that may radiate to the left arm, neck, jaw or shoulder blade.

A woman thing?

Any patient may experience atypical chest pain, but it's more common in women. (See *Atypical chest pain in women*.)

It hurts when I do this

Angina most frequently follows physical exertion but may also follow emotional excitement, exposure to cold or a large meal. Angina is commonly relieved by nitroglycerin and rest. It's less severe and shorter-lived than the pain of acute MI.

Four forms

Angina has four major forms:

 stable—predictable pain, in frequency and duration, which can be relieved with nitrates and rest

 unstable—increased pain, which is easily induced

Prinzmetal's or a variant—pain from unpredictable coronary artery spasm

microvascular—angina-like chest pain due to impairment of vasodilator reserve in a patient with normal coronary arteries.

Atypical chest pain in women

Women with coronary artery disease may experience typical chest pain, but commonly experience atypical chest pain, vague chest pain or a lack of chest pain. They're more likely than men to experience a toothache or pain in the arm, shoulder, jaw, neck, throat, back, breast or stomach.

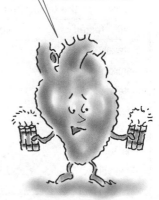

Somehow I don't think the practitioner had this formula in mind when they prescribed nitroglycerin for my angina.

My, my, MI pain

A patient with MI experiences severe, persistent chest pain that isn't relieved by rest or nitroglycerin. They may describe pain as crushing or squeezing. The pain is usually substernal, but may radiate to the left arm, jaw, neck or shoulder blades.

And many more

Other signs and symptoms of MI include:
- a feeling of impending doom
- fatigue
- nausea and vomiting
- shortness of breath
- cool extremities
- perspiration
- anxiety
- hypotension or hypertension
- palpable precordial pulse
- muffled heart sounds.

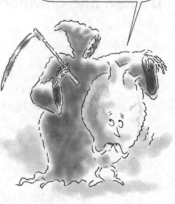

Besides physical signs and symptoms, a patient with MI may report a feeling of impending doom or anxiety.

What tests tell you

These tests are used to diagnose CAD:
- ECG during an anginal episode shows ischaemia. Serial 12-lead ECGs may be normal or inconclusive during the first few hours after an MI. Abnormalities include serial ST-segment depression in NSTEMI and ST-segment elevation and Q waves, representing scarring and necrosis, in STEMI. (See *Locating myocardial damage*.)
- Coronary angiography reveals coronary artery stenosis or obstruction and collateral circulation and shows the condition of the arteries beyond the narrowing.

Locating myocardial damage

After you've noted characteristic lead changes of an acute myocardial infarction, use this chart to identify the areas of damage. Match the lead changes in the second column with the affected wall in the first column and the artery involved in the third column. Column four shows reciprocal lead changes.

Wall affected	Leads	Artery involved	Reciprocal changes
Anterior	V_2 to V_4	Left coronary artery, left anterior descending (LAD) artery	II, III, aV_F
Anterolateral	I, aV_L, V_3 to V_6	LAD artery, circumflex artery	II, III, aV_F
Anteroseptal	V_1 to V_4	LAD artery	None
Inferior (diaphragmatic)	II, III, aV_F	Right coronary artery	I, aV_L
Lateral	I, aV_L, V_5, V_6	Circumflex artery, branch of left coronary artery	II, III, aV_F
Posterior	V_8, V_9	Right coronary artery, circumflex artery	V_1 to V_4
Right ventricular	V_4R, V_5R, V_6R	Right coronary artery	None

- Myocardial perfusion imaging with thallium-201 during treadmill exercise discloses ischaemic areas of the myocardium, visualised as 'cold spots'.
- With MI, serial serum cardiac marker measurements show elevated CK, especially the CK-MB isoenzyme (the cardiac muscle fraction of CK), troponin T and I, myoglobin and ischaemia-modified albumin.
- C-reactive protein (CRP) levels help measure cardiac risk. Patients with chest pain and a higher CRP level have an increased risk of CAD.
- With STEMI, echocardiography shows ventricular wall dyskinesia.

How it's treated

For patients with angina, the goal of treatment is to reduce myocardial oxygen demand or increase oxygen supply.

The following treatments are used to manage angina:
- Nitrates reduce myocardial oxygen consumption.
- Beta-adrenergic blockers may be administered to reduce the workload and oxygen demands of the heart.
- If angina is caused by coronary artery spasm, calcium channel blockers may be given.
- Antiplatelet drugs minimise platelet aggregation and the danger of coronary occlusion.
- Antilipemic drugs can reduce elevated serum cholesterol or triglyceride levels.
- Obstructive lesions may necessitate CABG or PTCA. Other alternatives include laser angioplasty, minimally invasive surgery, atherectomy or stent placement.

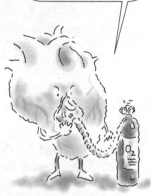

For patients with angina, the goal is to reduce oxygen demand or increase oxygen supply.

MI relief

The goals of treatment for MI are to relieve pain, stabilise heart rhythm, revascularise the coronary artery, preserve myocardial tissue and reduce cardiac workload.

Here are some guidelines for treatment:
- Thrombolytic therapy should be started within 6 hours of the onset of symptoms (unless contraindications exist). Thrombolytic therapy involves administration of streptokinase, alteplase or reteplase.
- PTCA and stent placement are options for opening blocked or narrowed arteries.
- Oxygen is administered to increase oxygenation of the blood.
- Nitroglycerin is administered sublingually to relieve chest pain, unless systolic blood pressure is less than 90 mmHg or heart rate is less than 50 or greater than 100 beats per minute.

Heart ache

- Morphine is administered as analgesia because pain stimulates the sympathetic nervous system, leading to an increase in heart rate and vasoconstriction.

- Aspirin and antiplatelet drugs are administered to inhibit platelet aggregation.
- I.V. heparin is given to patients who have received tissue plasminogen activator to increase the chances of patency in the affected coronary artery.
- Amiodarone, transcutaneous pacing patches (or a transvenous pacemaker), defibrillation or adrenaline may be used if arrhythmias are present.
- Physical activity is limited for the first 12 hours to reduce cardiac workload, thereby limiting the area of necrosis.
- I.V. nitroglycerin is administered for 24–48 hours in patients without hypotension, bradycardia or excessive tachycardia, to reduce afterload and preload and relieve chest pain.
- Glycoprotein IIb/IIIa inhibitors are administered to patients with continued unstable angina or acute chest pain, or following invasive cardiac procedures, to reduce platelet aggregation.
- I.V. beta-adrenergic blocker is administered early to patients with evolving acute MI; it's followed by oral therapy to reduce heart rate and contractibility and reduce myocardial oxygen requirements.
- ACE inhibitors are administered to those with evolving MI with ST-segment elevation or left bundle-branch block, to reduce afterload and preload and prevent remodelling.
- Laser angioplasty, atherectomy or stent placement may be initiated.
- Lipid-lowering drugs are administered to patients with elevated LDL and cholesterol levels.

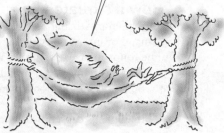

Physical activity is limited for the first 12 hours after MI to reduce the cardiac workload and limit necrosis. Time to catch some Z's!

What to do
- During anginal episodes, monitor blood pressure and heart rate. Take an ECG before administering nitroglycerin or other nitrates. Record duration of pain, amount of medication required to relieve it and accompanying symptoms.

CCU, ECG and more!

- On admission to the coronary care unit, monitor and record the patient's ECG, blood pressure, temperature and heart and breath sounds. Also, assess and record the severity, location, type and duration of pain.
- Obtain a 12-lead ECG and assess heart rate and blood pressure when the patient experiences acute chest pain.
- Monitor the patient's haemodynamic status closely. Be alert for indicators suggesting decreased CO, such as decreased blood pressure, increased heart rate, increased PAP, increased PAWP, decreased CO measurements and decreased right atrial pressure.
- Assess urine output hourly.
- Monitor the patient's oxygen saturation levels and notify the doctor if oxygen saturation falls below 94%.
- Check the patient's blood pressure after giving nitroglycerin, especially the first dose.

- During episodes of chest pain, monitor ECG, blood pressure and PA catheter readings (if applicable) to determine changes.
- Frequently monitor ECG rhythm strips to detect heart rate changes and arrhythmias.
- Obtain serial measurements of cardiac enzyme levels as ordered.
- Watch for respiratory crackles (if auscultation is one of your skills), cough, tachypnoea and oedema, which may indicate impending left-sided heart failure. Carefully monitor daily weight, intake and output, respiratory rate, serum enzyme levels, ECG waveforms and blood pressure.
- Prepare the patient for reperfusion therapy as indicated.
- Administer and titrate medications as ordered. Avoid giving I.M. injections; I.V. administration provides more rapid symptom relief.

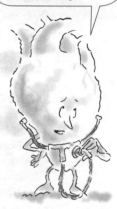

During episodes of chest pain, monitor ECG, blood pressure and PA catheter readings for changes.

I need a break

- Organise patient care and activities to allow rest periods. If the patient is immobilised, turn them often and use a pressure relieving mattress. Gradually increase the patient's activity level as tolerated.
- Provide a clear-liquid diet until nausea subsides. Anticipate a possible order for a low-cholesterol, low-sodium diet without caffeine.
- You may need to ask the doctor to prescribe a stool softener to prevent straining during defecation.

National framework for coronary heart disease

Coronary heart disease has been the topic of a national strategy (National Service Framework) to reduce morbidity and mortality. While this section outlines some of the specific clinical interventions for the disorders listed, there are some overarching principles and standards that should guide care within UK hospitals. These include:
- Assessment of the risks of heart disease in individual patients and their reduction where possible (e.g. smoking cessation, diet and exercise).
- Specific care and advice to promote health in those with established heart disease or those at significant risk.
- Those presenting with acute coronary syndromes (unstable angina and MI) should have access to prompt treatment by individuals who are appropriately trained and who are following evidence-based protocols to increase chances of survival.
- Those with stable angina should be investigated and managed to reduce pain and reduce the risk of coronary events.
- Those with increasing severity or frequency of angina should be referred to a cardiologist for assessment.
- There should be hospital-wide systems in place to ensure patients receive timely and appropriate care to reduce their risk of subsequent events and reduce symptoms.
- Those with suspected heart failure should be appropriately investigated (e.g. ECG and echocardiogram) to confirm or refute the diagnosis. If the

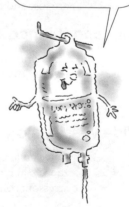

Remember, I.V. administration of medications provides more rapid relief from the patient's MI symptoms.

heart failure is diagnosed, treatment to reduce symptoms and risk of death should be offered.
• Patient with coronary heart disease should be offered secondary prevention through cardiac rehabilitation programmes.

Aortic aneurysm

An aortic aneurysm is a localised outpouching or an abnormal dilation in a weakened arterial wall. Aortic aneurysm typically occurs in the aorta between the renal arteries and the iliac branches, but the abdominal, thoracic or ascending arch of the aorta may be affected.

What causes it

The exact cause of an aortic aneurysm is unclear, but several factors place a person at risk, including:
• advanced age
• history of hypertension
• smoking
• atherosclerosis
• connective tissue disorders
• diabetes mellitus
• trauma.

How it happens

Aneurysms arise from a defect in the middle layer of the arterial wall (tunica media or medial layer). Once the elastic fibres and collagen in the middle layer are damaged, stretching and segmental dilation occur. As a result, the medial layer loses some of its elasticity, and it fragments. Smooth muscle cells are lost and the wall thins.

Thin and thinner

The thinned wall may contain calcium deposits and atherosclerotic plaque, making the wall brittle. As a person ages, the elastin in the wall decreases, further weakening the vessel. If hypertension is present, blood flow slows, resulting in ischaemia and additional weakening.

Wide vessel, slow flow

Once an aneurysm begins to develop, lateral pressure increases, causing the vessel lumen to widen and blood flow to slow. Over time, mechanical stressors contribute to elongation of the aneurysm.

Blood forces

Haemodynamic forces may also play a role, causing pulsatile stresses on the weakened wall and pressing on the small vessels that supply nutrients to the arterial wall. In aortic aneurysms, this causes the aorta to become bowed and tortuous.

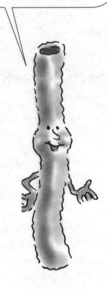

An aortic aneurysm arises from a defect in the middle layer of the arterial wall that causes stretching and segmental dilation, loss of elasticity and arterial wall thinning.

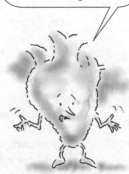

Most patients with aortic aneurysms are asymptomatic until an enlarging aneurysm compresses surrounding tissue.

What to look for

Most patients with aortic aneurysms are asymptomatic until the aneurysms enlarge and compress surrounding tissue.

A large aneurysm may produce signs and symptoms that mimic those of MI, renal calculi, lumbar disc disease and duodenal compression.

When symptoms arise

Usually, if the patient exhibits symptoms, it's because of rupture, expansion, embolisation, thrombosis or pressure from the mass on surrounding structures. Rupture is more common if the patient also has hypertension or if the aneurysm is larger than 6 cm.

Some of the classic symptoms of a thoracic aortic aneurysm include substernal pain, hoarseness or coughing, difficulty swallowing, difficulty breathing, aortic murmur and unequal blood pressure and pulses when measured in both arms.

Thoracic aortic aneurysm

If the patient has a suspected thoracic aortic aneurysm, the patient should be assessed for:
- complaints of substernal pain possibly radiating to the neck, back, abdomen or shoulders
- hoarseness or coughing
- difficulty swallowing
- difficulty breathing
- unequal blood pressure and pulse when measured in both arms
- aortic insufficiency murmur.

Acute expansion

When there's an acute expansion of a thoracic aortic aneurysm, the patient should be assessed for:
- severe hypertension
- neurological changes
- a new murmur of aortic sufficiency
- right sternoclavicular lift
- jugular vein distention
- tracheal deviation.

Abdominal aortic aneurysm

The patient with an abdominal aortic aneurysm may experience:
- dull abdominal pain
- lower back pain that's unaffected by movement
- gastric or abdominal fullness
- pulsating mass in the periumbilical area (if the patient isn't obese)
- systolic bruit over the aorta on auscultation of the abdomen
- hypotension (with aneurysm rupture).

What tests tell you

No specific laboratory test to diagnose an aortic aneurysm exists. However, these tests may be helpful:
• If blood is leaking from the aneurysm, leukocytosis and a decrease in haemoglobin and haematocrit may be noted.

Telltale TOE

• TOE allows visualisation of the thoracic aorta. It's commonly combined with Doppler flow studies to provide information about blood flow.
• Abdominal ultrasonography or echocardiography can be used to determine the size, shape and location of the aneurysm.
• Anteroposterior and lateral x-rays of the chest or abdomen can be used to detect aortic calcification and widened areas of the aorta.
• Computed tomography (CT) scan and magnetic resonance imaging (MRI) can disclose the aneurysm's size and effect on nearby organs.
• Serial ultrasonography at 6-month intervals reveals any growth of small aneurysms.
• ECG will be absent of any signs of MI.
• Aortography is used in determining the aneurysm's approximate size and patency of the visceral vessels.

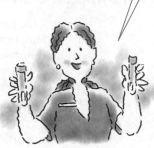

Unless blood is leaking from the aneurysm, there's no specific laboratory test to aid the diagnosis.

How it's treated

Aneurysm treatment usually involves surgery and appropriate drug therapy. Aortic aneurysms usually require resection and replacement of the aortic section using a vascular or Dacron graft. However, keep these points in mind:
• If the aneurysm is small and produces no symptoms, surgery may be delayed, with regular physical examination and ultrasonography performed to monitor its progression.
• Large or symptomatic aneurysms are at risk for rupture and need immediate repair.
• Endovascular grafting may be an option for a patient with an abdominal aortic aneurysm. This procedure, which can be done using local or regional anaesthesia, is a minimally invasive procedure whereby the walls of the aorta are reinforced to prevent expansion and rupture of the aneurysm.
• Medications to control blood pressure, relieve anxiety and control pain are also prescribed.

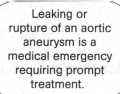

Leaking or rupture of an aortic aneurysm is a medical emergency requiring prompt treatment.

Rush to respond to rupture

A leaking or rupture of an aortic aneurysm is a medical emergency requiring prompt treatment. This may be rarely seen in the critical care unit as it is more common that the pathway of care takes the patient from the accident and emergency department to theatre. However, it is worthwhile knowing the preoperative treatment—which includes:
• resuscitation with fluid and blood replacement
• possibly I.V. Esmolol and/or Glyceryl trinitrate (GTN) if the patient is hypertensive—particularly in aortic dissection

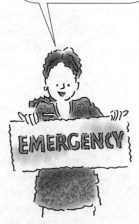

EMERGENCY

- analgesics to relieve pain
- an arterial line, central line and indwelling urinary catheter to monitor the patient's condition perioperatively.

What to do

- Assess cardiovascular status frequently, including heart rate, rhythm and ECG.
- Obtain blood samples to evaluate kidney function by assessing urea, creatinine and electrolyte levels. Measure intake and output, hourly if necessary, depending on the patient's condition.
- Monitor FBC for evidence of blood loss, including decreased haemoglobin, haematocrit and red blood cell (RBC) count.
- Send blood to the laboratory to be typed and cross-matched—usually the patient will need a blood transfusion.
- Obtain an arterial sample for ABG analysis and lactate in order to evaluate oxygenation, acidosis and shock.
- Observe the patient for signs of rupture and shock—acute blood loss: decreasing blood pressure; increasing pulse and respiratory rates; cool, clammy skin; restlessness; and decreased LOC.
- Prepare the patient for emergency surgery.

After surgery

Postoperatively patients who have had elective repair of their aneurysm or emergency repair due to leak or rupture will need critical care monitoring and organ support. Both groups can have similar problems—including acute myocardial infarction, acute renal failure, leaking from the vascular repair, pneumonia and surgical infections as well as emboli and subsequent ischaemia. Some will also suffer acute delirium. However, these complications occur more often following emergency repair. For all patients you should:

- Administer prescribed vasoactive drugs, inotropes or antihypertensive drugs and titrate to maintain a normotensive state.
- Provide analgesics to relieve pain.
- Administer anticoagulants, such as heparin, to help prevent formation of thrombi.
- Continue to monitor ECG for changes. Monitor the patient's haemodynamic status and report abnormalities to the doctor.
- Administer I.V. fluids as ordered.
- Monitor the patient for signs of bleeding, such as hypotension and decreased haemoglobin and haematocrit.
- Perform meticulous pulmonary hygiene measures, including suctioning, chest physiotherapy and deep breathing.
- Assess urine output hourly.
- Maintain NG tube patency to ensure gastric decompression.
- Assist with serial Doppler examination of all extremities to evaluate the adequacy of vascular repair and presence of embolisation.
- Assess for signs of poor arterial perfusion, such as pain, paraesthesia, pallor, pulselessness, paralysis and poikilothermy (coldness).

Remember the six signs of poor arterial perfusion: pain, paraesthesia, pallor, pulselessness, paralysis and poikilothermy. (Poikilothermy is the condition in which a person is unable to regulate temperature so is reliant on environment for temperature.)

Cardiac tamponade

Cardiac tamponade is a rapid, unchecked increase in pressure in the pericardial sac. This compresses the heart, impairs diastolic filling and reduces CO.

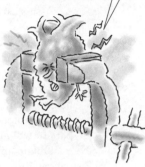

If I'm compressed, cardiac output decreases.

Pericardial pressure

The increase in pressure usually results from blood or fluid accumulation in the pericardial sac. Even a small amount of fluid (50–100 ml) can cause a serious tamponade if it accumulates rapidly.

If fluid accumulates rapidly, cardiac tamponade requires emergency lifesaving measures to prevent death. A slow accumulation and increase in pressure may not produce immediate symptoms because the fibrous wall of the pericardial sac can gradually stretch to accommodate as much as 1–2 L of fluid.

What causes it

Cardiac tamponade may result from:
* idiopathic causes (such as Dressler's syndrome)
* effusion (from cancer, bacterial infections, tuberculosis and, rarely, acute rheumatic fever)
* haemorrhage due to trauma (such as gunshot or stab wounds of the chest)
* haemorrhage due to nontraumatic causes (such as anticoagulant therapy in patients with pericarditis or rupture of the heart or great vessels (for example, following a CABG))
* viral or postirradiation pericarditis
* chronic renal failure requiring dialysis
* drug reaction
* connective tissue disorders (such as rheumatoid arthritis, systemic lupus erythematosus, rheumatic fever, vasculitis and scleroderma)
* acute MI.

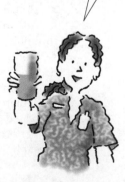

A patient with cardiac tamponade may not have immediate symptoms if fluid accumulates slowly. The fibrous wall of the pericardial sac can stretch gradually to accommodate as much as 1–2 L of fluid. Imagine that!

How it happens

In cardiac tamponade, accumulation of fluid in the pericardial sac causes compression of the heart chambers. This compression obstructs blood flow into the ventricles and reduces the amount of blood that can be pumped out of the heart with each contraction. (See *Understanding cardiac tamponade*, on page 241.)

What to look for

Cardiac tamponade has three classic features known as *Beck's triad*:

 elevated CVP with jugular vein distention

 muffled heart sounds

 drop in systolic blood pressure.

Understanding cardiac tamponade

The pericardial sac, which surrounds and protects the heart, is composed of several layers:

- The fibrous pericardium is the tough outermost membrane.
- The inner membrane, called the *serous membrane*, consists of the visceral and parietal layers.
- The visceral layer clings to the heart and is also known as the *epicardial layer* of the heart.
- The parietal layer lies between the visceral layer and the fibrous pericardium.

- The pericardial space—between the visceral and parietal layers—contains 10–30 ml of pericardial fluid. This fluid lubricates the layers and minimises friction when the heart contracts.

In cardiac tamponade, shown below right, blood or fluid fills the pericardial space, compressing the heart chambers, increasing intracardiac pressure, and obstructing venous return. As blood flow into the ventricles decreases, so does cardiac output. Without prompt treatment, low cardiac output can be fatal.

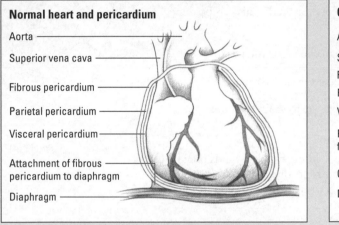

Normal heart and pericardium

Aorta

Superior vena cava

Fibrous pericardium

Parietal pericardium

Visceral pericardium

Attachment of fibrous pericardium to diaphragm

Diaphragm

Cardiac tamponade

Aorta

Superior vena cava

Fibrous pericardium

Parietal pericardium

Visceral pericardium

Pericardial space filled with excess fluid

Compressed heart

Diaphragm

That's not all

Other signs include:
- narrowed pulse pressure
- orthopnoea
- anxiety
- restlessness
- jugular vein distention with inspiration
- mottling
- clear breath sounds (this helps distinguish cardiac tamponade from heart failure).

What tests tell you

- Chest x-ray shows a slightly widened mediastinum and an enlarged cardiac silhouette.

• ECG may show low-amplitude QRS complex and electrical alternans, an alternating beat-to-beat change in amplitude of the P wave, QRS complex and T wave. Generalised ST-segment elevation is noted in all leads. An ECG is used to rule out other cardiac disorders; it may reveal changes produced by acute pericarditis.

• PA catheterisation discloses increased CVP, right ventricular diastolic pressure, PAWP and decreased CO/CI.

• Echocardiography may reveal pericardial effusion with signs of right ventricular and atrial compression.

• CT scan or MRI may be used to identify pericardial effusions or pericardial thickening caused by constrictive pericarditis.

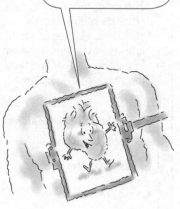

In cardiac tamponade, a chest x-ray reveals a widened mediastinum and enlarged cardiac silhouette.

How it's treated

The goal of treatment is to relieve intrapericardial pressure and cardiac compression by removing accumulated blood or fluid. This can be done in three different ways:

pericardiocentesis (needle aspiration of the pericardial cavity)

surgical creation of an opening, called a *pericardial window*

insertion of a drain into the pericardial sac to drain the effusion.

When pressure's low

If the patient is hypotensive, trial volume loading with I.V. fluids may be used to maintain systolic blood pressure. An inotropic drug, such as dobutamine, may be necessary to improve myocardial contractility until fluid in the pericardial sac can be removed.

Additional treatments

Additional treatments may be necessary, depending on the cause. Examples of such causes and treatments are:

• traumatic injury—blood transfusion or a thoracotomy to drain reaccumulating fluid or to repair bleeding sites

• heparin-induced tamponade—administration of the heparin antagonist protamine sulphate

• warfarin-induced tamponade—vitamin K administration

• renal failure–induced tamponade—haemodialysis.

To correct heparin-induced tamponade, administer the heparin antagonist protamine sulphate.

What to do

• Monitor the patient's cardiovascular status frequently, at least every hour, noting blood pressure and extent of jugular vein distention. Doctors may wish to assess heart sounds regularly.

• Assess haemodynamic status, including CVP, CO and any other parameters available from haemodynamic monitoring.

• Monitor for pulsus paradoxus.

• Be alert for ST-segment and T-wave changes on ECG. Note rate and rhythm and report evidence of any arrhythmias.

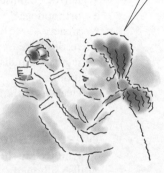

• Watch closely for signs of increasing tamponade, increasing dyspnoea and arrhythmias and report immediately.
• Infuse I.V. solutions and inotropic drugs, such as dobutamine, as prescribed to maintain the patient's blood pressure.
• Administer oxygen therapy as needed and assess oxygen saturation levels. Monitor the patient's respiratory status for signs of respiratory distress, such as severe tachypnoea and changes in the patient's LOC. Anticipate the need for ET intubation and mechanical ventilation if the patient's respiratory status deteriorates.
• Prepare the patient for pericardiocentesis or thoracotomy.

Under pressure

• If the patient has trauma-induced tamponade, assess for other signs of trauma and institute appropriate care, including the use of colloids, crystalloids and blood component therapy under pressure or by rapid volume infuser if massive fluid replacement is needed; administration of protamine sulphate for heparin-induced tamponade; and vitamin K administration for warfarin-induced tamponade.
• Assess renal function status closely, monitoring urine output every hour and notifying the doctor if output is less than 0.5 mg/kg/hour.
• Monitor capillary refill time, LOC, peripheral pulses and skin temperature for evidence of diminished tissue perfusion.

Cardiogenic shock

Cardiogenic shock is a condition of diminished CO that severely impairs tissue perfusion. It's sometimes called *pump failure*.

Shocking stats

Cardiogenic shock is a serious complication in nearly 15% of all patients hospitalised with acute MI. It typically affects patients whose area of infarction involves 40% or more of left ventricular muscle mass; in such patients, mortality may exceed 85%.

What causes it

Cardiogenic shock can result from any condition that causes significant left ventricular dysfunction with reduced CO, such as:
• MI (most common)
• myocardial ischaemia
• papillary muscle dysfunction
• cardiomyopathy
• chronic or acute heart failure.

Other offenders

Other causes include myocarditis and depression of myocardial contractility after cardiac arrest and prolonged cardiac surgery.

Administer oxygen and monitor for respiratory distress. And by all means, anticipate the need for ET and mechanical ventilation if the patient's respiratory status deteriorates.

Mechanical abnormalities of the ventricle, such as acute mitral or aortic insufficiency or an acutely acquired ventricular septal defect or ventricular aneurysm, may also result in cardiogenic shock.

How it happens

Regardless of the cause, here's what happens:
• Left ventricular dysfunction initiates a series of compensatory mechanisms that attempt to increase CO and, in turn, maintain vital organ function.
• As CO falls, baroreceptors in the aorta and carotid arteries initiate responses in the sympathetic nervous system. These responses, in turn, increase heart rate, left ventricular filling pressure and afterload to enhance venous return to the heart.
• These compensatory responses initially stabilise the patient but later cause the patient to deteriorate as the oxygen demands of the already compromised heart increase.

Lower and lower output

• The events involved in cardiogenic shock comprise a vicious cycle of low CO, sympathetic compensation, myocardial ischaemia and even lower CO.

What to look for

Cardiogenic shock produces signs of poor tissue perfusion, such as:
• cold, pale, clammy skin
• drop in systolic blood pressure to 30 mmHg below baseline or a sustained reading below 90 mmHg that isn't attributable to medication
• tachycardia
• rapid respirations
• oliguria (urine output less than 1/2 ml/kg/hour)
• anxiety
• confusion
• narrowing pulse pressure
• crackles heard in lungs
• neck vein distention.

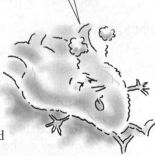

Compensatory mechanisms that increase cardiac output eventually cause the patient to deteriorate because of increased oxygen demands.

What tests tell you

• Haemodynamic monitoring reveals reduced CO (and CI) and increased CVP, PAP, PAWP and SVR, reflecting an increase in left ventricular end-diastolic pressure (preload) and heightened resistance to left ventricular emptying (afterload) caused by ineffective pumping and increased peripheral vascular resistance.
• Invasive arterial pressure monitoring shows systolic arterial pressure less than 90 mmHg caused by impaired ventricular ejection.
• ABG analysis may show metabolic acidosis reflecting poor tissue perfusion and elevated lactate; respiratory acidosis and hypoxia reflecting pulmonary congestion and impaired gas exchange.
• ECG demonstrates possible evidence of acute MI, ischaemia or ventricular aneurysm and arrhythmias.

- Echocardiography is used to determine left ventricular function and reveals valvular abnormalities.
- Serum enzyme measurements display elevated levels of CK, aspartate aminotransferase and alanine aminotransferase, which indicate MI or ischaemia and suggest heart failure or shock. CK-MB (an isoenzyme of CK that occurs in cardiac tissue) and troponin isoenzyme levels may confirm acute MI.
- Brain natriuretic peptide (BNP) levels are elevated, indicating ventricular overload.
- Cardiac catheterisation and echocardiography may reveal other conditions that can lead to pump dysfunction and failure, such as cardiac tamponade, papillary muscle infarct or rupture, ventricular septal rupture, pulmonary emboli, venous pooling (associated with vasodilators and continuous or intermittent positive-pressure ventilation), hypovolaemia and acute heart failure.

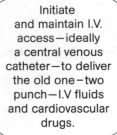

They tell me the signs of cardiogenic shock are as clear as the stars on a cloudless night, so I'm looking… looking… still looking…

How it's treated

The goal of treatment is to optimise cardiovascular status by increasing CO, improving myocardial perfusion and decreasing cardiac workload. Treatment consists of administering cardiovascular drugs and providing multisystem support to help prevent other organs from failing. In more extreme cases, and where technology is available, mechanically assisted techniques may be used.

Treatment ABCs

Treatment begins with these measures:
- maintaining a patent airway; preparing for intubation and mechanical ventilation if the patient develops respiratory distress
- providing supplemental oxygen to increase oxygenation
- cardiac monitoring to detect changes in heart rate and rhythm; administering antiarrhythmics, as necessary
- initiating and maintaining I.V. access—ideally a central venous catheter for fluid and drug administration and measurement of CVP
- using I.V. fluids, crystalloids, colloids or blood products, as necessary, to maintain intravascular volume.

Initiate and maintain I.V. access—ideally a central venous catheter—to deliver the old one–two punch—I.V fluids and cardiovascular drugs.

Cardiovascular drugs

Drug therapy may include I.V. dobutamine, noradrenaline and adrenaline. Dobutamine and adrenaline increase myocardial contractility, CO, blood pressure and blood flow to kidneys. Noradrenaline increases blood pressure by acting as a vasoconstrictor.

Decrease resistance and pressure

A vasodilator, usually GTN, may be used to further improve CO by decreasing afterload (SVR) and reducing left ventricular end-diastolic pressure (preload). However, the patient's blood pressure must be adequate to support nitroprusside therapy and must be monitored closely.

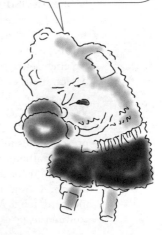

Overloaded and out of control

Diuretics also may be used to reduce preload (CVP and PAWP) in patients with relative fluid volume overload. Antiarrhythmics may also be used to prevent or control arrhythmias that may reduce CO.

Keeping things in balance

A range of drugs and therapies have been described above—some of which have opposite effects, for example, vasoconstrictors and vasodilators, fluid volume replacement and diuretics. The key to optimising the cardiovascular system when shock is present is close monitoring and then titration of drug and fluid therapy to achieve a balance of fluid volume status (preload), CO (contractility) and resistance (afterload).

Mechanical assistance

Treatment may also include mechanical assistance by IABP to improve coronary artery perfusion and decrease cardiac workload. The IABP is inserted through the femoral artery into the descending thoracic aorta. The balloon inflates during diastole to increase coronary artery perfusion pressure and deflates before systole (before the aortic valve opens) to reduce resistance to ejection (afterload) and therefore reduce cardiac workload.

Improved ventricular ejection significantly improves CO. Subsequent vasodilation in the peripheral vessels leads to lower preload volume and reduced workload of the left ventricle. This is because of decreasing SVR.

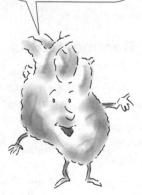

Improved ventricular ejection significantly improves cardiac output.

End-stage effort

When drug therapy and IABP insertion fail, a VAD may be inserted to assist the pumping action of the heart. When all other medical and surgical therapies fail, heart transplantation may be considered.

More measures

Additional treatment measures for cardiogenic shock may include:
• thrombolytic therapy or coronary artery revascularisation to restore coronary artery blood flow, if cardiogenic shock is due to acute MI
• emergency surgery to repair papillary muscle rupture or ventricular septal defect, if either is the cause of cardiogenic shock.

What to do

• Begin I.V. infusions of Normal saline or Hartmann's solution as prescribed using a large-bore (14G to 18G) peripheral cannula until a central venous catheter is inserted.
• Administer oxygen by face mask to ensure adequate oxygenation of tissues. Adjust the fraction of inspired oxygen according to ABG measurements. Many patients need 100% oxygen, and some require continuous positive airway pressure (CPAP) by mask or hood.

Monitor, record and then monitor more

- Monitor and record blood pressure, pulse, respiratory rate and peripheral pulses at least half hourly to hourly until the patient stabilises. Monitor cardiac rhythm continuously. Systolic blood pressure less than 80 mmHg usually results in inadequate coronary artery blood flow, cardiac ischaemia, arrhythmias and further complications of low CO.
- Use haemodynamic monitoring to monitor CVP, CO and SVR. If a PA catheter is inserted monitor PAPs and PAWPs. Report changes and parameters causing concern to medical staff.

Watch all those fluids

- Medical staff will determine how much fluid to give by checking blood pressure, urine output, CVP or PAWP and fluid intake and output charts. Whenever the fluid infusion rate is increased, watch for signs of fluid overload, such as an increase in CVP or PAWP. If the patient is hypovolaemic, preload may need to be increased, typically accomplished with I.V. fluids. However, I.V. fluids must be given cautiously, being increased gradually while haemodynamic parameters are closely monitored. In this situation, diuretics aren't given.
- Inscrt a urinary catheter to measure hourly urine output. If output is less than 1/2 ml/kg/hour report to medical staff and give increased fluid infusion rates as prescribed but watch for signs of fluid overload such as an increase in PAWP or CVP. Notify medical staff if urine output doesn't improve.
- Administer a diuretic, such as furosemide, as prescribed, to decrease preload and improve stroke volume and CO.
- Monitor ABG values, FBC, urea and creatinine and electrolyte levels. Administer electrolyte replacement therapy, such as potassium, as prescribed.
- During therapy, assess skin colour and temperature and note any changes. Cold, clammy skin may be a sign of continuing peripheral vascular constriction, indicating progressive shock.

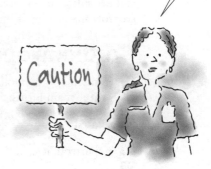

Report a high PAWP immediately. It indicates heart failure, increased systemic vascular resistance, decreased cardiac output and decreased cardiac index.

Don't move!

- If your patient is on the IABP, move them as little as possible. Never flex the patient's 'ballooned' leg at the hip because this may displace or fracture the catheter. Never place the patient in a sitting position for any reason (including chest x-rays) while the balloon is inflated; the balloon will tear through the aorta and result in immediate death.
- During use of the IABP, assess pedal pulses and skin temperature and colour to ensure adequate peripheral circulation. Check the dressing over the insertion site frequently for bleeding, and change it according to local policy. Also check the site for haematoma or signs of infection, and culture any drainage.

When to wean

- If the patient becomes haemodynamically stable, gradually reduce the frequency of balloon inflation to wean them from the IABP as prescribed.
- When weaning the patient from the IABP, watch for ECG changes, chest pain and other signs of recurring cardiac ischaemia as well as for shock.
- Prepare the patient for possible emergency cardiac catheterisation to determine eligibility for PTCA or CABG to reperfuse (restore blood flow to) areas with reversible injury patterns.
- To ease emotional stress, plan care measures to allow frequent rest periods and provide as much privacy as possible. Allow family members to visit and comfort the patient as much as possible.

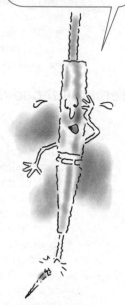

Never flex the patient's 'ballooned' leg at the hip—I may become displaced or break.

Cardiomyopathy

Cardiomyopathy generally refers to disease of the heart muscle fibres. It takes three main forms:

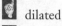 dilated

hypertrophic

restrictive (extremely rare).

Cardiomyopathy is the second most common direct cause of sudden death; CAD is first. Because dilated cardiomyopathy usually isn't diagnosed until its advanced stages, the prognosis is generally poor.

What causes it

Most patients with cardiomyopathy have idiopathic, or primary, disease, but some cases are secondary to identifiable causes. Hypertrophic cardiomyopathy is almost always inherited as a non-sex-linked autosomal dominant trait.

Males and those of Afro-Caribbean origin are at greatest risk for cardiomyopathy; other risk factors include hypertension, pregnancy, viral infections and alcohol use.

How it happens

The disease course in cardiomyopathy depends on the special type, as outlined here.

Dilated cardiomyopathy

Dilated cardiomyopathy primarily affects systolic function. It results from extensively damaged myocardial muscle fibres. Consequently, contractility in the left ventricle decreases.

I'm sorry to report that dilated cardiomyopathy usually isn't diagnosed until it's advanced, so the prognosis is generally poor.

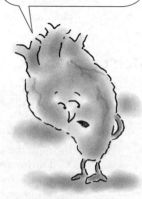

Poor compensation

As systolic function declines, stroke volume, ejection fraction and CO decrease. As end-diastolic volumes increase, pulmonary congestion may occur. The elevated end-diastolic volume is a compensatory response to preserve stroke volume despite a reduced ejection fraction.

The sympathetic nervous system is also stimulated to increase heart rate and contractility.

Kidneys kick in

The kidneys are stimulated to retain sodium and water to maintain CO, and vasoconstriction occurs as the renin–angiotensin system is stimulated. When these compensatory mechanisms can no longer maintain CO, the heart begins to fail.

Detrimental dilation

Left ventricular dilation occurs as venous return and SVR increase. The stretching of the left ventricle eventually leads to mitral insufficiency. Subsequently, the atria also dilate, as more work is required to pump blood into the full ventricles. Cardiomegaly is a consequence of dilation of the atria and ventricles. Blood pooling in the ventricles increases the risk of emboli.

Hypertrophic cardiomyopathy
Hypertrophic cardiomyopathy primarily affects diastolic function. The features of hypertrophic cardiomyopathy include:
- asymmetrical left ventricular hypertrophy
- hypertrophy of the intraventricular septum
- rapid, forceful contractions of the left ventricle
- impaired relaxation
- obstruction of left ventricular outflow.

Fouled-up filling

The hypertrophied ventricle becomes stiff, noncompliant and unable to relax during ventricular filling. Consequently, ventricular filling is reduced and left ventricular filling pressure rises, causing increases in left atrial and pulmonary venous pressures and leading to pulmonary venous congestion and dyspnoea.

The increase in venous pressures and venous congestion leads to tachycardia, which causes a decrease in left ventricular filling time. Reduced ventricular filling during diastole and obstruction to ventricular outflow lead to low CO.

Hypertrophy hazards

If papillary muscles become hypertrophied and don't close completely during contraction, mitral insufficiency occurs. Moreover, intramural coronary arteries are abnormally small and may not be sufficient to supply the

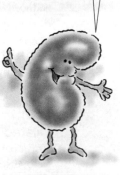

In dilated cardiomyopathy, I try to help maintain cardiac output by retaining water and sodium.

hypertrophied muscle with enough blood and oxygen to meet the increased needs of the hyperdynamic muscle.

Restrictive cardiomyopathy

Restrictive cardiomyopathy is characterised by stiffness of the ventricle caused by left ventricular hypertrophy and endocardial fibrosis and thickening. The ability of the ventricle to relax and fill during diastole is reduced. Furthermore, the rigid myocardium fails to contract completely during systole. As a result, CO decreases.

What to look for

Generally, for patients with dilated or restrictive cardiomyopathy, the onset is insidious. As the disease progresses, exacerbations and hospitalisations are frequent regardless of the type of cardiomyopathy.

Dilated cardiomyopathy

For a patient with dilated cardiomyopathy, signs and symptoms may be overlooked until left-sided heart failure occurs. Be sure to evaluate the patient's current condition and then compare it with that over the past 6–12 months. Signs and symptoms of dilated cardiomyopathy may include:
- shortness of breath, orthopnoea, dyspnoea on exertion, fatigue
- peripheral oedema, hepatomegaly, neck vein distention
- tachycardia, palpitations
- irregular pulse if atrial fibrillation exists
- crackles in lungs.

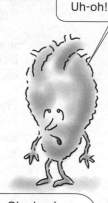

Unfortunately, signs and symptoms may be overlooked untill left-sided heart failure occurs.

Uh-oh!

Hypertrophic cardiomyopathy

Signs and symptoms vary widely among patients with hypertrophic cardiomyopathy. The presenting symptom is commonly syncope or sudden cardiac death. Other possible signs and symptoms include:
- angina
- dyspnoea and orthopnoea
- fatigue
- ventricular arrhythmias
- irregular pulse with atrial fibrillation, palpitations

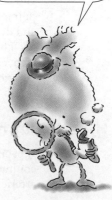

Oh, dear! The first clue to hypertrophic cardiomyopathy may be syncope or sudden cardiac death.

Restrictive cardiomyopathy

A patient with restrictive cardiomyopathy presents with signs of heart failure and other signs and symptoms, including:
- fatigue and weakness
- dyspnoea
- orthopnoea
- chest pain
- hepatomegaly
- peripheral oedema
- heart block.

What tests tell you
These tests are used to diagnose cardiomyopathy:

Dilated cardiomyopathy
• Chest x-ray shows an enlarged heart and pulmonary oedema.
• An ECG will show biventricular enlargement and, commonly, atrial fibrillation.
• Echocardiogram will show decreased ventricular movement and ejection fraction. It will also demonstrate an increase in atrial and ventricular chamber size and abdomen wall motion. It may also demonstrate mitral valve insufficiency.
• Haemodynamic monitoring will show an increased PAWP and PAP and a decreased CO/CI. In late stages, the CVP may also be elevated.
   Chest x-rays, ECGs, echocardiograms and haemodynamic monitoring can give a pretty good inside view of a patient's disease process.

Hypertrophic cardiomyopathy
• Chest x-ray shows an enlarged heart with pronounced left atrial dilation. Pulmonary congestion may also be seen.
• An ECG will show left atrial enlargement and left ventricular hypertrophy. ST and T-wave changes may be seen. Atrial fibrillation and ventricular arrhythmias, such as ventricular tachycardia and ventricular fibrillation are also common.
• An echocardiogram will show an enlarged left atrium and hypertrophy of the intraventricular septum. Left ventricular outflow narrowing, if present, can also be seen. Abnormal wall motion may also be present.
• Cardiac catheterisation with heart biopsy can provide definitive diagnosis.

Restricted cardiomyopathy
• Chest x-ray shows an enlarged heart and pulmonary oedema.
• An ECG will demonstrate low QRS-complex voltage. AV heart blocks are commonly seen.
• Echocardiogram will show atrial enlargement. The walls of the ventricles will be thickened but the interior chamber size will be decreased.
• Haemodynamic monitoring will show increased PAP and PAWP. Left and right end-diastolic pressures will also be elevated.

How it's treated
There's no known cure for cardiomyopathy. Treatment is individualised based on the type of cardiomyopathy and the patient's condition.

Dilated cardiomyopathy
For a patient with dilated cardiomyopathy, treatment may involve:
• management of the underlying cause, if it's known
• ACE inhibitors, and angiotensin II receptor blockers (ARBs), to reduce afterload through vasodilation and increase CO

- diuretics, taken with ACE inhibitors, to reduce fluid retention
- digoxin, for patients not responding to ACE inhibitor and diuretic therapy, to improve myocardial contractility
- isosorbide dinitrate to produce vasodilation
- beta-adrenergic blockers for patients with mild-to-moderate heart failure
- antiarrhythmics, such as amiodarone, used cautiously to control arrhythmias
- cardioversion to convert atrial fibrillation into sinus rhythm
- pacemaker insertion to correct arrhythmias
- anticoagulants to reduce the risk of emboli
- revascularisation, such as CABG surgery, if dilated cardiomyopathy is due to ischaemia
- valvular repair or replacement, if dilated cardiomyopathy is due to valve dysfunction
- lifestyle modifications such as smoking cessation; low-fat, low-sodium diet; physical activity; and abstinence from alcohol
- heart transplantation in patients resistant to medical therapy
- inotropes, such as dobutamine, to improve myocardial contractility and improve heart failure.

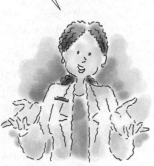

If the patient's condition doesn't improve with medical measures, a heart transplant may be needed.

Hypertrophic cardiomyopathy

For a patient with hypertrophic cardiomyopathy, treatment may involve:
- beta-adrenergic blockers to slow the heart rate, reduce myocardial oxygen demands and increase ventricular filling by relaxing the obstructing muscle, thereby increasing CO
- antiarrhythmic drugs, such as amiodarone, to reduce arrhythmias
- cardioversion to treat atrial fibrillation
- anticoagulation to reduce the risk of systemic embolism with atrial fibrillation
- verapamil and diltiazem to reduce ventricular stiffness and elevated diastolic pressures
- ablation of the AV node and implantation of a dual-chamber pacemaker (controversial), in patients with obstructive hypertrophic cardiomyopathy and ventricular tachycardias, to reduce the outflow gradient by altering the pattern of ventricular contraction
- ICD to correct ventricular arrhythmias
- ventricular myotomy or myectomy (resection of the hypertrophied septum) to ease outflow tract obstruction and relieve symptoms
- mitral valve replacement to correct mitral insufficiency
- heart transplantation for intractable symptoms.

Restrictive cardiomyopathy

For a patient with restrictive cardiomyopathy, treatment may involve:
- management of the underlying cause such as administering desferrioxamine to bind iron in restrictive cardiomyopathy due to haemochromatosis
- digoxin, diuretics and a restricted sodium diet to ease the symptoms of heart failure, although no therapy exists for patients with restricted ventricular filling
- oral vasodilators to control intractable heart failure.

What to do

- Administer drugs, as prescribed, to promote adequate heart function.
- Monitor haemodynamic status.
- Monitor intake and output closely and obtain daily weights; institute fluid restrictions as prescribed.
- Institute continuous cardiac monitoring to allow early identification of arrhythmias.

No sudden moves

- Assess the patient for possible adverse drug reactions, such as orthostatic hypotension associated with use of vasodilators, diuretics or ACE inhibitors. Urge the patient to change positions slowly.
- Be aware that patients with hypertrophic cardiomyopathy should not receive medication that may decrease preload (diuretics, nitrates) or dopamine or digoxin because the increase in myocardial contractility may worsen the outflow obstruction.
- Monitor vital signs for changes, especially a heart rate greater than 100 beats per minute, respiratory rate greater than 20 breaths per minute, and a systolic blood pressure less than 90 mm Hg, all of which suggest heart failure.
- Assist the patient with ADLs to decrease oxygen demand.

> Assess for orthostatic hypotension, a possible adverse effect with some cardiac medications. Urge the patient to change positions slowly.

Oxygen orders

- Administer supplemental oxygen as prescribed and monitor oxygen saturation levels using pulse oximetry. Assess for changes in LOC, such as restlessness or decreased responsiveness, indicating diminished cerebral perfusion.
- Organise care to promote periods of rest for the patient.
- Prepare the patient, as indicated, for insertion of pacemaker, ICD or IABP including transfer to specialist critical care units to facilitate these procedures.

Heart failure

Heart failure occurs when the heart can't pump enough blood to meet the metabolic needs of the body.

Heart failure results in intravascular and interstitial volume overload and poor tissue perfusion. An individual with heart failure experiences reduced exercise tolerance, a reduced quality of life and a shortened life span.

What causes it

The most common cause of heart failure is CAD, but it also occurs in infants, children and adults with congenital and acquired heart defects.

How it happens

Heart failure may be classified into four general categories:

 left-sided heart failure

right-sided heart failure

systolic dysfunction

diastolic dysfunction.

When the left loses its faculties

Left-sided heart failure is a result of ineffective left ventricular contractile function.

As the pumping ability of the left ventricle fails, CO drops. Blood is no longer effectively pumped out into the body; it backs up into the left atrium and then into the lungs, causing pulmonary congestion, dyspnoea and activity intolerance.

If the condition persists, pulmonary oedema and right-sided heart failure may result. Common causes include:
- left ventricular infarction
- hypertension
- aortic and mitral valve stenosis.

When right goes wrong

Right-sided heart failure results from ineffective right ventricular contractile function.

When blood isn't pumped effectively through the right ventricle to the lungs, blood backs up into the right atrium and into the peripheral circulation. The patient gains weight and develops peripheral oedema and engorgement of the kidney, liver and other organs.

Blame it on the left

Right-sided heart failure may be due to an acute right ventricular infarction or a pulmonary embolus. However, the most common cause is profound backward flow due to left-sided heart failure.

Other causes of right-sided heart failure include:
- arrhythmias
- volume overload
- mitral and pulmonary valve stenosis
- cardiomyopathy.

Just can't pump enough

Systolic dysfunction occurs when the left ventricle can't pump enough blood out to the systemic circulation during systole and the ejection fraction falls. Consequently, blood backs up into the pulmonary circulation and pressure

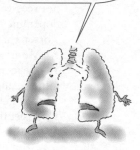

Uh-oh! Blood backs up into the left atrium and then into the lungs when the left ventricle can't pump well.

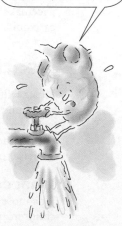

The most common cause of right-sided heart failure is profound backward flow due to left-sided heart failure. Does anybody know a good plumber?

increases in the pulmonary venous system. CO decreases; weakness, fatigue and shortness of breath may occur.

Causes of systolic dysfunction include:

- MI
- dilated cardiomyopathy
- arrhythmias
- aortic valve insufficiency
- acute rheumatic fever.

It all goes to swell from here

Diastolic dysfunction occurs when the ability of the left ventricle to relax and fill during diastole is reduced and the stroke volume falls. Therefore, higher volumes are needed in the ventricles to maintain CO. Consequently, pulmonary congestion and peripheral oedema develop.

Diastolic dysfunction may occur as a result of left ventricular hypertrophy, hypertension, cardiomyopathy, MI or cardiac tamponade.

This type of heart failure is less common than that due to systolic dysfunction, and treatment isn't as clear.

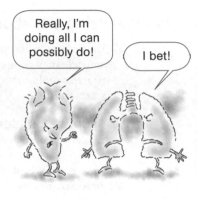

Really, I'm doing all I can possibly do!

I bet!

Compensatory mechanisms

All types of heart failure eventually lead to reduced CO, which triggers compensatory mechanisms that improve CO at the expense of increased ventricular work. The compensatory mechanisms include:

- increased sympathetic activity
- activation of the renin–angiotensin–aldosterone system
- ventricular dilation
- ventricular hypertrophy.

Increased sympathetic activity

Increased sympathetic activity—a response to decreased CO and blood pressure—enhances peripheral vascular resistance, contractility, heart rate and venous return. Signs of increased sympathetic activity, such as cool extremities and clamminess, may indicate impending heart failure.

Renin–angiotensin–aldosterone system

Increased sympathetic activity also restricts blood flow to the kidneys, causing them to secrete renin which, in turn, converts angiotensinogen into angiotensin I, which then becomes angiotensin II—a potent vasoconstrictor. Angiotensin causes the adrenal cortex to release aldosterone, leading to sodium and water retention and an increase in circulating blood volume.

This renal mechanism is helpful; however, if it persists unchecked, it can aggravate heart failure as the heart struggles to pump against the increased volume.

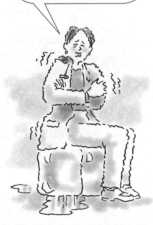

Such signs as cool extremities and clamminess may indicate impending heart failure.

Ventricular dilation

In ventricular dilation, an increase in end-diastolic ventricular volume (preload) causes increased stroke work and stroke volume during contraction.

This stretches cardiac muscle fibres so that the ventricle can accept the increased volume. Eventually, the muscle becomes stretched beyond optimum limits and contractility declines.

Ventricular hypertrophy

In ventricular hypertrophy, an increase in ventricular muscle mass allows the heart to pump against increased resistance to the outflow of blood, improving CO. However, this increased muscle mass also increases the myocardial oxygen requirements.

Compromising situation

An increase in the ventricular diastolic pressure necessary to fill the enlarged ventricle may compromise diastolic coronary blood flow, limiting the oxygen supply to the ventricle and causing ischaemia and impaired muscle contractility.

Counterregulatory substances

In heart failure, counterregulatory substances—prostaglandins, atrial natriuretic factor and BNP—are produced in an attempt to reduce the negative effects of volume overload and vasoconstriction caused by the compensatory mechanisms.

Kidneys' contributions

The kidneys release the prostaglandins prostacyclin and prostaglandin E2, which are potent vasodilators. These vasodilators also act to reduce volume overload produced by the renin–angiotensin–aldosterone system by inhibiting sodium and water reabsorption by the kidneys.

Counteracting hormones

Atrial natriuretic factor is a hormone that's secreted mainly by the atria in response to stimulation of the stretch receptors in the atria caused by excess fluid volume. This hormone works to counteract the negative effects of sympathetic nervous system stimulation and the renin–angiotensin–aldosterone system by producing vasodilation and diuresis.

   BNP is another hormone that's secreted by the ventricle in response to increased ventricular pressures. BNP works in the same manner as atrial natriuretic factor to help counteract the sympathetic nervous system and the renin–angiotensin–aldosterone system.

What to look for

Learn to recognise the signs and symptoms of both right- and left-sided heart failure to ensure that your patient receives attention promptly.

Left-sided heart failure

Look for these early and later signs of disease.

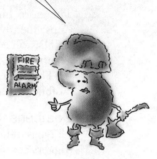

In heart failure, my job is to help the atria and ventricles control vasoconstriction and volume overload by releasing potent counterregulatory substances called *prostaglandins*. I guess you could call me a hero of sorts.

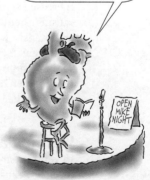

No need to tear up the floorboards to uncover the telltale signs of left- and right-sided heart failure. They're all written here for our edification.

Early bird specials

Early signs and symptoms of left-sided heart failure include:
- dyspnoea
- orthopnoea
- paroxysmal nocturnal dyspnoea
- fatigue
- nonproductive cough.

Late night leftovers

Later clinical manifestations of left-sided heart failure may include:
- crackles on auscultation
- haemoptysis
- displacement of the PMI (point of maximal impact) towards the left anterior axillary line
- tachycardia
- cool, cyanotic skin
- confusion.

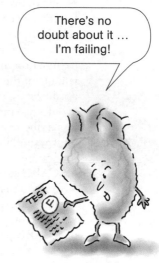

There's no doubt about it ... I'm failing!

Right-sided heart failure

Look for these clinical manifestations of right-sided heart failure:
- neck vein distention
- hepatojugular reflux and hepatomegaly
- right upper quadrant pain
- anorexia and nausea
- nocturia
- weight gain
- pitting oedema
- ascites or anasarca.

What tests tell you

These tests are used to diagnose heart failure:
- Chest x-ray shows increased pulmonary vascular markings, interstitial oedema or pleural effusion and cardiomegaly.
- ECG may indicate hypertrophy, ischaemic changes or infarction, and may also reveal tachycardia.
- Laboratory testing may reveal abnormal liver function, elevated urea and creatinine levels and elevated BNP levels.
- ABG analysis may reveal hypoxaemia from impaired gas exchange and respiratory alkalosis because the patient blows off more carbon dioxide as respiratory rate increases in compensation.
- Echocardiography may reveal left ventricular hypertrophy, dilation and abnormal contractility.
- Haemodynamic monitoring typically demonstrates elevated PAP and PAWP, left ventricular end-diastolic pressure and decreased CO/CI in left-sided heart failure and elevated right atrial pressure or CVP in right-sided heart failure.

How it's treated

The goal of therapy is to improve pump function. Correction of heart failure may involve:

- treatment of the underlying cause, if it's known
- diuretics to reduce fluid volume overload, venous return and preload
- ACE inhibitors for patients with left ventricle dysfunction to reduce production of angiotensin II, resulting in preload and afterload reduction
- beta-adrenergic blockers in patients with mild-to-moderate heart failure caused by left ventricular systolic dysfunction to prevent remodelling
- digoxin for patients with heart failure due to left ventricular systolic dysfunction to increase myocardial contractility, improve CO, reduce the volume of the ventricle and decrease ventricular stretch
- diuretics, nitrates, morphine and oxygen to treat pulmonary oedema
- lifestyle modifications to reduce symptoms of heart failure, such as weight loss if obese; limited sodium (to 2 g/day) and alcohol intake; reduced fat intake; smoking cessation; stress reduction; and development of an exercise programme
- CABG surgery or angioplasty for patients with heart failure due to CAD
- heart transplantation in patients receiving aggressive medical treatment but still experiencing limitations or repeated hospitalisations
- other surgery or invasive procedures, such as cardiomyoplasty, insertion of an IABP, partial left ventriculectomy, use of a mechanical VAD and implantation of an ICD or a biventricular pacemaker.

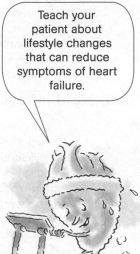

Teach your patient about lifestyle changes that can reduce symptoms of heart failure.

What to do

- Place the patient in semirecumbent position (45 degrees head elevation) to maximise chest expansion and give supplemental oxygen, as prescribed, to ease dyspnoea. Monitor oxygen saturation levels and ABGs as indicated. If respiratory status deteriorates, anticipate the need for ET intubation and mechanical ventilation.

Feel the rhythm

- If the patient develops a new arrhythmia, obtain a 12-lead ECG immediately.
- Monitor haemodynamic status, including CO, CI, pulmonary and systemic vascular pressures closely, noting trends.
- Administer medications as prescribed and evaluate their effects.
- Assess respiratory status frequently, at least every 1–2 hours. Auscultate lungs for abnormal breath sounds, such as crackles, wheezes and rhonchi. Encourage coughing and deep breathing.
- Obtain daily weights and observe for peripheral oedema.
- Assess hourly urine output. Also, monitor fluid intake, including I.V. fluids.
- Frequently monitor urea and serum creatinine, liver function tests, and serum potassium, sodium, chloride, magnesium levels daily.

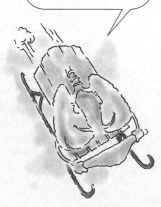

If the patient's respiratory status takes a downhill slide, be ready to institute intubation and mechanical ventilation.

Event planner

- Organise all activities to provide maximum rest periods. Assess for signs of activity intolerance, such as increased shortness of breath, chest pain, increased arrhythmias, heart rate greater than 120 beats per minute, and ST-segment changes, and have the patient stop activity.
- To prevent deep vein thrombosis caused by vascular congestion, assist the patient with limb exercises. Enforce bed rest and apply antiembolism stockings or intermittent compression devices.
- Prepare the patient for possible surgical intervention or insertion of IABP or ICD if indicated.

Pericarditis

Pericarditis is an inflammation of the pericardium, the fibroserous sac that envelops, supports and protects the heart. It occurs in acute and chronic forms. Acute pericarditis can be fibrinous or effusive, with purulent, serous or haemorrhagic exudate. Chronic constrictive pericarditis is characterised by dense fibrous pericardial thickening.

What causes it

Pericarditis may result from:
- idiopathic factors (most common in acute pericarditis)
- bacterial, fungal or viral infection (infectious pericarditis)
- neoplasms (primary disease or metastases from lungs, breasts or other organs)
- high-dose radiation to the chest
- uraemia
- hypersensitivity or autoimmune disease, such as acute rheumatic fever (the most common cause of pericarditis in children), systemic lupus erythematosis and rheumatoid arthritis
- previous cardiac injury, such as MI (Dressler's syndrome), trauma or surgery (postcardiotomy syndrome) that leaves the pericardium intact but causes blood to leak into the pericardial cavity.

How it happens

Here's what happens in pericarditis:
- Pericardial tissue damaged by bacteria or other substances results in the release of chemical mediators of inflammation (prostaglandins, histamines, bradykinins and serotonin) into the surrounding tissue, thereby initiating the inflammatory process.
- Friction occurs as the inflamed pericardial layers rub against each other.
- Histamines and other chemical mediators dilate vessels and increase vessel permeability. Vessel walls then leak fluids and protein (including fibrinogen) into tissues, causing extracellular oedema.
- Macrophages already present in the tissue begin to phagocytise the invading bacteria and are joined by neutrophils and monocytes.

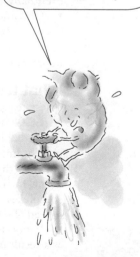

Pericardial effusion develops if fluid accumulates in the pericardial cavity.

- After several days, the area fills with an exudate composed of necrotic tissue and dead and dying bacteria, neutrophils and macrophages.
- Eventually, the contents of the cavity autolyse and are gradually reabsorbed into healthy tissue.
- Pericardial effusion develops if fluid accumulates in the pericardial cavity.
- Cardiac tamponade results when there's a rapid accumulation of fluid in the pericardial space, compressing the heart and preventing it from filling during diastole, and resulting in a drop in CO.
- Chronic constrictive pericarditis develops if the pericardium becomes thick and stiff from chronic or recurrent pericarditis, encasing the heart in a stiff shell and preventing the heart from properly filling during diastole. This causes an increase in both left- and right-sided filling pressures, leading to a drop in stroke volume and CO.

What to look for

- The patient with acute pericarditis typically complains of sharp, sudden pain, usually starting over the sternum and radiating to the neck, shoulders, back and arms. The pain is usually pleuritic, increasing with deep inspiration and decreasing when the patient sits up and leans forward. This decrease occurs because leaning forward pulls the heart away from the diaphragmatic pleurae of the lungs. A pericardial friction rub may be heard over the left lateral sternal border.

Cardiac complications

- Pericardial effusion, the major complication of acute pericarditis, may produce effects of heart failure, such as dyspnoea, orthopnoea and tachycardia. It may also produce ill-defined substernal chest pain and a feeling of chest fullness.
- If fluid accumulates rapidly, cardiac tamponade may occur, causing pallor, clammy skin, hypotension, pulsus paradoxus, jugular vein distention and, eventually, cardiovascular collapse and death.
- Chronic constrictive pericarditis causes a gradual increase in systemic venous pressure and produces symptoms similar to those of chronic right-sided heart failure, including fluid retention, ascites and hepatomegaly.

What tests tell you

These tests are used to diagnose pericarditis:
- ECG may reveal diffuse ST-segment elevation in the limb leads and most precordial leads that reflect the inflammatory process. Upright T waves are present in most leads. QRS size may be diminished when pericardial effusion exists. Arrhythmias, such as atrial fibrillation and sinus arrhythmias, may occur. In chronic constrictive pericarditis, there may be low-voltage QRS complexes, T-wave inversion or flattening and P mitral waves (wide P waves) in leads I, II and V_6.
- Laboratory testing may reveal an elevated erythrocyte sedimentation rate as a result of the inflammatory process or a normal or elevated WBC count,

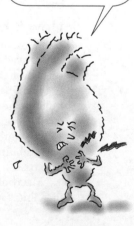

That hurts! A patient with acute pericarditis typically reports sharp, sudden pain, usually starting over the sternum and radiating to the neck, shoulders, back and arms.

especially in infectious pericarditis. Elevated urea may point to uraemia as a cause of pericarditis. C-reactive protein levels may be elevated, indicating inflammation.

- Blood cultures may be used to identify an infectious cause.
- Echocardiography may show an echo-free space between the ventricular wall and the pericardium, and reduced pumping action of the heart. It may also help identify if a pleural effusion is present.
- Chest x-rays may be normal with acute pericarditis. The cardiac silhouette may be enlarged, with a water bottle shape caused by fluid accumulation, if pleural effusion is present.

How it's treated
Treatment for a patient with pericarditis aims to:
- relieve symptoms
- prevent or correct pericardial effusion and cardiac tamponade
- manage the underlying disease.

Bed rest and drug therapy
In idiopathic pericarditis, post-MI pericarditis and post-thoracotomy pericarditis, treatment is twofold, including:
- bed rest as long as fever and pain persist
- administration of nonsteroidal antiinflammatory drugs to relieve pain and reduce inflammation.

If symptoms continue, corticosteroids may be prescribed to provide rapid and effective relief. Corticosteroids must be used cautiously because pericarditis may recur when drug therapy stops.

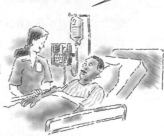

You should really be in an upright position to relieve dyspnoea and chest pain.

Further treatments
When infectious pericarditis results from disease of the left pleural space, mediastinal abscesses, or septicaemia, the patient requires antibiotics, surgical drainage or both.

If cardiac tamponade develops, the doctor may perform emergency pericardiocentesis and may inject antibiotics directly into the pericardial sac.

Heavy-duty treatments

Recurrent pericarditis may necessitate partial pericardiectomy, which creates a window that allows fluid to drain into the pleural space. In constrictive pericarditis, total pericardiectomy may be necessary to permit the heart to fill and contract adequately.

What to do
- Maintain the patient on bed rest until fever and pain diminish. Assist the patient with hygiene and daily needs to reduce myocardial oxygen demand.
- Place the patient in an upright position to relieve dyspnoea and chest pain. Administer supplemental oxygen as needed based on oxygen saturation or blood gases.

• Administer analgesics to relieve pain and nonsteroidal antiinflammatory drugs (NSAIDs), as prescribed to reduce inflammation. Administer steroids as prescribed if the patient fails to respond to NSAIDs.

• If your patient has a PA catheter, monitor haemodynamic status. Assess the patient's cardiovascular status frequently, watching for signs of cardiac tamponade.

• Administer antibiotics, as prescribed, on time to maintain consistent drug levels in the blood.

• Institute continuous cardiac monitoring to evaluate for changes in ECG. Look for the return of ST segments to baseline with T-wave flattening by the end of the first 7 days.

• Keep a pericardiocentesis set available if pericardial effusion is suspected, and prepare the patient for pericardiocentesis as indicated.

• Provide appropriate postoperative care, similar to that given after cardiothoracic surgery.

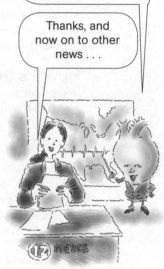

Look for a return of ST segments to baseline levels with T waves flattening by the end of the week, Joy.

Thanks, and now on to other news . . .

Valvular heart disease

In valvular heart disease, three types of mechanical disruption can occur:

1 stenosis, or narrowing, of the valve opening

2 incomplete closure of the valve

3 prolapse of the valve.

What causes it

Valvular heart disease in children and adolescents most commonly results from congenital heart defects. In adults, rheumatic heart disease is a common cause.

Other causes are grouped according to the type of valvular heart disease and include the following:

Mitral insufficiency
• Hypertrophic cardiomyopathy
• Papillary muscle dysfunction
• Left ventricle dilation from left ventricle failure

Mitral stenosis
• Endocarditis
• Left atrium tumours
• Mitral annulus calcification

Aortic insufficiency
• Calcification
• Endocarditis
• Hypertension
• Drugs, especially appetite suppressants

Aortic stenosis
• Calcification

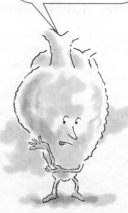

Valvular heart diseases are categorised according to the specific valves (mitral, aortic or pulmonic) and type of disorder (stenosis or insufficiency) the patient has.

Pulmonary stenosis
• Carcinoid syndrome

How it happens
Valvular heart disease may result from numerous conditions, which vary and are different for each type of valve disorder. Pathophysiology of valvular heart disease varies according to the valve and the disorder.

Mitral insufficiency
In mitral insufficiency, blood from the left ventricle flows back into the left atrium during systole, causing the atrium to enlarge to accommodate the backflow. As a result, the left ventricle also dilates to accommodate the increased volume of blood from the atrium and to compensate for diminishing CO.

Ventricular hypertrophy and increased end-diastolic pressure result in increased PAP, eventually leading to left-sided and right-sided heart failure.

Although the pathophysiology varies with the type of valve and specific disorder, the end result seems to be the same—some form of heart failure and pulmonary involvement.

Mitral stenosis
In mitral stenosis, the valve narrows as a result of valvular abnormalities, fibrosis or calcification. This obstructs blood flow from the left atrium to the left ventricle. Consequently, left atrial volume and pressure increase and the chamber dilates.

Greater resistance to blood flow causes pulmonary hypertension, right ventricular hypertrophy and right-sided heart failure. Also, inadequate filling of the left ventricle produces low CO.

Aortic insufficiency
In aortic insufficiency, blood flows back into the left ventricle during diastole, causing fluid overload in the ventricle which, in turn, dilates and hypertrophies. The excess volume causes fluid overload in the left atrium and, finally, the pulmonary system. Left-sided heart failure and pulmonary oedema eventually result.

Aortic stenosis
In aortic stenosis, elevated left ventricular pressure tries to overcome the resistance of the narrowed valvular opening. The added workload increases the demand for oxygen, and diminished CO causes poor coronary artery perfusion, ischaemia of the left ventricle and left-sided heart failure.

Pulmonic stenosis
In pulmonic stenosis, obstructed right ventricular outflow causes right ventricular hypertrophy in an attempt to overcome resistance to the narrow valvular opening. The ultimate result is right-sided heart failure.

What to look for
The history and physical examination findings vary according to the type of valvular defects.

Mitral insufficiency

Signs and symptoms of mitral insufficiency include:
- orthopnoea
- dyspnoea
- fatigue
- angina (rare)
- palpitations
- right-sided heart failure (jugular vein distention, peripheral oedema, hepatomegaly).

Mitral stenosis

Signs and symptoms of mitral stenosis include:
- dyspnoea on exertion, paroxysmal nocturnal dyspnoea, orthopnoea
- fatigue, weakness
- right-sided heart failure
- crackles on auscultation
- palpitations.

Aortic insufficiency

Signs and symptoms of aortic insufficiency include:
- dyspnoea
- cough
- left-sided heart failure
- pulsus biferiens (rapidly rising and collapsing pulses)
- chest pain with exertion
- crackles on auscultation.

Aortic stenosis

Signs and symptoms of aortic stenosis include:
- dyspnoea and paroxysmal nocturnal dyspnoea
- fatigue
- syncope
- angina
- palpitations and cardiac arrhythmias
- left-sided heart failure
- chest pain with exertion.

Pulmonary stenosis

Although a patient with pulmonary stenosis may be asymptomatic, possible signs and symptoms include:
- dyspnoea on exertion
- right-sided heart failure.

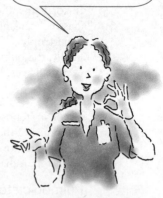

Be aware that a patient with pulmonary stenosis may have no symptoms at all.

What tests tell you

The diagnosis of valvular heart disease can be based on the results of:
- cardiac catheterisation
- chest x-rays
- echocardiography
- ECG.

How it's treated

Treatments for patients with valvular heart disease may include:
- digoxin, a low-sodium diet, diuretics, vasodilators and especially ACE inhibitors to correct left-sided heart failure
- oxygen administration in acute situations, to increase oxygenation
- anticoagulants to prevent thrombus formation around diseased or replaced valves
- prophylactic antibiotics before and after surgery or dental care to prevent endocarditis
- nitroglycerin to relieve angina in conditions such as aortic stenosis
- beta-adrenergic blockers or digoxin to slow the ventricular rate in atrial fibrillation or atrial flutter
- cardioversion to convert atrial fibrillation into sinus rhythm
- open or closed commissurotomy to separate thick or adherent mitral valve leaflets
- balloon valvuloplasty to enlarge the orifice of a stenotic mitral, aortic or pulmonary valve
- annuloplasty or valvuloplasty to reconstruct or repair the valve in mitral insufficiency
- valve replacement with a prosthetic valve for mitral and aortic valve disease.

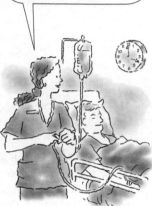

Treatment for valvular heart disease typically includes giving various combinations of medications and, in some cases, valve repair or replacement.

What to do

- Assess the patient's vital signs, ABG values, pulse oximetry, intake and output, daily weights, blood chemistry studies, chest x-rays and ECG.
- Place the patient in an upright position to relieve dyspnoea if needed. Administer oxygen to prevent tissue hypoxia as needed and indicated by ABGs and pulse oximetry.
- Institute continuous cardiac monitoring to evaluate for arrhythmias; if any occur, administer appropriate therapy according to prescription and local policies.
- For a patient with aortic insufficiency, observe the ECG for arrhythmias, which can increase the risk of pulmonary oedema, and for fever and infection.
- If the patient has mitral stenosis, watch closely for signs of pulmonary dysfunction caused by pulmonary hypertension, tissue ischaemia caused by emboli and adverse reactions to drug therapy.
- For a patient with mitral insufficiency, observe for signs and symptoms of left-sided heart failure, pulmonary oedema and adverse reactions to drug therapy.

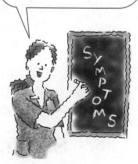

Watch those valves. If the patient has mitral stenosis, observe closely for signs and symptoms of pulmonary dysfunction, emboli and adverse reactions to drug therapy.

Quick quiz

1. Which sign is characteristic of cardiac tamponade?
   - A. Shortness of breath
   - B. Beck's triad
   - C. Palpitations
   - D. Bounding peripheral pulse

Answer: B. Beck's triad comprises the three classic signs of cardiac tamponade: elevated CVP with jugular vein distention, muffled heart sounds and a drop in systolic blood pressure.

2. Identify the arrhythmia in the rhythm strip below.

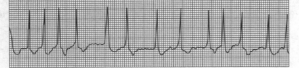

    A. Atrial flutter
    B. Sinus tachycardia
    C. AV junctional rhythm
    D. Atrial fibrillation

Answer: D. The rhythm strip reveals atrial fibrillation. No P waves are identifiable; ventricular rate is varied; QRS complexes are uniform in shape but occur at irregular intervals.

3. Which drug is indicated in hypotension especially septic shock?
    A. Noradrenaline
    B. Amiodarone
    C. Digoxin
    D. Milrinone

Answer: A. Noradrenaline is a vasopressor indicated in hypotension especially in septic shock.

4. Which parameter is elevated in right-sided heart failure?
    A. CVP
    B. Left ventricular end-diastolic pressure
    C. PAWP
    D. Cardiac output

Answer: A. CVP is elevated in right-sided heart failure.

5. ACE inhibitors correct heart failure by:
    A. increasing preload.
    B. causing vasoconstriction.
    C. increasing afterload.
    D. reducing afterload.

Answer: D. ACE inhibitors reduce afterload through vasodilation, thereby reducing heart failure.

Good job! Take a breather and then move on to the respiratory system.

Scoring

☆☆☆ If you answered all five questions correctly, you're all heart! (You'd have to be to make it through this cardiovascular workout!)

☆☆ If you answered four questions correctly, take heart. You have all the blood and gumption you need to succeed.

☆ If you answered fewer than four questions correctly, have yourself a heart-to-heart, then try again. You'll do better next time.

5 Respiratory system

Just the facts

In this chapter, you'll learn:

♦ structure and function of the respiratory system
♦ assessment of the respiratory system
♦ diagnostic tests and procedures for the respiratory system
♦ respiratory disorders and treatments.

Understanding the respiratory system

The respiratory system delivers oxygen to the bloodstream and removes excess carbon dioxide from the body.

Respiratory system structures

The structures of the respiratory system include the airways and lungs, bony thorax and respiratory muscles. (See *A close look at the respiratory system*, page 268.)

Airways and lungs

The airways of the respiratory system consist of two parts: the upper and lower airways. The two lungs are parts of the lower airway and share space in the thoracic cavity with the heart and great vessels, trachea, oesophagus and bronchi.

Upper airway

The upper airway warms, filters and humidifies inhaled air and then sends it to the lower airway. It also contains the structures that enable a person to make sounds. Upper airway structures include the nasopharynx (nose), oropharynx (mouth), laryngopharynx and larynx.

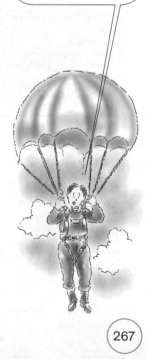

What a system the body has going! The upper airways warm, filter and humidify air before sending it to the lower airways.

A close look at the respiratory system

Get to know the basic structures and functions of the respiratory system so you can perform a comprehensive respiratory assessment and identify abnormalities. The major structures of the upper and lower airways are illustrated below. An alveolus is shown in the inset.

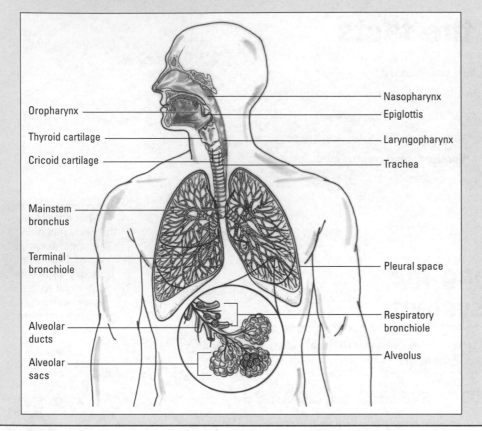

Oropharynx

Thyroid cartilage

Cricoid cartilage

Mainstem bronchus

Terminal bronchiole

Alveolar ducts

Alveolar sacs

Nasopharynx

Epiglottis

Laryngopharynx

Trachea

Pleural space

Respiratory bronchiole

Alveolus

In the zone

The larynx, which is located at the top of the trachea, houses the vocal cords. It's the transition point between the upper and lower airways.

The larynx is composed of nine cartilage segments. The largest is the shield-shaped thyroid cartilage. The cricoid cartilage, which is the only complete ring at the lower end of the larynx, attaches to the first cartilaginous ring of the trachea.

To flap and protect

The epiglottis is a flap of tissue that closes over the top of the larynx when the patient swallows. This protects the patient from aspirating food or fluid into the lower airways.

Lower airway

The lower airway includes the:
- trachea
- bronchi
- lungs.

Low-down on lower airway

The lower airway begins with the trachea, which divides at the carina to form the right and left mainstem bronchi of the lungs. The right mainstem bronchus is shorter, wider and more vertical than the left.

The mainstem bronchi branch out in the lungs, forming the:
- lobar bronchi
- tertiary bronchi
- terminal bronchioles
- respiratory bronchioles
- alveolar ducts
- alveoli.

Lungs and lobes

The right lung is larger and has three lobes: upper, middle and lower. The left lung is smaller and has only two lobes: upper and lower.

Plenty of pleura

Each lung is wrapped in a lining called the *visceral pleura* and all areas of the thoracic cavity that come in contact with the lungs are lined with parietal pleura.

A small amount of pleural fluid fills the area between the two layers of the pleura. This allows the layers to slide smoothly over each other as the chest expands and contracts. The parietal pleura also contain nerve endings that transmit pain signals when inflammation occurs.

All about alveoli

The alveoli are the gas exchange units of the lungs. The lungs in a typical adult contain about 300 million alveoli.

Alveoli consist of type I and type II epithelial cells:
- Type I cells form the alveolar walls, through which gas exchange occurs.
- Type II cells produce surfactant, a lipid-type substance that coats the alveoli. During inspiration, the alveolar surfactant allows the alveoli to expand uniformly. During expiration, the surfactant prevents alveolar collapse.

In circulation

Oxygen-depleted blood enters the lungs from the pulmonary artery of the right ventricle, then flows through the main pulmonary arteries into the smaller vessels of the pleural cavities and the main bronchi, through the arterioles and, eventually, to the capillary networks surrounding the alveoli.

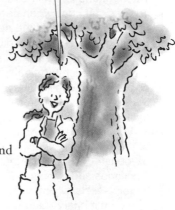

The mainstem bronchi branch out in the lungs to form smaller airways.

Trading gases

Gas exchange (oxygen and carbon dioxide diffusion) takes place in the alveoli. The factors that affect gas exchange are: the surface area available for gas exchange, the thickness of the alveolocapillary membrane and the difference in partial pressures of gases on either side of the membrane. After passing through the pulmonary capillaries, oxygenated blood flows through progressively larger vessels, enters the main pulmonary veins and, finally, flows into the left atrium. (See *Tracking pulmonary circulation*.)

Bony thorax

The bony thorax is composed of:
- clavicles
- sternum
- scapula
- 12 sets of ribs
- 12 thoracic vertebrae.

Imagine that!

Parts of the thorax and some imaginary vertical lines on the chest are used to describe the locations of pulmonary assessment findings. (See *Respiratory assessment landmarks*, page 271.)

> Hundreds of millions of tiny alveoli conduct gas exchange in the lungs.

Tracking pulmonary circulation

The right and left pulmonary arteries carry deoxygenated blood from the right side of the heart to the lungs. These arteries divide to form distal branches called *arterioles,* which terminate as a concentrated capillary network in the alveoli and alveolar sac, where gas exchange occurs.

Venules—the end branches of the pulmonary veins — collect oxygenated blood from the capillaries and transport it to larger vessels, which carry it to the pulmonary veins. The pulmonary veins enter the left side of the heart, where oxygenated blood is distributed throughout the body.

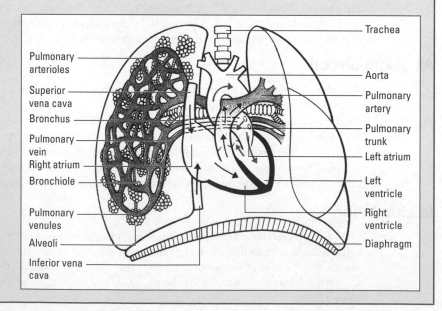

Labels: Pulmonary arterioles; Superior vena cava; Bronchus; Pulmonary vein; Right atrium; Bronchiole; Pulmonary venules; Alveoli; Inferior vena cava; Trachea; Aorta; Pulmonary artery; Pulmonary trunk; Left atrium; Left ventricle; Right ventricle; Diaphragm

Respiratory assessment landmarks

Use these figures to find the common landmarks used in respiratory assessment.

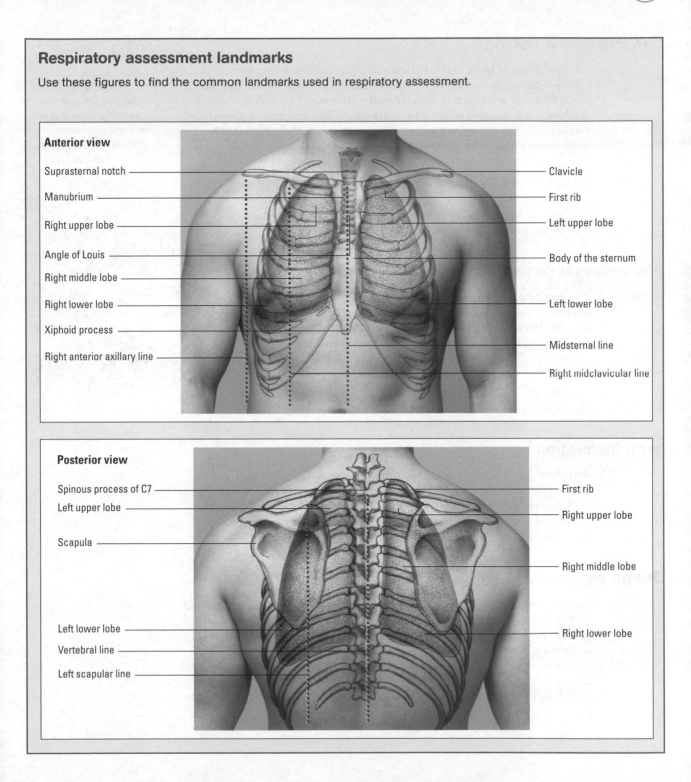

Anterior view

- Suprasternal notch
- Manubrium
- Right upper lobe
- Angle of Louis
- Right middle lobe
- Right lower lobe
- Xiphoid process
- Right anterior axillary line

- Clavicle
- First rib
- Left upper lobe
- Body of the sternum
- Left lower lobe
- Midsternal line
- Right midclavicular line

Posterior view

- Spinous process of C7
- Left upper lobe
- Scapula
- Left lower lobe
- Vertebral line
- Left scapular line

- First rib
- Right upper lobe
- Right middle lobe
- Right lower lobe

Can you take a ribbing?

Ribs are made of bone and cartilage and allow the chest to expand and contract during each breath. All ribs are attached to vertebrae. The first seven ribs also are attached directly to the sternum. The eighth, ninth and tenth ribs are attached to the ribs above them. The eleventh and twelfth ribs are called *floating ribs* because they aren't attached to any other bones in the front.

Respiratory muscles

The primary muscles used in breathing are the diaphragm and the external intercostal muscles. These muscles contract when the patient inhales and relax when the patient exhales.

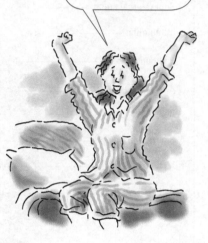

Ho-hum. The diaphragm and the external intercostal muscles contract on inhalation and relax on exhalation.

Brain—breath connection

The respiratory centre in the medulla initiates each breath by sending messages over the phrenic nerve to the primary respiratory muscles. Impulses from the phrenic nerve regulate the rate and depth of breathing, depending on the carbon dioxide and pH levels in the cerebrospinal fluid.

Accessory inspiratory muscles

Here's how other muscles assist in breathing:

In on inspiration

Accessory inspiratory muscles (the trapezius, sternocleidomastoid and scalenes) elevate the scapula, clavicle, sternum and upper ribs. This expands the front-to-back diameter of the chest when use of the diaphragm and intercostal muscles isn't effective enough, as in exercise or in respiratory failure because of poor gas exchange.

Out on expiration

Expiration occurs when the diaphragm and external intercostal muscles relax. If the patient has an airway obstruction, they may also use the abdominal muscles and internal intercostal muscles to exhale. (See *Understanding the mechanics of breathing*, page 273.)

Respiration

Effective respiration requires gas exchange in the lungs (external respiration) and in the tissues (internal respiration).

Understanding the mechanics of breathing

Mechanical forces, such as movement of the diaphragm and intercostal muscles, drive the breathing process. In these depictions, a plus sign (+) indicates positive pressure and a minus sign (–) indicates negative pressure.

At rest   **Inhalation**   **Exhalation**

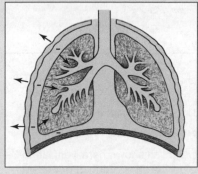 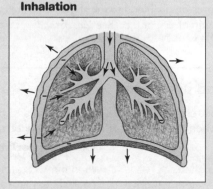 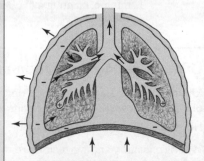

- Inspiratory muscles relax.
- Atmospheric pressure is maintained in the tracheobronchial tree.
- No air movement occurs.

- Inspiratory muscles contract.
- The diaphragm descends.
- Negative alveolar pressure is maintained.
- Air moves into the lungs.

- Inspiratory muscles relax, causing the lungs to recoil to their resting size and position.
- The diaphragm ascends.
- Positive alveolar pressure is maintained.
- Air moves out of the lungs.

O_2 to lungs

Three external respiration processes are needed to maintain adequate oxygenation and acid–base balance:

☝ Ventilation (gas distribution into and out of the pulmonary airways)

✌ Pulmonary perfusion (blood flow from the right side of the heart, through the pulmonary circulation and into the left side of the heart)

🤟 Diffusion (gas movement from an area of greater to lesser concentration through a semipermeable membrane).

O_2 to tissues

Internal respiration occurs only through diffusion, when the red blood cells (RBCs) release oxygen and absorb carbon dioxide.

Ventilation and perfusion

Gravity affects oxygen and carbon dioxide transport in a positive way by causing more deoxygenated blood to travel to the lower and middle lung lobes than to the upper lobes. That's why ventilation and perfusion differ in various parts of the lungs.

Match game

Areas where perfusion and ventilation are similar have a ventilation–perfusion ($\dot{V}/\dot{Q}$) match; gas exchange is most efficient in such areas.

For example, in normal lung function, the alveoli receive air at a rate of about 4 L/minute while the capillaries supply blood to the alveoli at a rate of about 5 L/minute, creating a ($\dot{V}/\dot{Q}$) ratio of 4:5, or 0.8. (See *Understanding ventilation and perfusion*.)

Understanding ventilation and perfusion

Effective gas exchange depends on the relationship between ventilation and perfusion, or the $\dot{V}/\dot{Q}$ ratio. The diagrams below show what happens when the $\dot{V}/\dot{Q}$ ratio is normal and abnormal.

Normal ventilation and perfusion

When ventilation and perfusion are matched, unoxygenated blood from the venous system returns to the right side of the heart and through the pulmonary artery to the lungs, carrying carbon dioxide (CO_2). The arteries branch into the alveolar capillaries. Gas exchange takes place in the alveolar capillaries.

Inadequate perfusion (dead-space ventilation)

When the $\dot{V}/\dot{Q}$ ratio is high, as shown here, ventilation is normal but alveolar perfusion is reduced or absent. Note the narrowed capillary, indicating poor perfusion. This commonly results from a perfusion defect, such as pulmonary embolism or a disorder that decreases cardiac output.

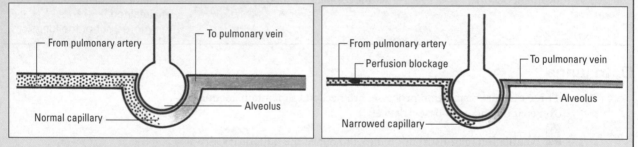

Inadequate ventilation (shunt)

When the $\dot{V}/\dot{Q}$ ratio is low, pulmonary circulation is adequate but not enough oxygen (O_2) is available to the alveoli for normal diffusion. A portion of the blood flowing through the pulmonary vessels doesn't become oxygenated.

Inadequate ventilation and perfusion (silent unit)

A silent unit indicates an absence of ventilation and perfusion to the lung area. A silent unit may help compensate for a $\dot{V}/\dot{Q}$ balance by delivering blood flow to better ventilated lung areas.

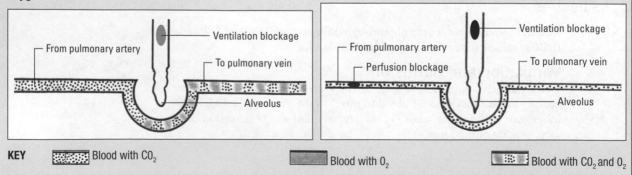

KEY ▨ Blood with CO_2 ▬ Blood with O_2 ▨ Blood with CO_2 and O_2

Mismatch mayhem

A (V̇/Q̇) mismatch, resulting from ventilation–perfusion dysfunction or altered lung mechanics, causes most of the impaired gas exchange in respiratory disorders.

Ineffective gas exchange between the alveoli and pulmonary capillaries can affect all body systems by changing the amount of oxygen delivered to living cells. Ineffective gas exchange causes three outcomes:

- *Shunting* (reduced ventilation to a lung unit) causes unoxygenated blood to move from the right side of the heart to the left side of the heart and into systemic circulation. Shunting may result from a physical defect that allows unoxygenated blood to bypass fully functioning alveoli. It may also result when airway obstruction prevents oxygen from reaching an adequately perfused area of the lung. Common causes of shunting include acute respiratory distress syndrome (ARDS), atelectasis, pneumonia and pulmonary oedema.
- *Dead-space ventilation* (reduced perfusion to a lung unit) occurs when alveoli don't have adequate blood supply for gas exchange to occur, such as with pulmonary emboli and pulmonary infarction.
- A *silent unit* (a combination of shunting and dead-space ventilation) occurs when little or no ventilation and perfusion are present, such as in cases of pneumothorax and severe ARDS.

> Gas exchange is most efficient where perfusion and ventilation match.

Oxygen transport

Almost all the oxygen collected in the lungs binds with haemoglobin to form oxyhaemoglobin. The extent to which oxygen is saturated with haemoglobin is measured by oxygen saturations—SaO_2. This is not the quantity of oxygen carried—since that measurement depends on haemoglobin levels—rather it tells us how well the available haemoglobin carries oxygen. However, a very small portion of the oxygen collected in the lungs dissolves in the plasma. The portion of oxygen that dissolves in the plasma can be measured as the partial pressure of arterial oxygen (PaO_2) in blood. Oxygen needs to dissolve in plasma before it can then bind to haemoglobin. Because of this, PaO_2 is a really good measure of how well oxygen diffuses across the alveolocapillary membrane. SaO_2 is affected by many other factors, including oxygen utilisation at the tissues, and therefore isn't as reflective of oxygen diffusion.

Riding the RBC express

After oxygen binds to haemoglobin, RBCs carry it by way of the circulatory system to tissues throughout the body. Internal respiration occurs by cellular diffusion when RBCs release oxygen and absorb the carbon dioxide produced by cellular metabolism. The RBCs then transport the carbon dioxide back to the lungs for removal during expiration.

Acid–base balance

Because carbon dioxide is 20 times more soluble than oxygen, it dissolves in the blood, where most of it forms bicarbonate (a base) and smaller amounts form carbonic acid.

Acid–base controller

The lungs control bicarbonate levels by converting bicarbonate to carbon dioxide and water for excretion. In response to signals from the medulla, the lungs can change the rate and depth of ventilation. This controls acid–base balance by adjusting the amount of carbon dioxide that's lost.

In metabolic alkalosis, which results from excess bicarbonate retention, the rate and depth of ventilation decrease so that carbon dioxide is retained. This increases carbonic acid levels.

In metabolic acidosis (resulting from excess acid retention or excess bicarbonate loss), the lungs increase the rate and depth of ventilation to exhale excess carbon dioxide, thereby reducing carbonic acid levels.

Off balance

Inadequately functioning lungs can produce acid–base imbalances. For example, *hypoventilation* (reduced rate and depth of ventilation) results in carbon dioxide retention, causing respiratory acidosis. Conversely, *hyperventilation* (increased rate and depth of ventilation) leads to increased exhalation of carbon dioxide and causes respiratory alkalosis.

> Poorly functioning lungs can produce acid–base imbalances.

Respiratory assessment

An important domain of the registered nurse's role is the assessment and monitoring of important physiological systems. However, this is usually a collaborative process reflected in the multidisciplinary approach which is a salient feature of critical care. When assessing and monitoring the respiratory system it is important to focus on the key physiological concepts outlined earlier.

This domain of practice involves thinking critically about how the system is functioning, what is 'normal' for the patient and how chronic or acute health problems might be affecting important functions.

It is perhaps best to think of assessment as a single episode of information gathering and critical thinking about the information in order to form a judgement about the patient. Monitoring on the other hand is a process of considering assessment findings over a period of time.

Respiratory monitoring is a major part of critical care nursing and will usually take place continually with parameters recorded on charts every one to two hours, though it could be more frequent in extreme situations where things are changing very quickly or life is in acute danger. The types of monitoring and their clinical use will be discussed later. First it is important to think about a framework for assessment.

Being systematic

Assessment of the respiratory system includes knowing:
- History of the present complaint
- Health history
- Clinical assessment and monitoring
- Results and significance of diagnostic tests and investigations

History of the present complaint

In essence you need to know why the patient has come into hospital and into critical care, to know any timescales and key events. In particular, find out any symptoms and how these relate to respiratory function.

Health history

Build your patient's health history by asking short, open-ended questions. Conduct the interview in several short sessions if you have to, depending on the severity of your patient's condition. Ask their family to provide information if your patient can't.

Respiratory disorders may be caused or exacerbated by obesity, smoking and workplace conditions so be sure to ask about these conditions.

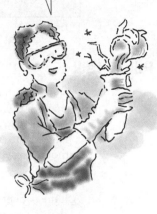

Respiratory disorders may be caused or worsened by obesity, smoking and workplace conditions.

Current health status

Begin by asking your patient about their current problem. Because many respiratory disorders are chronic, ask how the patient's latest acute episode compares with previous episodes and what relief measures are helpful and unhelpful.

Chronic complaint department

Patients with respiratory disorders commonly report such complaints as:
- shortness of breath
- cough
- sputum production
- wheezing
- chest pain
- sleep disturbance.

Shortness of breath

Assess your patient's shortness of breath by asking them to rate their usual level of dyspnoea on a scale of 0–10, in which 0 means no dyspnoea and 10 means the worst they have experienced. Then ask them to rate their current level of dyspnoea. Other scales grade dyspnoea as it relates to activity, such as climbing a set of stairs or walking up a hill. (See *Grading dyspnoea*, page 278.)

In addition to using a severity scale, ask these questions: What do you do to relieve the shortness of breath? How well does it usually work?

The number of pillows you need to sleep indicates the severity of your orthopnoea.

Pillow talk

A patient with *orthopnoea* (shortness of breath when lying down) tends to sleep with their upper body elevated. Ask this patient how many pillows they use. The answer reflects the severity of the orthopnoea. For instance, a patient who uses three pillows can be said to have 'three-pillow orthopnoea'.

Cough

Ask the patient with a cough these questions: At what time of day do you cough most often? Is the cough productive? Has it changed recently (if chronic)? If so, how? What makes the cough better? What makes it worse?

Sputum production

If a patient produces sputum, ask them to estimate the amount produced in teaspoons or some other common measurement. Also ask these questions: What's the colour and consistency of the sputum? Has it changed recently (if chronic)? If so, how? Do you cough up blood? If so, how much and how often?

Wheezing

If a patient wheezes, ask these questions: When does wheezing occur? What makes you wheeze? Do you wheeze loudly enough for others to hear it? What helps stop your wheezing?

Chest pain

If the patient has chest pain, ask these questions: Where is the pain? What does it feel like? Is it sharp, stabbing, burning or aching? Does it move to another area? How long does it last? What causes it? What makes it better?

Pain provocations

Chest pain due to a respiratory problem is usually the result of pleural inflammation, inflammation of the costochondral junctions or soreness of chest muscles because of coughing. It may also be the result of indigestion. Less common causes of pain include rib or vertebral fractures caused by coughing or osteoporosis.

Sleep disturbance

Sleep disturbances may be related to obstructive sleep apnoea or another sleep disorder requiring additional evaluation.

Daytime drowsiness

If the patient complains of being drowsy or irritable in the daytime, ask these questions: How many hours of continuous sleep do you get at night? Do you wake up often during the night? Does your family complain about your snoring or restlessness?

Previous health status

Look at the patient's health history, being especially watchful for:
- a smoking habit
- exposure to second-hand smoke
- allergies
- previous surgeries
- respiratory diseases, such as pneumonia and tuberculosis (TB).

Ask about current immunisations, such as a flu vaccination or pneumococcal vaccine. Also determine if the patient uses any respiratory equipment, such as oxygen or nebulisers, at home.

Family history

Ask the patient if they have a family history of cancer, sickle cell anaemia, heart disease or chronic illness, such as asthma or emphysema. Determine whether the patient lives with anyone who has an infectious disease, such as TB or influenza.

Lifestyle patterns

Ask about the patient's workplace because some jobs, such as coal mining and construction work, expose workers to substances that can cause lung disease.

Also ask about the patient's home, community and other environmental factors that may influence how they deal with their respiratory problems. For example, you may ask questions about interpersonal relationships, stress management and coping methods. Ask about any high risk habits or practices that might have put them at risk of acquiring AIDS—such as unprotected sex with multiple partners and intravenous drug use. This is important because

I guess your secret is finally out . . . you really *are* a pain in the chest!

Well, only sometimes!

Remember, ladies, snoring is a symptom of a respiratory disorder . . . it isn't a conspirancy to keep us from getting to sleep.

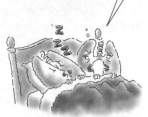

some pulmonary disorders, such as TB and *Pneumocystis carinii* pneumonia, are associated with AIDS.

Clinical assessment and monitoring

In most cases, you should begin the clinical examination after you take the patient's history. However, you may not be able to take a complete history if the patient develops an ominous sign such as acute respiratory distress. If your patient is in respiratory distress, establish the priorities of your nursing assessment, progressing from the most critical factors (airway, breathing and circulation [the ABCs]) to less critical factors. (See *Emergency respiratory assessment*.)

Advice from the experts

Emergency respiratory assessment

If your patient appears to have deteriorated or you are immediately concerned you should undertake a rapid assessment using an ABCDE approach:

Airway—Check the airway for patency and the patient's ability to maintain and protect the airway. Use a head tilt, chin lift manoeuvre and/or basic airway adjuncts (such oropharyngeal or nasopharyngeal airways) in a patient who does not have an artificial airway *in situ*. If the patient has an artificial airway—ensure this is patent—if in doubt—perform endotracheal suction to clear secretions and check patency.

Breathing—Check the effectiveness of breathing and gas exchange. Measure oxygen saturations, respiratory rate. Assess the rhythm and extent of chest excursion (normally 3–6 cm) as well as symmetry of excursion. Look for colour changes that might indicate hypoxia (pallor, central cyanosis) or hypercapnoea (e.g. facial flushing). Look for indicators of increased work of breathing (e.g. shoulder shrugging and use of sternocleidomastoid muscle). Look for intercostal recession and supraclavicular recession. Commence and titrate oxygen for acutely ill patients with increased work of breathing and/or decreased gas exchange (e.g. low SaO_2). Titrate oxygen to achieve $SaO_2 > 94\%$ (aim for 88–92% in patients at risk of hypercapnoea through chronic disease or morbid obesity).

Circulation—Check the adequacy of circulation. Check pulse rate, blood pressure, capillary refill time and presence of I.V. access. Fluid intake and output—including urine output. Consider fluid challenges as prescribed if there is hypotension and fluid overload is not present.

Disability (neurological disability)—rapidly assess neurological status. Use the AVPU scale to rate responsiveness: Alert, responds to Voice, responds to Pain only, is Unresponsive. Also note anxiousness, confusion, agitation (all possible signs of hypoxia). Check pupils for size and reaction to light. Check blood glucose (a common cause of reduced consciousness—along with hypoxia). Ensure the airway is kept patent.

Exposure—Expose the patient and undertake a general survey for anything abnormal. Maintain the patients dignity but be sure to look from top-to-toe (chest, abdomen, legs, feet, hands).

Setting priorities

Absence of signs of life means you should initiate immediate CPR and call the cardiac arrest team. Be sure to deal with problems identified with A before moving onto B, C, D and E and calling for help if you are concerned.

(Text continues on page 281)

Myocardial infarction

All infarcts have a central area of necrosis surrounded by an area of potentially viable hypoxic injury. This viable area can be salvaged if circulation is restored. If not, it may progress to necrosis. The zone of injury, in turn, is surrounded by viable ischaemic tissue.

Tissue destruction in myocardial infarction

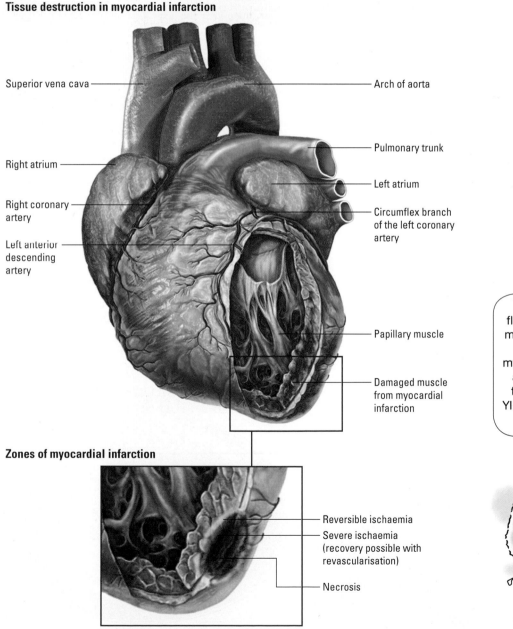

Superior vena cava

Arch of aorta

Pulmonary trunk

Right atrium

Left atrium

Right coronary artery

Circumflex branch of the left coronary artery

Left anterior descending artery

Papillary muscle

Damaged muscle from myocardial infarction

Zones of myocardial infarction

Reversible ischaemia

Severe ischaemia (recovery possible with revascularisation)

Necrosis

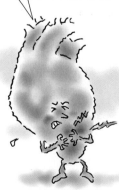

Reduced blood flow through one or more of my coronary arteries leads to myocardial ischaemia and necrosis. And that can lead to... YIKES!... myocardial infarction!

Alveolar changes in ARDS

Acute respiratory distress syndrome (ARDS) is a form of pulmonary oedema that can quickly lead to acute respiratory failure. Also known as *shock lung, stiff lung, white lung* or *wet lung,* ARDS may follow direct or indirect injury to the lung. However, diagnosis is difficult and death can occur within 48 hours of onset if ARDS isn't promptly diagnosed and treated.

In phase 1, injury reduces normal blood flow to the lungs. Platelets aggregate and release histamine (H), serotonin (S) and bradykinin (B).

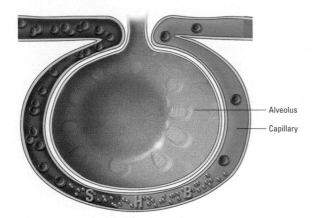

— Alveolus
— Capillary

In phase 2, those substances—especially histamine—inflame and damage the alveolocapillary membrane, increasing capillary permeability. Fluids then shift into the interstitial space.

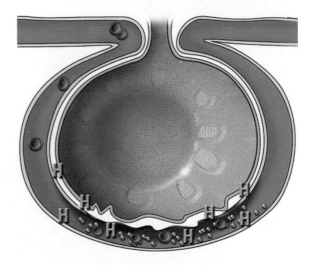

In phase 3, as capillary permeability increases, proteins and fluids leak out, increasing interstitial osmotic pressure and causing pulmonary oedema.

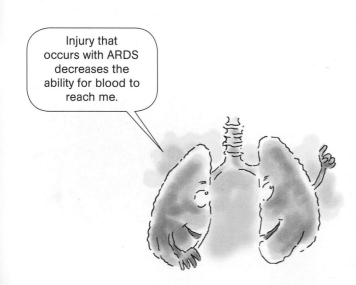

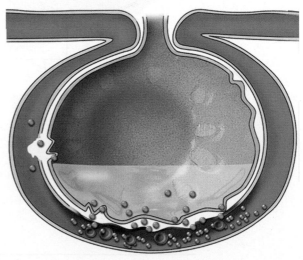

Gas exchange is impeded in ARDS due to factors such as fibrosis, shunting, collapse and oedema in the lungs.

In phase 5, sufficient oxygen (O₂) can't cross the alveolocapillary membrane, but carbon dioxide (CO₂) can and is lost with every exhalation. O₂ and CO₂ levels decrease in the blood.

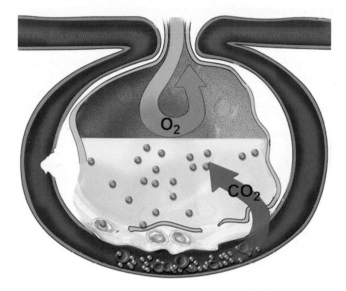

In phase 4, decreased blood flow and fluids in the alveoli damage surfactant and impair the cell's ability to produce more. As a result, alveoli collapse, impeding gas exchange and decreasing lung compliance.

In phase 6, pulmonary oedema worsens, inflammation leads to fibrosis and gas exchange is further impeded.

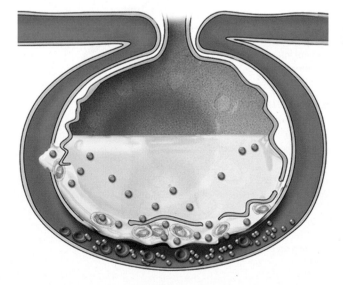

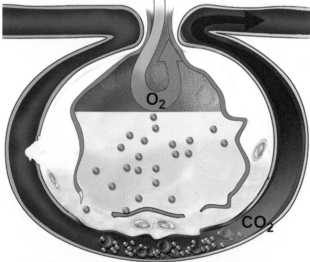

Stroke

Stroke occurs when cerebral circulation is suddenly impaired in one or more blood vessels that supply the brain. When circulation is impaired, oxygen supply to the brain is diminished or interrupted, causing damage or death in the brain tissues. The cause can be ischaemic or haemorrhagic.

Ischaemic stroke

With ischaemic stroke, thrombus and plaque form in the vessel, interrupting cerebral circulation.

Thrombi develop in different areas of the heart according to the underlying condition. They sometimes become dislodged, travelling to the cerebral circulation.

Common sites of cardiac thrombosis

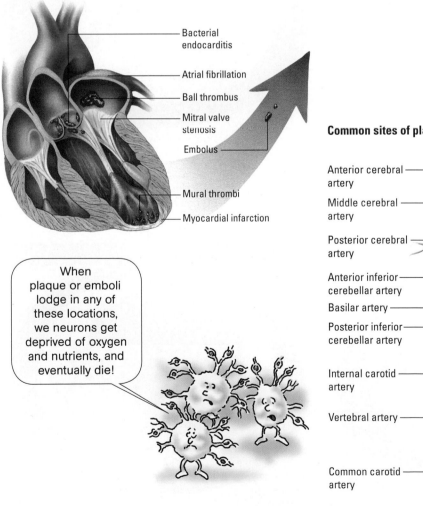

- Bacterial endocarditis
- Atrial fibrillation
- Ball thrombus
- Mitral valve stenosis
- Embolus
- Mural thrombi
- Myocardial infarction

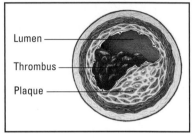

- Lumen
- Thrombus
- Plaque

When plaque or emboli lodge in any of these locations, we neurons get deprived of oxygen and nutrients, and eventually die!

Common sites of plaque formation, embolism, and infarction

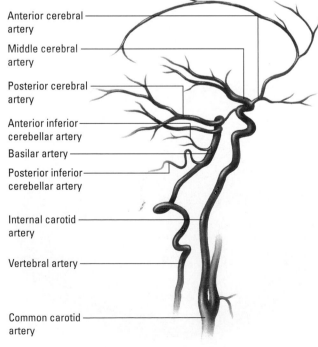

- Anterior cerebral artery
- Middle cerebral artery
- Posterior cerebral artery
- Anterior inferior cerebellar artery
- Basilar artery
- Posterior inferior cerebellar artery
- Internal carotid artery
- Vertebral artery
- Common carotid artery

Four steps

Use a systematic approach to detect subtle and obvious respiratory changes. The four steps for conducting a clinical examination of the respiratory system are:
- inspection
- palpation
- percussion
- auscultation.

Making introductions

Before you begin the examination, make sure the room is well lit and warm. Introduce yourself to the patient and explain why you're there.

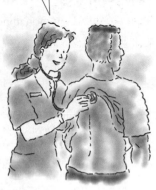

If possible, examine the back as well as the front, and always compare one side with the other, following a systematic sequence of inspection, palpation, percussion and auscultation.

Inspection

Make a few observations about the patient as soon as you approach the bedside and include these observations in your assessment. Note the patient's position in the bed. Do they appear comfortable? Are they sitting up or lying quietly or shifting about? Do they appear anxious? Are they having trouble breathing? Do they require oxygen? Are they on a ventilator?

Chest inspection

Help the patient achieve an upright or at least 45 degree incline if possible. Expose the chest to allow inspection. Inspect the patient's chest configuration, tracheal position, chest symmetry, skin condition and nostrils (for flaring), and look for accessory muscle use.

Beauty in symmetry

Look for chest wall symmetry. Both sides of the chest should appear equal at rest and expand equally as the patient inhales. The diameter of the chest, from front to back, should be about one-half of the width of the chest.

Your first observations of the patient are important parts of the assessment.

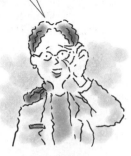

A new angle

Also, look at the angle between the ribs and the sternum at the point immediately above the xiphoid process. This angle, the costal angle, should be less than 90 degrees in an adult. The angle is larger if the chest wall is chronically expanded because of an enlargement of the intercostal muscles, as can happen with chronic obstructive pulmonary disease (COPD).

Muscles in motion

When the patient inhales, their diaphragm should descend and the intercostal muscles should contract. This dual motion causes the abdomen to push out and the lower ribs to expand laterally.

When the patient exhales, their abdomen and ribs return to their resting positions. The upper chest shouldn't move much. Accessory muscles may hypertrophy, indicating frequent use. This may be normal in some athletes, but for most patients it indicates a respiratory problem, especially when the patient purses their lips and flares their nostrils when breathing.

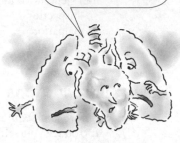

Hey, watch the elbows . . . we're all cramped in here!

Chest wall abnormalities

Inspect for chest wall abnormalities, keeping in mind that a patient with a deformity of the chest wall might have completely normal lungs that are cramped in the chest. The patient might have a smaller-than-normal lung capacity and limited exercise tolerance.

Barrels, pigeons and curves

Common abnormalities include:
* *Barrel chest*—A barrel chest looks like the name implies; it's abnormally round and bulging. Barrel chest may be normal in infants and elderly patients. In other patients, barrel chest occurs as a result of COPD due to lungs that have lost their elasticity. The patient typically uses accessory muscles to breathe and easily becomes breathless. Also note kyphosis of the thoracic spine.
* *Pigeon chest*—A patient with pigeon chest, or pectus carinatum, has a chest with a sternum that protrudes beyond the front of the abdomen. The displaced sternum increases the front-to-back diameter of the chest but is a minor deformity that doesn't require treatment.
* *Funnel chest*—A patient with funnel chest, or pectus excavatum, has a funnel-shaped depression on all of or part of the sternum. This may cause disruptions in respiratory or cardiac function. Compression of the heart and great vessels may cause murmurs.
* *Thoracic kyphoscoliosis*—The patient's spine curves to one side and the vertebrae are rotated. Because the rotation distorts lung tissues, it may be more difficult to assess respiratory status.

Raising a red flag

Watch for paradoxical, or uneven, movement of the patient's chest wall. Paradoxical movement may appear as an abnormal collapse of part of the chest wall when the patient inhales or an abnormal expansion when the patient exhales. In either case, such uneven movement indicates a loss of normal chest wall function.

The rate, rhythm and quality of respirations are key indicators of respiratory function.

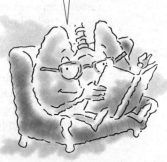

Breathing rate and pattern

Assess your patient's respiratory function by determining the rate, rhythm and quality of respirations.

Count on it

Adults normally breathe at a rate of 12–20 breaths per minute. To determine the patient's respiratory rate, count for a full minute, or longer if you note abnormalities. Don't tell the patient what you're doing or they might alter their natural breathing pattern.

The respiratory pattern should be even, coordinated and regular, with occasional sighs. The normal ratio of inspiration to expiration (I:E ratio) is about 1:2.

Abnormal respiratory patterns

Identifying abnormal respiratory patterns can be a great help in understanding the patient's respiratory status and overall condition.

Tachypnoea

Tachypnoea is a respiratory rate greater than 20 breaths per minute; the depth may be normal or shallow. It's commonly seen in patients with restrictive lung disease, pain, sepsis, obesity, anxiety and respiratory distress. Fever is another possible cause. The respiratory rate may increase by 4 breaths per minute for every 1°F (0.6°C) increase in body temperature.

Bradypnoea

Bradypnoea is a respiratory rate below 10 breaths per minute. It's commonly noted just before a period of apnoea or full respiratory arrest.

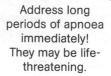

As your patient's body temperature increases with fever, respiratory rate also increases.

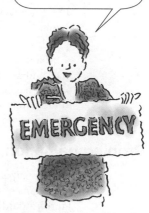

Depressed CNS

Patients with bradypnoea might have central nervous system (CNS) depression as a result of excessive sedation, tissue damage, diabetic coma or any situation in which the brain's respiratory centre is depressed. Increased intracranial pressure and metabolic alkalosis may also cause bradypnoea. Note that the respiratory rate is usually slower during sleep.

Apnoea

Apnoea is the absence of breathing. Periods of apnoea may be short and occur sporadically, such as in Cheyne–Stokes respirations or other abnormal respiratory patterns. This condition may be life-threatening if periods of apnoea last long enough, and should be addressed immediately.

Hyperpnoea

Hyperpnoea is characterised by deep breathing with either a normal or increased rate. It occurs during exercise or due to fever, hypoxia or acid–base imbalances.

Kussmaul's respirations

Kussmaul's respirations are rapid and deep, with sighing breaths. This type of breathing occurs in patients with metabolic acidosis, especially when associated with diabetic ketoacidosis, as the respiratory system tries to lower the carbon dioxide level in the blood and restore it to normal pH.

Cheyne–Stokes respirations

Cheyne–Stokes respirations have a regular cycle of change in the rate and depth of breathing. Respirations are initially shallow but gradually become deeper and deeper before becoming shallow again followed by a period of

Address long periods of apnoea immediately! They may be life-threatening.

apnoea, lasting 20–60 seconds, and the cycle starts again. This respiratory pattern is seen in patients with heart failure, kidney failure or CNS damage. Cheyne–Stokes respirations can be a normal breathing pattern during sleep in elderly patients.

Biot's respirations

Biot's respirations involve rapid deep breaths that alternate with abrupt periods of apnoea. They're an ominous sign of severe CNS damage.

Inspecting related structures

Inspect the patient's skin for pallor, cyanosis and diaphoresis.

Don't be blue

Skin colour varies considerably among patients, but a patient with a bluish tint to their skin, nail beds and mucous membranes is considered cyanotic. Cyanosis, which occurs when oxygenation to the tissues is poor, is a late sign of hypoxaemia. However, peripheral cyanosis may be seen when circulation to the extremities is reduced so it is more reliable to look for central cyanosis—best detected by inspecting mucous membranes.

Finger findings

When you inspect the fingers, assess for clubbing, a sign of long-standing respiratory or cardiac disease. The fingernail normally enters the skin at an angle of less than 180 degrees. When clubbing occurs, the angle is greater than or equal to 180 degrees.

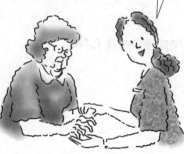

Inspect the fingers for clubbing—a sign of long-standing respiratory or cardiac disease.

Palpation

Palpation of the chest provides some important information about the respiratory system and the processes involved in breathing. (See *Palpating the chest*, page 285.)

Leaky lungs

The chest wall should feel smooth, warm and dry. Crepitus ('surgical emphysema' or 'subcutaneous emphysema'), which feels like puffed-rice cereal crackling under the skin, indicates that air is leaking from the airways or lungs.

   If a patient has an intercostal drain (pleural underwater-seal drain), you may find a small amount of subcutaneous air around the insertion site. If the patient has no chest tube, or the area of crepitus gets larger, alert the doctor immediately—there will probably be pneumothorax which if not treated may cause tension and be life-threatening.

You're positive you haven't been sneaking anymore late-night crispy rice cereal snacks? You're starting to feel more crackly to me.

Probing palpation pain

Gentle palpation shouldn't cause the patient pain. If the patient complains of chest pain, try to find a painful area on the chest wall. Here's a guide to assessing some types of chest pain:

Palpating the chest

To palpate the chest, place the palm of your hand (or hands) lightly over the thorax, as shown. Palpate for tenderness, alignment, bulging and retractions of the chest and intercostal spaces. Assess the patient for crepitus, especially around drainage sites. Repeat this procedure on the patient's back if the patient's condition allows.

Next, use the pads of your fingers, as shown, to palpate the front and back of the thorax. Pass your fingers over the ribs and any scars, lumps, lesions or ulcerations. Note the skin temperature, turgor and moisture. Also note tenderness and bony or subcutaneous crepitus. The muscles should feel firm and smooth.

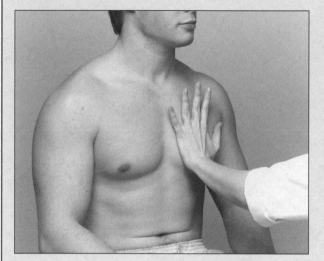
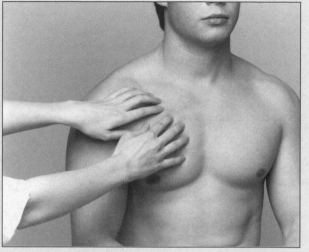

- Painful costochondral joints are typically located at the midclavicular line or next to the sternum.
- A rib or vertebral fracture is quite painful over the fracture.
- Sore muscles may result from protracted coughing.
- A collapsed lung can cause pain in addition to dyspnoea.
- A sharp pain on inspiration or on coughing may be because of an inflamed pleura—such as in lobar pneumonia.
- Cardiac chest pain—as in angina or MI is typically heavy and central.

Feeling for fremitus

Fremitus is a palpable vibration felt when the hands are placed on the chest wall. There are two types of fremitus you can feel. Firstly, there is rhonchial fremitus—the course bubbling feeling caused by secretions or fluid in the large upper airways. Secondly, there is vocal fremitus—the vibration of the voice transmitted to and palpable on the chest wall. Vocal fremitus is decreased over areas where pleural fluid collects, when the patient speaks softly, and with pneumothorax, atelectasis and emphysema.

Checking for tactile fremitus

When you check the back of the thorax for tactile fremitus, ask the patient to fold their arms across their chest, as shown here. This movement shifts the scapulae out of the way.

What to do

Check for tactile fremitus by lightly placing your open palms on both sides of the patient's back and front without touching their skin with your fingers, as shown. When checking for vocal fremitus, ask the patient to repeat 'ninety-nine' loud enough to produce palpable vibrations. Then palpate the front of the chest using the same hand positions.

What the results mean

Vibrations of vocal fremitus that feel more intense on one side than the other indicate tissue consolidation on that side. Less intense vibrations may indicate emphysema, pneumothorax or pleural effusion. Faint or no vibrations in the upper posterior thorax may indicate bronchial obstruction or a fluid-filled pleural space.

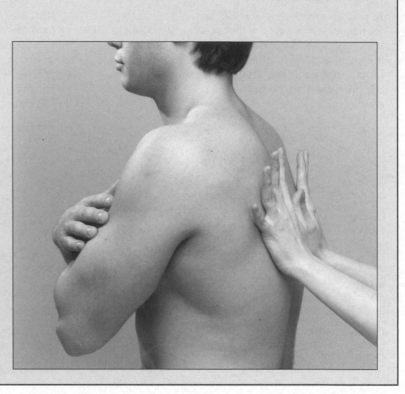

Vocal fremitus is increased abnormally over consolidated areas of lung and over areas in which alveoli are filled with fluid or exudates, as happens in pneumonia. (See *Checking for tactile fremitus*.)

Evaluating symmetry

To evaluate your patient's chest wall symmetry and expansion, place your hands on the front of the chest wall with your thumbs touching each other at the second intercostal space. As the patient inhales deeply, watch your thumbs. They should separate simultaneously and equally to a distance several centimetres away from the sternum.

Repeat the measurement at the fifth intercostal space. You may take the same measurement on the back of the chest near the ten rib.

Warning signs

The patient's chest may expand asymmetrically if they have:
- pleural effusion
- atelectasis

Asymmetry or abnormal chest expansion may be warning signs of diseases and disorders.

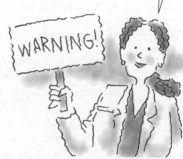

- pneumonia
- pneumothorax.

Chest expansion may be decreased at the level of the diaphragm if the patient has:

- emphysema
- respiratory depression
- diaphragm paralysis
- atelectasis
- obesity
- ascites.

And you thought I was just filled with hot air!

Percussion

Percuss the chest to:

- find the boundaries of the lungs
- determine whether the lungs are filled with air, fluid or solid material
- evaluate the distance the diaphragm travels between the patient's inhalation and exhalation. (See *Percussing the chest*.)

Sites and sounds

Listen for normal, resonant sounds over most of the chest. In the left front chest wall from the third or fourth intercostal space at the sternum to the third or fourth intercostal space at the midclavicular line listen for a dull sound; that's the space occupied by the heart. With careful percussion, you can identify the borders of the heart when lung tissue is normal. Resonance

---

Percussing the chest

To percuss the chest, hyperextend the middle finger of your left hand if you're right-handed or the middle finger of your right hand if you're left-handed. Place your hand firmly on the patient's chest. Use the tip of the middle finger of your dominant hand—your right hand if you're right-handed, left hand if you're left-handed—to tap on the middle finger of your other hand just below the distal joint (as shown here).

The movement should come from the wrist of your dominant hand, not your elbow or upper arm. Keep the fingernail you use for tapping short so you don't hurt yourself. Follow the standard percussion sequence over the front and back chest walls.

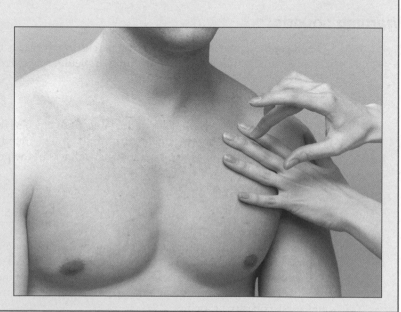

Percussion sequences

Follow these percussion sequences to distinguish between normal and abnormal sounds in the patient's lungs. Compare sound variations from one side with the other as you proceed. Carefully describe abnormal sounds you hear and note their locations. (Follow the same sequence for auscultation.)

Anterior

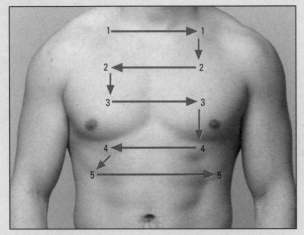

Posterior

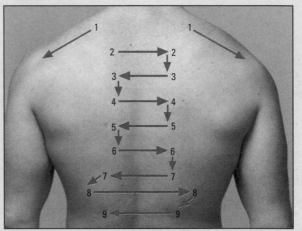

resumes at the sixth intercostal space. The sequence of sounds in the back is slightly different. (See *Percussion sequences*.)

Warning sounds

When you hear hyperresonance during percussion, it means you've found an area of increased air in the lung or pleural space. Expect to hear hyperresonance in your patients with:
- pneumothorax
- acute asthma
- *bullous emphysema* (large holes in the lungs from alveolar destruction).
  When you hear abnormal dullness, it means you've found areas of decreased air in the lungs. Expect abnormal dullness in the presence of:
- pleural fluid
- consolidation or atelectasis
- tumour.

Detecting diaphragm movement

Percussion also allows you to assess how much the diaphragm moves during inspiration and expiration. The normal diaphragm descends $1\frac{1}{8}$″ to $1\frac{7}{8}$″ (3–5 cm) when the patient inhales. The diaphragm doesn't move as far in patients with emphysema, respiratory depression, diaphragm paralysis, atelectasis, obesity or ascites.

> Hyperresonance indicates increased air in the lung or pleural space; dullness is a sign of decreased air in the lungs. I hear that!

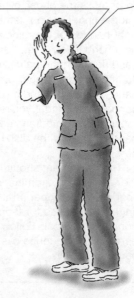

Auscultation

As air moves through the bronchi, it creates sound waves that travel to the chest wall. The sound produced by breathing changes as air moves from larger to smaller airways. Sounds also change if they pass through fluid, mucus or narrowed airways.

Auscultation preparation

Auscultation sites are the same as percussion sites. Listen to a full cycle of inspiration and expiration at each site, using the diaphragm of the stethoscope. Ask the patient to breathe through their mouth if it doesn't cause discomfort; nose-breathing alters the pitch of breath sounds.

When things get hairy

If the patient has abundant chest hair, mat it down with a damp washcloth so the hair doesn't make sounds that could be mistaken for crackles.

Be firm

To auscultate for breath sounds, press the diaphragm side of the stethoscope firmly against the skin. Remember that if you listen through clothing or chest hair, breath sounds won't be heard clearly, and you may hear unusual and deceptive sounds.

Normal breath sounds

During auscultation, listen for four types of breath sounds over normal lungs. (See *Locations of normal breath sounds*, page 290.)

Here's a run-down of the normal breath sounds and their characteristics:
• Tracheal breath sounds, heard over the trachea, are harsh, tubular in quality and discontinuous. They occur when the patient inhales or exhales.
• Bronchial breath sounds, usually heard next to the trachea just above or below the clavicle, are loud, high-pitched and discontinuous. They're loudest when the patient exhales.
• Bronchovesicular sounds are medium-pitched and continuous. They're best heard over the upper third of the sternum and between the scapulae when the patient inhales or exhales.
• Vesicular sounds, heard over the rest of the lungs, are soft and low-pitched. They're prolonged during inhalation and shortened during exhalation. (See *Qualities of normal breath sounds*, page 290.)

Interpreting breath sounds

Classify each breath sound you auscultate by its intensity, pitch, duration, characteristic and location. Note whether it occurs during inspiration, expiration or both.

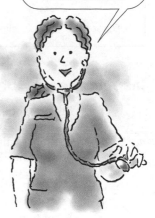

Can't decide between the mouth and the nose? When auscultating, have the patient breathe through their mouth, if possible. Nose-breathing can change the pitch of breath sounds.

Qualities of normal breath sounds

Use this chart as a quick reference for the qualities of normal breath sounds.

Breath sound	Quality	Inspiration: expiration ratio	Location
Tracheal	Harsh, high-pitched	I < E	Over trachea
Bronchial	Loud, high-pitched	I > E	Next to trachea
Bronchovesicular	Medium in loudness and pitch	I = E	Next to sternum, between scapula pitch
Vesicular	Soft, low-pitched	I > E	Remainder of lungs

Locations of normal breath sounds

These photographs show the locations of different types of normal breath sounds.

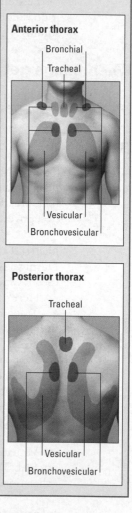

Anterior thorax

Bronchial
Tracheal
Vesicular
Bronchovesicular

Posterior thorax

Tracheal
Vesicular
Bronchovesicular

Inspect the unexpected

Breath sounds heard in an unexpected area are abnormal. For instance, if you hear bronchial sounds where you expect to hear vesicular sounds, the area you're auscultating might be consolidated, filled with fluid or exudates, as in pneumonia. The vesicular sounds you expect to hear in those areas are absent because no air is moving through the small airways.

Vocal fremitus

Vocal fremitus is the sound produced by chest vibrations as the patient speaks. Abnormal transmission of voice sounds can occur over consolidated areas because sound travels well through fluid. There are three common abnormal voice sounds:
• *Bronchophony*—Ask the patient to say 'ninety-nine' or 'blue moon'. Over normal tissue, the words sound muffled, but over consolidated areas, the words sound unusually loud.
• *Egophony*—Ask the patient to say 'E'. Over normal lung tissue, the sound is muffled, but over consolidated areas, it sounds like the letter A.
• *Whispered pectoriloquy*—Ask the patient to whisper '1, 2, 3'. Over normal lung tissue, the numbers are almost indistinguishable. Over consolidated tissue, the numbers sound loud and clear.

Abnormal breath sounds

Because solid tissue transmits sound better than air or fluid, breath sounds (as well as spoken or whispered words) are louder than normal over areas of consolidation. If pus, fluid or air fills the pleural space, breath sounds are quieter than normal. If a foreign body or secretions obstruct a bronchus, breath sounds are diminished or absent over lung tissue distal to the obstruction.

Adventitious sounds

Adventitious sounds are abnormal no matter where you hear them in the lungs. (See *Abnormal breath sounds*, page 292.)

There are five types of adventitious breath sounds:

Crackles are intermittent, nonmusical and brief crackling sounds caused by collapsed or fluid-filled alveoli popping open that are heard primarily when the patient inhales. They're classified as either fine or coarse and usually don't clear with coughing. If they do, they're most likely caused by secretions. (See *Types of crackles*, page 293.)

Wheezes are high-pitched sounds heard first when a patient exhales. They're caused by narrowed airways. As the severity of the block increases, they may also be heard on inspiration. Patients may wheeze as a result of asthma, infection, heart failure or airway obstruction from a tumour or foreign body. (See *When wheezing stops*, page 293.)

Rhonchi are low-pitched, snoring, rattling sounds that occur primarily when a patient exhales, although they may also be heard when the patient inhales. Rhonchi usually change or disappear with coughing. The sounds occur when fluid partially blocks the large airways.

Stridor is a loud, high-pitched crowing sound that's heard, usually without a stethoscope, during inspiration. It's caused by an obstruction in the upper airway and requires immediate attention.

Pleural friction rub is a low-pitched, grating, rubbing sound heard when the patient inhales and exhales. Pleural inflammation causes the two layers of pleura to rub together. The patient may complain of pain in areas where the rub is heard.

Results and significance of diagnostic tests and investigations

If your patient's history and the physical examination findings reveal evidence of pulmonary dysfunction, diagnostic testing is done to identify and evaluate the dysfunction. These tests include:
- blood and sputum studies
- endoscopy and imaging
- pulmonary angiography
- bedside testing procedures.

Prepping the patient

Diagnostic testing may be routine for you, but it can be frightening to the patient. Take steps to prepare the patient and their family for each procedure and monitor the patient during and after the procedure.

Some tests can be performed at the bedside in the critical care unit. Many others, however, must be performed in the imaging department; in these cases, you may need to accompany unstable patients who require monitoring.

Blood and sputum studies

Blood and sputum studies include arterial blood gas (ABG) analysis and sputum analysis.

ABG analysis

ABGs offer useful information about acid–base disorders in the body, as well as the ability of the respiratory system to exchange respiratory gases (oxygen and carbon dioxide) by measuring the partial pressures of gases dissolved in arterial blood.

The ABCs of ABGs

Arterial blood is used because it reflects how much oxygen is available to peripheral tissues. Together, ABG values tell the story of how well a patient is ventilating and whether they're developing acidosis or alkalosis.

Here's a summary of commonly assessed ABG values and what the findings indicate:
• pH measurement of the hydrogen ion (H^+) concentration is an indication of the blood's acidity or alkalinity. The greater the number of hydrogen ions the more acidic the blood. But pH is an inverse hydrogen measurement scale so higher hydrogen ion levels give lower pH values.
• Partial pressure of arterial carbon dioxide ($PaCO_2$) reflects the adequacy of ventilation of the lungs. There is an inverse relationship between lung ventilation and $PaCO_2$ levels. Hypoventilation leads to higher $PaCO_2$. Hyperventilation leads to lower $PaCO_2$.
• PaO_2 is the oxygen dissolved in the plasma after diffusing across alveolocapillary membrane in the lungs—thus it reflects gas exchange in the lungs.
• Bicarbonate is the metabolic component of ABG analysis. Bicarbonate (HCO_3^-) is the chief alkali (or 'base') that buffers acids in the blood. Bicarbonate falls when it is used up in buffering excess acids. It also falls when the kidneys fail and are unable to create bicarbonate.

The bicarbonate level reflects the activity of the kidneys in retaining or excreting bicarbonate. Your labs or blood gas analyser may report base excess or deficit (BE/BD). Since the chief base is bicarbonate this is simply a way of reporting whether there is a high (base excess $>+2$) or low (base deficit <-2) bicarbonate level in the arterial blood.
• Oxygen saturation (SaO_2) is the percentage of haemoglobin saturated with oxygen as a proportion of potential oxygen-carrying capacity of the haemoglobin. (See *Normal ABG values*, page 294.)

Abnormal breath sounds

Here's a quick guide to assessing abnormal breath sounds:

• *Crackles*— intermittent, nonmusical, crackling sounds heard during inspiration; classified as fine or coarse; common in elderly people when small sections of the alveoli don't fully aerate and secretions accumulate during sleep; alveoli reexpand or pop open when the patient takes deep breaths upon awakening
• *Wheezes*—high-pitched sounds caused by blocked airflow; heard on exhalation
• *Rhonchi*—low-pitched snoring or rattling sounds; heard primarily on exhalation
• *Stridor*—loud, high-pitched sound heard during inspiration
• *Pleural friction rub*—low-pitched, grating sound heard during inspiration and expiration; accompanied by pain.

Types of crackles

Here's how to differentiate fine crackles from coarse crackles, a critical distinction when assessing the lungs.

Fine crackles

The following characteristics distinguish fine crackles:

- They occur when the patient stops inhaling.
- They're usually heard in lung bases.
- They sound like a piece of hair being rubbed between the fingers or like Velcro being pulled apart.
- They occur in restrictive diseases, such as pulmonary fibrosis, asbestosis, silicosis, atelectasis, heart failure and pneumonia.

Coarse crackles

The following characteristics distinguish coarse crackles:

- They occur when the patient starts to inhale and may be present when the patient exhales.
- They may be heard through the lungs and even at the mouth.
- They sound more like bubbling or gurgling as air moves through secretions in the larger airways.
- They occur in chronic obstructive pulmonary disease, bronchiectasis, pulmonary oedema and in severely ill patients who can't cough.
- They're also called the 'death rattle'.

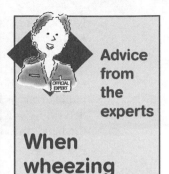

Advice from the experts

When wheezing stops

If you no longer hear wheezing in a patient having an acute asthma attack, the attack may be far from over. When bronchospasm and mucosal swelling become severe, little air can move through the airways. As a result, wheezing stops.

If all other assessment criteria—laboured breathing, prolonged expiratory time and accessory muscle use—point to acute bronchial obstruction (a medical emergency), maintain the patient's airway and give oxygen and medications as prescribed to relieve the obstruction. The patient may begin to wheeze again when the airways open more.

Interpreting ABG values

If interpretation of blood gases is a regular part of your role—you need a systematic way of interpreting them and lots of practice to enable you to understand the range of useful things that blood gases can help you find out about your patients' physiology. There are some simple relationships between the various parameters you'll need to know as well as the normal values. (See *Normal ABG values*, page 294.)

A five-step approach to interpretation of ABGs:

- Step 1—Oxygenation: Look at the PaO_2 (and SaO_2) and determine whether there is hypoxaemia, normal oxygenation or hyperoxaemia.
- Step 2—Acidity–alkalinity: Look at the pH (or H^+—both measure acidity) and decide whether there is an acidosis or alkalosis.
- Step 3—pH imbalance from respiratory problems: Look at the $PaCO_2$ and compare it with the pH; if they are moving in opposite directions the pH imbalance is of respiratory origin. (See *Understanding acid–base disorders*, page 295.)
- Step 4—pH imbalance from metabolic problems: Look at the HCO_3 (or BE/BD) and compare it with the pH; if they are moving in the same direction the imbalance is metabolic in origin. (See *Understanding acid–base disorders*, page 295.)
- Step 5—Compensation and mixed problems: Compare the $PaCO_2$ with the HCO_3 (or BXS); if they are moving in the same direction one system is attempting to compensate for the other (the clinical picture will indicate which is the failing system). If they are moving in opposite directions a mixed respiratory and metabolic imbalance is present.

Nursing considerations

• In critical care units arterial samples are usually drawn from an arterial line if the patient has one. If a percutaneous puncture must be done, the site must be chosen carefully. The most common site is the radial artery but the brachial or femoral arteries can be used. When a radial artery is used, an Allen's test is done before drawing the sample to determine whether the ulnar artery can provide adequate circulation to the hand, in case the radial artery is damaged. (See *Performing Allen's test*, page 296.)

• After a sample is obtained from percutaneous puncture, apply pressure to the puncture site for 5 minutes and tape a gauze pad firmly in place. Regularly monitor the site for bleeding and check the arm for signs of complications, such as swelling, discoloration, pain, numbness and tingling. (See *Obtaining an ABG sample*, page 296.)

• Note whether the patient is breathing room air or oxygen. If the patient is on oxygen via nasal cannula document the number of litres. If the patient is receiving oxygen by mask or mechanical ventilation, document the fraction of inspired oxygen (FIO_2).

• Examples of conditions that can interfere with test results are failure to properly heparinise the syringe before drawing a blood sample or exposing the sample to air. Venous blood in the sample may lower PaO_2 levels and elevate $PaCO_2$ levels. Make sure you remove all air bubbles in the sample syringe because air bubbles also alter results.

• Make sure the sample of arterial blood is kept cold if it is not to be analysed immediately, preferably on ice, and delivered as soon as possible to the laboratory for analysis. Some chemical reactions that alter findings continue to take place after the blood is drawn; rapid cooling and analysis of the sample minimises this.

Sputum analysis

Sputum analysis assesses sputum specimens (the material expectorated from a patient's lungs and bronchi during deep coughing or from endotracheal suction) to diagnose respiratory disease, identify the cause of pulmonary infection (including viral and bacterial causes), identify abnormal lung cells and manage lung disease.

Under the microscope

Most commonly sputum is cultured and any organisms grown tested for sensitivity to antibiotics. A negative culture may suggest a viral infection. Sputum specimens may also be stained and examined under a microscope.

Nursing considerations

• If the patient experiences difficulties expectorating sputum, or it is too tenacious to aspirate through endotracheal suction, give nebulised saline or humidification to facilitate sample collection.

Normal ABG values

Arterial blood gas (ABG) values provide information about the blood's acid–base balance and oxygenation.

Normal values are given here in kPa, the most common unit of measurement. (To convert to mmHg multiply by 7.5.)

• pH — 7.35 to 7.45
• H^+ — 35 to 45 nmol/L
• $PaCO_2$ — 4.6 to 6 kPa
• PaO_2 — 10 to 13 kPa
• HCO_3^- — 22 to 26 mEq/L
• BE/BD — −2 to +2
• SaO_2 — 95% to 100%

Keep it cold and be quick! Deliver the chilled arterial blood sample ASAP for analysis!

Understanding acid–base disorders

This chart provides an overview of selected acid–base disorders.

Disorder and ABG findings	Possible causes	Signs and symptoms
Respiratory acidosis		
(excess carbon dioxide retention) pH < 7.35 Bicarbonate (HCO_3^-) > 26 mEq/L (if compensating) Partial pressure of arterial carbon dioxide ($PaCO_2$) > 6 kPa	• Central nervous system depression from drugs, injury or disease • Respiratory arrest • Hypoventilation from pulmonary, cardiac or neuromuscular disease	*Early:* tachycardia, tachypnoea *Late:* bradypnoea, confusion, hypotension, lethargy, coma (very late sign)
Respiratory alkalosis		
(excess carbon dioxide excretion) pH > 7.45 HCO_3^- < 22 mEq/L (if compensating) $PaCO_2$ < 4.7 kPa	• Hyperventilation from anxiety, pain, or improper ventilator settings • Respiratory stimulation by drugs, disease, or fever • Gram-negative bacteraemia • Pulmonary embolism	Paraesthesias, confusion, light-headedness, anxiety, palpitations
Metabolic acidosis		
(bicarbonate loss, acid retention) pH < 7.35 HCO_3^- <22 mEq/L $PaCO_2$ <4.7 kPa (if compensating)	• HCO_3^- depletion from diarrhoea • Excessive production of organic acids from endocrine disorders, shock, or drug intoxication • Inadequate excretion of acids from renal disease	Fruity breath, headache, lethargy, nausea, vomiting, abdominal pain, tremors, confusion, coma (if severe)
Metabolic alkalosis		
(bicarbonate retention, acid loss) pH>7.45 HCO_3^- >26 mEq/L $PaCO_2$ >6 kPa (if compensating)	• Loss of hydrochloric acid from prolonged vomiting or gastric suctioning • Loss of potassium from increased renal excretion (as in diuretic therapy) or steroids • Excessive alkali ingestion • Hepatic disease	Slow breathing, hypertonic muscles, twitching, confusion, tetany, seizures, dizziness, coma (if severe)

• To prevent foreign particles from contaminating the specimen, instruct the patient not to eat, brush their teeth or use mouthwash before expectorating. They may rinse their mouth with water.

• When they're ready to expectorate, instruct the patient to take three deep breaths and force a deep cough, supporting any abdominal wounds and whilst sitting in an upright position if possible.

• If you're aspirating a sample for culture by endotracheal suction—be sure to use a sterile sputum trap.

• Before sending the specimen to the laboratory, make sure it's sputum, not saliva. Saliva has a thinner consistency and more bubbles (froth) than sputum.

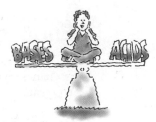

Performing Allen's test

Before obtaining an arterial blood gas sample from the radial artery, make sure you perform Allen's test to assess the patient's collateral arterial blood supply:

- Direct the patient to close their hand while you occlude the radial and ulnar arteries for 10–30 seconds, watching for the hand to blanch.

- Tell the patient to open their hand. Continue to hold pressure on the radial and ulnar arteries.

- Release pressure on the ulnar artery. Colour should return to the patient's hand in 15 seconds. If the colour doesn't return, select another site for an arterial puncture.

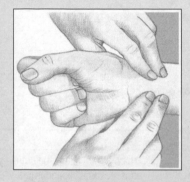 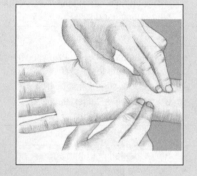 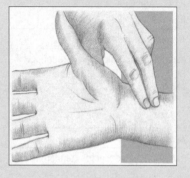

Obtaining an arterial blood gas (ABG) sample

Follow the steps below to obtain a sample for ABG analysis:

- After performing Allen's test, perform a cutaneous arterial puncture (or, if an arterial line is in place, draw blood from the arterial line).
- Use a heparinized blood gas syringe to draw the sample.
- Eliminate all air from the sample, place it on ice immediately, and transport it for analysis.

- Apply pressure to the puncture site for 3 to 5 minutes. If the patient is receiving anticoagulants or has a coagulopathy, hold the puncture site longer than 5 minutes, if necessary.
- Tape a gauze pad firmly over the puncture site. If the puncture site is on the arm, don't tape the entire circumference because this may restrict circulation.

Endoscopy and imaging

Endoscopy and imaging tests include bronchoscopy, chest x-ray, magnetic resonance imaging (MRI), thoracic computed tomography (CT) scan and V̇/Q̇ scan.

Bronchoscopy

Bronchoscopy allows direct visualisation of the larynx, trachea and bronchi through a fibre-optic bronchoscope, a slender flexible tube with mirrors and a light at its distal end. The flexible fibre-optic bronchoscope is

> Instruct your patient not to eat, brush their teeth or use mouthwash before sputum collection.

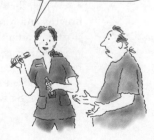

preferred to metal because it's smaller, allows a better view of the bronchi and carries less risk of trauma.

To remove and evaluate

The purpose of a bronchoscopy is to:
• remove foreign bodies, malignant or benign tumours, mucus plugs or excessive secretions from the tracheobronchial tree and control massive haemoptysis
• pass brush biopsy forceps or a catheter through the bronchoscope to obtain specimens for cytological evaluation.

Nursing considerations
• In the critically ill bronchoscopy will usually be performed at the bedside—so the equipment will be brought to the patient. Check what equipment is needed—your unit may have a checklist to help you prepare.
• Prepare the patient and family by explaining the procedure to the patient and their family and answering their questions.
• Monitor the patient throughout the procedure for complications such as desaturation or haemodynamic changes that may result from sedation.
• Obtain a chest x-ray as ordered, to detect pneumothorax and evaluate lung status.
• Keep resuscitative equipment available during the procedure and for 24 hours afterwards.

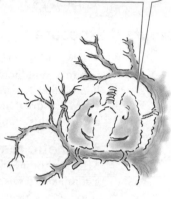

Bronchoscopy allows removal of tissue or foreign bodies from the tracheobronchial tree.

Chest x-ray
During chest radiography (commonly known as chest x-ray), x-ray beams penetrate the chest and react on specially sensitised film. Because normal pulmonary tissue is radiolucent, such abnormalities as infiltrates, foreign bodies, fluid and tumours appear dense (white) on the film.

More is better

A chest x-ray is most useful when compared with the patient's previous films, allowing the practitioner to detect changes.

By themselves, chest x-rays may not provide definitive diagnostic information. For example, they may not reveal mild-to-moderate obstructive pulmonary disease. However, they can show the location and size of lesions and can also be used to identify structural abnormalities that influence ventilation and diffusion.

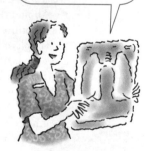

A chest x-ray is most useful when it's compared with previous films, allowing changes to be detected.

X-ray vision

Examples of abnormalities visible on x-ray include:
• pneumothorax
• fibrosis
• atelectasis
• pleural effusion
• consolidation
• infiltrates
• tumours.

Nursing considerations

• Patients in the critical care usually have chest x-rays performed at the bedside. Explain to the patient that someone will help them to a sitting position while a cold, hard film plate is placed behind their back. Ask them to take a deep breath and to hold it for a few seconds while the x-ray is taken. Instruct the patient to remain still for those few seconds.

Minimal exposure

• Provide reassurance that the amount of radiation exposure is minimal. Staff should leave the area when the technician takes the x-ray because they're potentially exposed to radiation many times per day.
• Make sure that female patients of childbearing age wear a lead apron. Males should have protection for the testes.

Magnetic resonance imaging

MRI is a noninvasive test that employs a powerful magnet, radio waves and a computer. It's used to diagnose respiratory disorders by providing high-resolution, cross-sectional images of lung structures and by tracing blood flow.

A view that's see-through

The greatest advantage of MRI is that it enables one to 'see-through' bone and delineate fluid-filled soft tissue in great detail, without using ionising radiation or contrast media. It's used to distinguish tumours from other structures such as blood vessels.

Nursing considerations

• All metal objects must be removed from the patient before entering the scanning room. The MRI suite will usually send a safety checklist to complete before the patient goes for the scan (See *MRI and metals don't mix*).
• The critically ill patient who is mechanically ventilated will be heavily sedated prior to the scan. If the patient is conscious and suffers from claustrophobia, sedation may be prescribed before the scan.
• The critically ill patient will need to be transported to the scanner and closely monitored in transit and throughout the procedure. Prepare and check the transport equipment needed for a critically ill mechanically ventilated patient. Check with the accompanying doctor for any special equipment or drugs that may be needed.
• If the patient is conscious tell the patient that they'll be asked to lie on a table that slides into an 8′ (2.4 m) tunnel inside the magnet. Some facilities can perform open MRIs, which are more tolerable for patients who are claustrophobic. The test usually takes 15–30 minutes.
• Explain that the machinery is noisy, with sounds ranging from an incessant ping to a loud bang. The patient may feel claustrophobic or bored. Encourage them to relax and to concentrate on breathing or a favourite subject or image.

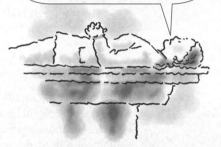

Advise the patient that each required x-ray will take only a few seconds, but that they must remain still and hold their breath during that time.

MRI and metals don't mix

Before your patient undergoes magnetic resonance imaging (MRI), make sure they don't have a pacemaker or surgically implanted joint, pin, clip, valve or pump containing metal. Such objects could be attracted to the strong MRI magnet.

Ask your patient whether they've ever worked with metals or have ever had metal in their eyes. Some facilities have a checklist that covers all pertinent questions regarding metals, clips, pins, pacemakers and other devices. If they have such an object or device, the test can't be done.

Also remember that pieces of medical equipment may have metal components—if in doubt check with the manufacturers.

Thoracic computed tomography scans

Thoracic CT scan provides cross-sectional views of the chest by passing an x-ray beam from a computerised scanner through the body at different angles and depths. A contrast agent is sometimes used to highlight blood vessels and allow greater visual discrimination.

CT in 3-D

Thoracic CT scan provides a three-dimensional image of the lung, allowing assessment of abnormalities in the configuration of the trachea or major bronchi and evaluate masses or lesions, such as tumours and abscesses, and abnormal lung shadows.

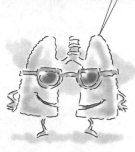

My very own 3-D images! This could be the start of a whole new career for me. Look out, Hollywood!

Nursing considerations

- Confirm that the patient isn't allergic to iodine or shellfish. A patient with these allergies may have an adverse reaction to the contrast medium.
- If a contrast medium is used, explain that it's injected into the existing I.V. line or that a new line may be inserted.
- Explain to the patient that they may feel flushed or notice a metallic or salty taste in their mouth when the contrast medium is injected.
- Explain that the CT scanner circles around the patient for a few minutes, depending on the procedure, and that the equipment may make them feel claustrophobic.
- Instruct the patient to lie still during the test.
- The contrast medium may discolour their urine for 24 hours.
- Encourage oral fluid intake to flush the contrast medium out of the patient's system, unless it's contraindicated or the patient is on nothing-by-mouth status. The rate of intravenous fluid infusion may be increased and/or N-acetyl-cysteine may be used to protect the kidneys in individuals at risk of contrast-induced nephropathy. Administer these as prescribed.
- The critically ill patient who is mechanically ventilated will be heavily sedated prior to the scan. If the patient is conscious and suffers from claustrophobia, sedation may be prescribed before the scan.
- The critically ill patient will need to be transported to the scanner and closely monitored in transit and throughout the procedure. Prepare and check the transport equipment needed for a critically ill mechanically ventilated patient. Check with the accompanying doctor for any special equipment or drugs that may be needed.

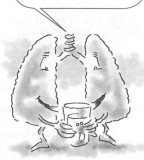

Remember to get plenty of fluid into your patient's system to flush the contrast medium.

Ventilation–perfusion scan

A V̇/Q̇ scan is used to:
- evaluate V̇/Q̇ mismatch
- detect pulmonary emboli
- evaluate pulmonary function, especially in patients with marginal lung reserves.

Although it's less reliable than pulmonary angiography, V̇/Q̇ scanning carries fewer risks.

Two-tined test

A V̇/Q̇ scan has two parts:

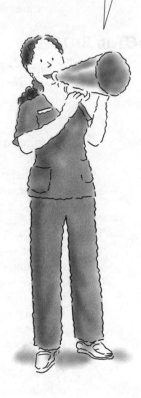

1 During the ventilation portion of the test, the patient inhales the contrast medium gas; ventilation patterns and adequacy of ventilation are noted on the scan.

2 During the perfusion scan, the contrast medium is injected I.V. and the pulmonary blood flow to the lungs is visualised.

A caveat

V̇/Q̇ scans aren't commonly used for patients on mechanical ventilators because the ventilation portion of the test is difficult to perform. (Pulmonary angiography is the preferred test for a critically ill patient with a suspected pulmonary embolus.)

Nursing considerations

• Explain the test to the patient and their family, telling them who performs the test and where it's done.
• Like pulmonary angiography, a V̇/Q̇ scan requires the injection of a contrast medium. Confirm that the patient doesn't have an allergy to the contrast material.
• Explain to the patient that the test has two parts. During the ventilation portion, a mask is placed over their mouth and nose and the patient breathes in the contrast medium gas mixed with air while the scanner takes pictures of their lungs. For the perfusion portion, the patient is placed in a supine position on a movable table as the contrast medium is injected into the I.V. line while the scanner again takes pictures of the lungs.
• After the procedure, maintain bed rest as ordered and monitor the patient's vital signs, oxygen saturation levels and heart rhythm.
• Monitor for adverse reactions to the contrast medium, which may include restlessness, tachypnoea and respiratory distress, tachycardia, urticaria and nausea and vomiting. Keep emergency equipment nearby in case of a reaction.

Pulmonary angiography

Pulmonary angiography, also called *pulmonary arteriography*, allows radiographic examination of the pulmonary circulation.

After injecting a radioactive contrast dye through a catheter inserted into the pulmonary artery or one of its branches, a series of x-rays is taken to detect blood flow abnormalities, possibly caused by emboli or pulmonary infarction.

More reliable, more risks

Pulmonary angiography yields more reliable results than a V̇/Q̇ scan, but carries higher risks for certain conditions, such as cardiac arrhythmias (especially ventricular arrhythmias due to myocardial irritation from passage of the catheter through the heart chambers). It may be the preferred test, especially if the patient is on a ventilator.

Nursing considerations
• Explain the procedure to the patient and their family and answer their questions. Tell them who performs the test, where it's done and how long it takes.

Preprocedure patient preparation
• Confirm that the patient isn't allergic to shellfish or iodine. Notify the doctor if the patient has such an allergy because the patient may have an adverse reaction to the contrast medium.
• Preprocedure testing should include evaluation of renal function (by serum creatinine levels and urea levels) and potential risk of bleeding (by prothrombin time, partial thromboplastin time [PTT] and platelet count). Notify the doctor of abnormal results.
• Instruct the patient to lie still for the procedure.
• Explain that they'll probably feel a flushed sensation in their face as the dye is injected.

Postprocedure procedures
• Maintain bed rest, as ordered, and monitor the patient's vital signs, oxygen saturation levels and heart rhythm.
• Keep a sandbag or femoral compression device over the injection site as ordered.
• After the procedure, check the pressure dressing for signs of bleeding. Monitor the patient's peripheral pulse in the arm or leg used for catheter insertion (mark the site), check the temperature, colour and sensation of the extremity and compare with the opposite side.
• Unless contraindicated, encourage the patient to drink more fluids to flush the dye or contrast medium from their system, or increase the I.V. flow rate as ordered.
• Check serum creatinine and urea levels after the procedure because the contrast medium can cause acute renal failure.
• Monitor for adverse reactions to the contrast medium, which may include restlessness, tachypnoea and respiratory distress, tachycardia, facial flushing, urticaria and nausea and vomiting. Keep emergency equipment nearby in case of a reaction.

Bedside testing procedures
Diagnostic tests used at the bedside to evaluate respiratory function include pulse oximetry, mixed venous oxygen saturation ($S\bar{v}O_2$) and end-tidal carbon dioxide ($ETCO_2$) monitoring.

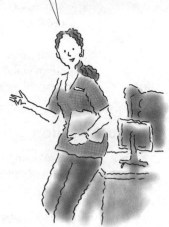

Pulmonary angiography may be preferred over $\dot{V}/\dot{Q}$ scanning, especially if your patient is on a ventilator.

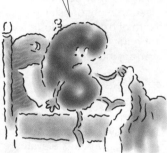

Maintain the patient on bed rest and be sure to check serum creatinine and urea levels because the contrast medium can cause acute renal failure.

Pulse oximetry

Pulse oximetry is a relatively simple procedure used to monitor arterial oxygen saturation noninvasively. It's performed either intermittently or continuously.

Shedding light on the subject

In this procedure, two diodes send red and infrared light through a pulsating arterial vascular bed such as the one in the fingertip.

A photodetector (also called a *sensor or transducer*) slipped over the finger measures the transmitted light as it passes through the vascular bed, detects the relative amount of each colour absorbed by arterial blood and calculates the saturation without interference from the venous blood, skin or connective tissue. The percentage expressed is the ratio of oxygen to haemoglobin. (See *A closer look at pulse oximetry.*)

Note denotation

In pulse oximetry, arterial oxygen saturation values are usually denoted with the symbol SpO_2. Arterial oxygen saturation values, which are measured invasively via ABG analysis, are denoted by the symbol SaO_2.

Nursing considerations

- Place the sensor over the finger or other site, such as the toe, or earlobe, so that the light beams and sensors are opposite each other.
- Protect the sensor from exposure to strong light, such as fluorescent lighting, because it interferes with results. Check the sensor site frequently to make sure the device is in place and to examine the skin for abrasion and pressure damage.
- The pulse oximeter displays the patient's pulse rate and oxygen saturation reading. The pulse rate on the oximeter must correspond to the patient's actual pulse. If the rates don't correspond, the saturation reading can't be considered accurate. You may need to reposition the sensor to obtain an accurate reading.

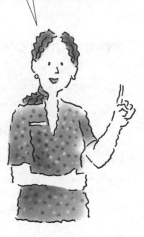

Place the sensor over a finger or other site so that the light beams and sensors are opposite each other.

A closer look at pulse oximetry

Oximetry may be intermittent or continuous and is used to monitor arterial oxyhaemoglobin saturation. Normal oxyhaemoglobin saturation levels are 95–100% for adults. Lower levels may indicate hypoxaemia and warrant intervention.

Interfering factors

Certain factors can interfere with the accuracy of oximetry readings. For example, an elevated bilirubin level may falsely lower oxyhaemoglobin saturation readings, whereas elevated carboxyhaemoglobin or methaemoglobin levels can falsely elevate oxyhaemoglobin saturation readings.

Certain intravascular substances, such as lipid emulsions and dyes, can also prevent accurate readings. Other interfering factors include excessive light (such as from phototherapy or direct sunlight), excessive patient movement, excessive ear pigment, hypothermia, hypotension and vasoconstriction.

Some acrylic nails and certain colours of nail polish (blue, green, black and brown-red) may also interfere with readings.

- Rotate the sensor site at least every 4 hours, or according to the manufacturer's instructions and your facility's policy for site rotation, to avoid skin irritation and pressure damage.
- If oximetry is done properly, the oxygen saturation readings are usually within 2% of ABG values. A normal reading is 95–100%.

Poisoning precludes pulse oximetry

- Pulse oximetry isn't accurate when carbon monoxide poisoning is suspected because the oximeter doesn't differentiate between oxygen and carbon monoxide bound to haemoglobin. An ABG analysis should be performed in such cases.

Mixed venous oxygen saturation monitoring

$S\bar{v}O_2$ reflects the oxygen saturation level of venous blood. It's determined by measuring the amount of oxygen extracted and used or consumed by the body's tissues.

$S\bar{v}O_2$ indications

In a healthy adult, the arterial oxygen saturation (SaO_2) is >95%; the tissues extract about 25% of the delivered oxygen—leaving a venous saturation ($S\bar{v}O_2$ of around 70%. When the $S\bar{v}O_2$ is lower than 70% it may indicate that the delivery of oxygen is low (low SaO_2 and/or low cardiac output) and/or that tissue oxygen extraction is high (e.g. sepsis of high fever).

Increased values greater than 80% may occur in states of increased oxygen delivery or may indicate decreased oxygen extraction by the tissues (when tissue hypoxia exists despite the availability of oxygen).

Drawing from the right location

The term mixed venous means that blood from the superior vena cava and inferior vena cava have mixed in the heart—thus the measurement is an average of the whole circulation. Ideally, the $S\bar{v}O_2$ sample is obtained from the most distal port of the pulmonary artery (PA) catheter, which contains the ideal mix of all venous blood in the heart. Samples may be drawn from a central catheter if a PA catheter isn't available. However, a central venous catheter will tend to reflect the superior vena caval blood because of its frequent positioning in the central veins above the right atrium. This will generally result in a reading that is approximately 5% higher than mixed venous. This is because slightly less oxygen is extracted in the head and arms (draining into the superior vena cava) than in the lower body (draining into the inferior vena cava). This should be considered when interpreting the results.

A calculating catheter

Continuous $S\bar{v}O_2$ monitoring is done using the $S\bar{v}O_2$ or oximetric PA catheter. This specialised PA catheter calculates oxygen saturation of haemoglobin by measuring the wavelengths of reflected light through fibre-optic bundles.

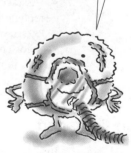

The patient's $S\bar{v}O_2$ level reflects the amount of oxygen extracted by the body's tissues. Hey, we all have needs!

The information is exhibited on a bedside computer and may be displayed numerically and graphically. The manufacturer's instructions for catheter calibration must be followed to ensure accurate readings.

Nursing considerations

- Explain the procedure to the patient and their family. Make sure they understand the expected outcomes and risks of the procedure related to catheter placement, pneumothorax, cardiac arrhythmias and infection.
- If you assist with catheter insertion, monitor the patient's vital signs and heart rhythm as you assess for changes in ventilatory function.
- Apply a sterile dressing or sterile transparent dressing over the catheter insertion site. Follow local policy for changing the dressing and pulmonary artery monitoring system (tubing and solution).
- Document the date and time of catheter insertion, initial $S\bar{v}O_2$ readings and any changes in the patient's condition. Monitor the pulmonary artery pressure (PAP) and $S\bar{v}O_2$ readings, and document hourly or according to local policy. (See *Normal and abnormal $S\bar{v}O_2$ waveforms*, page 305.)
- Closely monitor the patient's haemodynamic status. Troubleshoot the catheter for problems that can interfere with accurate testing, such as loose connections, balloon rupture or clot formation on the tip of the catheter.

End-tidal carbon dioxide monitoring

$ETCO_2$ is used to measure the carbon dioxide concentration at end expiration. An $ETCO_2$ monitor may be a separate monitor or part of the patient's bedside monitoring system.

Indications for $ETCO_2$ monitoring include:
- Assessment of ET tube placement. After intubation the tube placed in the oesophagus will generate no CO_2.
- Assessment of the patient with hypercapnoea in acute asthma.
- Close monitoring and titration of mechanical ventilation to control $PaCO_2$ in the patient with acute brain injury. (See Chapter 3).
- Monitoring the effectiveness of mechanical ventilation of patients during inter-hospital transport.

In-lightened

In $ETCO_2$ monitoring, a photodetector measures the amount of infrared light absorbed by the airway during inspiration and expiration. (Light absorption increases along with the carbon dioxide concentration.) The monitor converts these data to a carbon dioxide value and a corresponding waveform, or capnogram if capnography is used. (See *Understanding $ETCO_2$ monitoring*, page 306.)

Crunching the numbers

Values are obtained by monitoring samples of expired gas from an endotracheal (ET) tube or tracheostomy.

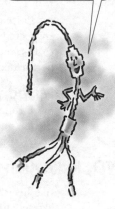

Follow the manufacturer's instructions for catheter calibration to ensure accurate readings.

Normal and abnormal S$\overline{\text{v}}$o$_2$ waveforms

This tracing represents a stable, normal S$\overline{\text{v}}$o$_2$ level: around 70%. Note the relatively constant line.

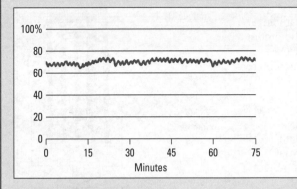

This waveform shows typical changes in the S$\overline{\text{v}}$o$_2$ level as a result of various activities.

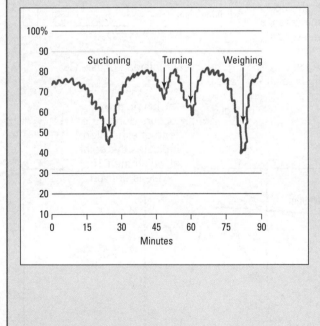

This tracing represents the patient's response to a muscle relaxant.

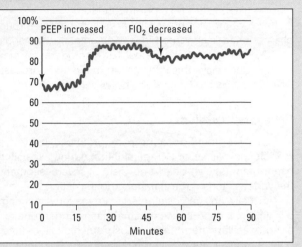

This waveform shows the patient's response to changes in ventilator settings. Note that increasing the positive end-expiratory pressure (PEEP) causes an increase in S$\overline{\text{v}}$o$_2$; therefore, the fraction of inspired oxygen (FIo$_2$) can be decreased.

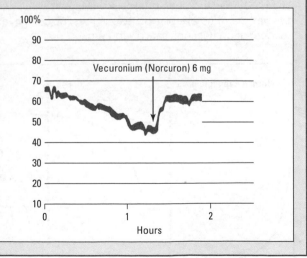

Understanding ETco₂ monitoring

The optical portion of an end-tidal carbon dioxide (ETco₂) monitor contains an infrared light source, a sample chamber, a special carbon dioxide (CO_2) filter and a photodetector.

In ETco₂ monitoring, the infrared light passes through the sample chamber and is absorbed in varying amounts, depending on the amount of CO_2 the patient just exhaled. The photodetector measures CO_2 content and relays this information to the microprocessor in the monitor, which displays the CO_2 value and waveform.

Capnogram reading

The CO_2 waveform, or capnogram, produced in ETco₂ monitoring reflects the course of CO_2 elimination during exhalation. A normal capnogram (shown below) consists of several segments, which reflect the various stages of exhalation and inhalation.

Normally, any gas eliminated from the airway during early exhalation is dead-space gas that hasn't undergone exchange at the alveolocapillary membrane. Measurements taken during this period contain no CO_2. As exhalation continues, CO_2 concentration increases sharply and rapidly. The sensor now detects gas that has undergone exchange, producing measurable quantities of CO_2.

The final stages of alveolar emptying occur during late exhalation. During the alveolar plateau phase, CO_2 concentration increases gradually because alveolar emptying is relatively constant.

The point at which the ETco₂ value is derived is the end of exhalation, when CO_2 concentration peaks. However, this value doesn't accurately reflect alveolar CO_2 if no alveolar plateau is present. During inhalation, the CO_2 concentration declines sharply to zero.

ETco₂ monitor

Exhaled CO_2

Infrared light source

Sample chamber

CO_2 filter

Photodetector

This peak that occurs during the end of exhalation indicates the point at which the ETco₂ value is derived.

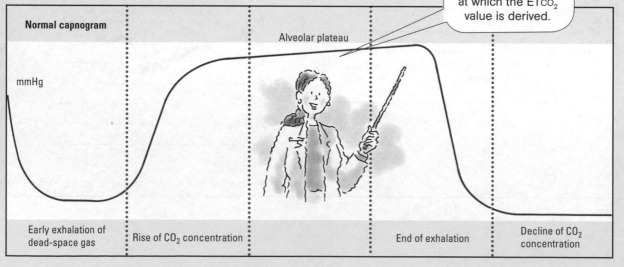

Normal capnogram

Alveolar plateau

mmHg

Early exhalation of dead-space gas

Rise of CO_2 concentration

End of exhalation

Decline of CO_2 concentration

In health the PaCO$_2$ values are usually around 0.5 kPa higher than the ETCO$_2$ values. However, this is when there is no ventilatory or gas exchange dysfunction. In the presence of airflow limiting disorders such as exacerbations of asthma or COPD there may be great differences between PaCO$_2$ and ETCO$_2$ of up to 5 kPa or more depending on the severity of the condition. The degree of disparity is an indication of severity and as the disparity resolves this is an indication of improvement. Capnographs and ETCO$_2$ monitoring reduce the need for frequent ABG sampling; however, it is important for the critical care nurse never to assume that differences between ETCO$_2$ and PaCO$_2$ are consistent or that changes in one will accurately reflect changes in the other.

Nursing considerations

- Explain the procedure to the patient and their family.
- Ensure you are familiar with how to calibrate and troubleshoot the equipment.
- Assess the patient's respiratory status, vital signs, oxygen saturation and ETCO$_2$ readings. Observe waveform quality and trends of ETCO$_2$ readings and take acute changes as a prompt to check an ABG.
- Chart the ETCO$_2$ readings with your regular observations and document trends in PaCO$_2$ on the chart as well to allow monitoring of changes in disparity between the two levels.
- Be aware that circuit disconnection, endotracheal suction and coughing will cause acute changes in the waveform (capnograph) and the numbers displayed until things settle.

Treatments

Respiratory disorders interfere with airway clearance, breathing patterns and gas exchange. If not corrected, they can adversely affect many other body systems and can be life-threatening.

Treatments for patients with respiratory disorders include oxygen and ventilatory therapy, drug therapy and surgery.

Oxygen and ventilatory therapy

This therapy involves methods to deliver supplemental oxygen, progressing through CPAP (continuous positive airway pressure) and NIV (noninvasive ventilation) through to mechanical ventilation for those with the most severe forms of respiratory failure. ET (endotracheal) intubation and appropriately managed weaning from ventilation are also key elements of respiratory management and are therefore also given consideration here.

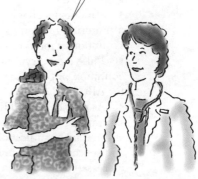

Notify the doctor if there's a sustained 10% increase or decrease in ETCO$_2$ readings.

Oxygen therapy

For patients with respiratory dysfunction oxygen therapy is the most common intervention. It is essential to prevent hypoxaemia and minimise the increased work of breathing that will be a natural response to deteriorating gas exchange.

Commencing and titrating oxygen

Ideally oxygen should be prescribed by a doctor or by a nonmedical prescriber. When oxygen is prescribed it is essential for the prescriber to state the target range for oxygen saturations. This is usually >94% (or 88–92% for those at risk of hypercapnic respiratory failure). An appropriate delivery device is then selected (see *Types of oxygen therapy*) according to how much oxygen is needed to achieve target oxygen saturations (or PaO_2). However, urgent situations will require prompt initiation of oxygen therapy to prevent hypoxaemia. You may not have time to get a formal prescription so knowing how to commence, titrate and evaluate oxygen therapy is important.

Important steps

When you are commencing oxygen here's what to do:
• If there are signs of hypoxaemia in a critically ill patient (e.g. cyanosis, tachypnoea, respiratory distress and shock) initiate oxygen immediately—give the highest concentration you can with the equipment to hand (usually a reservoir mask at 15 L/minute). Get medical help urgently. If there is feeble or slow respiratory effort or apnoea use a bag-valve-mask to hand ventilate the patient and call for immediate medical help.
• Others with acute illness who have oxygen saturations below the normal target range (>94%) will need supplemental oxygen via an appropriate device to achieve saturation within the target range. Those with saturations between 90 and 94% may need low levels of supplemental oxygen that can be delivered by 1–2 L/minute by a nasal cannula or by 24–28% venturi mask initially. However, those with oxygen saturations <85% should always be given oxygen at 15 L/minute via reservoir mask followed by urgent medical assessment.
• For those who are at risk of hypercapnic respiratory failure (e.g. severe COPD, morbid obesity, neuromuscular disorders and chest wall deformity) the target saturation should be 88–92%. Commence oxygen by a venturi mask at 24–28%, ask for a medical assessment and prepare equipment for ABG sampling.
• Prolonged oxygen therapy (longer than 4 hours), except where delivery is via nasal cannula, should be humidified.
• Patients should be helped to position themselves in an upright (at least 45° incline) position as supine laying will reduce lung capacity and impair gas exchange.
• Patients receiving continuous oxygen therapy should have regular monitoring of their oxygen saturations. If patients are critically ill oxygen saturations should be continuously monitored.
• Pulse oximetry is not a substitute for ABG analysis and any changes in condition or oxygen requirements should prompt consideration of the need for ABG analysis.
• As the acute condition resolves wean oxygen whilst maintaining oxygen saturations in the target range. This is an important point as oxygen is not without its complications—these include reduced mucocillary function and sputum retention, reduced lung immune function, tissue damage and increased atelectasis with high concentrations.

Types of oxygen therapy

Various types of devices are used to deliver oxygen therapy. Regardless of the type, always assess the patient closely and check the results of pulse oximetry immediately, or arterial blood gas analysis 20–30 minutes after adjusting the oxygen flow rate, percentage or delivery device.

Delivery device	Oxygen concentration administered	Administration guidelines
Nasal cannula	Low flow, 1–6 L/minute (24–44% oxygen but not fixed performance)	• May be used where fixed performance is not essential in patients who have relatively normal vital signs and/or low supplemental oxygen needs. • Ensure the cannulae are fitted as per manufacturer's instructions. • Nose is a physiological humidifier thus reducing complications of giving unhumidified oxygen.
Simple mask	2–10 L/minute (24–40% oxygen but not fixed performance)	• Place mask over the patient's nose, mouth, and chin, moulding the flexible metal edge to the bridge of their nose. • Adjust elastic to hold the mask firmly but comfortably in place. • Because the mask is not a fixed performance device the faster and/or deeper the patent breathes the greater the oxygen is diluted by air drawn into the mask. Thus accuracy when stating oxygen concentrations is not possible and when higher concentrations are needed or greater accuracy is needed this mask shouldn't be used. • Delivers dry oxygen—if administered over a prolonged period (hours) will cause drying of mucous membranes and secretions.
Nonrebreather mask (reservoir mask)	15 L/minute (approximately 85% oxygen—but not fixed performance)	• It should be used for the critically ill as a short-term means of giving a high concentration of oxygen. • Close the valve momentarily prior to applying to allow the reservoir to inflate. • Make sure the mask fits snugly and the one-way valves are secure and functioning. • Keep the reservoir bag from twisting or kinking and ensure free expansion of the bag by keeping it outside of the patient's gown and bedcovers.
Fixed performance venturi mask	2–15 L/minute (24–60%—fixed performance)	• Use this mask when precise oxygen concentration is important. • Ensure that the proper device is used and that the oxygen flow rate is set at the amount specified on each mask. • Make sure that the venturi valve is set for the desired F_{IO_2}. • Delivers dry oxygen—if administered over a prolonged period (hours) will cause drying of mucous membranes and secretions.
Aerosols (cold water humidifiers)	May have an adjustable venturi valve that allows for fixed performance	• Ensure that the proper device is used and that the oxygen flow rate and F_{IO_2} is set at the amount prescribed by the doctor. • Be alert for condensation build-up in the tubing; empty the tubing at frequent intervals. • Ensure that condensate doesn't enter the trachea. • When using a high-output nebuliser, watch for signs of overhydration, pulmonary oedema, crackles and electrolyte imbalances.

CPAP and NIV

CPAP (continuous positive airway pressure)

CPAP is often used when patients are hypoxaemic despite high levels of oxygen therapy. A breathing system is used to deliver high-flow oxygen via a circuit that includes a valve preventing full exhalation. The pressure the spring-loaded valve exerts maintains increased resting volume in the lungs (functional residual capacity), thus preventing collapse of dysfunctional alveoli at end of expiration. For this reason CPAP will also be used when there is alveolar collapse due to infection or underinflation of basal lung zones, in the postoperative patient for example. In order to achieve an airtight seal a tight fitting, cushioned, face mask or hood is used as the patient interface. (See *CPAP circuit and face mask*.).

You will also see CPAP used when patients are weaning from mechanical ventilation and still have an artificial airway. In this instance the airtight seal is made by attaching a T-piece to the ET or tracheostomy tube instead of using a CPAP mask or hood.

How it works

By maintaining a positive pressure in the airways at all times, CPAP essentially increases functional residual capacity (residual volume) in alveoli which would otherwise collapse.

CPAP circuit and face mask

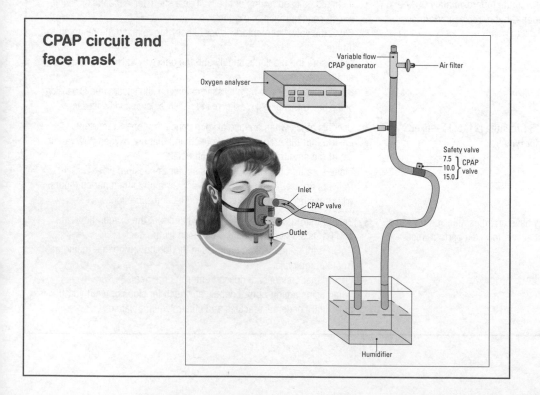

Alveoli that are already partly inflated take less effort to further inflate so applying CPAP improves lung compliance and therefore reduces the work of breathing.

In improving ventilation it improves gas exchange through a more efficient ventilation:perfusion ratio.

When CPAP is indicated

Type I respiratory failure where there is acute hypoxaemia (despite high levels of inspired oxygen) without carbon dioxide retention; that is, those patients having problems with oxygenation and not ventilation—for example:
- Acute pneumonia where the patient remains hypoxaemic despite high-flow oxygen
- Cardiogenic pulmonary oedema where the patient remains hypoxaemic despite maximum medical therapy
- Chest wall trauma where the patient remains hypoxaemic despite adequate analgesia
- Significant alveolar collapse (atelectasis), as in postoperative respiratory failure or pneumonia

It may be appropriate to attempt trials of CPAP as a means of preventing the need for intubation and mechanical ventilation. If this is the case then this should always be done within a critical care unit.

NIV (noninvasive ventilation)

NIV may also be referred to as BiPAP (bilevel or biphasic positive airway pressure). NIV is mechanical ventilation delivered via a face or nasal mask, or more recently by a hood.

How it works

The noninvasive ventilator is set to deliver positive-pressure breaths ending when a preset pressure in the circuit is reached. This pressure is referred to as IPAP (inspiratory positive airway pressure). A further pressure setting made on the noninvasive ventilator is EPAP (expiratory positive airway pressure).

EPAP helps increase FRC as in CPAP, whilst IPAP provides mechanical assistance during inspiration for those with reduced inspiratory effort or strength causing ventilatory failure. The overall effect is an increase in tidal volume and alveolar ventilation which results in greater carbon dioxide elimination.

When NIV is indicated

Type II respiratory failure where there is acute hypercapnia and respiratory acidosis. That is, those patients having problems with ventilation rather than oxygenation. Clinical application of NIV includes:
- Acute exacerbation of COPD where there is respiratory acidosis (pH < 7.35) despite controlled oxygen therapy achieving a target SpO_2 between 88 and 92%.
- Acute or acute-on-chronic hypercapnic respiratory failure due to chest wall deformity or neuromuscular disease.
- Postoperative respiratory failure.

- During weaning from mechanical ventilation when conventional strategies fail.
- In situations where mechanical ventilation might be avoided through short-term support with NIV within a critical care unit.

When to be cautious about CPAP and NIV

There are some situations where CPAP and NIV carry such a high risk that it should not be used. These include:
- Recent facial trauma
- Recent airway surgery
- Upper airway obstruction or inability of the patient to maintain and protect their own airway
- Vomiting

In other situation CPAP and NIV should only be used with extreme caution and only when supervised by expert medical and nursing staff. These include:
- Recent upper GI surgery
- Excessive respiratory secretions
- Acute confusion, agitation, combativeness
- Acute intestinal obstruction
- In the presence of a pneumothorax (this would usually be ruled out prior to commencing CPAP—or a pleural drain inserted if pneumothorax present).

What to do to ensure the success of CPAP and NIV

- Check for contraindications before you commence the treatment.
- Ensure the patient has had a chest x-ray and ABG analysis and these have been interpreted by a doctor.
- Prepare the patient for what to expect. Tell them that communication will be difficult, and that eating and drinking will not be possible during time when the mask or hood is sealed. But reassure them that they will have at least brief breaks for these activities according to their condition and as tolerated.
- Ensure the patient is assisted to achieve a position in which they can breathe most effectively—generally with the head of the bed elevated to at least 45 degrees.
- Set initial NIV pressures to 8–10 cmH$_2$O (IPAP) over 4–6 cmH$_2$O (EPAP) and titrate according to ABG results, chest expansion, patient comfort and tolerance.
- Commence CPAP at between 5 and 10 cmH$_2$O and titrate according to ABG results.
- Establish a target level for oxygen saturations and constantly monitor using pulse oximetry. Report any deterioration from agreed target range to medical staff.
- When commencing therapy fit the mask or hood whilst explaining to the patient what to expect.
- Ensure that there are no air leaks in the circuit—particularly around the face mask where leaking air may dry the corneas of the eye causing ulceration.

- Repeat ABG analysis approximately 1 hour after commencing CPAP or NIV and then after any changes in clinical condition or in levels of oxygen or pressure settings.
- Titrate inspired oxygen according to agreed target range for oxygen saturations and/or PaO_2.
- Titrate pressures/settings as prescribed to achieve target $PaCO_2$.
- Check the connections and patient interface for leaks and ensure that the CPAP valve is exposed and visible at all times to prevent obstruction. Make regular observations of the valve and ensure that air/oxygen flow is sufficient to keep the valve open through inspiration as well as expiration.
- Ensure adequate humidification of inspired air.
- Provide breaks for physiotherapy, mouth care, oral fluids and diet as tolerated.
- Provide pressure area care—especially around the face mask and head strapping.
- Ensure adequate hydration by I.V. route as prescribed if oral fluid intake is inadequate.
- Monitor cardiovascular and respiratory conditions regularly. Observe for indications of intolerance and for complications (sore eyes, dry mouth, dehydration, pressure damage to skin, sputum retention) and for deteriorating condition indicating the need for intubation and mechanical ventilation.

ET intubation

ET intubation involves insertion of a tube into the trachea through the mouth or nose to establish a patent airway. It protects patients from aspiration by sealing off the trachea from the digestive tract and permits removal of tracheobronchial secretions in patients who can't cough effectively. ET intubation also provides a route for mechanical ventilation and oxygen administration.

> ET intubation bypasses normal respiratory defences against infection. That's good news for me, but bad news for the patient!

Too good to be true?

Drawbacks of ET intubation are that it bypasses normal respiratory defences against infection, reduces cough effectiveness, may be uncomfortable and prevents verbal communication.

Potential complications of ET intubation include:
- bronchospasm or laryngospasm
- aspiration of blood, secretions or gastric contents
- tooth damage or loss
- injury to the lips, mouth, pharynx or vocal cords
- hypoxaemia (if attempts at intubation are prolonged or oxygen delivery interrupted)
- tracheal stenosis, erosion and necrosis
- cardiac arrhythmias.

Orotracheal intubation

With orotracheal intubation, the oral cavity is used as the route of insertion. It's preferred in emergency situations because it's easier and faster. However, maintaining exact tube placement is more difficult because the tube must be well secured to avoid kinking and prevent bronchial obstruction or accidental extubation. It's also uncomfortable for conscious patients because it stimulates salivation, coughing and the gag reflex.

The right size

The typical size for an oral ET tube is 7.0–8.0 mm (indicates the size of the lumen) for women and 7.5–9.0 mm for men.

Not for everyone

Orotracheal intubation is contraindicated in patients with orofacial injuries, acute cervical spinal injury and degenerative spinal disorders.

Nasal intubation

With nasal intubation, a nasal passage is used as the route of insertion. Nasal intubation is preferred for elective insertion when the patient is capable of spontaneous ventilation for a short period.

A conscious choice

Nasal intubation is more comfortable than oral intubation and is typically used for conscious patients who are at risk for imminent respiratory arrest or who have cervical spinal injuries. It's contraindicated for patients with facial or basilar skull fractures.

Difficult and damaging

Although it's more comfortable than oral intubation, nasal intubation is more difficult to perform. Because the tube passes blindly through

> On the downside, nasal intubation is more difficult to do than oral intubation, and causes more tissue damage.

Securing an ET tube

When securing an endotracheal (ET) tube, make sure the tube is immobile. Remember—Securing an ET tube is a two-person job.

When you're using a manufactured tube holder

- Follow the manufacturer's instructions on how to use.

When you're using ties

- Cut about 60 cm of a tracheostomy tie and place it under the patient's neck.
- Bring both ends up to the tube and cross them at the bottom of the tube near the patient's lips.
  Tie a double knot. Make sure the tie is not too tight—you should be able to pass two fingers beneath the tie.
- Bring the ends to the top of the tube and tie them in an overhand knot around the tube securing the tube to the tie.
- Bring the ends back to the bottom of the tube, tie another overhand knot and then secure the ties with a square knot (right over left and then left over right).
- Check the tie's regularly to ensure they are not causing pressure damage and that they haven't become too tight or loose.

the nasal cavity, it causes more tissue damage, increases the risk of infection by nasal bacteria introduced into the trachea and increases the risk of pressure necrosis of the nasal mucosa. For these reasons you'll rarely see nasal intubation in the critically ill.

Nursing considerations
• After intubation secure the ET tube. (See *Securing an ET tube*, page 314.)
• Auscultate breath sounds and watch for bilateral chest movement to ensure correct tube placement and full lung ventilation.
• A chest x-ray will be ordered to confirm tube placement.
• An $ETCO_2$ detector may be used to confirm correct placement in some circumstances where the intubation was difficult or there is doubt about the placement.
• Follow local infection prevention and control guidelines for suction through the ET tube.
• Perform suction through the ET tube as the patient's condition indicates, to clear secretions and prevent mucus plugs from obstructing the tube. If available, use a closed tracheal suctioning system, which permits the ventilated patient to remain on the ventilator during suctioning without loss of PEEP and avoidance of spray of respiratory secretions towards health care staff. (See *Closed tracheal suctioning*, page 316.)

Mechanical ventilation
Mechanical ventilation involves the use of a machine to move air into a patient's lungs. Mechanical ventilators used in critical care use positive pressure to push air into the patient's lungs.

When to ventilate

Indications for mechanical ventilation include:
• acute respiratory failure due to ARDS, pneumonia, acute exacerbations of COPD, heart failure, trauma or drug overdose
• respiratory centre depression due to stroke, brain injury or trauma
• neuromuscular disturbances caused by neuromuscular diseases, such as Guillain–Barré syndrome, multiple sclerosis and myasthenia gravis; trauma, including spinal cord injury; or CNS depression.

Accentuate the positive

Positive-pressure ventilators exert a positive pressure on the airway, which causes inspiration while increasing tidal volume (V_T).
The inspiratory cycles of these ventilators may be adjusted for volume, pressure or time:
• A volume-cycled ventilator, the type used most commonly, delivers a preset volume of air each time, regardless of the amount of lung resistance.

> Mechanical ventilation uses a machine to move air into the patient's lungs.

> Take a deep breath and join the oxygen movement

Closed tracheal suctioning

The closed tracheal suctioning system can ease removal of secretions and reduce patient complications. The system consists of a sterile suction catheter in a clear plastic sleeve. It permits the patient to remain connected to the ventilator during suctioning.

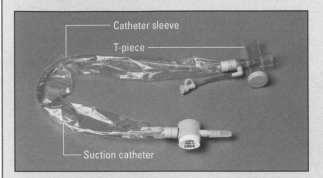

Catheter sleeve

T-piece

Suction catheter

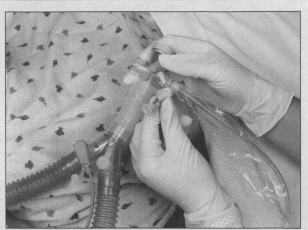

As a result, the patient can maintain the tidal volume, oxygen concentration and PEEP (positive end-expiratory pressure) delivered by the ventilator while being suctioned. In turn, this reduces the occurrence of suction-induced hypoxaemia.

Another advantage of this system is a reduced risk of infection, even when the same catheter is used many times. The caregiver doesn't need to touch the catheter and the ventilator circuit remains closed.

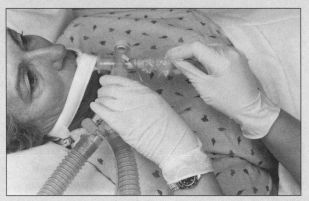

Performing the procedure

To perform the procedure, assemble the closed suction device as per manufacturer's instruction. Then, follow these steps:

- Depress the thumb suction-control valve and keep it depressed while setting the suction pressure to the desired level—usually in the medium range.
- Connect the T-piece to the ventilator breathing circuit, making sure that the irrigation port is closed; then connect the T-piece to the patient's endotracheal or tracheostomy tube (as shown).
- With one hand keeping the T-piece parallel to the patient's chin, use the thumb and index finger of the other hand to advance the catheter through the tube and into the patient's tracheobronchial tree (as shown).

- If necessary, gently retract the catheter sleeve as you advance the catheter.
- While continuing to hold the T-piece and control valve, apply intermittent suction and withdraw the catheter until it reaches its fully extended length in the sleeve. Repeat the procedure as necessary.
- After you finish suctioning, flush the catheter by maintaining suction while slowly introducing normal saline solution or sterile water into the irrigation port.
- Place the thumb control valve in the off position.
- Dispose off and replace the suction equipment and supplies according to your department's policy.
- Change the closed suction system according to your department's policy—usually daily.

Ventilator modes

Positive-pressure ventilators are categorised as volume or pressure ventilators and have various modes and options. Because manufacturers use different words to describe *their* version of common modes it is important to learn how each mode works then you can use different ventilators by just learning the specific mode name on each model. A brief overview is given here—we've tried to use generic terms but beware—these modes may have a different name on the ventilator in your unit.

Volume modes

Volume modes include controlled mandatory ventilation (CMV), and synchronised intermittent mandatory ventilation (SIMV).

CMV

In the CMV mode, the ventilator supplies all ventilation for the patient. The respiratory rate, tidal volume (V_T), inspiratory time, and positive end-expiratory pressure (PEEP) are preset. This mode is usually used when a patient can't initiate spontaneous breaths, such as when they're paralysed from a spinal cord injury or neuromuscular disease, or chemically paralysed with neuromuscular blocking agents.

SIMV

SIMV mode requires preset respiratory rate, V_T, inspiratory time, sensitivity and PEEP. Mandatory breaths are delivered at a set rate and V_T. In between the mandatory breaths, the patient can breathe spontaneously at their own rate and V_T. The V_T of these spontaneous breaths can vary because the breaths are determined by the patient's ability to generate negative pressure in their chest as well as any pressure-support set to assist the patient's breath. With SIMV, the ventilator synchronises the mandatory breaths with the patient's own inspirations.

Pressure modes

Pressure modes include pressure-support ventilation (PSV), pressure-controlled ventilation (PCV) and pressure-controlled/inverse ratio ventilation (PC/IRV).

PSV

The PSV mode augments inspiration for a spontaneously breathing patient. The inspiratory pressure level, PEEP and sensitivity are preset. When the patient initiates a breath, the breath is delivered at the preset pressure level and is maintained throughout inspiration. The patient determines the V_T, respiratory rate and inspiratory time.

PCV

In PCV mode, inspiratory pressure, inspiratory time, respiratory rate and PEEP are preset. V_T varies with the patient's airway pressure and compliance because reaching the preset pressure is the thing that ends the breath. PCV modes are generally referred to by manufacturers in terminology that describes the fact that two pressure levels are set (e.g. BiLevel or BiPAP).

PC/IVR

PC/IVR combines pressure-limited ventilation with an inverse ratio of inspiration to expiration. In this mode, the inspiratory pressure, respiratory rate, inspiratory time (1:1, 2:1, 3:1 or 4:1) and PEEP are preset. PCV and PC/IRV modes may be used in patients with acute respiratory distress syndrome.

- A pressure-cycled ventilator generates flow until the machine reaches a preset pressure, regardless of the volume delivered or the time required to achieve the pressure.
- A time-cycled ventilator generates flow for a preset amount of time.
  Several different modes of ventilatory control are found on the ventilator. The choice of mode depends on the patient's respiratory condition. (See *Ventilator modes*.)

Responding to ventilator alarms

This chart outlines the possible causes and the nursing interventions needed if a ventilator alarm sounds.

Signal	Possible cause	Interventions
Low-pressure alarm	Endotracheal (ET) tube disconnected from ventilator	Reconnect the tube to the ventilator.
	Tube displaced above vocal cords or tracheostomy tube displaced	Check the tube placement; reposition if needed. If extubation or displacement has occurred, ventilate the patient manually and call the doctor immediately.
	Leaking tidal volume from low cuff pressure (from an underinflated or ruptured cuff or a leak in the cuff or one-way valve)	Listen for a whooshing sound around the tube, indicating an air leak. If you hear one, check the cuff pressure. If you can't maintain pressure, call the doctor and prepare for reintubation.
	Ventilator malfunction	Disconnect the patient from the ventilator and ventilate them manually, if necessary. Obtain another ventilator.
	Leak in ventilator circuitry (from loose connection or hole in tubing, loss of temperature-sensitive device or cracked humidification chamber)	Make sure all connections are intact. Check for holes or leaks in the tubing and replace, if necessary. Check the humidification chamber and replace, if cracked.
High-pressure alarm	Increased airway pressure or decreased lung compliance caused by worsening disease	Auscultate the lungs for evidence of increasing lung consolidation, barotrauma or wheezing. Call the doctor if indicated.
	Patient biting on oral ET tube	Insert a bite block if needed or sedate the patient more deeply if not contraindicated.
	Secretions in airway	Look, listen and feel for secretions in the airway. To remove them, suction the patient or have them cough.
	Condensate in large-bore tubing	Check tubing for condensate and remove any fluid.
	Intubation of right mainstem bronchus	Check tube position and for evidence of expansion on the right side only. If it has slipped, call the doctor, who may need to reposition it.
	Patient coughing, gagging or attempting to talk	If the patient fights the ventilator, the doctor may order an increase in sedation.
	Chest wall resistance	Reposition the patient to see if doing so improves chest expansion. If repositioning doesn't help, administer the prescribed analgesic.
	Failure of high-pressure relief valve	Have the faulty equipment replaced.
	Bronchospasm	Assess the patient for the cause—indications might be wheeze. Report to the doctor and treat the patient, as prescribed.

Nursing considerations

• Provide emotional support to the patient during all phases of mechanical ventilation to reduce anxiety and promote successful treatment. Even if the patient is unresponsive, continue to explain all procedures and treatments.

Be alarmed

• Make sure the ventilator alarms are on at all times and are set to appropriate parameters to alert you to potentially hazardous conditions and changes in the patient's status.
• Assess cardiopulmonary status frequently, at least hourly or more, if indicated. Assess vital signs and auscultate breath sounds. Monitor pulse oximetry and $ETCO_2$ levels and haemodynamic parameters as ordered. Monitor intake and output and assess for fluid volume excess or dehydration.
• Be alert for the development of complications associated with mechanical ventilation. These complications include decreased cardiac output (especially with the use of PEEP), barotrauma, pneumothorax, atelectasis, oxygen toxicity, stress ulcers and ventilator-associated pneumonia (VAP). (See *Reducing complications in the critically ill and mechanically ventilated patient.*)
• Unless contraindicated, turn the patient from side to side every 1–2 hours to aid lung expansion and postural drainage which removes secretions. Perform active or passive limb exercises for all extremities to reduce the hazards of immobility.
• Place the call bell within the patient's reach and establish a method of communication (such as a communication board) because intubation and mechanical ventilation impair the patient's ability to speak.
• Administer a sedative and/or opiate as prescribed, to relax the patient or eliminate spontaneous breathing efforts that can interfere with the ventilator's action.

Be extra vigilant

• Remember that the patient receiving a neuromuscular blocking agent requires close observation because they can't breathe or communicate. In addition, if the patient is receiving a neuromuscular blocking agent, make sure they also receive adequate amounts of sedation. Neuromuscular blocking agents cause paralysis without altering the patient's LOC. Reassure the patient and their family that the paralysis is temporary. Signs that the patient may be 'awake' but paralysed include the usual thing you'd expect to see in someone who is frightened and anxious—tachycardia, elevated blood pressure and sweating.
• Remember that if there are any problems with the ventilator or airway the patient will be unable to breathe unaided—so you'll need to ensure that emergency equipment is to hand for all paralysed or deeply sedated patients. This includes a method of hand ventilating the patient with supplemental oxygen. Make sure you can use this device safely—you may need to do it urgently.

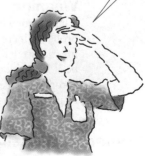

Stay alert! A patient receiving a neuromuscular blocking agent requires close observation because of their inability to breathe or communicate.

Reducing complications in the critically ill and mechanically ventilated patient

There are many significant complications that can arise during critical illness and mechanical ventilation. There is evidence that these are preventable and that the use of a 'care bundle'—a collection of interventions all consistently delivered can reduce complications significantly. Here are the regular standards of care that should be implemented to reduce complications.

Prophylaxis of DVT from immobility and critical illness

- Give thromboprophylaxis as prescribed

Prophylaxis of gastric ulcer from critical illness

- Give gastric ulcer prophylaxis as prescribed

Haemoglobin (Hb) trigger to reduce risk through modulation of immune system (if septic or ventilated)

- Unless there are other good reasons, such as ischaemia or active bleeding, don't transfuse blood unless the Hb is below 7 g/dl

Oral hygiene to prevent oropharyngeal bacterial overgrowth leading to VAP

- Routine oral hygiene including chlorhexidine gluconate for patients with an artificial airway

Elevation of the head of the bed to 45° to reduce the risk of ventilator-associated pneumonia (if ventilated)

- If head/brain injured—then aim for 30°
- If suspected/confirmed acute spinal injury—tilt whole bed to 30°
- If severe cardiovascular instability—aim for maximum workable head elevation

Appropriate humidification of inspired gas to prevent inspissation of secretions (if ventilated)

- Use heat-moisture exchanger (HME) or heated humidifier (HH)
- Consider addition of nebulised saline if secretions are tenacious or use of HME/HH is not possible.

Daily sedation holding to reduce duration of mechanical ventilation and VAP (if sedated and ventilated)

- Unless contraindicated stop sedation (excluding clonidine infusion) and sedating analgesia daily until patient is able to follow simple commands or is uncomfortable or agitated.

Suctioning of respiratory secretions as required (if ET/tracheostomy present)

- Wear apron and examination gloves, and decontaminate hands before and after procedure

Ventilator tubing management to prevent airway contamination (if ventilated)

- Replace when visibly soiled or mechanically malfunctioning
- Prevent condensate from entering patient's airway

> I'm fully weaned from the ventilation machine, but still dependent on oxygen. Not very stylish, but I'm not complaining.

Weaning

The patient who is mechanically ventilated will generally have pulmonary problems increasing the work required for breathing as well as loss of respiratory muscle strength and stamina. Anyone ventilated for longer than one week will be at high risk of being unable to sustain adequate breathing if ventilation is abruptly stopped. Thus ventilatory support is gradually weaned to allow the respiratory muscles to increase in strength and stamina and to assess progress with set goals.

Spontaneous strength

Successful weaning depends on a strong spontaneous respiratory effort, a stable cardiovascular system, sufficient respiratory muscle strength and level

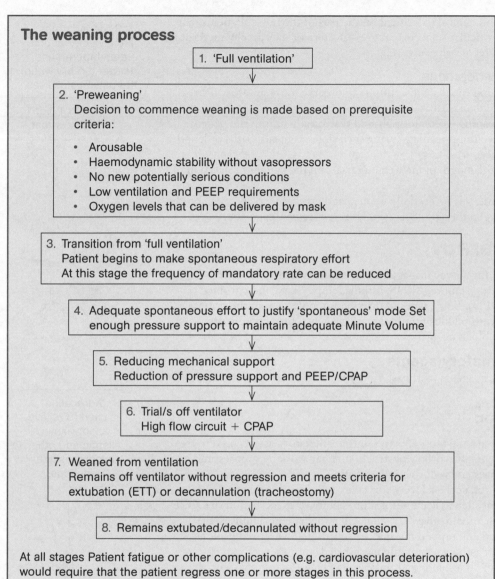

The weaning process

1. 'Full ventilation'

2. 'Preweaning'
Decision to commence weaning is made based on prerequisite criteria:

- Arousable
- Haemodynamic stability without vasopressors
- No new potentially serious conditions
- Low ventilation and PEEP requirements
- Oxygen levels that can be delivered by mask

3. Transition from 'full ventilation'
Patient begins to make spontaneous respiratory effort
At this stage the frequency of mandatory rate can be reduced

4. Adequate spontaneous effort to justify 'spontaneous' mode Set enough pressure support to maintain adequate Minute Volume

5. Reducing mechanical support
Reduction of pressure support and PEEP/CPAP

6. Trial/s off ventilator
High flow circuit + CPAP

7. Weaned from ventilation
Remains off ventilator without regression and meets criteria for extubation (ETT) or decannulation (tracheostomy)

8. Remains extubated/decannulated without regression

At all stages Patient fatigue or other complications (e.g. cardiovascular deterioration) would require that the patient regress one or more stages in this process.

of consciousness (LOC) to sustain spontaneous breathing. Certain criteria must be met before weaning can begin. (See *The weaning process*.)

The weaning process

Whilst not all patients are the same and practices vary from one critical care unit to another it is useful to consider the possible stage in the process of weaning a patient from a ventilator so that you can anticipate the next step and proactively care for your patient. (See *The weaning process*.) Weaning can be one of the most challenging aspects of care—at times requiring great patience, skill and clinical judgement on the part of the nurse. Patients may get stuck in a particular stage, may regress at times or may accelerate through or skip stages if recovering very well.

Nursing considerations
- When weaning the patient, continue to observe for respiratory distress, fatigue, hypoxaemia or cardiac arrhythmias.
- Schedule weaning to comfortably and realistically fit into the patient's daily routine, avoiding weaning during such times as meals, baths or lengthy therapeutic procedures.
- Document the length of the weaning trial and the patient's toleration of the procedure.
- After the patient is successfully weaned and extubated, place them on the appropriate oxygen therapy. (See *Types of oxygen therapy*, page 309.)

Drug therapy

Drugs are used for airway management in patients with such disorders as acute respiratory failure, ARDS, asthma, emphysema and chronic bronchitis (COPD). Some types of drugs commonly seen in the critical care environment include antiinflammatory agents, bronchodilators, neuromuscular blocking agents and sedatives.

Antiinflammatory agents
Antiinflammatory agents (corticosteroids) are used to reduce bronchial inflammation.

Reversing obstruction

Corticosteroids are the most effective antiinflammatory agents used to treat patients with reversible airflow obstruction. They work by suppressing immune responses and reducing inflammation.

Systemic drugs, such as Hydrocortisone, are given to manage an acute respiratory event such as acute respiratory failure or exacerbation of COPD. These drugs are initially given I.V. and, when the patient stabilises, the dosage is tapered and oral dosing may be substituted with prednisolone.

Patients with asthma commonly use inhaled steroids, such as beclomethasone, budesonide and fluticasone. These agents also work by suppressing the immune response and reducing airway inflammation. (See *Understanding corticosteroids*.).

Bronchodilators
Bronchodilators relax bronchial smooth muscles and are used to treat patients with bronchospasms. Here's how some types of bronchodilators are used:
- Short-acting inhaled beta$_2$-adrenergic agonists, such as salbutamol are used to relieve the acute symptoms in asthma and bronchospasm.
- Adrenaline acts on both alpha- and beta-adrenergic receptors. It's used to relieve anaphylactic, allergic and other hypersensitivity reactions. Its beta-adrenergic effects relax bronchial smooth muscle and relieve bronchospasm.

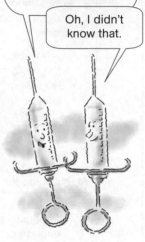

Systemic drugs are given I.V. at first, then tapered and delivered orally when the patient stabilises.

Oh, I didn't know that.

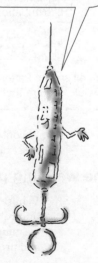

Adrenaline is used to relieve anaphylactic, allergic and other hypersensitivity reactions.

Understanding corticosteroids

Use this table to learn about the indications, adverse reactions and practice pointers associated with corticosteroids.

Drugs	Indications	Adverse reactions	Practice pointers
Systemic steroids			
• Hydrocortisone • Prednisolone	• Antiinflammatory for acute respiratory failure, acute respiratory distress syndrome and chronic obstructive pulmonary disease • Antiinflammatory and immunosuppressor for asthma	• Heart failure • Arrhythmias • Oedema • Circulatory collapse • Thromboembolism • Pancreatitis • Peptic ulcer • Insomnia • Acute delirium • Hyperglycaemia • Hypokalaemia • Acute adrenal insufficiency (at withdrawal)	• Use cautiously in patients with recent myocardial infarction, hypertension, renal disease and GI ulcer. • Monitor blood pressure and blood glucose levels.
Inhaled steroids			
• Beclomethasone • Budesonide • Fluticasone	• Long-term asthma control	• Hoarseness • Dry mouth • Wheezing • Bronchospasm • Oral candidiasis • Headache	• Don't use for treatment of acute asthma attack. • Use a spacer to reduce adverse effects. • Rinse the patient's mouth after use to prevent oral fungal infection.

• Anticholinergic agents, such as ipratropium (Atrovent), act by inhibiting the action of acetylcholine at bronchial smooth-muscle receptor sites and thus produce bronchodilation. (See *Understanding bronchodilators*, page 324.)

Neuromuscular blocking agents

Patients on mechanical ventilation may require neuromuscular blocking agents to eliminate spontaneous breathing efforts that can interfere with the ventilator's function or adversely affect lung compliance. Neuromuscular blocking agents cause paralysis without altering the patient's LOC so sedation is also needed. (See *Understanding neuromuscular blocking agents*, page 325.)

Sedatives

Within critical care propofol, and the benzodiazepine midazolam, are the drugs most frequently used to relieve anxiety and promote sedation in patients on mechanical ventilators, especially those receiving

Understanding bronchodilators

Use this table to learn about the indications, adverse reactions and practice pointers associated with bronchodilators.

Drugs	Indications	Adverse reactions	Practice pointers
Beta₂-adrenergic agonists			
Salbutamol	• Provide short-acting relief of acute symptoms with asthma and bronchospasm • Prevent exercise-induced bronchospasm	• Paradoxical bronchospasm • Tachycardia • Palpitations • Tremor • Hyperactivity	• Warn patient about possibility of paradoxical bronchospasm. If it occurs, stop drug and seek medical treatment. • Be aware that elderly patient may require a lower dose. • Monitor respiratory status, vital signs and heart rhythm.
Epinephrine	• Relax bronchial smooth muscle by stimulating beta₂-adrenergic receptors; used for bronchospasm, hypersensitivity reaction, anaphylaxis, acute asthma	• Ventricular fibrillation • Palpitations • Tachycardia • Hypertension	• Use cautiously in elderly patients and those with long-standing asthma and emphysema with degenerative heart disease. • Monitor respiratory status, vital signs and heart rhythm. • Be aware of contraindication in patients with angle-closure glaucoma, coronary insufficiency and cerebral arteriosclerosis.
Anticholinergic agents			
Ipratropium	• Reduce bronchospasm associated with chronic bronchitis and emphysema (COPD)	• Bronchospasm • Palpitations • Nervousness	• Because of delayed onset of bronchodilation, the drug isn't recommended for acute respiratory distress. • Use cautiously in patients with closed angle glaucoma, bladder neck obstruction and prostatic hypertrophy. • Monitor respiratory status, vital signs and heart rhythm.

neuromuscular blocking agents. Neuromuscular blocking agents cause paralysis without altering the patient's LOC, which—without sedation—is frightening for the patient. (See *Understanding sedatives*, page 327.)

Surgery

If drugs or other therapeutic modes fail to maintain the patient's airway patency and protect healthy tissues from disease, surgery may be necessary. Some types of respiratory surgeries are formation of a tracheostomy, chest tube insertion, thoracotomy and lung transplant.

Understanding neuromuscular blocking agents

Use this table to learn about the indications, adverse reactions and practice pointers associated with neuromuscular blocking agents.

Drugs	Indications	Adverse reactions	Practice pointers
Depolarising			
Suxamethonium	• Used as adjunct to anaesthesia to induce skeletal muscle relaxation • Facilitate endotracheal (ET) intubation and mechanical ventilation especially in rapid sequence induction of anaesthesia	• Bradycardia, arrhythmias, cardiac arrest • Postoperative muscle pain • Respiratory depression, apnoea, bronchoconstriction • Malignant hyperthermia, increased intraocular pressure, flushing • Anaphylaxis	• Be aware that the drug is contraindicated in patients with a history of malignant hyperthermia, acute closed angle glaucoma and penetrating eye injuries. • Monitor the patient for histamine release and resulting hypotension and flushing. • Be sure to have emergency resuscitation and ventilation equipment available.
Nondepolarising			
Atracurium	• Used as adjunct to general anaesthesia to facilitate ET intubation and to provide skeletal muscle relaxation during surgery or mechanical ventilation when a short-to-intermediate acting agent is required.	• Flushing, bradycardia • Prolonged dose-related apnoea • Anaphylaxis	• Keep in mind that the drug doesn't affect consciousness or relieve pain. Be sure to keep the patient sedated and administer analgesics, if appropriate. • Be aware that the drug has little or no effect on heart rate and doesn't counteract or reverse the bradycardia caused by anaesthetics or vagal stimulation. Thus, bradycardia is seen more frequently with atracurium than with other neuromuscular blocking agents. Pretreatment with anticholinergics (atropine or glycopyrrolate) is advised. • Use this drug only if ET intubation, administration of oxygen under positive pressure, artificial respiration and assisted or controlled ventilation are immediately available. • Use a peripheral nerve stimulator to monitor responses during critical care unit administration; it may be used to detect residual paralysis during recovery and to avoid atracurium overdose.
Vecuronium	• Used as adjunct to anaesthesia to facilitate intubation and to provide skeletal muscle relaxation during surgery or mechanical ventilation when an intermediate acting agent is required.	• Respiratory insufficiency or apnoea • Skeletal muscle weakness	• Administer by rapid I.V. injection or I.V. infusion; don't give I.M. • Prepare for a recovery time that may double in patients with cirrhosis or cholestasis. • Assess baseline serum electrolyte levels, acid–base balance and renal and hepatic function before administration.

(continued)

Understanding neuromuscular blocking agents (continued)

Drugs	Indications	Adverse reactions	Practice pointers
Nondepolarising			
Pancuronium	• Used as adjunct to anaesthesia to induce skeletal muscle relaxation and facilitate intubation and ventilation when a long acting agent is required.	• Residual muscle weakness • Prolonged, dose-related respiratory insufficiency or apnoea • Allergic or idiosyncratic hypersensitivity reactions • Tachycardia	• If using suxamethonium, allow its effects to subside before giving pancuronium. • Don't mix this drug in the same syringe or give through same needle with barbiturates or other alkaline solutions. • Be aware that large doses may increase frequency and severity of tachycardia.

Tracheostomy formation

This involves a surgical procedure to create an opening into the trachea, called a *tracheostomy*, which allows insertion of an indwelling tube to keep the patient's airway open.

The tracheostomy tube may be made of plastic, polyvinyl chloride or metal and comes in various sizes, lengths and styles depending on the patient's needs. A patient receiving mechanical ventilation needs a cuffed tube to prevent loss of minute volume from the ventilator through air leaking around the tube. A cuffed tracheostomy tube also prevents an unconscious or a paralysed patient from aspirating food or secretions. (*See Comparing tracheostomy tubes*, page 328.)

Emergency or planned procedure

In emergency situations, such as laryngeal oedema with anaphylactic shock or foreign body obstruction, tracheostomy formation may be done at the bedside. More commonly, it's a planned procedure that's done in theatre or in the critical care unit by percutaneous dilational technique when a patient is likely to need prolonged mechanical ventilation.

Nursing considerations

• Know what equipment your critical care unit keeps to use in the case of an emergency tracheostomy. Find out where it is kept and how to prepare for the procedure—you'll need to do it quickly if it is needed.
• Before a scheduled tracheostomy, explain the procedure and the need for anaesthesia to the patient and their family. If possible, mention whether the tracheostomy is permanent or temporary. Tell them the patient is monitored in the critical care unit before and after the procedure.
• Ensure that samples for ABG analysis and other diagnostic tests have been collected and that the patient or a responsible family member has signed a consent form.

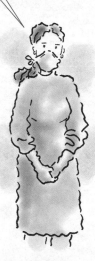

Surgery may be necessary if drugs or other treatment measures fail.

Understanding sedatives

Use this table to learn about the indications, adverse reactions and practice pointers associated with sedatives.

Drugs	Indications	Adverse reactions	Practice pointers
Midazolam	• Preoperative sedation (to induce sleepiness or drowsiness and relieve apprehension) • Conscious sedation before short diagnostic or endoscopic procedures • Continuous infusion for sedation of intubated and mechanically ventilated patients as a component of anaesthesia or during treatment in a critical care setting	• Pain at injection site • Cardiac arrest • Nausea • Hiccups • Decreased respiratory rate • Apnoea • Hypotension • Amnesia	• Be aware that the drug is contraindicated in patients with acute angle-closure glaucoma and in those experiencing shock, coma or acute alcohol intoxication. • Use cautiously in patients with uncompensated acute illnesses, in elderly or debilitated patients. • Closely monitor cardiopulmonary function; continuously monitor patients who have received midazolam to detect potentially life-threatening respiratory depression.
Propofol	• Induce and maintain anaesthesia • Sedate mechanically ventilated patients	• Hypotension • Bradycardia • Hyperlipidaemia • Apnoea	• Laryngospasm and bronchospasm, although rare, may occur. • The major haemodynamic effect in patients maintaining spontaneous ventilation is hypotension (blood pressure can decrease as much as 30%) with little or no change in heart rate and cardiac output. However, significant depression of cardiac output may occur in patients undergoing positive-pressure ventilation. • Keep in mind that the drug is contraindicated in patients hypersensitive to propofol or components of the emulsion, including soybean oil, egg lecithin and glycerol. Because drug is administered as an emulsion, administer cautiously to patients with a disorder of lipid metabolism (such as pancreatitis, primary hyperlipoproteinaemia and diabetic hyperlipidaemia). Use cautiously if the patient is receiving lipids as part of a total parenteral nutrition infusion; I.V. lipid dose may need to be reduced. Use cautiously in elderly or debilitated patients and in those with circulatory or seizure disorders. • The lipids may interfere with coagulation tests—giving a falsely prolonged result. • Change the infusion bottle and tubing every 12 hours.

Comparing tracheostomy tubes

Tracheostomy tubes are made of plastic or metal and come in uncuffed, cuffed and fenestrated varieties. Tube selection depends on the patient's condition and the practitioner's preference. Make sure you're familiar with the advantages and disadvantages of these commonly used tracheostomy tube.

Uncuffed (plastic or metal)

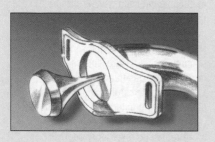

Advantages

- Free flow of air around tube and through larynx
- Reduced risk of tracheal damage
- Mechanical ventilation possible in patient with neuromuscular disease

Disadvantages

- Increased risk of aspiration in adults due to lack of cuff
- Adapter possibly needed for ventilation

Plastic cuffed (low pressure and high volume)

Advantages

- Disposable
- Cuff bonded to tube (won't detach accidentally inside trachea)
- Low cuff pressure that's evenly distributed against tracheal wall (no need to deflate periodically to lower pressure)
- Reduced risk of tracheal damage

Disadvantages

- Possibly more expensive than other tubes

Fenestrated

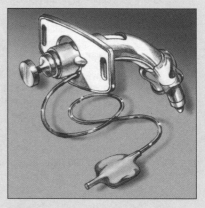

Advantages

- Speech possible through upper airway when external opening is capped and cuff is deflated
- Breathing by mechanical ventilation possible with inner cannula in place and cuff inflated
- Easy removal of inner cannula for cleaning

Disadvantages

- Possible occlusion of fenestration
- Possible dislodgment of inner cannula
- Cap removal necessary before inflating cuff

Afterwards ward

- After the procedure, assess the patient's respiratory status, breath sounds, oxygen saturation level, vital signs and heart rhythm. Note any crackles, rhonchi, wheezes or diminished breath sounds.
- Assess the patient for complications that can occur within the first 48 hours after tracheostomy tube insertion, including haemorrhage, oedema into tracheal tissue causing airway obstruction, aspiration of secretions, hypoxaemia and introduction of air into surrounding tissue causing subcutaneous emphysema.

Advice from the experts

Emergency tracheostomy equipment

Make sure you keep emergency tracheostomy equipment at the patient's bedside, including:

- sterile tracheal dilator
- sterile obturator that fits the tracheostomy tube
- extra sterile tracheostomy tube and obturator in the appropriate size
- suction equipment and supplies.

Keep the emergency equipment in full view at the patient's bedside at all times for easy access in case of emergency. Consider taping a wrapped, sterile tracheostomy tube to the head of the bed for easy access. If your patient coughs or pulls the tracheostomy tube out, you may use a sterile tracheal dilator to keep the stoma open and the airway patent until a new tube can be inserted.

- Keep appropriate equipment at the bedside for immediate use in an emergency. (See *Emergency tracheostomy equipment*.)
- Perform tracheostomy care at least every 8 hours or as needed. Change the dressing as often as needed because a wet dressing with exudate or secretions predisposes the patient-to-skin excoriation, breakdown and infection.
- Don't change the tracheostomy ties unnecessarily during the immediate postoperative period (usually 4 days) to avoid accidentally dislodging the tube.
- Document the procedure, the amount, colour and consistency of secretions, stoma and skin conditions, the patient's respiratory status, the duration of any cuff deflation and cuff pressure readings with inflation.

Chest drain insertion

Chest drain insertion may be needed when treating patients with pneumothorax, haemothorax, empyema, pleural effusion or chylothorax. The tube, which is inserted into the pleural space, allows blood, fluid, pus or air to drain and allows the lung to reinflate.

Gotta have some negative pressure

The tube restores negative pressure to the pleural space through an underwater-seal drainage system. The water in the system prevents air from being sucked back into the pleural space during inspiration and effectively works as a one-way valve. If a leak occurs through the bronchi and can't be sealed, a bronchopleural fistula—suction applied to the underwater-seal system—removes air from the pleural space faster than it can collect and helps to keep the lung inflated.

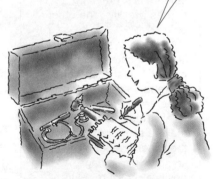

If your patient requires an emergency bedside tracheostomy, gather the necessary supplies or a tracheostomy kit quickly.

Put a valve on it

A one-way flutter valve, such as the Heimlich valve, is sometimes used instead of an underwater-seal drainage system. The one-way valve is connected to the end of the chest tube and allows accumulated air to escape, but not enter. This type of valve allows portability for patients who need long-term chest tube placement or during transport between hospitals.

Nursing considerations

- Explain the procedure to the patient and their family.
- Obtain baseline vital signs.
- Collect necessary equipment, including a chest drain insertion tray and an underwater-seal drainage system. Prepare lignocaine for local anaesthesia as directed. The doctor will clean the insertion site with chlorhexidine gluconate and alcohol solution. Set up the underwater-seal drainage system according to the manufacturer's instructions and place it at the bedside. (See *Closed chest drainage system*.)

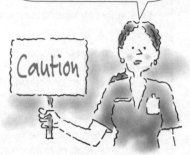

To avoid dislodging the tube, don't change your patient's tracheostomy ties unnecessarily and make sure they are secure.

Closed chest drainage system

One-piece, disposable plastic drainage systems often contain three chambers. The drainage chamber with calibrated columns that display the amount of drainage collected. When the first column fills, drainage carries over into the other columns.

The water-seal chamber is often located in the centre. The suction-control chamber is filled with water to achieve various suction levels. Rubber diaphragms may be provided to change the water level or remove samples of drainage. A positive-pressure relief valve at the top of the water-seal chamber vents excess pressure into the atmosphere, preventing pressure build-up.

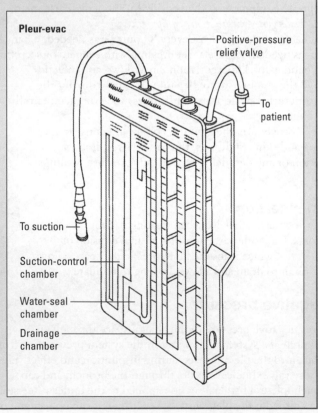

Pleur-evac

- Positive-pressure relief valve
- To patient
- To suction
- Suction-control chamber
- Water-seal chamber
- Drainage chamber

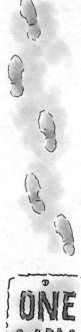

ONE WAY

- Assess respiratory function and obtain vital signs and oxygen saturation levels immediately after insertion. Routinely assess chest tube function. Describe and record the amount of drainage at least every 8 hours. Notify the doctor immediately if there is fresh blood more than 200 ml in 1 hour (indicates bleeding).
- The fluid in the water-seal chamber typically rises on inspiration and decreases on expiration. If the patient is receiving positive-pressure ventilation, the opposite is normal.
- Avoid creating dependent loops, kinks or pressure in the tubing. Don't lift the drainage system above the patient's chest because fluid may flow back into the pleural space.
- If the drainage collection chamber fills, replace it according to local policy. To do so, kink and nip the tubing close to the insertion site then exchange the system.
- To prevent tension pneumothorax (which can occur when clamping stops air and fluid from escaping), avoid using clamps.
- Notify the doctor immediately if the patient develops cyanosis, rapid or shallow breathing, subcutaneous emphysema, chest pain or excessive bleeding.

Thoracotomy

Thoracotomy, a surgical incision into the thoracic cavity, is done to locate and examine abnormalities, such as tumours, bleeding sites or thoracic injuries; to perform a biopsy; or to remove diseased lung tissue. It's most commonly done to remove part or all of a lung to spare healthy lung tissue from disease. It is also performed to give access to the oesophagus during oesophagectomy.

Lung excisions

Types of lung excisions include pneumonectomy, lobectomy, segmental resection and wedge resection:

Bye-bye lung

A pneumonectomy is the excision of an entire lung. It's usually performed to treat patients with bronchogenic cancer, but may be used to treat those with TB, bronchiectasis, lung abscess or lung damaged in trauma. Pneumonectomy is used only when a less radical approach would fail to remove all diseased tissue. After a pneumonectomy, chest cavity pressures stabilise and, over time, fluid fills the cavity where lung tissue was removed, preventing significant mediastinal shift.

One out of five lobes

A lobectomy is the removal of one of the five lung lobes. It's used to treat patients with bronchogenic cancer, TB, lung abscess, emphysematous blebs, benign tumours or localised fungal infections. After this surgery, the remaining lobes expand to fill the entire pleural cavity.

> Thoracotomy is usually done to remove part or all of a lung.

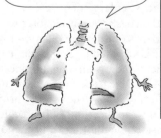

Checking for chest tube leaks

When trying to locate a leak in your patient's chest drain system, try:

- briefly kinking the tube at various points along its length, beginning at the tube's proximal end and working down towards the drainage system
- paying special attention to the seal around the connections
- pushing any loose connections back together and taping them securely with a lattice to allow visualisation of the connections; avoid using sleak which obscures the connections from view.

Bubble may mean trouble

The bubbling of the system stops when the tube is kinked between an air leak and the water seal. If you kink along the tube's entire length and the bubbling doesn't stop, you probably need to replace the drainage unit because it may be cracked.

How do you like your resection?

A segmental resection is the removal of one or more lung segments. This procedure preserves more functional tissue than lobectomy; it's commonly used to treat patients with bronchiectasis.

A wedge resection is removal of a small portion of the lung without regard to segments. It preserves the most functional tissue of all the surgeries but is used only when the patient has a small, well-circumscribed lesion. Remaining lung tissue should be then reexpand.

Other thoracic surgeries

Here are some other types of thoracic surgeries:
• Exploratory thoracotomy is used to examine the chest and pleural space in evaluating chest trauma and tumours.
• Decortication is used to help reexpand the lung in a patient with empyema. It involves removing or stripping the thick, fibrous membrane covering the visceral pleura.
• Thoracoplasty is performed to remove part or all of one rib and to reduce the size of the chest cavity. It decreases the risk of mediastinal shift when TB has reduced lung volume.
• Bronchoplastic (sleeve) reduction involves the excision of one lobar bronchus along with part of the right or left bronchus. The distal bronchus is then reanastomosed to the proximal bronchus or trachea.
• Lung reduction surgery is used to treat patients with emphysema. Giant bullae are excised, thereby reducing lung volume and allowing compressed alveoli to reexpand.
• Video-assisted thoracic surgery is a minimally invasive technique used to treat patients with some pulmonary conditions, perform open lung biopsies and to stage and diagnose some lung cancers.

Nursing considerations

• Explain the procedure to the patient and their family. Tell them that, after surgery, the patient may have a chest tube and an oxygen delivery system in place.
• After thoracic surgery, assess vital signs, oxygen saturation levels, breath sounds and cardiopulmonary and haemodynamic status. Monitor for cardiac arrhythmias. Atrial arrhythmias, especially atrial fibrillation, commonly occur after pneumonectomy due to pulmonary vasculature blood flow changes and atrial enlargement.
• Monitor the chest drain insertion site and assess and record the amount and characteristics of drainage. Suction isn't used after a pneumonectomy and the chest tube is attached to gravity drainage only.
• If the patient underwent a pneumonectomy, position them only on their operative side or their back until stabilised. This prevents fluid from draining into the unaffected lung if the sutured bronchus opens.
• Monitor for complications of thoracotomy, including haemorrhage, infection, tension pneumothorax, bronchopleural fistula and empyema.

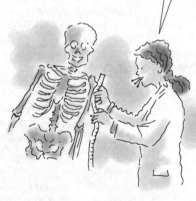

With thoracoplasty, part or all of a rib is removed to reduce the size of the chest cavity. Yes, I think we can take it in another inch or two.

Lung transplantation

Lung transplantation involves the replacement of one or both lungs with that from a donor. Cystic fibrosis is the most common underlying disease that necessitates lung transplantation; others include bronchopulmonary dysplasia, pulmonary hypertension and pulmonary fibrosis.

In some cases, only one lobe may be involved in transplantation. Single-lung transplantation is considered for patients with end-stage COPD. Typically, the patient has a life expectancy of less than 2 years. One-year survival rate after transplantation is about 80% and about 60% after 4 years.

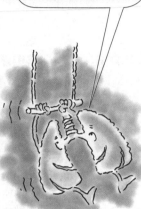

To qualify for lung transplantation, I thought I would have to jump through hoops, not swing from a trapeze. What gives?

So, who qualifies?

The qualifications for lung transplantation vary based on the underlying disease process. The patient must have significant pulmonary complications as well as other specific criteria.

Not gonna happen

Lung transplantation is absolutely contraindicated in cases of:
• major organ dysfunction, especially involving the renal or cardiovascular system
• human immunodeficiency virus infection
• active malignancy
• hepatitis C with positive biopsy for liver damage
• positive testing for hepatitis B antigen.
Relative contraindications include symptomatic osteoporosis.

TKO for transplant

Lung transplantation is performed under general anaesthesia. Bilateral anterior thoracotomy incisions and a transverse sternotomy provide access to the thoracic cavity. After removal of the patient's lungs, the donor lungs are implanted with anastomoses to the patient's bronchus.

Cardiopulmonary bypass is commonly used during the transplantation procedure.

Complications

The major complication after lung transplantation is organ rejection, which occurs because the recipient's body responds to the implanted tissue as a foreign body and triggers an immune response. This leads to fibrosis and scar formation.

Secondary snags

Another major complication after lung transplantation is infection due to immunosuppressive therapy.

Other possible complications include haemorrhage and reperfusion oedema. Long-term complications (typically occurring after 3 years) include obliterative bronchiolitis and posttransplant lymphoproliferative disorder. Either may be fatal.

Nursing considerations

Provide care before and after transplantation.

Educate and administer

- Answer all questions about the transplantation and what the patient can expect. Explain postoperative care (intubation, for example), equipment used in the acute postoperative phase and availability of analgesics for pain.
- Administer medications and obtain laboratory testing as ordered.

Keep on assessing

- Assess cardiopulmonary status frequently (every 5–15 minutes in the immediate postoperative period) until the patient is stabilised. Be alert for cardiac index less than 2.2, hypotension, fever higher than 37.5°C, crackles or rhonchi and decreased oxygen saturation.
- Assess respiratory status and ventilatory equipment frequently and suction secretions as necessary. Expect frequent ABG analyses and daily chest x-rays to evaluate the patient's readiness to wean from the ventilator.
- Assess chest drainage for amount, colour and characteristics. Assess for bleeding. Notify the doctor according to the hospital's and surgeon's parameters for normal drainage.
- Closely monitor fluid intake and output. If the patient becomes haemodynamically unstable, administer vasoactive and inotropic agents as prescribed and titrate the dose to achieve the desired response.
- After extubation, assess the patient often for shortness of breath, tachypnoea, dyspnoea, malaise and increased sputum production; these suggest acute rejection.
- After a single-lung transplantation, the newly implanted lung is denervated, but the patient's remaining lung continues to send messages to the brain indicating poor oxygenation. The patient may complain of shortness of breath and dyspnoea even with oxygen saturation levels greater than 90%.
- Maintain strict infection control precautions such as meticulous hand washing.
- Inspect surgical dressings for bleeding in the early postoperative phase. Inspect the surgical incisions later for redness, swelling and other signs of infection.

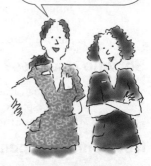

> Check the patient's ABG levels and chest x-rays daily to determine if they can be weaned from the ventilator.

> After a single-lung transplantation, the remaining lung continues to send messages to the brain that it's oxygen-starved, even though oxygen saturation is over 90%.

Disorders

Common respiratory disorders you'll encounter in the critical care unit include:
- acute respiratory failure
- asthma
- COPD

- pneumonia
- ARDS
- pneumothorax
- pulmonary embolism
- pulmonary hypertension.

Acute respiratory failure

Acute respiratory failure results when the lungs can't adequately oxygenate blood or eliminate carbon dioxide. There are two types of respiratory failure.
- *Type 1 failure* is defined by a PaO_2 of <8 kPa with a normal or low $PaCO_2$.
- *Type 2 failure* is defined by a PaO_2 of <8 kPa and a $PaCO_2$ of >6 kPa.

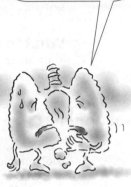

Uh-oh! When I can't oxygenate blood or remove carbon dioxide, acute respiratory failure results.

What causes it

Type 1 respiratory failure is generally caused by conditions that affect lung tissue and gas exchange (V/Q mismatch or right-to-left shunting). These include:
- pneumonia
- pulmonary oedema
- pulmonary emboli
- pneumothorax
- atelectasis
- ARDS

Type 2 respiratory failure is generally a result of ventilatory failure (alveolar hypoventilation)—from conditions that affect the mechanics of breathing or the passage of air through the airways in the lungs. These include:
- acute COPD exacerbation
- obesity
- anaesthesia
- sleep apnoea
- CNS disease (such as myasthenia gravis, Guillain–Barré syndrome and amyotrophic lateral sclerosis)
- head trauma
- CNS depressants
- respiratory fatigue.

Poor oxygenation

Blood that passes through the lungs but isn't oxygenated due to alveolar hypoventilation is called shunted blood. Alveolar ventilation that takes place in the absence of blood flow to lung areas is referred to as dead-space ventilation. Blood flow in the lung can be impaired by obstruction or hypovolaemia. Obstruction is the most acute form, and is most commonly caused by pulmonary emboli. Respiratory failure may result from either dead-space ventilation or shunting or a mix of both.

Lots of lactic acid

As tissue hypoxaemia develops, anaerobic metabolism occurs within the hypoxic tissues, which results in a build-up of lactic acid (a by-product of anaerobic metabolism) and thus metabolic acidosis. This takes longer to develop than respiratory acidosis, but the result is increasing acidity of the blood, which interferes with normal function of all body systems.

What to look for

Your patient's history may reveal an underlying respiratory condition or an acute process leading to respiratory failure (such as sepsis, drug overdose or trauma).

Got no time

There's usually little time to collect a thorough history and the patient typically can't give the history himself. Their family members or medical records may be the main sources of such information.

Time is of the essence

Physical assessment findings vary depending on the duration and severity of the condition. On inspection, note ashen skin and cyanosis of the oral mucosa, lips and nail beds. The patient may use accessory muscles of respiration to breathe and sit bolt upright or slightly hunched over. They may be agitated or highly anxious. In later stages, as the patient's LOC decreases due to hypoxaemia, they may lie down and appear confused and disoriented.

If pneumothorax is present, you may observe asymmetrical chest movement, a deviated trachea or be able to palpate subcutaneous emphysema.

Finding failure

Look for these physical signs of respiratory failure:
• Tachypnoea increases the patient's respiratory rate so it's greater than the normal range of 16–20 breaths per minute.
• Tachycardia is a heart rate greater than 100 beats per minute. You may not see this in patients with heart disease who are taking medications that prevent tachycardia. The pulse may be strong and rapid initially, but thready and irregular in later stages.
• Cold, clammy skin and frank diaphoresis are apparent, especially around the forehead and face.
• Percussion reveals hyperresonance in patients with COPD, asthma or pneumothorax. In patients with atelectasis or pneumonia, percussion sounds are dull or flat.
• Lung auscultation usually reveals diminished breath sounds. In patients with pneumothorax, breath sounds are absent over the affected lung tissue. In other cases of respiratory failure, adventitious breath sounds, such as wheezes

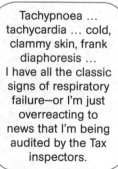

Let's see … nothing too acidic today. I'm lactic acid-intolerant, you know.

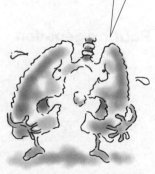

Tachypnoea … tachycardia … cold, clammy skin, frank diaphoresis … I have all the classic signs of respiratory failure—or I'm just overreacting to news that I'm being audited by the Tax inspectors.

(in asthma) and rhonchi (in bronchitis), may be heard. If you auscultate fin crackles, suspect pulmonary oedema as the cause of respiratory failure. Course crackles are heard in pneumonia.

What tests tell you

• ABG analysis indicates early respiratory failure when PaO_2 is low (usually less than 8 kPa) and $PaCO_2$ is high (greater than 6 kPa) and the HCO_3^- level is normal. The pH is also low. ABG levels in patients with COPD may be difficult to interpret, so compare them with earlier ABG values.
• Chest x-ray is used to identify pulmonary diseases, such as emphysema, atelectasis, pneumothorax, infiltrates and effusions.
• Electrocardiogram (ECG) can demonstrate arrhythmias, commonly found with heart failure and myocardial hypoxia.
• Pulse oximetry reveals a decreasing SpO_2 level.
• WBC count aids detection of an underlying infection. Blood cultures, sputum cultures and Gram stain may also be used to identify pathogens.
• Abnormally low haemoglobin and haematocrit levels signal blood loss, indicating decreased oxygen-carrying capacity.
• Haemodynamic monitoring may be used to distinguish pulmonary causes from cardiovascular causes of acute respiratory failure, and to monitor responses to treatment.

How it's treated

The primary goal of treatment is to restore adequate gas exchange. The secondary goal is to correct the underlying cause and development of respiratory failure.

Go to the O_2

Oxygen therapy is initiated immediately to optimise oxygenation of pulmonary blood. You may instruct the patient to try pursed-lip breathing to prevent alveolar collapse. If the patient can't breathe adequately on their own, ET intubation and mechanical ventilation are instituted.

Oh, and drug therapy, too

Various drug therapies may be prescribed:
• Reversal agents such as naloxone are given if drug overdose is suspected.
• Bronchodilators are given to open airways.
• Antibiotics are given to combat infection.
• Corticosteroids may be given to reduce inflammation.
• Continuous I.V. solutions of positive inotropic agents may be given to increase cardiac output, and vasopressors may be given to induce vasoconstriction to improve or maintain blood pressure. Fluid resuscitation is often needed as patients rapidly become dehydrated.
• Diuretics may be given to reduce fluid overload and pulmonary oedema.

To prevent alveolar collapse, instruct the patient to try pursed-lip breathing. There will be no time for lipstick though.

What to do

• Assess the patient's respiratory status hourly or more often, as indicated. Observe for a positive response to oxygen therapy, such as improved breathing, colour and oximetry and ABG values.

• Position the patient for optimal breathing ideally with head of bed elevated to 45 degrees. Put the call bell within easy reach to reassure the patient and prevent unnecessary exertion when they need to call the nurse.

• Maintain a normothermic environment and give antipyretics to reduce the patient's temperature, thus reducing oxygen demand.

• Monitor vital signs, heart rhythm and fluid intake and output to identify fluid overload or impending dehydration or hypovolaemia.

• After intubation, auscultate the lungs to check for accidental intubation of the right mainstem bronchus. Be alert for aspiration, broken teeth, nosebleeds and vagal reflexes causing bradycardia, arrhythmias and hypotension.

• Don't suction too often without identifying the underlying cause of an equipment alarm. Use strict sterile technique during suctioning. ET intubation bypasses many of the body's normal barriers to infection, so the patient is at high risk during this procedure.

• Watch oximetry and capnography values because these are important indicators of changes in the patient's condition.

• Note the amount and quality of lung secretions and look for changes in the patient's status.

• Check cuff pressure on the ET tube to prevent erosion from an overinflated cuff. Normal cuff pressure is about 20 mmHg.

• Administer gastric ulcer prophylaxis and be alert for GI bleeding. Inspect gastric secretions for blood, especially if the patient has a nasogastric (NG) tube or reports or shows evidence of epigastric or abdominal tenderness. Decreasing haemoglobin level and haematocrit and occult blood in the stools are other indicators of GI bleeding.

• Provide a means of communication for patients who are intubated and alert. Institutions use different approaches, based on signs and signals, or communication boards. Explain all procedures to the patient and their family.

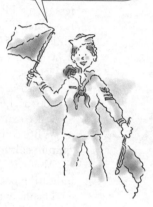

Be sure to provide a means of communication for patients who are intubated and alert.

Asthma

Acute asthma necessitating critical care can present as acute severe or life-threatening severity. It begins with impaired gas exchange and—without rapid intervention—may lead to respiratory failure and, eventually, death.

Asthma overview

Asthma is a chronic inflammatory airway disorder that causes episodic airway obstruction and hyperreactive airways in response to multiple stimuli. It results from bronchospasms, increased mucous secretion and mucosal oedema. If left untreated or if the patient doesn't respond to drug therapy after 24 hours, the patient's life is in danger.

Making things worse

Asthma exacerbations are acute or subacute episodes of worsening shortness of breath, coughing and wheezing, with measurable decreases in expiratory airflow.

What causes it
Many asthmatics, especially children, have intrinsic and extrinsic asthma.

Outside factors

Extrinsic, or *atopic*, asthma begins in childhood. Patients are typically sensitive to specific external allergens. Extrinsic allergens that can trigger an asthma attack include such elements as pollen, animal dander, house dust or mould, feather pillows, food additives containing sulphites and other sensitising substances.

Extrinsic asthma in childhood is commonly accompanied by other hereditary allergies, such as eczema and allergic rhinitis.

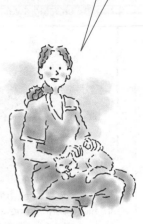

Extrinsic allergens, such as pollen and pet dander, can trigger an asthma attack.

Factors within

Patients with *intrinsic*, or *nonatopic*, asthma react to internal, nonallergenic factors. Intrinsic factors that can trigger an asthma attack include emotional stress, fatigue, endocrine changes, temperature variations, humidity variations, exposure to noxious fumes, anxiety, coughing or laughing and genetic factors.

Most episodes occur after a severe respiratory tract infection, especially in adults.

Irritants in the workplace

Many adults acquire an allergic form of asthma or exacerbation of existing asthma from exposure to agents in the workplace. Such irritants as chemicals in flour, acid anhydrides and excreta of dust mites in carpet are a few such agents that trigger asthma.

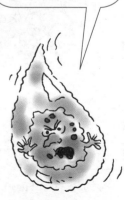

Hah! Most intrinsic asthma attacks in adults follow severe respiratory tract infection.

Genetic messes

Asthma is associated with two genetic influences, including:
• the ability to develop asthma because of an abnormal gene (atopy)
• the tendency to develop hyperresponsive airways (without atopy).

A potent mix

Environmental factors interact with inherited factors to cause asthmatic reactions with associated bronchospasms.

How it happens
Status asthmaticus begins with an asthma attack. In asthma, bronchial linings overreact to various stimuli, causing episodic smooth-muscle spasms that severely constrict the airways. (See *Understanding asthma*, page 340.)

Understanding asthma

Asthma is an inflammatory disease of the airways. The inflammation causes hyperreactiveness (to various stimuli) and bronchospasms. Here's how an asthma attack progresses:

Histamine attaches to receptor sites in larger bronchi, causing swelling of the smooth muscles.

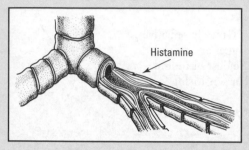

Leukotrienes attach to receptor sites in the smaller bronchi and cause swelling of smooth muscle there. Leukotrienes also cause prostaglandins to travel via the bloodstream to the lungs, where they enhance histamine's effects.

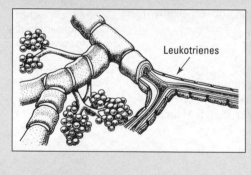

Histamine stimulates the mucous membranes to secrete excessive mucus, further narrowing the bronchial lumen. On inhalation, the narrowed bronchial lumen can still expand slightly; however, on exhalation, the increased intrathoracic pressure closes the bronchial lumen completely.

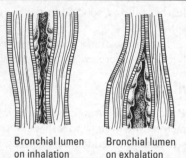

Bronchial lumen on inhalation   Bronchial lumen on exhalation

Mucus fills lung bases, inhibiting alveolar ventilation. Blood is shunted to alveoli in other parts of the lungs, but it still can't compensate for diminished ventilation.

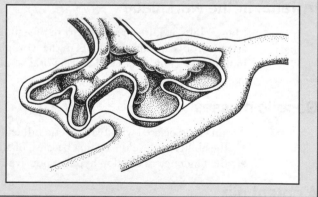

Here's how asthma develops into status asthmaticus:
- Immunoglobulin (Ig) E antibodies attached to histamine-containing mast cells and receptors on cell membranes initiate intrinsic asthma attacks.
- When exposed to an antigen, such as pollen, the IgE antibody combines with the antigen.
- On subsequent exposure to the antigen, mast cells degranulate and release mediators.

- Mast cells in the lung are stimulated to release histamine and the slow-reacting substance of anaphylaxis.
- Histamine attaches to receptor sites in the larger bronchi, where it causes swelling in smooth muscles.
- Mucous membranes become inflamed, irritated and swollen. The patient may experience dyspnoea, prolonged expiration and an increased respiratory rate.
- Leukotrienes attach to receptor sites in the smaller bronchi and cause local swelling of the smooth muscle.
- Leukotrienes also cause prostaglandins to travel by way of the bloodstream to the lungs, where they enhance the effect of histamine. A wheeze may be audible during coughing; the higher the pitch, the narrower is the bronchial lumen.
- Histamine stimulates the mucous membranes to secrete excessive mucus, further narrowing the bronchial lumen.

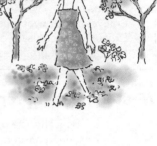

When exposed to antigens such as pollen, mast cells in the lung release histamine, which causes swelling in smooth muscles.

Got goblet?

- Goblet cells secrete viscous mucus that's difficult to cough up, resulting in coughing, rhonchi, increased-pitch wheezing and increased respiratory distress. Mucosal oedema and thickened secretions further block the airways.
- On inhalation, the narrowed bronchial lumen can still expand slightly, allowing air to reach the alveoli. On exhalation, increased intrathoracic pressure closes the bronchial lumen completely. Air enters but can't escape.
- When status asthmaticus occurs, hypoxaemia worsens and expiratory rate and volume decrease even further.
- Obstructed airways impede gas exchange and increase airway resistance. The patient labours to breathe.
- With fatigue and hypoxaemia the patient's respiratory rate drops to normal, $PaCO_2$ levels rise and the patient hypoventilates from exhaustion.
- Respiratory acidosis develops as $PaCO_2$ increases.
- The situation becomes life-threatening when no air is audible on auscultation (a silent chest) and $PaCO_2$ rises to over 9 kPa.
- Without treatment, the patient experiences acute respiratory failure.

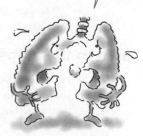

As mucous membranes become inflamed, irritated and swollen, the patient may experience dyspnoea, prolonged expiration and increased respiratory rate.

What to look for

An asthma attack may begin slowly or dramatically. Progressive cyanosis, confusion and lethargy may indicate that the acute asthma attack has progressed to status asthmaticus. In status the severity of the asthma may range from acute severe to life-threatening. (See *Severity of asthma seen in the critically ill patient*, page 342.) The degree of severity may be due to the degree of airway obstruction or the ability of the patient to compensate for the increased work of breathing imposed by airway obstruction. Thus a patient with a lesser degree of obstruction may still have a life-threatening attack of asthma if they are unable to compensate for the increased work of breathing. A prolonged attack even if moderate may also result in a life-threatening situation as fatigue sets in.

Severity of asthma seen in the critically ill patient

Features of acute severe asthma

- Cannot complete sentences in one breath.
- Use of accessory muscles.
- Respirations ⩾25 breaths per minute.
- Pulse >110 beats per minute.
- Peak expiratory flow (PEF) ⩽50% of predicted or best.

Features of a life-threatening asthma

- Silent chest, or feeble respiratory effort
- Cyanosis
- Bradycardia or hypotension
- Exhaustion, confusion or coma
- PEF < 33% of predicted or best

Histamine stimulates the secretion of excessive mucus, narrowing the bronchial lumen.

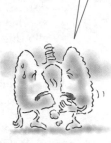

What the patient reports

Typically, the patient reports exposure to a particular allergen followed by a sudden onset of dyspnoea, wheezing and tightness in the chest accompanied by a cough that produces thick clear or yellow sputum.

The patient may complain of feeling suffocated, appear visibly dyspnoeic and be able to speak only a few words before pausing to catch their breath.

What you may find

Mental status is a sensitive indicator of oxygen deprivation, and the patient may initially be irritable or anxious. As hypoxaemia progresses, the patient becomes confused and increasingly lethargic, a sign of impending respiratory failure.

The patient's heart rate is elevated and commonly irregular. Respiratory rate is also well above normal. When the patient begins to tire, their respiratory rate begins to slow, which may be another sign of impending respiratory failure if the patient is also confused and lethargic.

On inspection, you may see intercostal retractions. During an attack, the patient's face may appear pale and diaphoretic. The patient generally sits bolt upright or leans forward slightly.

On percussing the chest wall, you may find hyperresonance; palpation may reveal reduced tactile vocal fremitus.

Your patient's mental status is a sensitive indicator of oxygen deprivation that may signal impending respiratory failure.

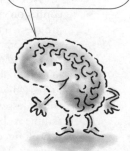

Listen to the lungs

When you listen to the lungs, you may hear harsh respirations with inspiratory and expiratory wheezes and, possibly, reduced breath sounds over some areas of the lung. The expiratory phase of respiration is prolonged. Marked wheezing may develop due to increased oedema and mucus in the lower airways.

Breath sounds and wheezing may suddenly stop (status asthmaticus) because of severe bronchoconstriction and oedema.

What tests tell you

These tests are used to establish the diagnosis:

• Pulmonary function tests reveal decreased vital capacity and increased total lung and residual capacities during an acute attack. Peak and expiratory flow rate measurements are less than 50% of baseline in acute severe asthma.

• Pulse oximetry commonly shows that oxygen saturation is less than 90%.

• Chest x-ray may show hyperinflation with areas of atelectasis and flat diaphragm due to increased intrathoracic volume. Chest x-ray is a priority in the baseline assessment of anyone with acute severe asthma as they may have developed a spontaneous pneumothorax. This should be ruled out as an exacerbating factor as part of the priority treatment and investigation.

• ABG analysis reveals decreasing PaO_2 and increasing $PaCO_2$. Even normal $PaCO_2$ in the presence of tachypnoea is abnormal as you should expect reduced $PaCO_2$. So a normal or increased $PaCO_2$ indicates decreased gas exchange. When $PaCO_2$ rises above 7 kPa this is usually an indication to admit the patient to critical care and prepare for ET intubation and mechanical ventilation.

• ECG shows sinus tachycardia during an attack.

• Sputum analysis may indicate increased viscosity, mucous plugs, presence of Curschmann's spirals (casts of airways), Charcot–Leyden crystals and eosinophils; culture may disclose causative organisms if infection is the trigger.

• A full blood count with differential shows an increased eosinophil count secondary to inflammation and an elevated WBC count and granulocyte count if an acute infection is present.

How it's treated

In acute status asthmaticus, the patient is monitored closely for respiratory failure. Oxygen, inhaled and intravenous bronchodilators, and corticosteroids may be prescribed. The patient may be intubated and placed on mechanical ventilation if $PaCO_2$ increases or if respiratory arrest occurs. Magnesium sulphate may be prescribed as an adjunct to standard bronchodilator therapy. Magnesium acts as a smooth-muscle relaxant in the airways. In addition, the more severe attacks, resulting in mechanical ventilation, may be treated with low-dose inhaled volatile anaesthetic agents.

Addressing asthma

Correcting asthma typically involves:

• prevention by identifying and avoiding precipitating factors, such as environmental allergens or irritants

• desensitisation to specific antigens if the stimuli can't be removed entirely, which decreases the severity of asthma attacks with future exposure

• bronchodilators (such as salbutamol or adrenaline) to decrease bronchoconstriction, reduce bronchial airway oedema and increase pulmonary ventilation

• anticholinergics to increase the effects of bronchodilators
• corticosteroids (such as methylprednisolone) to decrease bronchoconstriction, reduce bronchial airway oedema and increase pulmonary ventilation
• mast cell stabilisers (cromolyn) in patients with atopic asthma who have seasonal disease; when given prophylactically, they block the acute obstructive effects of antigen exposure by inhibiting the degranulation of mast cells, thereby preventing the release of chemical mediators responsible for anaphylaxis
• leukotriene-receptor modifiers given prophylactically to help block the inflammatory actions in asthma.

Calling for high humidity

• Humidified oxygen to correct hypoxaemia and to maintain an oxygen saturation greater than 94%
• Mechanical ventilation, which is necessary if the patient doesn't respond to initial supplemental oxygen and drugs or develops respiratory failure

What to do

• Conduct careful and frequent assessment of the patient's respiratory status, especially if the patient isn't intubated. Check the respiratory rate, auscultate breath sounds and monitor oxygen saturation.
• Be alert for a patient who was wheezing but suddenly stops wheezing and continues to show signs of respiratory distress. In this case the absence of wheezing may be due to severe bronchial constriction that narrows the airways severely during inhalation and exhalation. As a result, so little air passes through the narrowed airways that no sound is made. This is a sign of imminent respiratory collapse; the patient needs ET intubation and mechanical ventilation. Reassure the patient and stay with them. Help them to relax as much as possible.
• Assess the patient's mental status for confusion, agitation or lethargy.
• Assess the patient's heart rate and rhythm. Be alert for cardiac arrhythmias related to bronchodilator therapy or hypoxaemia.
• Obtain requested tests and report results promptly.
• Administer medications as prescribed. I.V. fluids are commonly ordered to replace insensible fluid loss from hyperventilation.
• When the acute phase is over, position the patient for maximum comfort, usually in semirecumbent position with the head of the bed elevated to 45 degrees. Encourage coughing to clear secretions. Offer emotional support and reassurance.

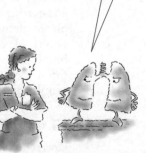

No, it's not a staring contest. I need to watch them closely for signs of imminent respiratory collapse.

Chronic obstructive pulmonary disease

COPD results from emphysema or chronic bronchitis, or a combination of these disorders. It's the most common chronic lung disease in the UK.

Out...

COPD is a chronic condition that can usually be managed on an outpatient basis even in advanced disease, when a patient may require continuous oxygen therapy.

...or in

Exacerbations of COPD that necessitate hospitalisation are caused by various factors that place additional demand on the respiratory system, such as infection, heart failure and exposure to allergens.

What causes it

Common causes of COPD include:

- cigarette smoking or exposure to cigarette smoke
- recurrent or chronic respiratory tract infections
- air pollution
- allergies.

Familial and hereditary factors, such as alpha$_1$-antitrypsin deficiency paired with cigarette smoking, are also responsible for emphysema.

How it happens

Patients with COPD have decreased gas exchange ability due to alveolar damage caused by exposure to smoke or chemical irritants over a long period.

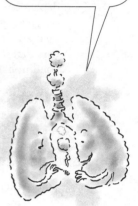

There's no getting around the fact that cigarette smoking or exposure to cigarette smoke is a leading cause of COPD—the most common chronic lung disease in the UK.

Quit it!

Smoke inhalation impairs ciliary action and macrophage function and causes inflammation in the airways and increased mucous production. Early inflammatory changes may be reversed if the patient stops smoking before lung disease becomes extensive.

Air trap

In chronic bronchitis, mucous plugs and narrowed airways cause air trapping. Air trapping also occurs with asthma and emphysema. In emphysema, permanent enlargement of the alveoli is accompanied by destruction of the alveolar walls. Obstruction and air trapping result from tissue changes rather than mucous production.

Here's what happens in air trapping: hyperinflation of the alveoli occurs on expiration. On inspiration, airways enlarge, allowing air to pass beyond the obstruction; on expiration, airways narrow and prevent gas flow.

Pressure pockets

As the alveolar walls are destroyed, they're no longer separate, but coalesce into large air pockets that put additional pressure on surrounding tissues. This affects the lung's blood supply as well, because it increases the pressure needed to push blood through the lungs. This form of high blood pressure is known as pulmonary hypertension.

Overwhelming work

Eventually, the high workload overwhelms the right side of the heart and hypertrophy and right-sided failure (cor pulmonale) result. Patients commonly have supraventricular arrhythmias such as atrial fibrillation, which increase the danger of thrombus formation.

Because gas exchange is impaired, hypercapnia ($PaCO_2$ above 6 kPa) becomes the norm for those patients with severe COPD. The respiratory centre of the brain, which stimulates breathing when $PaCO_2$ rises, becomes dependent instead on low PaO_2. This is an important consideration when oxygen is given for hypoxaemia and a fixed performance device should always be used. Some professionals regard this is a myth but it is not! It is however, true that it is only seen in patients with severe COPD (and some other conditions where hypoventilation is a feature such as motor neurone disease).

What to look for

Your patient most likely has a history of COPD and may be able to identify the precipitating cause (cigarette smoking, for example).

Tachy and not-so-tachy finds

Your patient is also likely to have tachycardia and an irregular heart rhythm as well as tachypnoea and dyspnoea on exertion. Fever may be present in the case of infection, but if the patient takes steroids regularly, the immune response is suppressed.

When you inspect the chest, you may notice that the anteroposterior diameter is increased (barrel chest), and the patient may appear generally cachectic. They may be coughing, with copious sputum production, if they have chronic bronchitis, or they may be wheezing.

When you listen to breath sounds, listen for a prolonged expiratory phase, perhaps crackles or rhonchi, and generally some decreased air movement.

Time will tell

Patients with COPD have abnormal breath sounds to begin with, and it may be hard to tell at first what's baseline and what's newly abnormal. As you listen over several hours or days abnormal breath sounds eventually become apparent.

What tests tell you

Stable COPD patients exhibit these abnormal diagnostic test results, which may be considered their baseline values:
• Pulmonary function tests show increased residual volume, with decreased vital capacity and amount of air exhaled in the first second of expiration (FEV_1). (See *Severity of COPD*.).
• Chest x-ray shows increased bronchovascular markings and overaeration of the lungs. In advanced disease, the diaphragm is flattened and bronchovascular markings may be reduced.

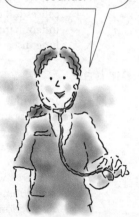

Your patient with COPD may have abnormal baseline breath sounds.

Severity of COPD

Severity	Signs and symptoms	FEV$_1$ (% predicted)
Mild	No abnormal signs	60–80%
	Smokers cough	
	Little or no breathlessness	
Moderate	Breathlessness (with or without wheeze) on moderate exertion. Cough (with or without sputum). Variable abnormal signs. Possible reduction in breath sounds, presence of wheeze.	40–59%
Severe	Breathlessness on exertion and at rest. Wheeze and cough often prominent. Lung overinflation usual; cyanosis, peripheral oedema and polycythaemia in advanced disease, espesially during exacerbations.	Below 40%

- ABG analysis may show reduced PaO$_2$ and normal or increased PaCO$_2$. In advanced COPD, it isn't uncommon for baseline PaCO$_2$ levels to be 7 kPa or higher.
- ECG may show atrial arrhythmias and, in advanced disease, right ventricular hypertrophy.
- Full blood count reveals elevated haemoglobin levels.

When it worsens

During an exacerbation, diagnostic tests may yield the following additional results:
- ABG analysis shows PaO$_2$ below the patient's baseline. PaCO$_2$ may be low, normal or high, depending on the patient's baseline. A rising PaCO$_2$ usually indicates respiratory fatigue.
- Chest x-ray may show infiltrates if pneumonia is present.
- ECG may show sinus tachycardia with supraventricular and, sometimes, ventricular arrhythmias.

How it's treated

Provide supportive treatments for your patients with COPD. Bronchodilators are useful in maintaining open airways. Steroids are often given to reduce airway inflammation—a contributory factor in airway obstruction. Continuous oxygen supplementation is needed to prevent hypoxia. When patients have chronically elevated PaCO$_2$ and rely on a relatively low PaO$_2$ they may experience further CO$_2$ retention and respiratory acidosis if SpO$_2$ levels are allowed to rise above 92%. However if SpO$_2$ levels are too low tissue hypoxia will develop. Therefore oxygen should be titrated to achieve SpO$_2$ in the range of 88–92% in those with known severe COPD.

Address the effects, then treat the cause

During exacerbations, management is twofold. First, respiratory support is given to avoid respiratory failure and cardiac arrest. Equally important is treatment addressing the underlying cause of the exacerbation.
• The first step is supplemental oxygen to avoid hypoxia and yet prevent hypercapnia
• If the patient becomes fatigued and develops respiratory acidosis, NIV may be used to prevent further fatigue and prevent the need for mechanical ventilation
• Bronchodilators and steroids to reduce inflammation are given early
• Antibiotics are given if infection is suspected or evident
• If respiratory failure is imminent, ET intubation and mechanical ventilation are needed.
• Diuretic agents may be given to reduce oedema if cardiac failure is present.
• Many patients will need fluid resuscitation or at least I.V. hydration.
• Antiarrhythmic medications may be given to control arrhythmias. The patient will usually need continuous ECG monitoring for observation of the heart rate and rhythm.
• If pneumothorax is present, a chest tube will be inserted.

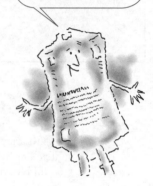

I.V. corticosteroids are given to reduce inflammation when COPD is exacerbated.

What to do

• Assess respiratory status, auscultate breath sounds, monitor oxygen saturation and ABG values and observe for a positive response to oxygen therapy, such as improved breathing, colour or oximetry and ABG values. Anticipate the need for intubation and mechanical ventilation.
• Assess frequently and carefully. Changes can be subtle and rapid. Be sure to assess mental status because it's an early and sensitive indicator of respiratory status. New onset of confusion and agitation are red flags, as is lethargy.
• Monitor vital signs and heart rhythm and observe for arrhythmias, which may indicate hypoxaemia, right-sided heart failure or an adverse effect of bronchodilator use.
• Obtain laboratory tests as ordered and report results promptly.
• Offer emotional support. Keep the environment as calm as possible. The patient may not be able to speak easily because of shortness of breath, so explain what's happening and try to anticipate their needs.

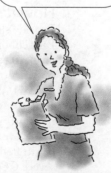

Frequent and careful assessment is the key to care because changes can be subtle and develop rapidly.

Pneumonia

Pneumonia is an acute infection of the lung parenchyma that commonly impairs gas exchange.

Those at risk

The prognosis is good for patients with pneumonia who are otherwise healthy. Debilitated patients are at much greater risk; bacterial pneumonia is

Senior moments

Pneumonia in older adults

Older adults are at greater risk for developing pneumonia because their weakened chest musculature reduces their ability to clear secretions. Those in long-term care facilities are especially susceptible.

Bacterial pneumonia is the most common type found in older adults; viral pneumonia is the second most common type. Aspiration pneumonia results from impaired swallowing ability and a diminished gag reflex due to stroke or prolonged illness.

And presenting ...

An older adult with pneumonia may present with fatigue, slight cough and a rapid respiratory rate and acute confusion. Pleuritic pain and fever may be present. An absence of fever doesn't mean absence of infection in an older adult; many older adults develop a subnormal body temperature in response to infection.

a leading cause of death among such individuals. Pneumonia occurs in both sexes and in all ages, but older adults are at greater risk for developing it. (See *Pneumonia in older adults*.)

What starts it

Infectious agents may be bacterial, viral, mycoplasmal, rickettsial, fungal, protozoal or mycobacterial. Bacterial pneumonia tends to be considered as 'typical' pneumonia whereas pneumonia caused by other organisms are less common and may be referred to as 'atypical' pneumonia.

Where it infects

Types of pneumonia based on location of the infection include:
- bronchopneumonia, involving distal airways and alveoli
- lobular pneumonia, involving part of a lobe
- lobar pneumonia, involving an entire lobe.

Get it here, there or anywhere

Pneumonia may be classified as community-acquired, hospital-acquired (nosocomial) or ventilator-associated pneumonia. (See *Types of pneumonia* page 350.)

Shared with the community

As the name implies, community-acquired pneumonia occurs in the community setting or within the first 48 hours of admission to hospital because of community exposure.

Types of pneumonia

Here's an overview of the various types of pneumonia, including their causative agents and common assessment findings.

Type	Causative agent	Assessment findings
Ventilator-associated pneumonia	Aspiration of gastric or oropharyngeal contents into trachea or lungs • *Pseudomonas aeruginosa* • Enteric gram-negative bacilli	• Fever • Crackles • Deterioration in gas exchange • Hypotension • Tachycardia • Chest x-ray with infiltrates
Community-acquired pneumonias		
Streptococcal pneumonia (pneumococcal pneumonia)	*Streptococcus pneumoniae*	• Sudden onset of rigour • Fever 38.9–40°C • History of previous upper respiratory infection • Pleuritic chest pain • Severe cough • Rust-coloured sputum • Areas of consolidation on chest x-ray (usually lobar) • Elevated white blood cell (WBC) count • Sputum culture possibly positive for gram-positive *S. pneumoniae*
Haemophilus influenza	*Haemophilus influenzae*	• Insidious onset • History of upper respiratory tract infection 2–6 weeks earlier • Fever • Chills • Dyspnoea • Productive cough • Chest x-ray with infiltrates in one or more lobes
Mycoplasma pneumonia	*Mycoplasma pneumoniae*	• Insidious onset • Sore throat • Ear pain • Headache • Low-grade fever • Pleuritic pain • Erythema rash • Dry cough • Myalgia

(continued)

Types of pneumonia (continued)

Type	Causative agent	Assessment findings
Viral pneumonia	Influenza virus, type A	• Initially beginning as upper respiratory infection • Cough (initially nonproductive; later purulent sputum) • Low-grade fever • Chills • Malaise • Dyspnoea • Frontal headache • Chest x-ray with diffuse bilateral bronchopneumonia radiating from hilus • Normal to slightly elevated WBC count • Fatigue
Legionnaires' disease	*Legionella pneumophila*	• Flulike symptoms • Malaise • Headache within 24 hours • Fever • Shaking chills • Fatigue • Mental confusion • Anorexia • Nausea, vomiting • Myalgia • Chest x-ray with patchy infiltrates, consolidation and possible effusion
Hospital-acquired pneumonias		
Klebsiella pneumonia	*Klebsiella pneumoniae*	• Fever • Recurrent chills • Rusty, bloody viscous sputum • Deterioration in gas exchange • Severe pleuritic chest pain • Chest x-ray typically with consolidation in upper lobe • Elevated WBC count • Sputum culture and Gram stain possibly positive for gram-negative cocci, *Klebsiella*

(*continued*)

Types of pneumonia (continued)

Type	Causative agent	Assessment findings
Pseudomonas pneumonia	*Pseudomonas aeruginosa*	• Fever • Chills • Dyspnoea • Cyanosis • Green foul-smelling sputum • Chest x-ray with diffuse consolidation
Staphylococcal pneumonia (may also be community-acquired)	*Staphylococcus aureus* (including methicillin-resistant *Staphylococcus aureus*—MRSA)	• Cough • Chills • High fever 38.9–40°C • Pleuritic pain • Progressive dyspnoea • Bloody sputum • Tachypnoea • Hypoxaemia • Chest x-ray with multiple abscesses and infiltrate; empyema • Elevated WBC count • Sputum culture and Gram stain possibly positive for gram-positive staphylococci

Not-so-comical pneumonia

Hospital-acquired pneumonia refers to the development of pneumonia 48 hours after admission to a hospital. For example, pneumonia following a general anaesthetic and surgical procedure.

What causes it

Primary pneumonia results from inhalation of a pathogen, such as bacteria or virus. Examples are pneumococcal and viral pneumonia. Clinically significant infections occur where a virulent pathogen is inhaled and/or when the host has compromised defences, for example, haematological malignancy, AIDS, postoperative patients, elderly or debilitated patients; those receiving NG tube feedings; and those with an impaired gag reflex, poor oral hygiene or a decreased LOC. Chronic disease such as heart failure and COPD also impair immunity.

Secondary pneumonia may follow initial lung damage from a noxious chemical (e.g. gastric acid aspirated into the lungs) or other insult (superinfection) or may result from haematogenous spread of bacteria from a distant area.

Yes, it's true. It's possible to develop pneumonia by acquiring an infection after being admitted to the hospital.

Yikes!

How it happens

The disease process varies among bacterial, viral and aspiration pneumonia.

• In bacterial pneumonia, which can affect any part of the lungs, an infection initially triggers alveolar inflammation and oedema. Capillaries become engorged with blood, causing stasis. As the alveolocapillary membrane breaks down, the alveoli fill with blood and inflammatory exudates, resulting in atelectasis.

• Viral pneumonia more commonly attacks bronchiolar epithelial cells, causing interstitial inflammation and desquamation. It then spreads to the alveoli. In advanced infection, a hyaline (fibrous) membrane may form, further compromising gas exchange.

• Aspiration pneumonia triggers similar inflammatory changes in the affected area, and also inactivates surfactant over a large area, leading to alveolar collapse. Acidic gastric contents may directly damage the airways and alveoli, and small particles may cause obstruction. The resulting inflammation makes the lungs susceptible to secondary bacterial pneumonia.

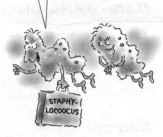

We get around! Bacterial pneumonia can move through the bloodstream to the lungs.

What to look for

Signs and symptoms of pneumonia include pleuritic chest pain, cough and fever, a change in sputum colour or quantity of production, as well as deterioration in gas exchange.

Sounds, sights and sensations

Your patient's cough may be dry, as in mycoplasma pneumonia, or very productive as in some bacterial bronchopneumonias. The sputum may be creamy yellow (staphylococcus), green (pseudomonas), or rust-coloured (pneumococcus).

In advanced cases of all types of pneumonia, percussion reveals dullness over the affected area of the lung. Auscultation may disclose crackles, wheezes or rhonchi over the affected areas as well as decreased breath sounds and decreased tactile vocal fremitus.

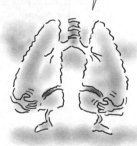

Oh, the pain of it all! The classic signs and symptoms of pneumonia are pleuritic chest pain, cough and fever. I've got them all!

What tests tell you

• Chest x-rays disclose infiltrates, confirming the diagnosis.

• Sputum specimen for Gram stain and culture and sensitivity testing may reveal inflammatory cells as well as bacterial cells.

• WBC count and differential may indicate the presence and type of infection. Elevated polymorphonucleocytes may indicate bacterial infection; in viral or mycoplasmal pneumonia, though, WBC count may not be elevated at all.

• ABG analysis is done to determine the extent of respiratory compromise due to alveolar inflammation.

• Bronchoscopy or bronchoalveolar lavage and aspiration allows the collection of material for cultures to identify the specific infectious organism. Pleural fluid may also be sampled for culture and Gram stain.

• Pulse oximetry may show a reduced oxygen saturation level and indicate the need for oxygen supplementation.

How it's treated

Because the cause is commonly infectious and, in cases of secondary and aspiration pneumonia, bacterial secondary infections are a risk, antimicrobial therapy is started immediately. The type of antibiotic used depends on the infectious agent.

More oxygen, please

Your patient will usually need supplemental oxygen, by mask in mild-to-moderate cases and with more severe pneumonia the patient may need CPAP by mask or hood (for type 1 failure), or NIV (for type 2 failure). If these do not prevent fatigue and hypoxia ET intubation and mechanical ventilation are necessary, or it may be necessary if deterioration is rapid.

Add-ons

Other treatment measures may include:
* bronchodilator therapy
* high-calorie diet/nutritional supplement and adequate hydration
* physiotherapy, positioning, humidification and suction to facilitate clearance of pulmonary
* secretions
* bed rest
* analgesics to relieve pleuritic chest pain and reduce fever.

What to do

* Maintain a patent airway and oxygenation. Position the patient with head of bed elevated to 45 degrees to maximise chest expansion and give supplemental oxygen as needed. Monitor oxygen saturation continuously and ABG levels as indicated.
* Assess respiratory status often, at least every 2 hours. Auscultate the lungs for abnormal breath sounds, such as crackles, wheezes or rhonchi. Encourage coughing and deep breathing.
* If your patient's respiratory status deteriorates, anticipate the need for ET intubation and mechanical ventilation.
* Adhere to local policy for infection prevention and control, depending on the causative organism.
* Institute cardiac monitoring to detect the development of arrhythmias secondary to hypoxaemia. Atrial fibrillation is very common in the elderly with pneumonia.
* Reposition your patient to maximise chest expansion, allow rest and reduce discomfort and anxiety.
* Obtain diagnostic tests as requested by medical staff and report results promptly.
* Administer drug therapy as prescribed.
* Carefully monitor your patient's fluid intake and output to allow early identification of dehydration, fluid overload and accurate tracking of nutritional status.

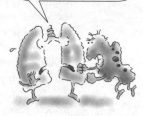

I hope they gave me the right antibiotic to fight off this microbe. He means business!

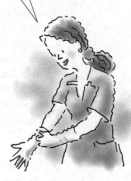

Adhere to infection prevention and control measures, depending on the causative organism.

Acute respiratory distress syndrome

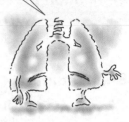

ARDS can quickly lead to acute respiratory failure, so know the clinical signs.

ARDS is a type of pulmonary oedema not related to heart failure. It's also known as *shock*, *white* or *wet lung*. ARDS may follow direct or indirect lung injury and can quickly lead to acute respiratory failure.
The three hallmark features of ARDS are:

 bilateral patchy infiltrates on chest x-ray

no signs or symptoms of heart failure

no improvement in PaO_2 despite increasing oxygen delivery.

The prognosis for patients with ARDS varies depending on the cause and the patient's age and health status before developing ARDS.

What causes it
Some of the most common predisposing factors for ARDS are:
- sepsis
- lung injury from trauma such as chest contusion
- pulmonary embolism (air, fat, amniotic fluid or thrombus)
- shock (any type)
- disseminated intravascular coagulation
- pancreatitis
- massive blood transfusions
- burns
- cardiopulmonary bypass
- drug overdose
- aspiration of stomach contents
- pneumonitis
- near drowning
- pneumonia
- inhalation of noxious gases (such as ammonia or chlorine).

How it happens
In ARDS, the tissues lining the alveoli and the pulmonary capillaries are injured, either directly by aspiration of gastric contents or inhalation of noxious gases, or indirectly, by chemical mediators released into the bloodstream in response to systemic disease and inflammatory response.

Inflammation follows injury

The injured tissues release cytokines and other molecules that cause inflammation as white blood cells (WBCs) collect at the site and swelling occurs. The tissues become more permeable to fluid and proteins, and the hydrostatic pressure gradient between the alveoli and the capillaries is reversed.

Memory jogger

To remember the progression of **ARDS,** use this mnemonic.

Assault to the pulmonary system

Respiratory distress

Decreased lung compliance

Severe respiratory failure

Impaired exchange

Proteins and fluid begin to move from the capillaries into the alveoli. When this happens, gas exchange is impaired in the affected alveoli. As the process continues, the alveoli collapse (atelectasis), and gas exchange becomes impossible.

Ventilation prevention

The fluid that accumulates in the interstitial spaces, alveolar spaces and small airways causes the lungs to stiffen, preventing air from moving into the lungs (ventilation).

Shunt stunts

As alveoli fill with fluid or collapse, the capillaries surrounding the alveoli fail to absorb oxygen. The body responds by shunting blood away from these alveoli, a process called *right-to-left shunting*.

Responses to the big build-up

As fluid builds up in the alveoli, the patient develops thick, frothy sputum and marked hypoxaemia with increasing respiratory distress. As pulmonary oedema worsens, inflammation leads to fibrosis, further impeding gas exchange.

Off-line alkaline

Early in the process or ARDS tachypnoea due to respiratory distress causes alkalosis as carbon dioxide levels decrease. However, as hypoxaemia develops anaerobic metabolism adds to the acidosis.

Unless gas exchange is restored and this process is reversed, acidosis and tissue hypoxia worsens until all organ systems are affected and fail.

What to look for

ARDS occurs in four stages, each with these typical signs and symptoms:

1 Stage I involves dyspnoea, especially on exertion. Respiratory and heart rates are normal to high. Auscultation may reveal diminished breath sounds, particularly when the patient is tachypnoeic. Stage I develops usually within the first 12 hours after the initial injury in response to decreasing oxygen levels in the blood.

2 Stage II is marked by greater respiratory distress. Respiratory rate is high, and the patient may use accessory muscles to breathe. They may appear restless, apprehensive and mentally sluggish, or agitated. They may have a dry cough or frothy sputum. The heart rate is elevated and the skin is cool and clammy. Lung auscultation may reveal basal crackles. The symptoms at this stage are sometimes incorrectly attributed to trauma.

3 Stage III involves obvious respiratory distress, with tachypnoea, use of accessory breathing muscles, and decreased mental acuity. The patient exhibits tachycardia with arrhythmias (usually premature ventricular contractions) and labile blood pressure. The skin is pale and cyanotic. Auscultation may disclose

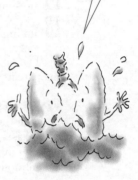

Fluid in the interstitial spaces, alveolar spaces and small airways prevents air from moving into the lungs.

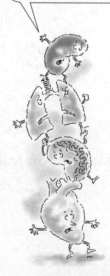

Uh-oh! Unless gas exchange is restored, increasing hypoxia and acidosis could be the downfall of all the organ systems.

diminished breath sounds, basal crackles and rhonchi. This stage generally requires ET intubation and mechanical ventilation.

Stage IV is characterised by decreasing respiratory and heart rates. The patient's mental status nears loss of consciousness. The skin is cool and cyanotic. Breath sounds are severely diminished to absent. (See *Understanding ARDS*.)

What tests tell you

These test results are used to diagnose ARDS:
• ABG analysis initially shows decreased PaO_2 despite oxygen supplementation. Because of tachypnoea, $PaCO_2$ is also decreased, causing an increase in blood pH (respiratory alkalosis).

Understanding ARDS

Here's how acute respiratory distress syndrome (ARDS) progresses:

1. Injury reduces normal blood flow to the lungs. Platelets aggregate and release histamine (H), serotonin (S) and bradykinin (B).

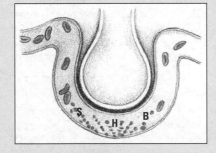

2. The released substances inflame and damage the alveolar capillary membrane, increasing capillary permeability. Fluids then shift into the interstitial space.

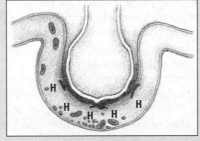

3. Capillary permeability increases and proteins and fluids leak out, increasing interstitial osmotic pressure and causing pulmonary oedema.

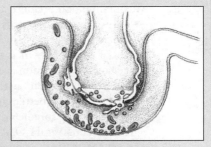

4. Decreased blood flow and fluids in the alveoli damage surfactant and impair the cell's ability to produce more. The alveoli then collapse, thus impairing gas exchange.

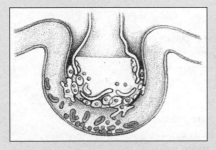

5. Oxygenation is impaired, but carbon dioxide (CO_2) easily crosses the alveolar capillary membrane and is expired. Blood oxygen (O_2) and CO_2 levels are low.

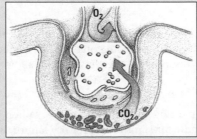

6. Pulmonary oedema worsens and inflammation leads to fibrosis. Gas exchange is further impeded.

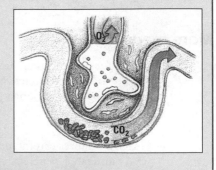

- As ARDS worsens, $PaCO_2$ increases and pH decreases as the patient becomes acidotic. This is worsened by metabolic acidosis caused by a lack of oxygen that comes from anaerobic metabolism.
- Initially, chest x-rays may be normal. Basal infiltrates begin to appear in about 24 hours. In later stages, lung fields have a ground glass appearance and, eventually, as fluid fills the alveoli, white patches appear. These may eventually cover both lung fields entirely in later stages of ARDS.
- Haemodynamic monitoring will help in differentiating whether the cause of the pulmonary oedema is heart failure or ARDS or other causes.
- A differential diagnosis must be done to rule out cardiogenic pulmonary oedema, pulmonary vasculitis and diffuse pulmonary haemorrhage. Tests used to determine the causative agent may include sputum analysis, blood cultures toxicology tests and serum amylase levels (to rule out pancreatitis).

How it's treated

The goal of therapy is to correct the underlying cause, if possible, and provide enough oxygen to allow normal body processes to continue until the lungs begin to heal. The most common cause of ARDS is sepsis.
- Antibiotics may be administered to fight infection and steroids to minimise inflammation in the later fibroproliferative stages of ARDS.
- Diuretics may be needed to reduce interstitial and pulmonary oedema. In later stages of ARDS, however, vasopressors are usually prescribed to maintain blood pressure and blood supply to critical tissues.
- Respiratory support is most important. Humidified oxygen delivery through a CPAP mask or hood may be adequate (if the condition is a mild form of ARDS known as ALI—acute lung injury) but ET intubation and mechanical ventilation are commonly required.
- Research has demonstrated that patients with ARDS, who are mechanically ventilated, have a better chance of survival if they receive tidal volumes of around 6 ml/kg (predicted body weight) and inspiratory plateau pressures no greater than $30 \, cmH_2O$. A moderate amount of PEEP should also be set to prevent atelectasis at end expiration. It is thought that continuous collapse and reinflation of alveoli causes sheer forces that further damage the lungs.
- Prone positioning may improve the patient's oxygenation though as yet there is no evidence that it improves chances of survival as a result. Those who do respond by having improved oxygenation usually improve within the first hour. (See *Prone positioning*, page 359.)

More meds

Additional medications are generally required when intubation and mechanical ventilation are instituted. Sedatives, including opioids and, sometimes, neuromuscular blocking agents, minimise restlessness and allow ventilation.

What to do

ARDS requires careful monitoring and supportive care. When your patient isn't intubated, watch carefully for signs of respiratory failure, which can happen quickly and necessitate intubation and mechanical ventilation.

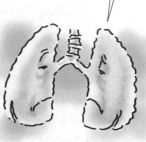

Patients with stage III ARDS generally require ET intubation and mechanical ventilation.

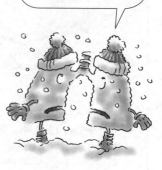

Either I'm entering the later stages of ARDS or we're in for one heck of a blizzard!

Prone positioning

Prone positioning (also known as *proning*) is a therapeutic manoeuvre to improve oxygenation and pulmonary function in patients with acute respiratory distress syndrome (ARDS). It involves physically turning a patient face down, which shifts blood flow to regions of the lung that are better ventilated.

The criteria for prone positioning commonly include:

- acute onset of acute respiratory failure
- hypoxaemia, specifically a partial pressure of arterial oxygen/fraction of inspired oxygen (PaO_2/FIO_2) ratio of 27 or less for ARDS
- radiological evidence of diffuse bilateral pulmonary infiltrates.

Equipment innovations

Innovative equipment, such as a lightweight, cushioned frame that straps to the front of the patient before turning, minimises the risks associated with moving patients and keeping them prone for several hours at a time.

With the right equipment, prone positioning may aid movement of the diaphragm by allowing the abdomen to expand more fully. It's usually used for 6 or more hours per day, for up to 10 days, until the patient's need for a high concentration of inspired oxygen resolves.

Pro-prone positioning

Prone positioning is indicated to support mechanically ventilated patients with ARDS, who require high concentrations of inspired oxygen. In patients who respond, prone positioning may correct severe hypoxaemia and aid maintenance of adequate oxygenation (PaO_2 greater than 60%) in patients with ARDS, while avoiding ventilator-induced lung injury. It isn't clear whether patients' survival rates are increased.

No prone positioning

Prone positioning is contraindicated for patients whose heads can't be supported in a face down position or who can't tolerate a head down position. Relative contraindications include increased intracranial pressure, spinal instability, unstable bone fractures, multiple trauma, left-sided heart failure (nonpulmonary respiratory failure), shock, abdominal compartment syndrome, abdominal surgery, extreme obesity (weight greater than 300 lb [136.1 kg]) and pregnancy. Haemodynamically unstable patients (systolic blood pressure less than 90 mmHg) despite aggressive fluid resuscitation and vasopressors should be thoroughly evaluated before being placed in the prone position.

- Assess the patient's respiratory status hourly or more often, if indicated. Note respiratory rate, rhythm and depth. Report the presence of dyspnoea and accessory muscle use.
- Administer oxygen as prescribed. Monitor SaO_2 levels.
- Auscultate lungs bilaterally for added or diminished breath sounds. Inspect the colour and character of sputum; clear, frothy sputum indicates pulmonary oedema. To maintain PEEP, suction only as needed using a closed suction system.
- Check and record ventilator settings and measured values. Monitor serial ABG levels; document and report changes in oxygen saturation as well as metabolic and respiratory acidosis and PaO_2 changes.

It's vital

- Monitor vital signs. Institute cardiac monitoring and observe for arrhythmias that may result from hypoxaemia, acid–base disturbances or electrolyte imbalance.
- Monitor the patient's LOC, noting confusion or mental sluggishness.
- Be alert for signs of treatment-induced complications, including arrhythmias, disseminated intravascular coagulation, GI bleeding, infection, malnutrition, paralytic ileus, pneumothorax, pulmonary fibrosis, renal failure, thrombocytopaenia and tracheal stenosis.

- Be alert for the development of multiple organ dysfunction syndrome. Monitor renal, GI and neurological system function.
- Give sedatives as prescribed to reduce restlessness. Administer sedatives and analgesics by continuous I.V. infusion if the patient on mechanical ventilation is receiving neuromuscular blocking agents.
- Provide routine eye care and instil artificial tears to prevent corneal drying and abrasion from the loss of the blink reflex in mechanically ventilated patients receiving neuromuscular blocking agents.
- Administer antiinfective agents as ordered if the underlying cause is sepsis or an infection.
- Place the patient in a comfortable position that maximises gas exchange and prevents complications such as ventilator-acquired pneumonia from microaspiration–ideally 45 degree head of bed elevation.

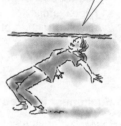

Place the patient in a comfortable position that maximises lung excursion and gas exchange, such as semierect at 45 degrees. This would not be comfortable!

Take a break!

- Allow for periods of rest to prevent fatigue and reduce oxygen demand.
- If your patient has a PA catheter in place, know the desired PAWP level and check readings as indicated. Watch for decreasing $S\bar{v}O_2$. Because PEEP may reduce cardiac output, check for hypotension, tachycardia and decreased urine output.
- Evaluate the patient's serum electrolyte levels frequently as ordered. Measure urine output hourly to ensure adequate renal function. Monitor intake and output. Weigh the patient daily if possible.
- Record caloric intake. Administer tube feedings and parenteral nutrition as prescribed.
- Perform passive movement exercises to maintain joint mobility. Provide meticulous skin care to prevent breakdown.

Pneumothorax

Pneumothorax is an accumulation of air in the pleural cavity that leads to partial or complete lung collapse. The amount of air trapped in the intrapleural space determines the degree of lung collapse. In some cases, venous return to the heart is impeded, causing a life-threatening condition called *tension pneumothorax*.

Pneumothorax can be classified as either traumatic or spontaneous. *Traumatic pneumothorax* may be further classified as open or closed. (Note that an open [penetrating] wound may cause closed pneumothorax.) *Spontaneous pneumothorax*, which is also considered closed, is most common in older patients with COPD but can occur in young, healthy patients as well, especially asthmatics. In fact it is a key thing to exclude when an asthmatic patient with COPD deteriorates suddenly. Patients on mechanical ventilators are also at risk due to positive pressure and you should be aware of the location and contents of your unit's chest drain trolley/kit.

What causes it
The causes of pneumothorax vary according to classification.

Traumatic pneumothorax

Causes of open pneumothorax include:
- penetrating chest injury (stab or gunshot wound)
- insertion of a central venous catheter, especially by subclavian vein route which lies close to the apical pleura
- chest surgery
- transbronchial biopsy
- thoracentesis or closed pleural biopsy.
  Causes of closed pneumothorax include:
- blunt chest trauma
- air leakage from ruptured blebs or bullae
- rupture resulting from barotrauma caused by high intrathoracic pressures during mechanical ventilation
- tubercular or cancerous lesions that erode into the pleural space
- interstitial lung disease such as eosinophilic granuloma.

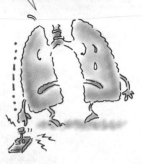

Accumulation of air in the pleural cavity can cause partial or complete lung collapse.

Spontaneous pneumothorax

Spontaneous pneumothorax is usually caused by the rupture of a subpleural bleb (a small cystic space) at the surface of a lung.

Tension pneumothorax

Causes of tension pneumothorax include:
- penetrating chest wound treated with an airtight dressing
- fractured ribs
- mechanical ventilation
- high-level PEEP that causes alveolar blebs to rupture
- chest tube occlusion or malfunction.

How it happens

The pathophysiology of pneumothorax also varies according to classification.

Traumatic pneumothorax

Open pneumothorax occurs when atmospheric air flows directly into the pleural cavity (under negative pressure). As the air pressure in the pleural cavity becomes positive, the lung on the affected side collapses, causing decreased total lung capacity. As a result, the patient develops a $\dot{V}/\dot{Q}$ imbalance that leads to hypoxia.

Closed pneumothorax occurs when an opening is created between the intrapleural space and the parenchyma (tissues and airways) of the lung. Air enters the pleural space from within the lung, causing increased pleural pressure and preventing lung expansion during inspiration.

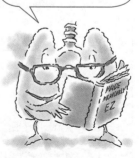

In my book, pneumothorax spells trouble for me.

Spontaneous pneumothorax

In spontaneous pneumothorax, the rupture of a subpleural bleb causes air leakage into the pleural spaces, which causes the lung to collapse. Hypoxia results from decreased total lung capacity, vital capacity and lung compliance.

Tension pneumothorax

Tension pneumothorax results when air in the pleural space is under higher pressure than air in the adjacent lung. Here's what happens:

• Air enters the pleural space from the site of pleural rupture, which acts as a one-way valve. Thus, air enters the pleural space on inspiration but can't escape as the rupture site closes on expiration.

• More air enters with each inspiration and air pressure begins to exceed barometric pressure.

• The air pushes against the recoiled lung, causing compression atelectasis, and pushes against the mediastinum, compressing and displacing the heart and great vessels.

• The mediastinum eventually shifts away from the affected side, affecting venous return and putting ever-greater pressure on the heart, great vessels, trachea and contralateral lung.

Without immediate treatment, this emergency can rapidly become fatal. (See *Understanding tension pneumothorax*.)

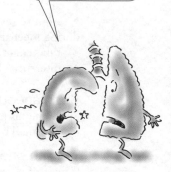

Depending on the severity of pneumothorax, your patient may have sudden, sharp pleuritic pain that exacerbates with movement, breathing or coughing. Oh, that one hurt!

What to look for

Assessment findings depend on the severity of the pneumothorax. Spontaneous pneumothorax that releases a small amount of air into the pleural space may cause no signs and symptoms. Generally, tension pneumothorax causes the most severe respiratory signs and symptoms.

Every breath hurts

Your patient's history reveals sudden, sharp, pleuritic chest pain. The patient may report that chest movement, breathing and coughing exacerbate the pain. They may also report shortness of breath.

Understanding tension pneumothorax

In tension pneumothorax, air accumulates intrapleurally and can't escape. As intrapleural pressure increases, the lung on the affected side collapses.

On inspiration, the mediastinum shifts towards the unaffected lung, impairing ventilation.

On expiration, the mediastinal shift distorts the vena cava and reduces venous return and consequently cardiac output.

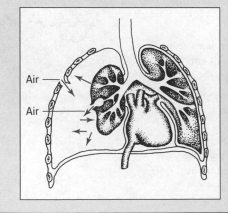

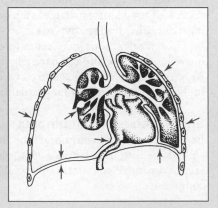

Further findings

Inspection reveals asymmetrical chest wall movement with overexpansion and rigidity on the affected side. The skin may be cool and clammy and cyanotic. Palpation of the chest wall may reveal crackling beneath the skin (subcutaneous emphysema) and decreased vocal fremitus.

In addition, percussion may reveal hyperresonance on the affected side, auscultation may disclose decreased or absent breath sounds on the affected side and vital signs may follow the pattern of respiratory distress seen with respiratory failure.

Did we mention the tension?

Tension pneumothorax also causes:
- hypotension and tachycardia due to decreased cardiac output
- tracheal deviation to the opposite side (a late sign)
- distended jugular veins due to high intrapleural pressure, mediastinal shift and reduced cardiac output.

What tests tell you
- Chest x-rays reveal air in the pleural space and a mediastinal shift that confirm pneumothorax.
- ABG analysis reveals hypoxaemia, usually with elevated $PaCO_2$ and normal bicarbonate ion levels in the early stages.
- ECG may reveal decreased QRS amplitude, precordial (V1-6) T-wave inversion, rightward shift of frontal QRS axis and small precordial (V1-6) R voltage.

How it's treated
Treatment of pneumothorax depends on the cause and severity.

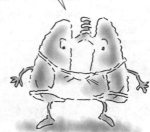

Open or traumatic pneumothorax may require surgical repair of affected tissues and pleural drain placement. See you in theatre.

With trauma

Open or traumatic pneumothorax may necessitate surgical repair of affected tissues, followed by placement of a pleural drain (chest drain) with an underwater seal.

With less lung collapse

Spontaneous pneumothorax with less than 30% lung collapse, no signs of increased pleural pressure and no dyspnoea or indications of physiological compromise may be corrected with:
- bed rest to preserve energy
- monitoring of vital signs to detect physiological compromise
- oxygen administration to improve hypoxia
- aspiration of air from the intrapleural space with a large-bore needle attached to a syringe to restore negative pressure within the pleural space.

With more lung collapse

Greater than 30% lung collapse may necessitate other measures, such as:
• placing a pleural drain in the second or third intercostal space in the mid-clavicular line to reexpand the lung by restoring negative intrapleural pressure
• connecting the pleural drain to an underwater seal or low-pressure suction to reexpand the lung.

I wonder if this is the kind of low-level suctioning they had in mind.

With tension

Treatment for your patient with tension pneumothorax typically involves:
• immediate large-bore needle insertion into the pleural space through the second intercostal space in the midclavicular line to reexpand the lung, followed by insertion of a pleural drain if large amounts of air escape through the needle after insertion
• analgesics to promote comfort and encourage deep breathing and coughing. (See *Combating tension pneumothorax*.)

What to do
• Assess the patient's respiratory status, including auscultation of bilateral breath sounds, at least every hour until stable. Monitor oxygen saturation levels closely for changes; obtain ABG analysis as indicated or requested.
• Monitor haemodynamic parameters frequently as appropriate and indicated; anticipate the need for cardiac monitoring because hypoxaemia can predispose the patient to arrhythmias.

Take charge!

Combating tension pneumothorax

Tension pneumothorax, the entrapment of air within the pleural space, can be fatal without prompt treatment.

What causes it?

An obstructed or dislodged pleural drain is a common cause of tension pneumothorax. Other causes include blunt chest trauma or high-pressure mechanical ventilation. In such cases, increased positive pressure within the patient's chest cavity compresses the affected lung and the mediastinum, shifting them towards the opposite lung. This impairs venous return and cardiac output and may cause the lung to collapse.

Telltale signs

Suspect tension pneumothorax if the patient develops dyspnoea, chest pain, an irritating cough, vertigo, syncope or anxiety after a blunt chest trauma or if the patient has a chest tube in place. Is their skin cold, pale and clammy? Are their respiratory and pulse rates unusually rapid? Does the patient have equal bilateral chest expansion?

If you note these signs and symptoms, palpate the patient's neck, face and chest wall for subcutaneous emphysema, and palpate their trachea for deviation from midline. Auscultate the lungs for decreased or absent breath sounds on one side. Then percuss them for hyperresonance. If you suspect tension pneumothorax, notify the doctor immediately and help identify the cause.

- Watch for complications, signalled by pallor, gasping respirations and sudden chest pain. Carefully monitor vital signs at least every hour for indications of shock, increasing respiratory distress or mediastinal shift. If your patient's respiratory status deteriorates, anticipate the need for ET intubation and mechanical ventilation and assist as necessary.
- Assist with the pleural drain insertion and connect to suction, as prescribed. Monitor your patient for possible complications associated with chest tube insertion.
- Check chest tube devices frequently for drainage and proper functioning. Document oscillation, bubbling and amount of drainage on the charts.
- Reposition your patient to promote comfort and drainage.

Pulmonary embolism

Pulmonary embolism is an obstruction of the pulmonary arterial bed. It occurs when a mass lodges in a pulmonary artery branch, partially or completely obstructing blood flow distal to it. This causes a $\dot{V}/\dot{Q}$ mismatch, resulting in hypoxaemia and intrapulmonary shunting.

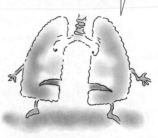

Pulmonary embolism causes a V/Q mismatch that results in hypoxaemia and intrapulmonary shunting.

What causes it

The most common source of pulmonary embolism is a dislodged thrombus that originated in the deep veins of the leg or, less commonly, in the pelvic, renal or hepatic veins, or right side of the heart. Other emboli arise from fat, air, amniotic fluid, tumour cells or a foreign object, such as a needle, catheter part or talc (from drugs intended for oral administration that are injected I.V. by addicts).

Risky red flags

Risk factors for developing pulmonary embolism include:
- predisposing disorders, including lung disorders, cardiac disorders (valvular disease and arrhythmias, such as atrial fibrillation), infection, diabetes, history of thromboembolism, sickle cell disease and polycythaemia
- venous stasis in those who are on prolonged bed rest, immobile, obese, burn victims, older than age 40 or in orthopaedic casts
- venous injury caused by surgery (especially of the legs, pelvis, abdomen and thorax), long-bone or pelvic fractures, I.V. drug abuse, I.V. therapy or manipulation or disconnection of central lines
- increased blood coagulability resulting from cancer, high oestrogen hormonal contraceptive use (particularly in women older than age 40 who smoke cigarettes) or pregnancy (which involves hypercoagulability, decreased mobility, oedema and decreased venous return).

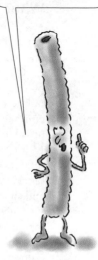

A dislodged thrombus originating in the deep veins of the leg is the most common cause of a pulmonary embolism.

The skinny on fat and air

Fat embolism risk factors include osteomyelitis, long-bone fractures, burns and adipose tissue or liver trauma. Risk factors for air embolism include cardiopulmonary bypass, haemodialysis, deep vein catheter insertion and endoscopy.

How it happens

Here's what happens when pulmonary embolism develops:
- A thrombus forms as a result of trauma to the vascular wall, venous stasis or hypercoagulability of the blood.
- Further trauma, clot dissolution, sudden muscle spasm, pressure changes or a change in peripheral blood flow can cause the thrombus to loosen or fragment.
- After it's dislodged, the thrombus becomes an embolus and floats through the venous system to the right side of the heart and onto the pulmonary vasculature, where it lodges in a small vessel and occludes blood flow beyond the occlusion.
- A $\dot{V}/\dot{Q}$ mismatch results in hypoxaemia that's commonly irreversible.

What to look for

Your patient's history may reveal a predisposing condition or another risk factor for pulmonary embolism.

The large and small of it

Other symptoms depend on the size of the embolus and if it's a fat or air embolism.
- A small embolism may not cause any signs or symptoms.
- An embolism that occludes less than 50% of the pulmonary artery bed may cause shortness of breath, anxiety, chest pain, S_3 or S_4 heart sound and crackles on auscultation.
- An embolism that occludes more than 50% of the artery bed may cause a sense of impending doom, dyspnoea, tachycardia, confusion, right-sided heart failure, hypotension and PEA (pulseless electrical activity).
- A fat embolism may produce no symptoms for up to 24 hours. Symptoms may include restlessness, confusion, shortness of breath, petechiae on the chest, wheezing and hypoxaemia.
- An air embolism may cause palpitations, weakness, tachycardia and hypoxia.

What tests tell you

- $\dot{V}/\dot{Q}$ scan demonstrates a mismatch, indicating abnormal perfusion. Though this is the traditional test used it is not possible in the critically ill due to dyspnoea. It is also less sensitive than CTPA.
- CT pulmonary angiogram (CT scan with contrast) may reveal a pulmonary vessel filling defect or an abrupt vessel ending, indicating pulmonary embolism. CTPA is a highly reliable test for pulmonary embolus. However, due to the need to give contrast agent it may not be possible in allergy, renal failure and pregnancy.
- ECG results distinguish pulmonary embolism from myocardial infarction (MI) and show right axis deviation, right bundle-branch block, tall, peaked P waves, depressed ST segments, T-wave inversions and supraventricular arrhythmias.
- Chest x-ray is used to rule out other pulmonary diseases, but it's inconclusive within 1–2 hours of the embolic event. It may also indicate areas of atelectasis, an elevated diaphragm, pleural effusion, a prominent pulmonary artery and, occasionally, the characteristic wedge-shaped infiltrate that suggests pulmonary infarction.

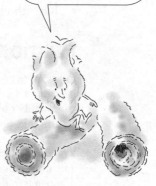

A dislodged thrombus, or an embolus, can float through the venous system to the heart and lungs and become stuck in a small vessel, occluding blood flow beyond that point.

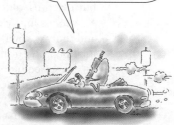

The signs and symptoms of pulmonary embolism vary with the size of the embolus and with other factors such as whether it's caused by a thrombus, fat or air.

- ABG analysis reveals hypoxaemia and possibly hypocapnia due to tachypnoea.
- PA catheterisation may reveal an elevated central venous pressure and PAP and a normal PAWP.
- MRI is used to identify the embolus or blood flow changes indicating an embolus.

How it's treated

The goal of treatment is to allow adequate gas exchange until the obstruction can be removed or resolves on its own. Oxygen therapy is the primary initial treatment to prevent hypoxaemia and its sequelae.

In addition to oxygen therapy, the following treatment measures may be indicated:
- For patients with blood clots, anticoagulation with heparin inhibits the formation of more thrombi. It's followed by warfarin for 3–6 months, depending on risk factors.
- Patients with massive pulmonary embolism and shock may need thrombolysis therapy to enhance fibrinolysis of the pulmonary emboli and remaining thrombi.
- Embolism from other sources may necessitate other therapy to dissolve the embolus, depending on its nature. Septic embolism, for example, calls for antibiotic therapy rather than anticoagulation.
- If hypotension occurs, vasopressors may be required to maintain blood pressure.

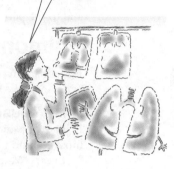

Pulmonary angiogram is a highly reliable test for diagnosing a pulmonary embolism, even though there is risk of complications.

Surgical salvation

- Surgery is indicated for patients who can't take anticoagulants because of recent surgery or other risks of bleeding or who have recurrent emboli during anticoagulant therapy. Surgery, which shouldn't be performed without angiographic evidence of pulmonary embolism, consists of vena caval ligation, plication or insertion of a filter device to filter blood returning to the heart and lungs.

What to do

- Monitor your patient's respiratory status, oxygen saturation and breath sounds, and administer oxygen therapy as prescribed. If breathing is severely compromised, anticipate the need for ET intubation and mechanical ventilation.
- Monitor vital signs and heart rhythm to detect arrhythmias secondary to hypoxaemia. Because many signs and symptoms of pulmonary embolism mimic those of MI, obtain a 12-lead ECG to rule out MI.
- Obtain laboratory tests as ordered and report results promptly.
- Monitor APTT regularly for patients on anticoagulation therapy. Effective heparin therapy increases PATT to about 2 to 2½ times normal.
- Keep antidotes for anticoagulants readily available. These include protamine sulphate for heparin and vitamin K for warfarin. Blood products may be needed in case of life-threatening bleeding.
- During anticoagulant therapy, assess your patient for epistaxis, petechiae and other signs of abnormal bleeding. Apply pressure over venous puncture

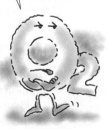

It's about time I got top billing as *the primary treatment.* I'm important you know!

sites for 5–10 and 15–20 minutes for arterial sites, until bleeding stops. Avoid giving I.M. injections.

• Avoid giving aspirin and other nonsteroidal antiinflammatory drugs (NSAIDs) if the patient is taking anticoagulants.

• Promote your patient's comfort by repositioning them often and administering analgesics for pain. Encourage leg movement if the patient is alert. Never vigorously massage the lower extremities.

• Monitor nutritional intake to ensure adequate calorie and fluid intake.

• Explain all procedures to the patient, even if their mentation is altered, and to the patient's family when present.

Pulmonary hypertension

Pulmonary hypertension refers to chronically elevated PAP, over 30 mmHg, and a mean PAP over 18 mmHg.

What causes it

Primary, or idiopathic, pulmonary hypertension has no known cause. It's most common in women between ages 20 and 40 and is usually fatal within 3–4 years. Mortality is highest in pregnant women.

Prefaced with heart or lung disease

Secondary pulmonary hypertension results from existing cardiac or pulmonary disease, or both. Cardiac causes include:
• left-sided heart failure
• ventricular septal defect
• patent ductus arteriosus.

Pulmonary causes include COPD and vasoconstriction of the arterial bed due to hypoxaemia and acidosis.

How it happens

In primary pulmonary hypertension, the intimal lining of the pulmonary arteries thickens, narrowing the lumen of the artery, impairing distensibility and increasing vascular resistance.

Alveolar hypoventilation can result from diseases causing alveolar destruction or diseases that prevent the chest wall from expanding sufficiently to allow air into the alveoli. The resulting decreased ventilation increases pulmonary vascular resistance.

Hypoxaemia resulting from the V̇/Q̇ mismatch causes vasoconstriction, further increasing vascular resistance and resulting in pulmonary hypertension.

Sans treatment

If a patient with pulmonary hypertension doesn't receive treatment, here's what happens:
• Hypertrophy occurs in the medial smooth-muscle layer of the arterioles, worsening nondistensibility.
• Increased pressure in the lungs is transmitted to the right ventricle (which supplies the pulmonary artery).

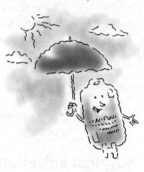

If your patient can't take anticoagulants or has recurrent emboli while on anticoagulant therapy, they may need a filter (e.g. umbrella filter) to prevent clots from travelling to the heart and lungs.

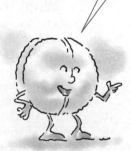

Avoid giving aspirin and other NSAIDs if your patient is taking anticoagulants.

- The ventricle becomes hypertrophic and eventually fails (cor pulmonale).
- Impaired distensibility due to hypertrophy can cause arrhythmias.

What to look for

Patients with pulmonary hypertension typically report increasing dyspnoea on exertion, weakness, syncope and fatigue.

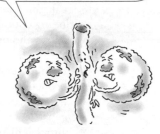

Sorry, guys. You'll get no more oxygen from me. You'll find I can be most resistant when I want to be.

Look, touch and listen

Look for the signs of pulmonary hypertension, including:
- tachycardia
- tachypnoea with mild exertion
- decreased blood pressure
- changes in mental status, from restlessness to agitation or confusion
- signs of right-sided heart failure, such as ascites and jugular vein distention
- a reduced carotid pulse
- possible peripheral oedema
- decreased diaphragmatic excursion and respiration
- point of maximal impulse (apex of heart) displaced beyond the midclavicular line.

What tests tell you
- ABG analysis reveals hypoxaemia.
- ECG changes commensurate with right ventricular hypertrophy include right axis deviation and tall or peaked P waves in inferior leads.
- PA catheterisation reveals increased PAP, with systolic pressure above 30 mmHg. It may also show an increased PAWP if the underlying cause is left atrial myxoma, mitral stenosis or left-sided heart failure; otherwise, PAWP is normal.
- Pulmonary angiography is used to detect filling defects in pulmonary vasculature.
- Pulmonary function studies may show decreased flow rates and increased residual volume in underlying obstructive disease. In underlying restrictive disease, they may show reduced total lung capacity.
- Radionuclide imaging reveals abnormal right and left ventricular functions.
- Echocardiography allows assessment of ventricular wall motion and possible valvular dysfunction. It's also used to identify right ventricular enlargement, abnormal septal configuration and reduced left ventricular cavity size.
- Perfusion lung scanning may yield normal results or multiple patchy and diffuse filling defects not consistent with pulmonary embolism.

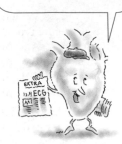

Let me paint a picture of a patient with pulmonary hypertension … someone who reports increasing dyspnoea on exertion, weakness, syncope and fatigue.

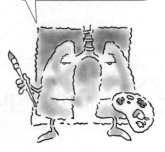

Don't forget me! Read up on how ECG changes indicate right ventricular hypertrophy.

How it's treated
Treatment measures include:
- oxygen therapy to correct hypoxaemia
- fluid restriction to decrease preload and minimise workload of the right ventricle.

In severe cases with irreversible changes, heart–lung transplantation may be necessary.

Diverse drugs

Your patient may receive:
- inotropic medications such as digoxin to increase cardiac output
- diuretics to decrease intravascular volume and venous return
- calcium channel blockers, ACE inhibitors and other vasodilators (possibly including continuous vasodilator infusion therapy) to reduce myocardial workload and oxygen consumption
- Prostaglandins to relax smooth muscles in the pulmonary vasculature (including epoprostenol intravenously and inhaled iloprost)
- bronchodilators to relax smooth muscles and increase airway patency
- beta-adrenergic blockers to reduce cardiac workload and improve oxygenation
- anticoagulant therapy in case of concurrent hypercoagulability.

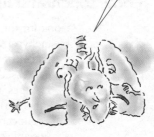

Get hold of yourself! In severe cases with irreversible changes, heart–lung transplantation may be necessary.

What to do

- Assess cardiopulmonary status. Auscultate breath sounds, being alert for crackles indicative of heart failure. Monitor vital signs, oxygen saturation and heart rhythm.
- Assess haemodynamic status, including PAP and PAWP hourly or more often, depending on the patient's condition, and report any changes.
- Monitor intake and output closely and obtain daily weights. Institute fluid restriction as prescribed.
- Administer medications as prescribed to promote adequate heart and lung functions. Assess for potential adverse reactions, such as postural hypotension with diuretics and beta-adrenergic blockers.
- Administer supplemental oxygen as ordered and organise care to allow rest periods.

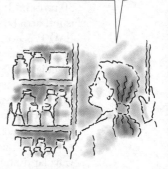

Administer drugs as prescribed to promote adequate heart and lung functions.

Quick quiz

1. When auscultating a patient's lungs, you hear crackles. These are caused by:
   A. secretions blocking the bronchial airways.
   B. collapsed or fluid-filled alveoli snapping open.
   C. a foreign body obstructing the trachea.
   D. consolidation.

Answer: B. Crackles are caused by alveoli opening and are usually associated with fluid in the alveolar space.

2. Which ABG analysis results would you expect to find in a patient with acute type 2 respiratory failure?
   A. pH 7.25, PaO_2 6.4, $PaCO_2$ 7.3
   B. pH 7.40, PaO_2 10.9, $PaCO_2$ 5.9
   C. pH 7.50, PaO_2 8, $PaCO_2$ 4
   D. pH 7.40, PaO_2 11.3, $PaCO_2$ 6.1

Answer: A. The patient with a PaO_2 less than 8, a decreased pH and elevated $PaCO_2$ is hypoxaemic and in respiratory acidosis—the hallmarks of acute type 2 respiratory failure.

3. Which option isn't a method of weaning a patient from mechanical ventilation?
   A. Synchronised intermittent mandatory ventilation
   B. Pressure-support ventilation
   C. Spontaneous breathing trials with T-piece
   D. Controlled mandatory ventilation

Answer: D. Controlled mandatory ventilation is used when the patient can't initiate spontaneous breaths, such as a patient paralysed because of a spinal cord injury. It isn't an acceptable weaning method.

4. ET tubes have inflatable cuffs to:
   A. measure pressure on tracheal tissues.
   B. drain gastric contents.
   C. prevent backflow of oxygen and aspiration of pooled pharyngeal secretions.
   D. treat laryngeal oedema.

Answer: C. ET tube cuffs prevent backflow of oxygen so that it's delivered fully to the lungs and aspiration of pooled pharyngeal secretions into the lungs.

5. A patient diagnosed with status asthmaticus who was previously wheezing suddenly stops wheezing and continues to show signs of respiratory distress. Your assessment findings would indicate that:
   A. their condition is slowly improving.
   B. they're in imminent danger of respiratory collapse.
   C. they aren't as sick as you thought because they stopped wheezing.
   D. you need more information because wheezing isn't a sensitive indicator of asthma.

Answer: B. Wheezing that stops suddenly when signs of respiratory distress continue indicates severe bronchial constriction with little air movement during inspiration and expiration. This is a dangerous event, requiring immediate intervention to prevent respiratory collapse.

Scoring

☆☆☆ If you answered all five questions correctly, breathe a big sigh of relief. You're a respiratory mastermind!

☆☆ If you answered four questions correctly, don't wait to exhale. You're an inspiration!

☆ If you answered fewer than four questions correctly, don't panic–you aren't on the verge of expiration. Take a deep breath and dive back into the chapter.

6 Gastrointestinal system

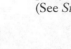

Just the facts

In this chapter, you'll learn:

♦ structure and function of the GI system

♦ assessment of the GI system

♦ diagnostic tests and treatments

♦ GI disorders and related nursing care.

Understanding the GI system

The GI system has two major components: the alimentary canal (also called the GI tract) and accessory organs of digestion.

GI function

The two major functions of the GI tract are:
- digestion, or breaking down food and fluid into simple chemicals that can be absorbed into the bloodstream and transported through the body
- elimination of wastes through excretion of stool.

GI failure

The GI system has a profound effect on a person's overall health. When a GI process malfunctions, the patient can experience problems ranging from loss of appetite to acid–base imbalance.

Alimentary canal

The alimentary canal is a hollow muscular tube that begins in the mouth and extends to the anus. It includes the pharynx, oesophagus, stomach and small and large intestines. (See *Structures of the GI system*, page 373.)

> The GI system has a profound effect on overall health. Can someone point me to the alimentary canal?

Structures of the GI system

The GI system includes the GI tract (pharynx, oesophagus, stomach and small and large intestines) and the accessory organs (liver, biliary duct system and pancreas). These structures are illustrated below.

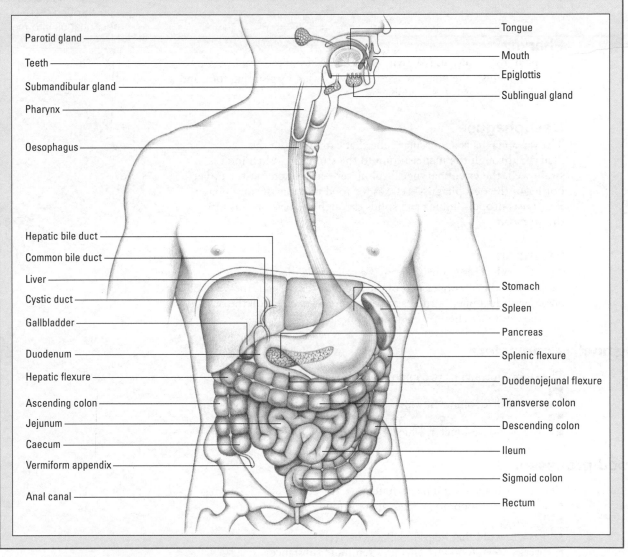

Parotid gland

Teeth

Submandibular gland

Pharynx

Oesophagus

Hepatic bile duct

Common bile duct

Liver

Cystic duct

Gallbladder

Duodenum

Hepatic flexure

Ascending colon

Jejunum

Caecum

Vermiform appendix

Anal canal

Tongue

Mouth

Epiglottis

Sublingual gland

Stomach

Spleen

Pancreas

Splenic flexure

Duodenojejunal flexure

Transverse colon

Descending colon

Ileum

Sigmoid colon

Rectum

Mouth

Digestion begins in the mouth with chewing, salivating and swallowing. The tongue provides a person's sense of taste. Saliva moistens food during chewing and is produced by three pairs of glands:

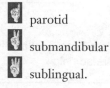 parotid

submandibular

sublingual.

Pharynx

The pharynx, or throat, is a cavity that extends from the oral cavity to the oesophagus. The pharynx assists in swallowing by grasping food and propelling it towards the oesophagus.

Oesophagus

The oesophagus is a muscular tube that extends from the pharynx through the mediastinum to the stomach. When food is swallowed, the cricopharyngeal sphincter—a sphincter at the upper border of the oesophagus—relaxes for food to enter the oesophagus. Peristalsis propels liquids and solids through the oesophagus into the stomach.

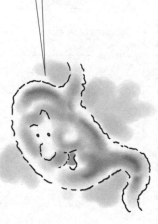

How perfect! Peristalsis propels liquids and solids through the oesophagus into me!

Stomach

The stomach, a reservoir for food, is a collapsible, pouchlike structure in the left upper part of the abdominal cavity, just below the diaphragm. Its upper border is attached to the lower end of the oesophagus, and the exit is attached to the duodenum.

Distinctive sphincters

The stomach contains two important sphincters:

the cardiac sphincter, which protects the entrance to the stomach

the pyloric sphincter, which guards the exit.

Food processor

The stomach has several major functions. It:
- serves as a temporary storage area for food
- begins digestion
- has a low pH that helps to kill any bacteria
- breaks down food into chyme, a semifluid substance
- moves the gastric contents into the small intestine.

Small intestine

The small intestine is about 20 feet (6 m) long and is named for its diameter, not its length. Nearly all digestion and nutrient absorption takes place in the small intestine.

There are three major divisions of the small intestine:

 duodenum, the longest and most superior division

jejunum, the middle and shortest segment

ileum, the most inferior portion.

Absorptive wall

The intestinal wall has several structural features that increase its absorptive surface area, including:
• plicae circulares, which are circular folds of the intestinal mucosa
• villi, which are fingerlike projections on the mucosa
• microvilli, which are tiny cytoplasmic projections on the surface of epithelial cells.

The small intestine also contains:
• intestinal crypts of Lieberkühn, which are simple glands lodged in the grooves separating villi
• Peyer's patches, which are collections of lymphatic tissue within the submucosa
• Brunner's glands, which secrete mucus.

Small intestine functions, no small feat

The small intestine functions by:
• completing food digestion
• absorbing food molecules, water and vitamins through its wall into the circulatory system, which then delivers them to cells throughout the body
• secreting hormones that control the secretion of bile, pancreatic juices and intestinal juice.

Large intestine

The large intestine, or colon, has six segments:

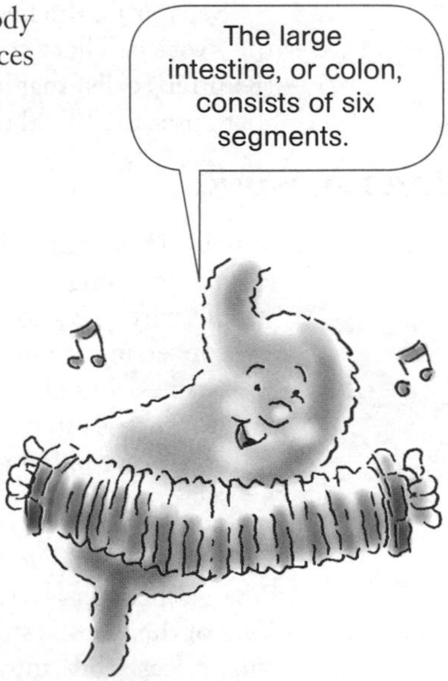

The caecum, a saclike structure, makes up the first few inches. It's connected to the ileum of the small intestine by the ileocaecal pouch.

The ascending colon rises on the right posterior abdominal wall and then turns sharply under the liver at the hepatic flexure.

The transverse colon is situated above the small intestine, passing horizontally across the abdomen and below the liver, stomach and spleen. At the left colic flexure, it turns downwards.

The descending colon starts near the spleen and extends down the left side of the abdomen into the pelvic cavity.

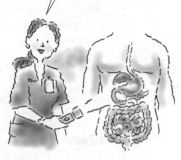

There's nothing small about the job of the small intestine. It does most of the digesting and absorbing!

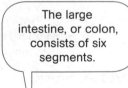

The large intestine, or colon, consists of six segments.

The sigmoid colon descends through the pelvic cavity, where it becomes the rectum.

The rectum, the last few inches of the large intestine, terminates at the anus.

Food's finale

The functions of the large intestine include absorbing excess water and electrolytes, storing food residue and eliminating waste products in the form of faeces.

Accessory organs of digestion

The accessory organs of the GI tract are the liver, gallbladder and pancreas. They contribute hormones, enzymes and bile, which are vital to digestion.

Liver

The liver is located in the right upper quadrant under the diaphragm. It has four lobes:
- left lobe
- right lobe
- caudate lobe (behind the right lobe)
- quadrate lobe (behind the left lobe).

Liver's lobule

The liver's functional unit is called the lobule. It consists of hepatic cells, or hepatocytes, that encircle a central vein and radiate outwards.

Separating the hepatocytes' plates from each other are sinusoids, the liver's capillary system. Reticuloendothelial macrophages (Kupffer's cells) that line the sinusoids remove bacteria and toxins that enter the blood through the intestinal capillaries.

Liver at work

The liver's functions include:
- metabolising carbohydrates, fats and proteins
- detoxifying various endogenous and exogenous toxins in plasma
- converting ammonia into urea for excretion
- synthesising plasma proteins, nonessential amino acids and vitamin A
- storing essential nutrients, such as iron and vitamins D, K and B12
- regulating blood glucose levels
- secreting bile.

Gallbladder

The gallbladder is a small, pear-shaped organ that lies halfway under the right lobe of the liver. It stores and concentrates bile produced by the liver and then releases bile into the common bile duct for delivery to the duodenum in response to the contraction and relaxation of the sphincter of Oddi.

> I may be considered an accessory, but my role is important.

Memory jogger

To remember the difference between exocrine and endocrine, just remember exocrine refers to external, so endocrine refers to internal.

Bile talk

Bile is a greenish liquid composed of water, cholesterol, bile salts and phospholipids. It has several functions, including emulsifying (breaking down) fat and promoting intestinal absorption of fatty acids, cholesterol and other lipids.

Pancreas

The pancreas lies horizontally in the abdomen behind the stomach. Its head and neck extend into the curve of the duodenum and its tail lies against the spleen. The pancreas performs exocrine and endocrine functions. (See *A look at the biliary tract.*)

Exocrine function and enzymes

The pancreas's exocrine function involves scattered cells that secrete more than 1,000 ml of digestive enzymes every day. Vagal stimulation and release of the hormones secretin and cholecystokinin control the rate and amount of pancreatic secretion.

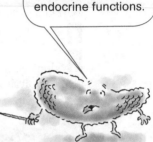

I'm a multifunctional little organ! I perform exocrine and endocrine functions.

A look at the biliary tract

Together, the gallbladder and pancreas constitute the biliary tract. The illustration below shows the parts of the biliary tract.

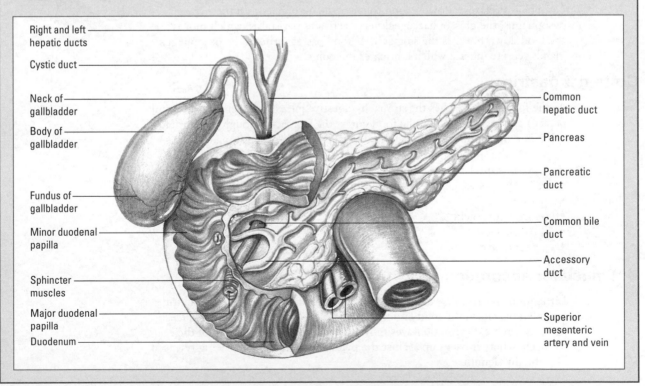

Right and left hepatic ducts

Cystic duct

Neck of gallbladder

Body of gallbladder

Fundus of gallbladder

Minor duodenal papilla

Sphincter muscles

Major duodenal papilla

Duodenum

Common hepatic duct

Pancreas

Pancreatic duct

Common bile duct

Accessory duct

Superior mesenteric artery and vein

Clustered lobules and lobes of enzyme-producing cells release their secretions into the pancreatic duct. The pancreatic duct runs the length of the pancreas and joins the bile duct from the gallbladder before entering the duodenum.

Endocrine function and hormones

The endocrine function of the pancreas involves the islets of Langerhans, located between the lobes. Over 1 million of these islets house two cell types:

☝ beta cells, which secrete insulin to promote carbohydrate metabolism

✌ alpha cells, which secrete glucagon, a hormone that stimulates glycogenolysis in the liver.

Insulin and glucagon flow directly into the blood. Blood glucose levels stimulate their release.

Digestion and elimination

Digestion starts in the oral cavity, where chewing (mastication), salivating (the beginning of starch digestion) and swallowing (deglutition) all take place.

Down it goes!

When a person swallows, the hypopharyngeal sphincter in the upper oesophagus relaxes, allowing food to enter the oesophagus. In the oesophagus, the glossopharyngeal nerve activates peristalsis, which moves the food down towards the stomach. As food passes through the oesophagus, glands secrete mucus, which lubricates the bolus.

Gotta get gastrin

As the food bolus reaches the stomach, digestive juices (hydrochloric acid and pepsin) are secreted. When the food enters the stomach through the cardiac sphincter, the stomach wall stretches. This distention of the stomach wall stimulates the stomach to release gastrin.

Gastrin stimulates the stomach's motor functions and secretion of gastric juices by the gastric gland. These digestive secretions consist mainly of:
• pepsin
• hydrochloric acid
• intrinsic factor
• proteolytic enzymes.

Not much for absorption

Little food absorption, except for alcohol, occurs in the stomach. Peristaltic contractions churn the food into tiny particles and mix it with gastric juices, forming chyme. Peristaltic waves move the chyme into the antrum of the stomach, where it backs up against the pyloric sphincter before being released into the duodenum.

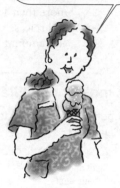

Yum! Digestion starts with chewing, salivation and swallowing.

Digestion and absorption powerhouse

The small intestine performs most of the work of digestion and absorption. Intestinal contractions and various digestive secretions break down carbohydrates, proteins and fats, actions that enable the intestinal mucosa to absorb these nutrients into the bloodstream (along with water and electrolytes).

Small to large

By the time chyme passes through the small intestine and enters the ascending colon of the large intestine, it has been reduced to mostly indigestible substances.

Journey through the large intestine

The food bolus begins its journey through the large intestine where the ileum and caecum join with the ileocaecal pouch. Then the bolus moves up the ascending colon, past the right abdominal cavity, to the liver's lower border. It crosses horizontally below the liver and stomach by way of the transverse colon and descends through the left abdominal cavity to the iliac fossa through the descending colon.

From there, the bolus travels through the sigmoid colon to the lower midline of the abdominal cavity, then to the rectum, and finally to the anal canal. The anus opens to the exterior through two sphincters:
• The internal sphincter contains thick, circular smooth muscle under autonomic control.
• The external sphincter contains skeletal muscle under voluntary control.

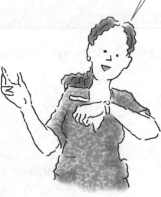

By the time chyme enters the large intestine, it's mostly indigestible.

All about absorption

The large intestine produces no hormones or digestive enzymes; it continues the absorptive process. Through blood and lymph vessels in the submucosa, the proximal half of the large intestine absorbs all but about 100 ml of the remaining water in the colon. It also absorbs large amounts of sodium and chloride.

Harbouring the enemy?

The large intestine harbours the bacteria *Escherichia coli*, *Enterobacter aerogenes*, *Clostridium perfringens* and *Lactobacillus bifidus*. All of these bacteria aid in synthesising vitamin K and breaking down cellulose into a usable carbohydrate. Bacterial action also produces flatus, which helps propel stool towards the rectum.

Lube job

In addition, the mucosa of the large intestine produces alkaline secretions. This alkaline mucus lubricates the intestinal walls and protects the mucosa from acidic bacterial action.

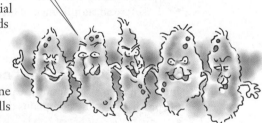

We're not all bad! Some bacteria help break down cellulose into a usable carbohydrate.

Elimination round

In the lower colon, long and relatively sluggish contractions cause propulsive waves. Normally occurring several times per day, these movements propel intestinal contents into the rectum and produce the urge to defecate. Defecation normally results from the defecation reflex, a sensory and parasympathetic nerve-mediated response, along with the voluntary relaxation of the external anal sphincter.

Key physiological principles

- Blood supply—Because a key function of the GI tract is absorption of food and fluid, it requires a good blood supply so that nutrients can be transported through the body and utilised.
- Fluid—Digestion and absorption functions mean that the GI tract both secretes and absorbs a large amount of fluid every day.
- Protection—A key mechanism of the GI tract is preventing infection. Potential ingestion of bacteria in food and the colonisation of the large intestine with essential flora cause risks of infection. By having a low pH in the stomach many bacteria will be destroyed at this point, the vomiting reflex and the constant motility in the gut (peristalsis) aid removal of bacteria. The mucus produced and the lymphatic tissue lining in the small intestine also protect the lining from penetration by bacteria that manages to enter.

GI assessment

Being able to identify subtle changes in a patient's GI system can mean all the difference between effective and ineffective care. GI signs and symptoms can have many baffling causes. Ask yourself the following questions:
- Is there an acute GI problem?
- Is there an underlying chronic GI problem?
- Is there potential for GI deterioration?

If the critically ill patient requires immediate stabilising treatment always use an ABCDE approach, otherwise begin with a thorough assessment adopting this structured approach:
- History of the present complaint
- Health history and medication
- Clinical assessment and monitoring
- Results and significance of diagnostic tests and investigations

History

History of the present complaint

Include information about the patient's chief complaint. The patient with a GI problem usually complains of:
- pain
- heartburn

- nausea
- vomiting
- altered bowel habits.

To investigate these and other signs and symptoms, ask about the onset, duration and severity of each. Also, inquire about the location of the pain, precipitating factors, alleviating factors and associated symptoms. (See *Asking the right questions*, page 382.) Conduct this part of the assessment as privately as possible because the patient/relatives may feel embarrassment when talking about GI functions.

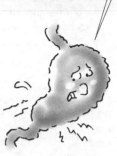

Listen up! Your patient is likely to report pain, heartburn and other GI-related signs and symptoms.

Health history and medication

In the health history ask about previous illnesses, medications used, family history and social history. To determine if the patient's problem is new or recurring, ask about GI illnesses, such as an ulcer, gallbladder disease, inflammatory bowel disease or GI bleeding. Also, ask if they have had abdominal surgery or trauma.

Further questions

Ask the patient additional questions, such as:
- Are you allergic to any foods or medications?
- Have you noticed a change in the colour, amount, frequency and appearance of your stool? Have you ever seen blood in your stool?
- Have you recently travelled abroad? (If the patient presents with diarrhoea, because diarrhoea, hepatitis and parasitic infections can result from ingesting contaminated food or water.)
- Ask them about their appetite, ability to swallow and any weight loss.
- Ask them about their dental history. Poor dentition may impair their ability to chew and swallow food.

Don't forget the drugs

Ask the patient if they're taking medication. Several drugs, including aspirin, sulphonamides, nonsteroidal antiinflammatory drugs (NSAIDs), analgesics and some antihypertensives, can cause nausea, vomiting, diarrhoea, constipation and other GI signs and symptoms. Be sure to ask about laxative use because habitual intake can cause constipation.

Family history can be important because some GI disorders are hereditary.

Family history

Because some GI disorders are hereditary, ask the patient whether anyone in their family has had a GI disorder. Disorders with a familial link include:
- ulcerative colitis
- colon cancer
- stomach ulcers
- diabetes
- alcoholism
- Crohn's disease.

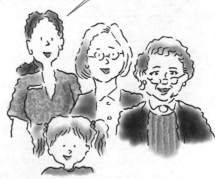

Asking the right questions

When assessing a patient with GI-related signs and symptoms, be sure to ask the right questions. To establish a baseline for comparison, ask about the patient's current state of health, including questions about the onset, duration, quality, severity and location of problems as well as precipitating factors, alleviating factors and associated symptoms.

Onset

How did the problem start? Was it gradual or sudden and with or without previous symptoms? What was the patient doing when they noticed it? If they have diarrhoea, had they been travelling? If so, when and where?

Duration

When did the problem start? Did the patient have the problem before? Did they have any abdominal surgery? If yes, when? If they're in pain, find out when the problem began. Is the pain continuous, intermittent or colicky (cramplike)?

Quality

Ask the patient to describe the problem. Did they ever have it before? Was it diagnosed? If they're in pain, find out whether the pain feels sharp, dull, aching or burning.

Severity

Ask the patient to describe how badly the problem bothers them—for example, have them rate it on a pain scale of 0–10. Does it keep them from their normal activities? Has it improved or worsened since they first noticed it? Does it wake them at night? If they're in pain, do they double over from it?

Location

Where does the patient feel the problem? Does it spread, radiate or shift? Ask them to point to where they feel it the most.

Precipitating factors

Does anything seem to bring on the problem? What makes it worse? Does it occur at the same time each day or with certain positions? Does the patient notice it after eating or drinking certain foods or after certain activities?

Alleviating factors

Does anything relieve the problem? Does the patient take any prescribed or over-the-counter medications for relief? Have they tried anything else for relief?

Associated symptoms

What else bothers the patient when they have the problem? Have they had nausea, vomiting, diarrhoea, constipation, bloating or flatulence? Have they lost their appetite or lost or gained any weight? If so, how much? When was the patient's last bowel movement? Was it unusual? Have they seen blood in their vomit or stool? Have their stool changed in size or colour or included mucus? Ask the patient whether they can eat normally and hold down foods and liquids. Also, ask about alcohol consumption.

Lifestyle patterns

Psychological and sociologic factors can profoundly affect health. To determine factors that may have contributed to your patient's problem, ask about their occupation, home life, financial situation, stress level and recent life changes.

Be sure to ask about alcohol, illegal drug, caffeine and tobacco use as well as food consumption, exercise habits and oral hygiene. Also ask about sleep patterns, such as hours of sleep and whether sleep is restful.

Cultural factors may affect a patient's dietary habits, so ask about any dietary restrictions the patient has such as following a vegetarian diet.

Clinical assessment and monitoring

Clinical assessment of the GI system usually includes evaluation of the mouth, abdomen, liver and rectum. Before beginning your examination, explain the techniques you'll be using and warn the patient that some procedures might be uncomfortable. Perform the examination in a private, quiet, warm and well-lighted room.

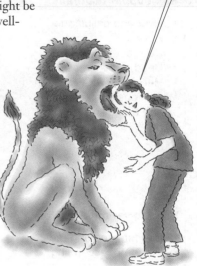

You should inspect and palpate your patient's mouth, as part of your physical examination.

Assessing the mouth

Use inspection and palpation to assess the oral cavity:
- Inspect the patient's mouth for obvious abnormality.
- Examine the tongue and mucous membranes for signs of dehydration, infection, thrush and ulceration.
- Note unusual breath odours.

Assessing the abdomen

When assessing the abdomen, observe for distension, discolouration and scars or stomas. Listen for the presence of bowel sounds. Assess painful areas last to avoid the patient becoming tense. An aid to inspecting the abdomen is to mentally divide it into four quadrants. (See *Identifying abdominal landmarks*, page 384.)

General inspection

Begin by performing a general inspection of the patient:
- Observe the skin, oral mucosa, nail beds and sclera for jaundice or signs of anaemia.
- Stand at the foot of the bed and observe the abdomen for symmetry, checking for bumps, bulges or masses. A bulge may indicate bladder distention or hernia.
- Note the patient's abdominal shape and contour. The abdomen should be flat to rounded in people of average weight. A protruding abdomen may be caused by obesity, pregnancy, ascites or abdominal distention.
A slender person may have a slightly concave abdomen.
- Next, inspect the abdominal skin, which normally appears smooth and intact. Striae, or stretch marks, can be caused by pregnancy, excessive weight gain or ascites. New striae are pink or blue; old striae are silvery white. In patients with darker skin, striae may be dark brown. Note dilated veins. Record the presence of any surgical scars on the abdomen.
- Note abdominal movements and pulsations. Usually, waves of peristalsis aren't visible unless the patient is very thin, in which case they may be visible as slight wavelike motions. Marked visible rippling may indicate bowel obstruction; report it immediately. In a thin patient,

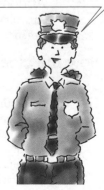

Keep in mind that obesity, pregnancy, ascites or abdominal distention can make the patient's abdomen protrude.

Identifying abdominal landmarks

To aid accurate abdominal assessment and documentation of findings, you can mentally divide the patient's abdomen into regions. Use the quadrant method—the easiest and most commonly used method—to divide the abdomen into four equal regions using two imaginary perpendicular lines crossing above the umbilicus.

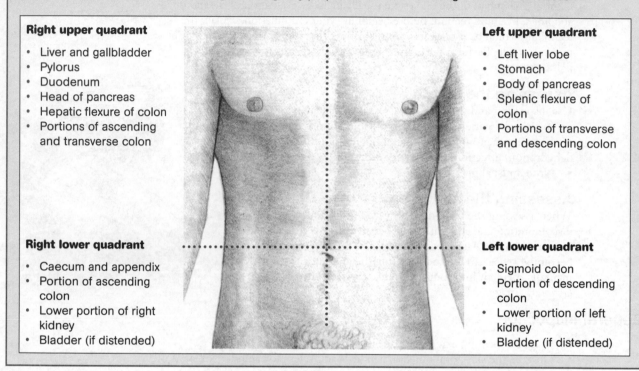

Right upper quadrant

- Liver and gallbladder
- Pylorus
- Duodenum
- Head of pancreas
- Hepatic flexure of colon
- Portions of ascending and transverse colon

Left upper quadrant

- Left liver lobe
- Stomach
- Body of pancreas
- Splenic flexure of colon
- Portions of transverse and descending colon

Right lower quadrant

- Caecum and appendix
- Portion of ascending colon
- Lower portion of right kidney
- Bladder (if distended)

Left lower quadrant

- Sigmoid colon
- Portion of descending colon
- Lower portion of left kidney
- Bladder (if distended)

pulsation of the aorta is visible in the epigastric area. Marked pulsations may occur with hypertension, aortic insufficiency and other conditions causing widening pulse pressure.

Abdominal auscultation

Auscultation provides information about bowel motility and the underlying organs.

Follow the clock

Use a stethoscope to auscultate for bowel and vascular sounds. Lightly place the stethoscope diaphragm in the right lower quadrant, slightly below and to the right of the umbilicus. Auscultate in a clockwise fashion in each of the four quadrants, spending at least 2 minutes in each area. Note the character and quality of bowel sounds in each quadrant. In some cases, you may need to auscultate for 5 minutes before you hear sounds. Be sure to allow enough time to listen in each quadrant before you decide that bowel sounds are absent.

Tube tip

Before auscultating the abdomen of a patient with a nasogastric (NG) tube or another abdominal tube connected to suction, briefly clamp the tube or turn off the suction. Suction noises can obscure or mimic actual bowel sounds.

Sound class

Bowel sounds are classified as normal, hypoactive or hyperactive:
• Normal bowel sounds are high-pitched, gurgling noises caused by air mixing with fluid during peristalsis. The noises vary in frequency, pitch and intensity and occur irregularly from 5 to 34 times per minute. They're loudest before mealtimes. Borborygmus, or stomach growling, is the loud, gurgling, splashing sound heard over the large intestine as gas passes through it.
• Hypoactive bowel sounds are associated with ileus, bowel obstruction or peritonitis and indicate diminished peristalsis. Paralytic ileus, torsion of the bowel or the use of narcotics and other medications can decrease peristalsis.
• Hyperactive bowel sounds are loud, high-pitched, tinkling sounds that occur frequently and may be caused by diarrhoea, constipation or laxative use.

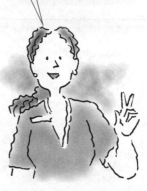

Auscultate for at least 2 minutes in each of the four abdominal quadrants.

Abdominal palpation

Abdominal palpation includes light and deep touch to determine the size, shape, position and tenderness of major abdominal organs and to detect masses and fluid accumulation. Palpate all four quadrants, leaving painful and tender areas for last.

Use light palpation to identify muscle resistance and tenderness. Deep palpation may evoke rebound tenderness when you suddenly withdraw your fingertips, a possible sign of peritoneal inflammation. (See *Eliciting abdominal pain*, page 386.)

Assessing the liver

The doctor can estimate the size and position of the liver through percussion and palpation.

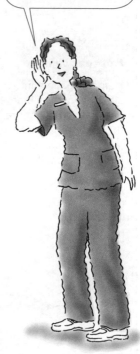

Listen for normal, hypoactive or hyperactive bowel sounds.

Interpreting abnormal abdominal sounds

Sound and description	Location	Possible cause
Abnormal bowel sounds		
Hyperactive sounds (unrelated to hunger)	Any quadrant	Diarrhoea, laxative use or early intestinal obstruction
Hypoactive, then absent sounds	Any quadrant	Paralytic ileus or peritonitis
High-pitched tinkling sounds	Any quadrant	Intestinal fluid and air under tension in a dilated bowel
High-pitched rushing sounds coinciding with abdominal cramps	Any quadrant	Intestinal obstruction

Eliciting abdominal pain

Rebound tenderness and the iliopsoas and obturator signs can indicate such conditions as appendicitis and peritonitis. You can elicit these signs of abdominal pain, as illustrated below.

Rebound tenderness

Help the patient into a supine position with their knees flexed to relax the abdominal muscles. Place your hands gently on the right lower quadrant. Slowly and deeply dip your fingers into the area, then release the pressure in a quick, smooth motion. Pain on release—rebound tenderness—is a positive sign. The pain may radiate to the umbilicus.

Caution: To minimise the risk of rupturing an inflamed appendix, don't repeat this manoeuvre.

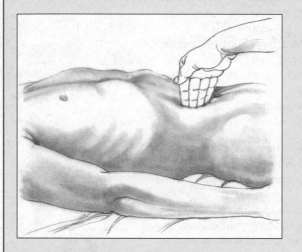

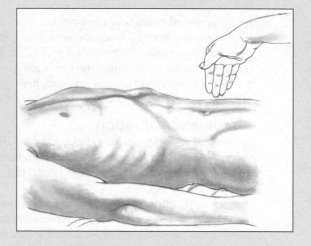

Iliopsoas sign

Help the patient into a supine position with their legs straight. Instruct them to raise their right leg upwards as you exert slight pressure with your hand. Repeat the manoeuvre with the left leg. When testing either leg, increased abdominal pain is a positive result, indicating irritation of the psoas muscle.

Obturator sign

Help the patient into a supine position with their right leg flexed 90 degrees at the hip and knee. Hold the leg just above the knee and at the ankle, then rotate the leg laterally and medially. Pain in the hypogastric region is a positive sign, indicating irritation of the obturator muscle.

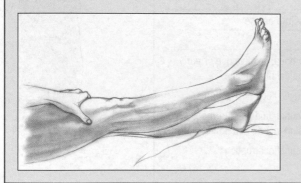

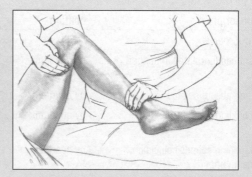

Percussing the liver allows you to estimate its size. Hepatomegaly is commonly associated with hepatitis and other liver disease. It's usually impossible to palpate the liver in an adult patient. If palpable, the liver border feels smooth and firm, with a rounded, regular edge. A palpable liver may indicate hepatomegaly.

Assessing the rectum

In any complaints of constipation, a rectal examination should be part of your GI assessment. Explain the procedure to reassure the patient.

Perianal is primary

To perform a rectal examination, first inspect the perianal area following these steps:
• Put on gloves and spread the buttocks to expose the anus and surrounding tissue, checking for fissures, lesions, scars, inflammation, discharge, rectal prolapse and external haemorrhoids.
• Ask the patient to strain as if they're having a bowel movement; this may reveal internal haemorrhoids, polyps or fissures.

Rectum is next

After examining the perianal area, palpate the rectum:
• Apply a water-soluble lubricant to your gloved index finger. Tell the patient to relax and explain to them that they'll feel some pressure.
• Insert your finger into the rectum towards the umbilicus. To palpate, rotate your finger. The walls should feel soft and smooth without masses, faecal impaction or tenderness.
• Remove your finger from the rectum and inspect the glove for stool, blood or mucus. Test faecal material adhering to the glove for occult blood.

Monitoring

Essential monitoring for critically ill patients with GI disorders as well as standard observations should include fluid balance, oral/NG intake, nausea and vomiting, bowel motion recording, drain and stoma output and pain scores.

Diagnostic tests and investigations

Many tests provide information used to guide your care of the patient with a GI problem. Even if you don't participate in testing, you should know why the test was ordered, what the results mean and what your responsibilities are before, during and after the test.

Diagnostic tests commonly ordered for patients with known or suspected GI disorders include endoscopy, laboratory tests, nuclear imaging scans and radiographic tests.

Endoscopy

The doctor can directly view hollow visceral linings by using a fibre optic endoscope. This test is used to diagnose inflammatory, ulcerative and infectious diseases; benign and malignant neoplasms; and other oesophageal, gastric and intestinal mucosal lesions. Endoscopy can also be used for therapeutic interventions or to obtain a biopsy.

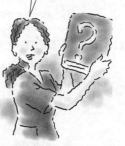

Know why a test was requested, what the results mean and what your responsibilities are before, during and after testing.

Bedside or not

The endoscopic procedure is commonly done at the bedside in the critical care unit. However, if it's performed in the procedure suite, you may accompany an unstable patient who requires monitoring.

Colonoscopy

Colonoscopy, also referred to as lower GI endoscopy, is used to:
- diagnose inflammatory and ulcerative bowel disease
- pinpoint lower GI bleeding
- detect lower GI abnormalities, such as tumours, polyps, haemorrhoids and abscesses.

Nursing considerations
- Explain the procedure and its purpose, and tell the patient they'll receive I.V. premedication and conscious sedation for the procedure.
- Make sure that an informed consent form has been signed.
- Withhold all fluids and food for at least 6–8 hours before the test.
- Administer bowel preparation, as ordered, such as a clear liquid diet and bowel cleaning solution with electrolyte lavage. If the patient can't swallow or is unconscious, administer electrolyte lavage solution through a feeding tube or an NG tube.
- To decrease the risk of aspiration in a patient receiving electrolyte lavage solution through an NG tube, ensure proper tube placement and elevate the head of the bed or position the patient on their side. Have suction equipment available. (See *Increased risk in elderly patients*).
- Advise the patient that they may feel the urge to defecate when the scope is inserted; encourage slow, deep breathing through the mouth, as appropriate.
- If the procedure is to be performed at the bedside, have necessary equipment for the procedure available, including emergency equipment and suction.
- Initiate an I.V. line if one isn't already in place for a patient who'll be receiving sedation.
- Obtain the patient's baseline vital signs and oxygen saturation levels. Monitor cardiac rhythm.
- Administer medications, as ordered, such as midazolam for sedation. Provide supplemental oxygen, as ordered.
- During the procedure, monitor the patient's vital signs, airway patency, oxygen saturation, cardiac rhythm, skin colour, abdominal distention, level of consciousness (LOC) and pain tolerance.

Senior moment

Increased risk in elderly patients

Elderly patients are at increased risk for experiencing adverse effects from gastric lavage, including nausea, vomiting, abdominal cramps, abdominal fullness, dizziness and fluid and electrolyte imbalances. What's more, elderly patients may have difficulty ingesting the required amount of solution because of these adverse effects.

Assess, administer, document

After colonoscopy

- Assess your patient's vital signs and cardiopulmonary status, breath sounds, oxygen saturation and LOC every 15 minutes for the first hour, every 30 minutes for the next hour and then hourly until the patient stabilises.
- Administer supplemental oxygen, as ordered and as indicated by oxygen saturation levels.
- Watch for adverse effects of sedation, such as respiratory depression, apnoea, hypotension, excessive diaphoresis, bradycardia and laryngospasm. Notify the doctor if any occur.
- Assess the patient's stool for evidence of frank or occult bleeding.
- Monitor the patient for signs and symptoms of perforation, such as vomiting, severe abdominal pain, abdominal distention or rigidity and fever. Notify the doctor if any occur.
- Document the procedure, interventions and assessment findings.

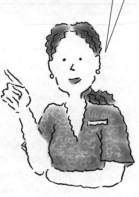

Remember good bowel prep is important to ensure successful colonoscopy.

OGD

Oesophagogastroduodenoscopy (OGD), also called *upper GI endoscopy*, is used to identify abnormalities of the oesophagus, stomach and small intestine, such as oesophagitis, inflammatory bowel disease, Mallory–Weiss syndrome, lesions, tumours, gastritis and polyps.

Bypass the surgery

OGD eliminates the need for extensive exploratory surgery and can be used to detect small or surface lesions missed by radiography. It can also be used for sclerotherapy or to remove foreign bodies by suction (for small, soft objects) or electrocautery, snare, or forceps (for large, hard objects).

Nursing considerations

Before endoscopy

- Explain the procedure and its purpose to the patient.
- Tell them the procedure takes about 30 minutes and that they'll receive I.V. premedication and sedation during the procedure as required as well as a local anaesthetic spray in their mouth and nose.
- Restrict food and fluids for at least 6 hours before the test.
- Make sure that an informed consent form has been signed.
- If the test is an emergency procedure, expect to insert an NG tube to aspirate contents and minimise the risk of aspiration.
- Make sure that the patient's dentures and eyeglasses are removed before the test.
- If the procedure is to be performed at the bedside, have the necessary equipment available for the procedure, including suction and emergency equipment (medications such as atropine, a monitor defibrillator and ET intubation equipment) and insertion of an I.V. line if one isn't already in place.

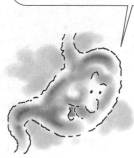

OGD is A-OK! It can even eliminate the need for extensive exploratory surgery.

• Monitor the patient before and throughout the procedure, including airway patency, vital signs, oxygen saturation, cardiac rhythm, abdominal distention, LOC and pain tolerance.

After it's over

After endoscopy
• Monitor your patient's vital signs, oxygen saturation, cardiac rhythm and LOC every 15 minutes for the first hour, every 30 minutes for the next hour and then hourly until the patient stabilises.
• Administer oxygen therapy, as ordered.
• Place the patient in a side-lying position with the head of the bed flat until sedation wears off.
• Withhold all food and fluids until your patient's gag reflex returns. After it returns, offer ice chips and sips of water, gradually increasing the patient's intake as tolerated and allowed.
• Observe for adverse effects of sedation, such as respiratory depression, apnoea, hypotension, excessive diaphoresis, bradycardia and laryngospasm. Notify the doctor if any occur.
• Monitor the patient for signs and symptoms of perforation, such as difficulty swallowing, pain, fever or bleeding as evidenced by black stools or bloody vomitus.
• Document the procedure, interventions and assessment findings.

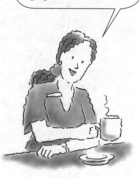

After endoscopy, withhold all food and fluids until your patient's gag reflex returns.

Laboratory tests

Common laboratory tests used to diagnose GI disorders include studies of stool and peritoneal contents. Percutaneous liver biopsy may also be done.

Faecal studies

Normal stool appears brown and formed but soft. These abnormal findings may indicate a problem:
• Narrow, ribbonlike stool signals spastic or irritable bowel, partial bowel obstruction or rectal obstruction.
• Constipation may be caused by diet or medications.
• Diarrhoea may indicate spastic bowel or viral infection.
• Mixed with blood and mucus, soft stool can signal bacterial infection; mixed with blood or pus, colitis.
• Yellow or green stool suggests severe, prolonged diarrhoea; black stool suggests GI bleeding or intake of iron supplements or raw-to-rare meat. Tan or white stool shows hepatic duct or gallbladder-duct blockage, hepatitis or cancer. Red stool may signal colon or rectal bleeding; however, drugs and foods can also cause this coloration.
• Most stool contains 10–20% fat. A higher fat content can turn stool pasty or greasy, a possible sign of intestinal malabsorption or pancreatic disease.

Nursing considerations
- Collect the stool specimen in a clean, dry container and immediately send it to the laboratory.
- Don't use stool that has been in contact with toilet-bowl water or urine.
- Use commercial faecal occult blood slides as a simple method of testing for blood in stool.
- Remember certain medications and foods can interfere with test results.

Peritoneal fluid analysis

Peritoneal fluid analysis includes examination of gross appearance, erythrocyte and leucocyte counts, cytologic studies, microbiological studies for bacteria and fungi and determinations of protein, glucose, amylase, ammonia and alkaline phosphatase levels.

Peritoneal through paracentesis

Abdominal paracentesis is a bedside procedure involving aspiration of fluid from the peritoneal space through a needle, trocar or cannula inserted in the abdominal wall.

Paracentesis is used to:
- diagnose and treat massive ascites resistant to other therapy
- detect intra-abdominal bleeding after traumatic injury
- obtain a peritoneal fluid sample for laboratory analysis
- decrease intra-abdominal pressure and alleviate dyspnoea.

> Aspiration of peritoneal fluid can be done at the bedside.

Nursing considerations
- Explain the procedure to the patient and obtain consent if required.
- Empty the bladder. Usually, an indwelling urinary catheter is inserted.
- Record the patient's baseline vital signs, weight, intra-abdominal pressure and abdominal girth. Indicate the abdominal area measured with a felt-tipped marking pen.
- Insert the trocar with the patient supine. After insertion, assist the patient to sit up in bed. (See *Positioning for abdominal paracentesis*, page 392.)
- Remind the patient to remain as still as possible during the procedure.
- During the procedure, monitor the patient's vital signs, oxygen saturation and cardiac rhythm every 15 minutes and observe for tachycardia, hypotension, dizziness, pallor, diaphoresis and increased anxiety, especially if more than 1,500 ml of peritoneal fluid is aspirated at one time.
- If the patient shows signs of hypovolaemic shock, slow the drainage rate by raising the collection container vertically so it's closer to the height of the needle, trocar or cannula. Stop the drainage if necessary. Limit aspirated fluid to between 1,500 and 2,000 ml.
- After the doctor removes the needle, trocar or cannula and, if necessary, sutures the incision, apply a dry sterile pressure dressing.

Positioning for abdominal paracentesis

When positioning a patient for abdominal paracentesis, help them sit up in bed or allow them to sit on the edge of the bed with additional support for their back and arms. In sedated patients elevate to 45 degrees head up.

In this position, gravity causes fluid to accumulate in the lower abdominal cavity. The internal organs provide counterresistance and pressure to aid fluid flow.

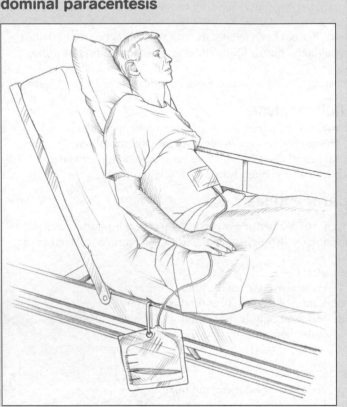

After it's over

After the procedure
• Monitor the patient's vital signs, oxygen saturation and cardiac rhythm, and check the dressing for drainage every 15 minutes for the first hour, every 30 minutes for the next 2 hours, every hour for 4 hours and then every 4 hours for 24 hours.
• Observe the patient for signs of haemorrhage or shock, such as hypotension, tachycardia, pallor and excessive diaphoresis. These signs may indicate puncture of the inferior epigastric artery, haematoma of the anterior caecal wall or rupture of the iliac vein or bladder. Observe for haematuria.
• Observe the patient for signs of a perforated intestine, such as increasing pain or abdominal tenderness.
• Document the procedure, and record the patient's daily weight, intra-abdominal pressure and abdominal girth to detect recurrent ascites.

Abdominal paracentesis is a bedside procedure that's used to aspirate fluid from the peritoneal space.

Nuclear imaging

Magnetic resonance imaging

Magnetic resonance imaging (MRI) is used to examine the liver and abdominal organs. It's useful in evaluating liver disease by characterising tumours, masses or cysts found on previous studies. An image is generated by energising protons in a strong magnetic field. Radio waves emitted as protons return to their former equilibrium and are recorded. No ionising radiation is transmitted during the scan.

MRI mire

Disadvantages of MRI include the closed tubelike space required for the scan. Newer MRI centres offer a less confining 'open-MRI' scan. In addition, the test can't be performed on patients with implanted metal prostheses or devices, and the monitoring, I.V. pumps and ventilators for critically ill patients must be MRI compatible.

Nursing considerations

- Explain the procedure to the patient and the need to remove metal objects before the procedure.
- Prepare for the scan lasting at least 1 hour.
- Generally, you'll have to accompany the patient to the MRI suite and will have to liase with staff regarding equipment.

Stress the need to remove metal objects before MRI scanning.

Radiographic tests

Radiographic tests include abdominal x-rays, various contrast media studies and CT scans.

Abdominal x-rays

An abdominal x-ray or *kidney–ureter–bladder radiography* is used to detect and evaluate tumours, kidney stones, abnormal gas collection and other abdominal disorders.

Reading the rays

On x-ray, air appears black, fat appears grey and bone appears white. Although a routine x-ray doesn't reveal most abdominal organs, it does show the contrast between air and fluid. For example, intestinal blockage traps large amounts of detectable fluids and air inside organs. When an intestinal wall tears, air leaks into the abdomen and becomes visible on x-ray.

Nursing considerations

- Explain the procedure to the patient. Radiography requires no special pre- or post-test care. It's usually done at the bedside using portable x-ray equipment.

CT scan

In CT scanning, a computer translates multiple x-ray beams into three-dimensional oscilloscope images of the patient's biliary tract, liver and pancreas.

Scores of scans

CT scanning is used to:
- distinguish between obstructive and nonobstructive jaundice
- identify abscesses, cysts, haematomas, tumours and pseudocysts
- evaluate the cause of weight loss and look for occult malignancy
- diagnose and evaluate pancreatitis.

The test can be done with or without a contrast medium, but contrast is preferred unless the patient is allergic to contrast media.

Nursing considerations

- Explain the procedure to the patient and tell them that they should lie still, relax and breathe normally during the test. Explain that if the doctor orders an I.V. contrast medium, they may experience discomfort from the needle puncture and a localised feeling of warmth on injection.
- Restrict food and fluids after midnight before the test, but continue any drug regimen as ordered.
- Confirm if the patient has an allergy to iodine or shellfish. Report immediately any adverse reactions, such as nausea, vomiting, dizziness, headache and urticaria.
- If the patient has nil-by-mouth status, increase the I.V. fluid rate as ordered after the procedure to flush the contrast medium from their system. Monitor creatinine and urea levels for signs of acute renal failure, which may be caused by the contrast medium. Patients with impaired renal function may be prescribed an I.V. acetylcysteine regime pre- and postcontrast to reduce nephrotoxic effects.

Ultrasound scans

An ultrasound scan provides basic imaging of many intra-abdominal structures. These scans are non-invasive with no potential side effects and can easily be performed at the bedside.

Abdominal ultrasound

An abdominal ultrasound scan may be used to detect kidney stones, gall stones, thickened gall bladder, pancreatic inflammation, abnormal gas collections and other abdominal disorders as well as stages of pregnancy. Procedures like drain insertion or fluid aspiration can be performed under ultrasound guidance.

Sounding it out

Although an abdominal ultrasound does not provide such detail as a CT scan it can be a useful starting point in diagnosis. Indeed many critical care doctors may be able to perform preliminary ultrasound scans using scanning equipment available on the units for guiding central line insertion.

Nursing considerations

Explain the procedure to the patient. Assist the patient into a suitable position as guided by the sonographer. Views are improved in dim lighting. It requires no special pre- or post-test care. It's usually done at the bedside using portable equipment.

Intra-abdominal pressure monitoring

Why do it?

If patients have extreme abdominal distension there may be intra-abdominal hypertension which means there is a high risk of them developing intra-abdominal compartment syndrome (IACS). This means that the abdominal contents become so compressed circulation is compromised and the bowel and internal organs become ischaemic. The only treatment for severe IACS is decompressive laparotomy. Abdominal girth measurements will allow you to recognise whether distension is increasing, but intra-abdominal pressure monitoring will give you a number equating to the pressure inside the abdominal cavity.

How to do it?

It is usually performed indirectly via a urinary catheter or occasionally directly via a peritoneal catheter. For more information on when and how to do it and what the measurements mean see 'Intra-abdominal hypertension' in the 'GI disorders' section (page 426).

Treatments

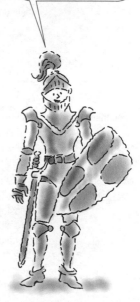

Treatment measures for GI disorders may include drug therapy, surgery, intubation and nutritional support.

GI dysfunctions present many treatment challenges because they stem from various mechanisms occurring separately or simultaneously, including tumours, hyperactivity and hypoactivity in the bowel, malabsorption, infection and inflammation, vascular disorders, intestinal obstruction and degenerative disease. Treatment options include drug therapy, surgery, GI intubation and nutritional support.

Drug therapy

Drug therapy may be used for such disorders as acute GI bleeding, peptic ulcer disease and hepatic failure. Some of the most commonly used drugs in critical care include anti-emetics, histamine-2 (H_2) receptor antagonists, proton pump inhibitors and ammonia detoxicants.

How fast?

Some of these drugs, such as anti-emetics, provide relief immediately. Other drugs, such as H_2-receptor antagonists, may take several days or longer to alleviate the problem. (See *Common GI drugs*.)

Common GI drugs

Drugs	Indications	Adverse reactions	Practice pointers
Ammonia detoxicant			
Lactulose	• To prevent and treat portosystemic encephalopathy in patients with severe hepatic disease (increasing clearance of nitrogenous products and decreasing serum ammonia levels through laxative effects) • Laxative to treat constipation	Abdominal cramps, diarrhoea, flatulence	• After administration through a nasogastric (NG) tube, flush tube with water. • Monitor patient's serum ammonia levels. • Neomycin and other antibiotics may decrease effectiveness. • Aim for three to four soft stools per day.
Antidiuretic hormone			
Vasopressin	• Injection administered I.V. or intra-arterially into the superior mesenteric artery used as treatment in acute, massive GI haemorrhage (such as peptic ulcer disease, ruptured oesophageal varices and Mallory–Weiss syndrome)	Angina, cardiac arrhythmias (bradycardia, heart block), cardiac arrest, water intoxication, seizures, bronchospasms, coronary thrombosis, possibly mesenteric and small bowel infarction with mesenteric artery intra-arterial infusion	• Intra-arterial injection into superior mesenteric artery requires angiographic catheter placement. • Monitor intake and output closely. • Monitor for water intoxication (drowsiness, headache, confusion, anuria). • Monitor cardiac rhythm. • Use cautiously in patients with coronary artery disease, heart failure, renal disease, asthma or a seizure disorder. • Use is contraindicated in patients with chronic nephritis. • Use cautiously in elderly, preoperative or postoperative patients.
Antiemetics			
Ondansetron	• Prevention and treatment of postoperative nausea and vomiting and in conjunction with cancer chemotherapy.	Diarrhoea, arrhythmias, electrocardiogram changes (prolonged PR and QT intervals and widened QRS complex), liver test abnormalities, pruritus	• Monitor cardiac rhythm. • Use cautiously in patients with prolonged QT intervals or with congenital QT syndrome. • Monitor liver function.
Metoclopramide	• Prevention and treatment of postoperative nausea and vomiting and in conjunction with cancer chemotherapy • Delayed gastric emptying secondary to diabetic gastroparesis	Restlessness, anxiety, depression, suicidal ideas, seizures, bradycardia, bronchospasm, transient hypertension	• Use cautiously in patients with GI haemorrhage or mechanical obstruction and patients with phaeochromocytoma seizures, depression or hypertension. • Monitor for onset of extrapyramidal symptoms.

(continued)

Common GI drugs (continued)

Drugs	Indications	Adverse reactions	Practice pointers
Histamine-2 receptor antagonists			
Ranitidine	• Treatment of duodenal and gastric ulcers, gastro-oesophageal reflux disease • Prevention of gastric stress ulcers • Prophylaxis for gastric stress ulcer (in very high risk critically ill patients)	Malaise, reversible confusion, depression or hallucinations, blurred vision, jaundice, leukopenia, angioedema	• Antacids decrease ranitidine absorption; give 1 hour apart. • Use cautiously in patients with renal disease. • Monitor renal and liver tests.
Proton pump inhibitors			
Lansoprazole	• Treatment of duodenal and gastric ulcers, erosive oesophagitis, gastro-oesophageal reflux disease and *Helicobacter pylori* eradication	Diarrhoea, abdominal pain, nausea, constipation, chest pain, dizziness, hyperglycaemia	• Use cautiously in patients with severe liver disease.
Omeprazole	• Prophylaxis for gastric stress ulcer (in critically ill patients)		• Monitor liver function values and blood glucose.
Pantoprazole			

Surgery

Surgery may be used to treat the patient with massive bleeding who hasn't responded to medical treatments (such as gastric lavage or sclerotherapy via endoscopy), also to remove tumours and ischaemic bowel and to repair perforated or infected sections of the GI tract. Be ready to provide special postoperative support for your patient after GI surgery because they may have to make permanent and difficult lifestyle changes. Some of the surgical procedures for GI disorders are liver transplantation and bowel resection +/− stoma formation. There are a large number of other surgical procedures affecting the GI tract (for example, gastrectomy, oesophagogastrectomy, hernia repair and cholecystectomy); all these cannot be detailed, but the principles of patient management can be adapted from these as detailed below.

Liver transplantation

For a patient with a life-threatening liver disorder who doesn't respond to other treatments, a liver transplant may be the best hope. Candidates include patients with:

- congenital biliary abnormalities
- chronic hepatitis
- inborn errors of metabolism
- end-stage liver disease (primary biliary cirrhosis, excess alcohol, paracetamol overdose).

Who's the candidate?

Criteria for referring a patient for transplantation include:
- a patient with advanced hepatic failure with expected survival time less than 2 years
- the unavailability of other medical or surgical therapies that offer long-term survival
- the absence of contraindicated conditions, such as cardiopulmonary disease, metastatic disease, acquired immunodeficiency syndrome and active alcohol or drug addiction
- the patient and family members who understand all aspects of the transplant process.

Nursing considerations

When caring for a patient undergoing a liver transplantation, concentrate on preparing the patient and their family physically and emotionally for the procedure, including instructing the patient about the procedure and events after. Also, take steps to prevent postoperative complications. (See *Managing liver transplantation complications*, page 399.)

Before it begins

Before transplantation

- Instruct the patient and their family about the transplant, necessary diagnostic tests, immunosuppressant medications and rejection risk.
- Review information about the equipment and procedures, such as cardiac monitoring, endotracheal tube, NG tube, indwelling urinary catheter and arterial lines. Reassure the patient that the equipment will be removed as soon as possible.
- Administer prescribed medications such as immunosuppressant agents.
- Make sure that an informed consent form has been signed.

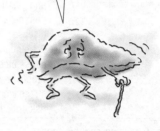

A liver transplant may be the last and best hope for a patient with a life-threatening liver disorder.

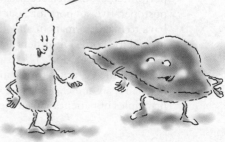

Teach the patient and their family all about the transplant process, testing, drugs and risks.

Managing liver transplantation complications

Check this table to find possible complications of liver transplantation and assessment and nursing interventions for each complication.

Complication	Assessment and intervention
Haemorrhage and hypovolaemic shock	• Assess the patient's vital signs and other indicators of fluid volume hourly and note trends indicating hypovolaemia; hypotension; weak, rapid, irregular pulse; oliguria; decreased level of consciousness; and signs of peripheral vasoconstriction. • Monitor the patient's haematocrit and haemoglobin levels daily. • Maintain patency of all I.V. lines, and reserve 2 units of blood in case the patient needs a transfusion.
Vascular obstruction	• Be alert for signs and symptoms of acute vascular obstruction in the right upper quadrant—cramping pain or tenderness, nausea and vomiting. Notify the doctor immediately if any occur. • As ordered, prepare for emergency thrombelectomy. Maintain I.V. infusions, check and document the patient's vital signs and maintain airway patency.
Wound infection or abscess	• Assess the incision site daily, and report any inflammation, tenderness, drainage or other signs and symptoms of infection. • Change the dressing daily or as needed. • Note and report any signs or symptoms of peritonitis or abscess, including fever, chills, leukocytosis (or leukopenia with bands) and abdominal pain, tenderness and rigidity. • Take the patient's temperature every 4 hours. • Collect abdominal drainage for culture and sensitivity studies. Document the colour, amount, odour and consistency of drainage. • Assess the patient for signs of infection in other areas, such as the urinary tract, respiratory system and skin. Document and report any signs of infection.
Pulmonary insufficiency or failure	• Maintain ventilation at prescribed levels. • Monitor the patient's arterial blood gas levels daily, and change ventilator settings, as ordered. • Auscultate for abnormal breath sounds every 2–4 hours. • Suction the patient, as needed.
Effects of immunosuppressant therapy	• Note any signs or symptoms of opportunistic infection, including fever, tachycardia, chills, leucocytosis, leucopenia and diaphoresis. • Maintain reverse isolation. • Report adverse reactions to drugs. • Check the patient's weight regularly.
Hepatic failure	• Monitor nasogastric tube drainage for upper GI bleeding. • Frequently assess the patient's neurovascular status. • Note development of peripheral oedema and ascites. • Monitor the patient's renal function by checking urine output, blood urea, creatinine and potassium levels. • Monitor serum amylase levels daily.

- Instruct family members in measures to control infection and minimise rejection after transplantation and advise them to have all their immunisations up-to-date.
- Provide emotional support to the patient and their family.

After it's over

After liver transplantation

- Assess the patient's cardiopulmonary and haemodynamic status, including vital signs, oxygen saturation and cardiac rhythm as indicated by their condition.
- Monitor the patient's temperature frequently for fever and signs of infection. (See *What does fever mean?*)
- Monitor laboratory tests, especially liver enzymes, bilirubin, electrolytes, coagulation screen and FBC.
- Assess insertion sites for indications of bleeding. If the patient has an NG tube, assess drainage colour at least every 2 hours.
- Institute strict infection control precautions.
- Administer prophylactic antibiotics and postoperative drugs, such as corticosteroids and immunosuppressants, as ordered.
- Assist with extubation as soon as possible and administer supplemental oxygen as needed. Encourage coughing, deep breathing and incentive spirometry.
- Monitor the patient's intake and output at least hourly, and notify the doctor if output is less than 30 ml/hour. Maintain fluids at 2,000–3,000 ml/ day, or as ordered, to prevent fluid overload.
- Maintain the patient on nil-by-mouth status with NG drainage until bowel sounds return.
- Change the patient's position at least every 2 hours, getting them out of bed and to the chair within 24 hours if their condition is stable.
- Continually assess the patient for signs and symptoms of acute rejection, such as malaise, fever, graft enlargement and diminished graft function (typically 7–14 days after the transplant).
- To ease emotional stress, plan care to allow rest and provide as much privacy as possible. Allow family members to visit and comfort the patient as much as possible.
- Teach the patient about danger signs and symptoms and the need to report these immediately.

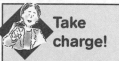

Stick with it. Continually assess the patient for signs and symptoms of acute rejection.

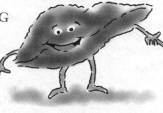

Take charge!

What does fever mean?

A sudden onset of high fever and an increase in liver enzymes suggest hepatic artery thrombosis. If your patient exhibits a fever and infection is suspected, be ready to obtain cultures of all body fluids, x-rays of the chest and abdomen and a Doppler ultrasound of the hepatic vessels.

Bowel resection with or without stoma formation

This procedure may be performed as elective or emergency surgery. It varies in name according to the section of bowel that has been removed. Candidates include patients with:

- cancer of the bowel
- chronic inflammatory conditions (Crohn's disease, ulcerative colitis)

(*Text continues on page 401*)

Acute pancreatitis

Pancreatitis, inflammation of the pancreas, occurs in acute and chronic forms. Acute pancreatitis, a life-threatening emergency, may be either oedematous (interstitial) or necrotising:
• Oedematous pancreatitis, the more common type (75% of cases), results in fluid accumulation and swelling. Prognosis for patients with oedematous pancreatitis is fairly good (the disease is self-limiting and subsides within 1 week after treatment in about 85% of patients).
• Necrotising pancreatitis, which occurs in about 25% of pancreatitis cases, causes cell death and tissue damage. Mortality is higher in cases of necrotising pancreatitis due to cellular necrosis, extensive fat necrosis and haemorrhage within the pancreas. If infection occurs concomitantly, mortality may be as high as 60%.

How it happens

Normally, the acini in the pancreas secrete inactive enzymes. Inappropriate activation of these enzymes results in autodigestion of the pancreas and tissue necrosis, resulting in acute pancreatitis. The mechanism that triggers this activation is unknown; however, several conditions are associated with it. The most common include biliary tract obstruction by gallstones and alcohol abuse (alcohol increases stimulation of pancreatic secretions).

What to do

Acute pancreatitis requires meticulous supportive care and continuous monitoring of vital systems. Complications of untreated disease include massive haemorrhage, shock, pseudocyst, biliary and duodenal obstruction, portal vein thrombosis, diabetes mellitus and acute respiratory failure.

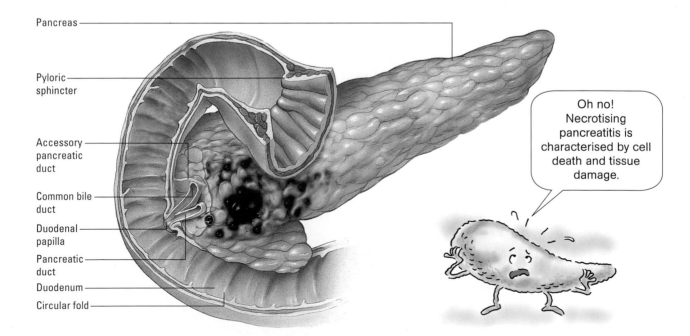

Pancreas

Pyloric sphincter

Accessory pancreatic duct

Common bile duct

Duodenal papilla

Pancreatic duct

Duodenum

Circular fold

Oh no! Necrotising pancreatitis is characterised by cell death and tissue damage.

Diabetes mellitus

Diabetes is a chronic disease that affects the way the body uses food to make the energy necessary for life. Primarily, diabetes is a disruption of carbohydrate (sugar and starch) metabolism that also affects fats and proteins. There are two main forms of diabetes (type 1 and type 2) as well as conditions of glucose intolerance, gestational diabetes and diabetes caused by pancreatic disorders. Regardless of the form, metabolic control under the care of a doctor is essential for good health.

What is insulin?

Insulin is an essential hormone that's produced in the pancreas and released into the bloodstream. Insulin attaches itself to cells at places called *insulin receptors*. When attached, insulin allows sugar or glucose from food to enter the body's liver, fat and muscle cells, where it's used for energy.

Type 1 diabetes mellitus

In type 1 diabetes, the pancreas makes little or no insulin. Without insulin, sugar can't enter cells to be used for energy. The body's tissues are starved and blood glucose levels grow dangerously high. The disorder usually begins in youth, but it may also occur in older adults. Type 1 diabetes occurs in 5–10% of patients with diabetes; these patients require insulin therapy for treatment.

Type 2 diabetes mellitus

In type 2 diabetes, the pancreas produces some insulin, but it's either too little or it isn't effective. In addition, insulin receptors that control the transport of sugar into cells may not work properly or are reduced in number. Type 2 diabetes typically develops in people older than age 40. Most newly diagnosed patients with type 2 diabetes are overweight but can control their diabetes through diet and weight loss. Some patients may require oral medications or insulin injections to achieve glucose control.

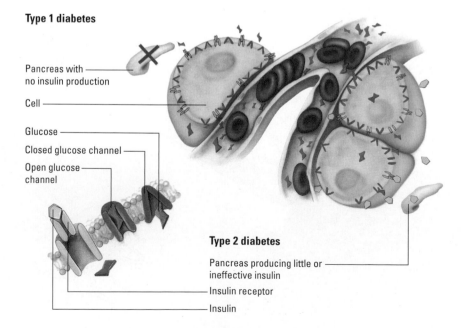

Type 1 diabetes

Pancreas with no insulin production

Cell

Glucose

Closed glucose channel

Open glucose channel

Type 2 diabetes

Pancreas producing little or ineffective insulin

Insulin receptor

Insulin

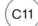

Long-term health problems

High plasma glucose levels caused by diabetes may damage small and large blood vessels and nerves. Diabetes may also reduce the body's ability to fight infection. As a result, people with diabetes are more likely to have serious eye problems, kidney disease, heart attacks, strokes, high blood pressure, poor circulation, tingling in hands and feet, sexual problems, amputations and infections. Good diabetes control may help prevent these problems or make them less serious.

Loss of vision

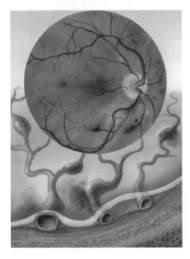

Nerve damage

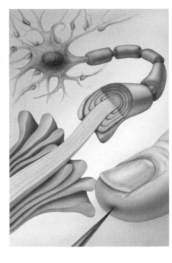

Poor circulation

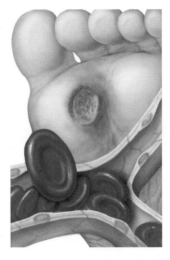

Heart disease

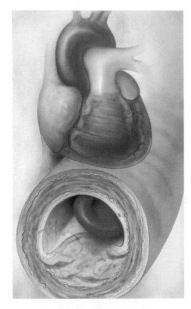

Kidney failure

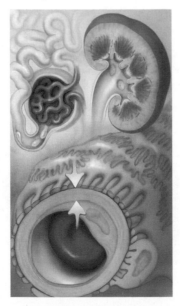

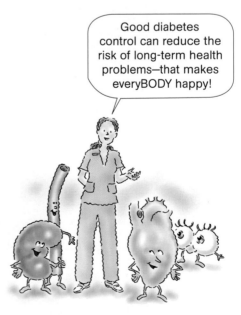

Good diabetes control can reduce the risk of long-term health problems—that makes everyBODY happy!

Cirrhosis

Cirrhosis is a chronic liver disease that's characterised by widespread destruction of hepatic cells. The destroyed cells are replaced by fibrotic cells in a process called *fibrotic regeneration*. As necrotic tissue yields to fibrosis, regenerative nodules form and the liver parenchyma undergo extensive and irreversible fibrotic changes. The disease alters normal liver structure and vasculature, impairs blood and lymphatic flow and, ultimately, causes hepatic insufficiency.

Therapy for cirrhosis aims to remove or alleviate the underlying cause, prevent further liver damage and prevent or treat complications.

It looks like cirrhosis has already begun to develop.

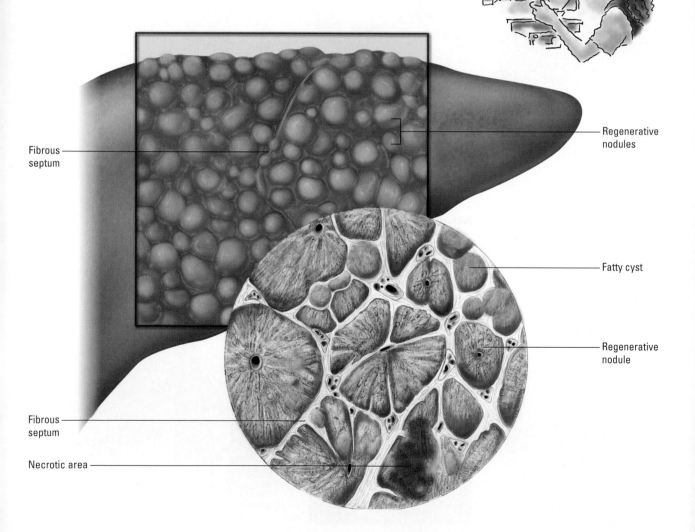

Fibrous septum

Regenerative nodules

Fatty cyst

Regenerative nodule

Fibrous septum

Necrotic area

- perforation of the bowel
- ischaemic bowel (strangulated hernias, poor perfusion or clotted vessels).

Who's the candidate?

Criteria for a patient to have bowel resection include:
- presentation with acutely distended abdomen, pain and suspicion of perforation/ischaemia
- removal of known carcinoma after diagnostic investigations or to bypass untreatable cancers
- uncontrolled inflammation in the bowel causing excessive diarrhoea/bleeding/high risk of infection
- elective stoma formation to divert faeces and prevent wound/burns contamination.

Nursing considerations

When caring for a patient undergoing a bowel resection, preparation will depend on whether it is an elective or emergency procedure. In elective cases concentrate on preparing the patient and their family physically and emotionally for the procedure, including instructing the patient about the procedure and events after. In emergency cases the patient is likely to have increased critical illness and may need stabilising preoperatively. In all cases take steps to prevent postoperative complications. If the bowel has been resected but a stoma has not been formed, the bowel will have been connected internally creating an 'anastamosis'. The anastamosis will need time and the right conditions to heal so good oxygenation, perfusion and hydration are important things to think about and the patient will usually remain nil by mouth for a longer period of time.

Before it begins

Before bowel resection

- Instruct the patient and their family about the procedure.
- Review information about the equipment and procedures, such as cardiac monitoring, pre-op ECG and x-ray, endotracheal tube, NG tube, indwelling urinary catheter and arterial lines. Reassure the patient/family that the equipment will be removed as soon as possible.
- Administer prescribed medications such as bowel preparation to empty the bowel.
- Make sure that an informed consent form has been signed.
- Make sure that all necessary blood tests have been performed, U&E, FBC, coagulation screen, X-match for blood if required.
- In elective cases if stoma formation is expected, the patient should have been seen preoperatively by the stoma nurse and the stoma site should have been planned. Whether the stoma is permanent or temporary (bowel can be reanastomosed at a later date) should have been discussed with the patient.
- Make sure that a plan for post-op analgesia has been decided, usually epidural in elective cases, this may not be possible in emergency cases.

- In emergency surgery NG tube insertion, fluid resuscitation and commencement of inotropes and vasoconstrictors may form part of the pre-op preparation according to severity of condition.
- Provide emotional support to the patient and their family.

After it's over

After bowel resection

- Assess the patient using an ABCDE approach to gain a holistic view of their condition.
- Monitor the patient's observations at least hourly as the patient is at high risk of infection from bacterial contamination, high risk of respiratory failure from basal collapse and sputum retention, high risk of dehydration from fluid depletion and high risk of arrhythmias from electrolyte abnormalities.
- Monitor blood tests, especially U&Es, coagulation screen, FBC, liver function tests and arterial blood gases.
- Assess pain score and sedation score to ensure adequate analgesia without adverse side effects. The large abdominal laparotomy wound stretching vertically down the abdomen is the usual method of opening and this can cause significant pain. Monitor observations specific to the analgesia being given, e.g. level of sensory and motor block and site assessment for epidurals.
- Monitor blood tests, especially U&Es, coagulation screen, FBC, liver function tests and arterial blood gases.
- Assess wound site, stoma and drains for indications of bleeding. If the patient has an NG tube, assess drainage colour at least every 2 hours.
- Monitor for abdominal distension which may indicate internal bleeding in early stages or paralytic ileus and anastamotic breakdown later.
- Monitor stoma site for formation, perfusion and functioning. An unvented clear post-op stoma bag should be used in the initial days so that any passing of flatus can be recognised and the stoma can be assessed regularly. Assessment is to check the stoma is pink and well perfused with no signs of ischaemia and is not protruding or retracting. The stoma may be an ileostomy (liquid stool) or colostomy (formed stool) depending on where in the bowel it is situated.
- Institute strict infection control precautions.
- Administer prophylactic antibiotics and postoperative drugs as prescribed. Discuss with medical staff if oral medication needs to be transferred via I.V. routes.
- Assist with extubation as soon as possible and administer supplemental oxygen as needed. Encourage coughing, deep breathing and incentive spirometry.
- Monitor the patient's intake and output at least hourly, and notify the doctor if output is less than 30 ml/hour. Maintain fluids at 2,000–3,000 ml/ day, or as prescribed, to prevent dehydration.
- Maintain the patient on nil-by-mouth status with NG drainage until bowel sounds return.
- Provide nutrition according to medical and dietetic advice, this may be enteral or parenteral feed or via I.V. fluids if oral diet is to recommence shortly.

• Change the patient's position at least every 2 hours, getting them out of bed and to the chair within 24 hours if their condition is stable.
• To ease emotional stress, plan care to allow rest and provide as much privacy as possible. Allow family members to visit and comfort the patient as much as possible.

GI intubation

NG and other specialised tubes may be used in treating the patient with impaired GI motility, acute intestinal obstruction, bleeding, oesophageal varices or another GI dysfunction. NG tubes are routinely inserted in sedated mechanically ventilated patients to reduce incidence of vomiting and aspiration and facilitate enteral feeding. The principles of GI intubation are ensuring the tube is positioned correctly in the stomach and it has not migrated into the patient's lung or mouth. This can be confirmed with x-ray initially, following this aspirates should be tested on pH paper to ensure pH is 5 or less. The tube should be well secured and the position documented. Patency must be maintained by regular flushing and aspiration.

Gastric lavage

Gastric lavage is an emergency treatment for the patient with GI haemorrhage caused by peptic ulcer disease or ruptured oesophageal or gastric varices and as emergency treatment for some drug overdoses.

It involves GI intubation with a large-bore, single or double lumen tube; instillation of irrigating fluid; and aspiration of gastric contents. In some cases of bleeding, a vasoconstrictor may be added to the irrigating fluid to enhance this action.

Rarities

Complications can include:
• vomiting and aspiration
• fluid overload
• electrolyte imbalance or metabolic acidosis
• bradycardia.

Nursing considerations
• Explain the procedure to the patient.
• Determine the length of the tube for insertion. (See *Measuring nasogastric tube length*, page 404.)
• Lubricate the end of the tube with a water-soluble lubricant and insert it into the patient's mouth or nostrils, as ordered. Advance the tube through the pharynx and oesophagus and into the stomach.
• Check the tube for placement by attaching a syringe, check the pH of tube aspirate to confirm correct placement of the tube. Gastric aspirate is acidic, with a pH ranging from 0 to 5. An alkaline pH of 6 or greater can indicate that the tube is in the respiratory tract.

• When the tube is in place, lower the head of the bed to 15 degrees and reposition the patient on their left side, if possible.

• Fill the syringe with 30–50 ml of irrigating solution and begin instillation. Instil about 250 ml of fluid, wait 30 seconds, and then begin to withdraw the fluid into the syringe. If you can't withdraw any fluid, allow the tube to drain into a vomit bowl.

• If the doctor prescribes a vasoconstrictor to be added to the irrigating fluid, wait for the prescribed period before withdrawing fluid to allow absorption of the drug into the gastric mucosa.

• Carefully measure and record fluid return. If the volume of fluid return doesn't at least equal the amount of fluid instilled, abdominal distention and vomiting result.

• Continue lavage until return fluid is clear or as instructed. Remove the tube or secure it, as ordered. If appropriate, send specimens to the laboratory for toxicology studies.

• Never leave the patient alone during gastric lavage.

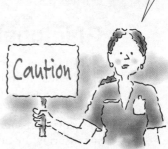

Never leave the patient alone during gastric lavage.

Caution

Measuring nasogastric tube length

To determine how long the nasogastric tube must be to reach the stomach, hold the end of the tube at the tip of the patient's nose. Extend the tube to the patient's earlobe and then down to the xiphoid process.

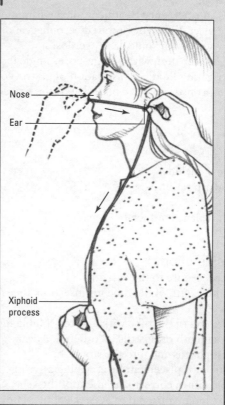

Nose

Ear

Xiphoid process

- Monitor the patient's cardiac rhythm and observe for possible complications, such as bradycardia, hypovolaemia, vomiting and aspiration.
- Monitor the patient's vital signs and oxygen saturation every 30 minutes until their condition stabilises.
- Document the procedure and appropriate interventions.

Multilumen oesophageal tube placement

In oesophagogastric tamponade, an emergency treatment, a multilumen oesophageal tube is inserted to control oesophageal or gastric haemorrhage resulting from ruptured varices. It's usually an emergency holding measure until sclerotherapy can be done. (See *Comparing oesophageal tubes*, page 406.)

How it's done

The tube is inserted through a nostril, or sometimes the mouth, and then passed into the stomach. The tube's oesophageal and gastric balloons are inflated to exert pressure on the varices to stop bleeding, while a lumen allows oesophageal and gastric contents to be aspirated.

Balloon inflation for longer than 48 hours may cause pressure necrosis, which can lead to further haemorrhage. Follow your unit's policy and procedure for balloon inflation and deflation.

Nursing considerations

Before the procedure
- Describe the procedure to the patient. Explain that a weight may be used to apply traction to keep balloon pressure at the gastro-oesophageal junction. Place the patient on their left side, with the head of the bed elevated to 15 degrees. An unresponsive patient will also require endotracheal intubation.
- Tape a pair of scissors to the head of the bed in case of acute respiratory distress.
- Check tube balloons for air leaks and patency before insertion.
- Never leave the patient alone during tamponade.

After it's over

After the procedure
- Closely monitor the patient's condition and lumen pressure. If the pressure changes or decreases, check for bleeding and notify the doctor immediately.
- Monitor the patient's cardiac rhythm, vital signs and oxygen saturation every 30–60 minutes. A change may indicate new bleeding.
- Monitor the patient's respiratory status and observe for respiratory distress. If respiratory distress develops, have someone notify the doctor. If the airway is obstructed, cut both balloon ports and remove the tube. Notify the doctor immediately.
- Maintain suction on the ports. Irrigate the gastric aspiration port to prevent clogging.
- Deflate the oesophageal balloon for about 30 minutes every 12 hours or according to your unit's policy and procedure.

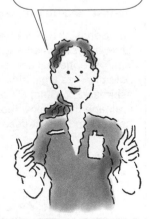

After your patient's bleeding is under control, assist the doctor with tube removal.

Comparing oesophageal tubes

Three types of oesophageal tubes include the Linton tube, the Minnesota oesophagogastric tamponade tube and the Sengstaken–Blakemore tube.

Linton tube

The Linton tube, a three-lumen, single-balloon device, has ports for oesophageal and gastric aspiration. Because the tube doesn't have an oesophageal balloon, it isn't used to control bleeding for oesophageal varices.

Minnesota oesophagogastric tamponade tube

The Minnesota oesophagogastric tamponade tube has four lumens and two balloons. It has pressure-monitoring ports for both balloons.

Sengstaken–Blakemore tube

The Sengstaken–Blakemore tube, a three-lumen device with oesophageal and gastric balloons, has a gastric aspiration port that allows drainage from below the gastric balloon and is also used to instil medication.

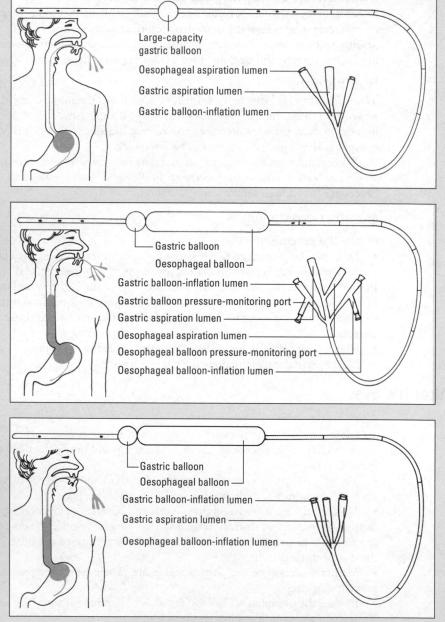

Large-capacity gastric balloon
Oesophageal aspiration lumen
Gastric aspiration lumen
Gastric balloon-inflation lumen

Gastric balloon
Oesophageal balloon
Gastric balloon-inflation lumen
Gastric balloon pressure-monitoring port
Gastric aspiration lumen
Oesophageal aspiration lumen
Oesophageal balloon pressure-monitoring port
Oesophageal balloon-inflation lumen

Gastric balloon
Oesophageal balloon
Gastric balloon-inflation lumen
Gastric aspiration lumen
Oesophageal balloon-inflation lumen

- Observe the patient for signs of oesophageal rupture, such as shock, increased respiratory difficulty and increased bleeding. Notify the doctor if such signs are present.
- Keep the patient warm, comfortable and as still as possible.
- When bleeding has been controlled, assist with tube removal.

Nutritional support

A patient with a GI problem who can't eat or otherwise ingest enough food may require enteral or parenteral nutrition.

Enteral nutrition

Enteral nutrition is used to deliver nutrients to the GI tract using a tube. The upper GI tract is bypassed and pureed food or a special liquid enteral formula is delivered directly into the stomach, duodenum or jejunum. Most commonly in critical care this will be via an NG tube—either via a standard NG tube that can be used for drainage or feeding, or once feeding is established via a fine bore tube. Nasojejunal tubes tend to be used for patients with particular GI problems, especially pancreatitis, to reduce stimulation and thus secretions from the stomach and pancreas. For patients requiring long-term enteral nutrition, a gastrostomy or jejunostomy tube may be inserted through the abdominal wall. Enteral feed can be administered on an intermittent bolus regime or as a continuous, slow infusion.

Who needs it?

Enteral nutrition delivery is indicated for the patient with a functional GI tract who can't adequately take food by mouth, such as a patient with:
- endotracheal intubation
- tracheostomy *in situ* and difficulty swallowing
- head and neck injuries
- neurological disease
- stroke
- oral cancers
- a psychiatric disorder.

Who can't have it?

Tube feeding is contraindicated in the patient with suspected intestinal obstruction, absent bowel sounds, perforated bowel or recent GI anastamosis until authorised by surgeons.

Nursing considerations

Before the procedure
- Explain the procedure to the patient and obtain the prescribed feed.
- Assess the patient's abdomen for bowel sounds and distention. Check placement of the feeding tube to ensure it hasn't slipped out since the last

feeding. Never commence tube feeding until you're sure the tube is properly positioned in the patient's stomach as confirmed by x-ray or pH testing. Administering feed through a misplaced tube can lead to aspiration.
• Check gastric aspirates to assess gastric emptying; aspirate and measure gastric residual contents. Withhold feedings if residual volume is more than the amount specified in your local policy (usually 200 ml). Reinstil any aspirate obtained. Increase feed volumes according to prescription and patient tolerance.
• When delivering the feeding, elevate the patient to 45 degrees head up to prevent aspiration and promote digestion.
• Irrigate the tube, administer the feeding as prescribed and then flush the tube when feeding finishes. Continuous feeding improves stability of blood glucose but requires constant patient connection to an infusion device and does not allow stomach pH to drop increasing risks of bacterial growth. Bolus feeding allows more freedom but may cause blood sugars to fluctuate. Both methods can cause patient diarrhoea.

After it's over

After the procedure
• Record the volume of feed ingested. Note the patient's tolerance of tube feeding.
• Weigh the patient regularly and monitor blood results.
• Provide meticulous mouth and tube care with good attention to hygiene in feed and equipment to prevent introduction of bacteria.

Parenteral nutrition

When a patient can't meet their nutritional needs by oral or enteral feedings, they may require I.V. nutritional support or parenteral nutrition.

Who needs it?

The patient's diagnosis, history and prognosis are used to determine the need for parenteral nutrition. Generally, this treatment is prescribed for any patient who can't absorb nutrients through the GI tract for more than 10 days.
More specific indications include:
• debilitating illness lasting longer than 2 weeks
• loss of 10% or more of pre-illness weight
• low serum albumin levels
• excessive nitrogen loss from wound infection, fistulas or abscesses
• renal or hepatic failure
• severe burns
• nonfunctioning GI tract for 5–7 days in a severely catabolic patient.

Delivery route

Parenteral nutrition may be given through a peripheral or central venous (CV) line. Depending on the solution, parenteral nutrition

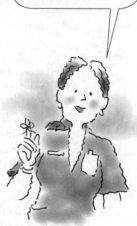

Never commence tube feeding until you're sure the tube is properly positioned in the patient's stomach.

Parenteral nutrition is prescribed for any patient who can't absorb nutrients through the GI tract for more than 10 days.

boosts the patient's calorie intake or surpasses their calorie requirements. There are two types of parenteral nutrition:

• *Total parenteral nutrition* refers to any nutrient solution, including lipids, given through a CV line and is more commonly used.

• *Peripheral parenteral nutrition* (PPN) is delivered through a peripheral line. PPN is used to supply the patient's full calorie needs while avoiding the risks that accompany a CV line. (See *Types of parenteral nutrition*, page 410.)

Nursing considerations

• Explain the procedure to the patient.

• Be sure to check the solution against the prescription for correct patient name, expiration date and formula components.

• Throughout the procedure, maintain sterile technique. Ensure the TPN is administered on a dedicated lumen of the line, changing the set every 24 hours when the solution is changed.

• Follow local policies and procedures and administer using an infusion pump with the pump tubing and micron filter. Infuse at a constant rate without interruption to avoid blood glucose fluctuations.

• Monitor the patient's vital signs at least every 2–4 hours, or more often if necessary. Watch them for increased temperature, an early sign of catheter sepsis and a common complication of TPN administration.

• Check the patient's blood glucose level 1 hour after commencing, then at least every 6 hours.

• Monitor the patient's intake and output and routine laboratory tests (U&Es, calcium, magnesium, phosphate, FBC and albumin).

• Monitor the patient's liver and kidney functions, the high nitrogen load can cause liver and renal impairment.

• Weigh the patient regularly if possible.

• Change the dressing using aseptic technique ensuring a clean dry intact semiocclusive dressing *in situ* at all times. Inspect the site daily for signs of infection and document findings. Monitor the catheter site for swelling, which may indicate infiltration.

• When discontinuing parenteral nutrition, decrease the infusion rate slowly, depending on the patient's current glucose intake, to minimise the risk of hyperinsulinaemia and resulting hypoglycaemia.

GI disorders

Critically ill patients can suffer from a variety of GI disorders as a complication of their primary critical illness, e.g. paralytic ileus secondary to shock states, GI bleeding caused by stress ulceration, diarrhoea or constipation from a variety of causes. Key principles of caring for patients with these disorders are try to remove/alleviate the cause, aim to maintain adequate supply of oxygenated blood to the GI tract, monitor fluid losses and replace fluids according to patient needs, and follow strict infection control to reduce bacterial transmission.

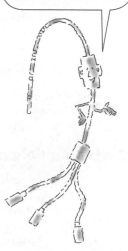

Monitor the catheter site for swelling, which may indicate infiltration.

Types of parenteral nutrition

Type	Solution components per litre	Uses
Total parenteral nutrition by central venous (CV) catheter or peripherally inserted central catheter into the superior vena cava through the supraclavicular vein, internal jugular vein or antecubital fossa	• $D_{15}W$ to $D_{25}W$ (1 L dextrose 25% = 850 nonprotein calories) • Crystalline amino acids 2.5–8.5% • Electrolytes, vitamins, trace elements as prescribed • Lipid emulsion 10–20%	• When needed for 1 week or more • For a patient with large calorie and nutrient needs • Provides calories, restores nitrogen balance and replaces essential vitamins, electrolytes, minerals and trace elements • Promotes tissue synthesis, wound healing and normal metabolic function • Allows bowel rest and healing; reduces activity in the gallbladder, pancreas and small intestine • Improves tolerance of surgery
Peripheral parenteral nutrition by peripheral catheter	• D_5W to $D_{10}W$ • Crystalline amino acids 2.5–5% • Electrolytes, minerals, vitamins and trace elements, as prescribed • Lipid emulsion 10–20% (1 L dextrose 10% and amino acids 3.5%infused at the same time as 1 L of lipid emulsion = 1,440 nonprotein calories)	• When needed for 1 week or less • Provides up to 2,000 calories/day • Maintains adequate nutritional status in a patient who can tolerate relatively high fluid volume, one who usually resumes bowel function and oral feedings after a few days and one susceptible to infections associated with the CV catheter

Primary abdominal disorders commonly encountered in a critical care unit include acute GI bleeding, acute pancreatitis, bowel infarction or perforation, cirrhosis, hepatic failure and hepatic encephalopathy and intra-abdominal hypertension.

Acute GI bleeding

GI bleeding can occur anywhere along the GI tract. Although GI bleeding stops spontaneously in most patients, acute bleeding accounts for significant morbidity and mortality.

Maybe multiple morbidities

Many patients requiring care in the critical care unit have upper GI bleeding. Additionally, they may have underlying comorbidities that contribute to the risk of upper GI bleeding, such as:
• coronary artery disease
• history of myocardial infarction (MI)

Special considerations

Basic solution

- Nutritionally complete
- Requires minor surgical procedure for CV line insertion
- Highly hypertonic solution
- May cause pneumothorax (typically during catheter insertion), phlebitis, thrombus formation, air embolus, high risk of infection, sepsis and metabolic complications (glucose intolerance, electrolyte imbalance, essential fatty acid deficiency)
- Must be delivered in a vein with high blood flow rate because glucose content may be increased beyond the level a peripheral vein can handle (commonly six times more concentrated than blood)

I.V. lipid emulsion

- May not be used effectively in a severely stressed patient (especially a patient with burns)
- May interfere with immune mechanisms; in a patient suffering from respiratory compromise, reduces carbon dioxide buildup
- Given by way of CV line

- Nutritionally complete for a short time
- Can't be used in a nutritionally depleted patient
- Can't be used in a volume-restricted patient
- Doesn't cause weight gain
- Avoids insertion and care of the CV line, but requires adequate venous access site; must be changed every 72 hours
- May cause phlebitis and increases risk of metabolic complications
- Less chance of metabolic complications than with CV line
- To avoid venous sclerosis, must contain no more than 10% dextrose, so patient must tolerate large fluid volume to meet nutritional needs

- As effective as dextrose for calorie source
- Diminishes phlebitis if infused at the same time as basic nutrient solution
- Irritates vein in long-term use
- Reduces carbon dioxide buildup when pulmonary compromise is present

---

- renal failure
- history of chronic liver damage secondary to alcohol abuse or hepatitis
- history of radiation therapy
- chronic pain condition, such as arthritis, requiring treatment with NSAIDs.

What causes it

Upper GI bleeding includes bleeding in the oesophagus, stomach and duodenum. Bleeding below this is considered lower GI bleeding; the most common site is in the colon.

Upper causes

The causes of upper GI bleeding include:
- peptic ulcer disease
- rupture of oesophageal varices
- oesophagitis
- Mallory–Weiss tear
- erosive gastritis

- angiodysplasias
- arteriovenous malformations
- increased stress and acid production in critical illness

Lower causes

The most common causes of lower GI bleeding include:
- diverticulitis
- inflammatory bowel disease
- polyps
- haemorrhoids
- neoplasm
- arteriovenous malformations.

The results are

The patient experiences a loss of circulating blood volume, regardless of the cause of bleeding.

What happens

Because the arterial blood supply near the stomach and oesophagus is extensive, bleeding can lead to a rapid loss of large amounts of blood, subsequent hypovolaemia, and shock. Here's what else happens:
- Loss of circulating blood volume leads to a decreased venous return.
- Cardiac output and blood pressure decrease, causing poor tissue perfusion. In response, the body compensates by shifting interstitial fluid to the intravascular space.
- The sympathetic nervous system is stimulated, resulting in vasoconstriction and increased heart rate.
- The renin–angiotensin–aldosterone system is activated, leading to fluid retention and increased blood pressure.
- If blood loss continues, cardiac output decreases, leading to cellular hypoxia. Eventually, all organs fail due to hypoperfusion.

What to look for

Because GI bleeding can occur anywhere along the GI tract, assessment is crucial in determining the amount and possible location of bleeding.

Source signs

The appearance of blood in tube drainage, vomitus and stool indicates the source of GI bleeding:
- Haematemesis—bright red blood in NG tube drainage or vomit— typically indicates an upper GI source. However, if the blood has spent time in the stomach where it was exposed to gastric acid, the drainage or vomit resembles coffee grounds.
- Haematochezia—bright red blood from the rectum—typically indicates a lower GI source of bleeding. It also may suggest an upper GI source if the transit time through the bowel was rapid.

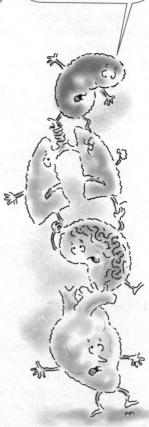

With continued bleeding, all organs eventually fail due to hypoperfusion.

- Melaena—black, tarry and sticky stool—usually indicates an upper GI bleeding source. However, it can result from bleeding in the small bowel or proximal colon.

Signs and symptoms

Typically, the patient exhibits signs and symptoms based on the amount and rate of bleeding. It is important to be suspicious because it is not until the blood loss is greater than 30% of the person's blood volume that they exhibit signs and symptoms of hypovolaemic shock, including:
- cool, clammy skin
- pallor
- restlessness
- apprehension
- tachycardia
- diaphoresis
- hypotension
- syncope.

What tests tell you

These findings aid in diagnosing acute GI bleeding:
- Upper GI endoscopy reveals the source of oesophageal or gastric bleeding.
- FBC reveals the amount of blood loss.
- Arterial blood gas (ABG) analysis can indicate metabolic acidosis from hypoperfusion.
- 12-lead electrocardiogram (ECG) may reveal evidence of cardiac ischaemia secondary to hypoperfusion.
- Abdominal x-ray may indicate air under the diaphragm, suggesting ulcer perforation.
- Angiography may aid in visualising the bleeding site.

How it's treated

Treatment goals include stopping the bleeding and providing fluid replacement while maintaining the patient's function. Treatment may include:
- fluid volume replacement with crystalloid solutions initially, followed by colloids and blood component therapy
- respiratory support
- gastric intubation with gastric lavage (unless the patient has oesophageal varices) and gastric pH monitoring
- drug therapy, such as antacids, H2-receptor antagonists and proton pump inhibitors
- endoscopic or surgical repair of bleeding sites.

What to do

- Type and cross-match at least 2 units of blood.
- Start at least two large-bore I.V. lines (16G or 18G preferred). Assess the patient for blood loss and begin fluid replacement therapy as ordered, initially delivering crystalloid solutions, such as normal saline or Hartmann's solution, followed by blood component products.

> Watch for signs and symptoms of hypovolaemic shock in patients with acute GI bleeding.

• Use an ABCDE approach. Ensure your patient's patent airway. Monitor cardiac and respiratory status and assess GCS at least every 15 minutes until they stabilise and then every 2–4 hours, as indicated by their status. Assist with insertion of haemodynamic monitoring devices, and assess haemodynamic parameters.
• Administer supplemental oxygen as ordered. Monitor oxygen saturation levels.
• Monitor the patient's skin colour and capillary refill for signs of hypovolaemic shock.
• Obtain serial haemoglobin, haematocrit levels and clotting screens. Administer blood or clotting products as prescribed.
• Monitor the patient's intake and output closely, including all losses from the GI tract. Check all stools and gastric drainage for occult blood.
• Assist with or insert an NG tube.
• Assess the patient's abdomen for bowel sounds and gastric pH, as ordered. Expect to resume enteral or oral feedings after bowel function returns and there's no evidence of further bleeding.
• Provide appropriate emotional support to the patient.
• Prepare the patient for endoscopic repair or surgery, if indicated.

Acute pancreatitis

Pancreatitis, inflammation of the pancreas, occurs in acute and chronic forms and may be due to oedema, necrosis or haemorrhage. In men, this disease is more commonly associated with alcoholism, trauma or peptic ulcers; in women, with biliary tract disease.

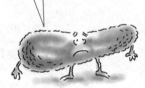

Pancreatitis occurs in acute and chronic forms. It may be caused by oedema, necrosis or haemorrhage.

What causes it
Causes of pancreatitis may include:
• biliary tract disease
• alcoholism
• abnormal organ structure
• metabolic or endocrine disorders, such as high cholesterol levels and hyperparathyroidism
• pancreatic cysts or tumours
• penetrating peptic ulcers
• blunt or surgical trauma
• drugs, such as glucocorticoids, sulphonamides, thiazides, procainamide, tetracycline and NSAIDs
• kidney failure or transplantation
• endoscopic examination of the bile ducts and pancreas.

Pathophysiology
Acute pancreatitis occurs in two forms:

 oedematous (interstitial) pancreatitis, which causes fluid accumulation and swelling

 necrotising pancreatitis, which causes cell death and tissue damage.

Damage and destruction

The inflammation that occurs with both types of pancreatitis is caused by premature activation of enzymes, which lead to tissue damage. If pancreatitis damages the islets of Langerhans, diabetes mellitus may result. Sudden severe pancreatitis can cause massive haemorrhage and total destruction of the pancreas, manifested as diabetic acidosis, shock or coma.

Association affects outcome

The prognosis is good for a patient with pancreatitis associated with biliary tract disease but poor when associated with alcoholism. Mortality is as high as 60% when pancreatitis is associated with necrosis and haemorrhage.

Rating mortality

Risk of death from pancreatitis can be calculated using the Balthazar score which examines CT scan results. The severity of pancreatitis is predicted using Ranson's criteria. If the patient meets fewer than three of the criteria, the mortality rate is less than 1%. When three or four of the criteria are met, the mortality rate increases to 15–20%. With five or six criteria, the mortality rate is 40%. (See *Ranson's criteria and Balthazar score*.)

What to look for

Commonly, the patient describes intense epigastric pain centred close to the umbilicus and radiating to the back. They typically report that the pain is aggravated by:
- eating fatty foods
- consuming alcohol
- lying in a recumbent position.

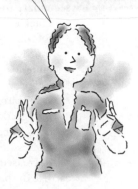

Good news! The prognosis is good when pancreatitis is associated with biliary tract disease.

Ranson's criteria and Balthazar score

The severity of your patient's acute pancreatitis is determined by the existence of certain characteristics. The more criteria met by the patient, the more severe the episode of pancreatitis and, therefore, the greater the risk of mortality.

On admission

Admission criteria include:

- age over 55
- white blood cell count greater than 16,000 per µl
- serum glucose greater than mmol/ml
- lactate dehydrogenase greater than 350 IU/L
- aspartate aminotransferase greater than 250 U/L.

After admission

During the first 48 hours after admission, criteria include:

- 10% decrease in haematocrit
- blood urea increase greater than 5 mg/dl
- serum calcium less than 2 mmol/L
- base deficit greater than 4 mEq/L
- partial pressure of arterial oxygen less than 8 kpa
- estimated fluid sequestration greater than 6 L.

Add in Balthazar score.

Take notes

During the physical examination, you may note:
- persistent vomiting (in a severe attack) from hypermotility or paralytic ileus
- abdominal distention (in a severe attack) from bowel hypermotility and fluid accumulation in the peritoneal cavity
- diminished bowel activity (in a severe attack), suggesting altered motility secondary to peritonitis
- crackles at lung bases (in a severe attack) secondary to heart failure
- left pleural effusion
- mottled skin
- jaundice
- ascites
- tachycardia
- low-grade pyrexia
- cold, sweaty extremities
- restlessness related to pain
- decreased cardiac output due to haemorrhage or dehydration; elevated cardiac output and decreased systemic vascular resistance if systemic inflammation or sepsis present.

What tests tell you

Findings that aid in diagnosing acute pancreatitis include:
- serum amylase and lipase levels elevated three to five times normal
- urine amylase increased for 1–2 weeks
- elevated white blood cell (WBC) count; haemoglobin and haematocrit decreased with haemorrhage and increased with dehydration; increased coagulation times
- decreased serum calcium
- other elevated results, including serum bilirubin levels, aspartate aminotransferase (AST), alanine aminotransferase (ALT), lactate dehydrogenase (LD) and alkaline phosphatase
- abdominal and chest x-rays showing pleural effusions and bowel dilation and ileus
- CT scan and ultrasonography showing an enlarged pancreas with fluid collection, cysts, abscess, masses and pseudocysts
- endoscopic pancreatography showing swelling and ductal system abnormalities
- ABG values that may reveal metabolic acidosis and raised lactate, decreased partial pressure of arterial oxygen, mild respiratory alkalosis and decreased oxygen saturation.

How it's treated

Treatment for the patient with acute pancreatitis may include:
- I.V. replacement of fluids, protein and electrolytes to treat shock
- fluid volume replacement and blood transfusions

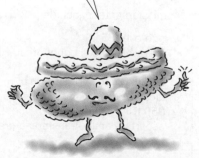

Treatment for pancreatitis may include I.V. fluids, drugs and peritoneal lavage.

- withholding oral food and fluids to rest the pancreas, commencing nasojejunal feeding or TPN
- analgesia, morphine is usually used for the severe pain caused, although because it causes more spasm in the sphincter of Oddi than other opioids some doctors favour pethidine
- NG tube suctioning
- drugs, such as antacids, H2-receptor antagonists, antibiotics, anticholinergics and insulin
- peritoneal lavage
- surgical drainage for a pancreatic abscess or pseudocyst
- laparotomy (if biliary tract obstruction causes acute pancreatitis) to remove the obstruction.

What to do

- Use an ABCDE approach. Ensure a patent airway, and assess the patient's respiratory status at least every hour or more often. Assess oxygen saturation levels and breath sounds for added or diminished breath sounds.
- Closely monitor the patient's cardiac and haemodynamic status at least every hour or more often, as ordered.
- Place the patient in a comfortable position that maximises air exchange, such as 45 degrees head up.
- Allow for periods of rest and activity.
- If the patient develops acute respiratory distress syndrome, anticipate the need for additional therapies such as CPAP via mask, mechanical ventilation or prone positioning.
- Initiate I.V. fluid replacement therapy. Monitor serum laboratory values (haematology, coagulation and biochemistry) for changes.
- Be especially alert for signs and symptoms of hypokalaemia (hypotension, muscle weakness, apathy, confusion and cardiac arrhythmias), hypomagnesaemia (hypotension, tachycardia, confusion, tremors, twitching, tetany and hallucinations) and hypocalcaemia (positive Chvostek's—spasm of facial muscles and Trousseau's signs—carpal spasm by compressing the upper arm, seizures and prolonged QT interval on ECG). Have emergency equipment readily available.
- Monitor the patient's intake and output closely and notify the doctor if urine output is less than 0.5 ml/kg/hour. Weigh the patient as able.
- Monitor the patient's neurological status, noting confusion or lethargy.
- Maintain your patient in a normothermic state to reduce the body's demand for oxygen.
- Assess the patient's pain level and administer analgesics, as prescribed.
- Administer antibiotics and monitor serum peak and trough levels, as appropriate.
- Withhold oral fluids and food to prevent stimulation of pancreatic enzymes.

- Insert an NG tube, as ordered. Check placement at least every 4 hours. Irrigate with water for patency. Monitor drainage for frank bleeding. Monitor vomit and stool for bleeding.
- Assess the patient's abdomen for distention and bowel sounds; measure their abdominal girth or intra-abdominal pressure as indicated.
- Administer nasojejunal enteral nutrition or parenteral nutrition therapy, as ordered. Monitor blood glucose levels. Administer insulin, as ordered.
- When bowel sounds become active, anticipate switching to NG or oral feedings.
- Perform passive exercises to maintain joint mobility.
- Perform meticulous skin care.
- Provide emotional support to the patient.
- Prepare the patient for surgery, as indicated.

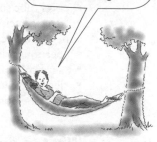

Place the patient in a comfortable position that maximises air exchange.

Bowel infarction

Bowel infarction is a decreased blood flow to the major mesenteric vessels. It leads to vasoconstriction and vasospasm of the bowel and contracted bowel with mucosal ulceration.

What causes it

Bowel infarction can be caused by:
- thrombosis after an MI
- cholesterol plaques in the aorta that become dislodged
- emboli in patients with endocarditis or atrial fibrillation
- arteriosclerosis
- cirrhosis of the liver
- hypercoagulation as seen in polycythaemia or after splenectomy
- reduced perfusion from heart failure, shock states or cardiac arrest
- reduced perfusion following GI or vascular surgery.

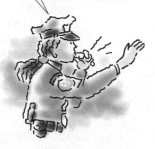

Hold it! Withhold all oral fluids and food to prevent stimulation of pancreatic enzymes.

Pathophysiology

Here's what happens with bowel infarction:
- Decreased blood flow to the mesenteric vessels leads to spasms.
- When the spasms subside, the muscles of the bowel are fatigued and unable to receive essential oxygen and nutrients.
- The bowel becomes oedematous and cyanotic, and necrosis can occur.
- As pressure in the lumens of the bowel increases, perforation can occur, leading to peritonitis or abscess formation.

What to look for

Look for signs and symptoms that may occur with bowel infarction, including:
- acute abdominal pain, more excessive than expected if following elective surgery
- vomiting
- bloody, offensive smelling diarrhoea

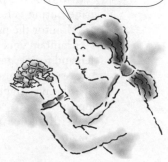

Infarction leads to vasoconstriction and vasospasm of the bowel.

- weight loss
- abdominal distention with tenderness and guarding
- absent or hypoactive bowel sounds
- signs and symptoms of shock.

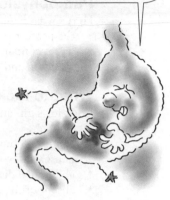

Abdominal distention with tenderness and guarding may indicate bowel infarction.

What tests tell you

These test results may aid in the diagnosis of bowel infarction:
- Abdominal x-rays reveal dilated loops of bowel.
- Barium studies show the infarction location.
- Angiography reveals the infarction location.
- Faecal occult blood tests are positive for blood.
- CT scan may reveal the area of infarction.
- Serum phosphate, haematocrit and serum osmolality levels are elevated.
- Sigmoidoscopy reveals an ischaemic bowel.

How it's treated

Treatment for your patient with bowel infarction may include:
- vasodilators for perfusion and pain relief
- angiograms
- anticoagulation
- surgery that may include bowel resection, endarterectomy, thrombectomy and aortomesenteric bypass grafting.

What to do

- Use ABCDE assessment. Monitor the patient's vital signs, oxygen saturation, cardiac rhythm and cardiopulmonary status.
- Assess the patient's abdomen for bowel sounds, and monitor their abdominal girth or intra-abdominal pressures.
- Monitor skin temperature and capillary refill.
- Administer fluid replacement, as ordered.
- Administer vasoactive agents, such as noradrenaline as prescribed.
- Prepare the patient for surgical repair, as indicated.
- Monitor the patient's intake and output.
- Administer analgesics to control pain and antibiotics, as ordered.
- Observe electrolytes and glucose levels for imbalances.
- Provide nutritional support, as ordered.

Bowel perforation

Bowel perforation is a hole in the bowel, resulting in leakage and contamination of the peritoneal cavity. It leads to septicaemia and carries a high risk of mortality.

What causes it

Bowel perforation can be caused by:
- blunt or penetrating abdominal trauma
- cancers

- ulcers
- infarcted bowel
- diverticular disease
- Crohn's disease or ulcerative colitis
- complications during elective surgery.

Pathophysiology

Here's what happens with bowel perforation:
- the protective mechanisms in the bowel are breached.
- faecal contamination of the peritoneal cavity causes peritonitis.
- infection and systemic inflammation cause severe sepsis and septic shock.

What to look for

Look for signs and symptoms that may occur with bowel perforation, including:
- acute abdominal pain, especially rebound tenderness
- nausea and vomiting
- abdominal distension and guarding
- absent or hypoactive bowel sounds
- signs and symptoms of shock
- signs and symptoms of infection.

What tests tell you

These test results may aid in the diagnosis of bowel perforation:
- Abdominal x-rays reveal air-dilated loops of bowel.
- Barium studies show the infarction location.
- Angiography reveals the infarction location.
- Faecal occult blood tests are positive for blood.
- CT scan may reveal the area of infarction.
- Serum phosphate, haematocrit and serum osmolality levels are elevated.
- Sigmoidoscopy reveals an ischaemic bowel.

How it's treated

Treatment for your patient with bowel infarction may include:
- vasodilators for perfusion and pain relief
- angiograms
- anticoagulation
- surgery that may include endarterectomy, thrombectomy and aortomesenteric bypass grafting.

What to do

- Monitor the patient's vital signs, oxygen saturation, cardiac rhythm and cardiopulmonary status.
- Assess the patient's abdomen for bowel sounds, and monitor their abdominal girth and weight daily.
- Monitor skin temperature and capillary refill.
- Administer fluid replacement, as ordered.

- Administer vasoactive agents, such as noradrenaline, as prescribed.
- Prepare the patient for surgical repair, as indicated.
- Monitor the patient's intake and output.
- Administer analgesics to control pain and antibiotics as prescribed.
- Observe electrolytes and glucose levels for imbalances.
- Provide nutritional support, as ordered.

Cirrhosis

Cirrhosis is a chronic disorder marked by diffuse destruction and fibrotic regeneration of hepatic cells. As necrotic tissue yields to fibrosis, this disease damages liver tissue and normal vasculature, impairs blood and lymph flow and ultimately causes hepatic insufficiency.

What causes it

There are several types of cirrhosis, including:
- portal (Laënnec's), caused by malnutrition and chronic alcohol ingestion
- biliary, caused by bile duct disease that suppresses bile flow
- postnecrotic, caused by various types of hepatitis
- pigment, caused by haemochromatosis (excess iron absorption)
- cardiac, caused by liver damage from right-sided heart failure.

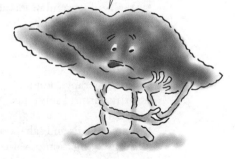

There are several types of cirrhosis, including portal, biliary, postnecrotic, pigment and cardiac.

Pathophysiology

Cirrhosis is characterised by irreversible chronic injury of the liver, extensive fibrosis and nodular tissue growth. The changes result from liver cell death (hepatocyte necrosis), collapse of the liver's supporting structure (the reticulin network), distortion of the vascular bed and nodular regeneration of remaining liver tissue.

What to look for

Assess your patient for these signs and symptoms, which are the same regardless of the cause:
- GI—anorexia, indigestion, nausea and vomiting, constipation or diarrhoea and dull abdominal ache
- respiratory—pleural effusion, limited thoracic expansion
- central nervous system (CNS)—lethargy, mental changes, slurred speech, asterixis, peripheral neuritis, hallucinations, coma
- haematological—bleeding tendencies, anaemia
- endocrine—testicular atrophy, menstrual irregularities, loss of chest and axillary hair
- skin—severe pruritus, extreme dryness, poor tissue turgor, abnormal pigmentation, spider angiomas, possible jaundice
- hepatic—jaundice, hepatomegaly, ascites, oedema of the legs
- miscellaneous—musty breath, muscle atrophy, pain in the right upper quadrant, palpable liver or spleen.

What tests tell you

The following findings aid in diagnosing cirrhosis:
- Liver biopsy confirms cirrhosis.
- Liver scan shows abnormal thickening and a liver mass.

These help, too

Other helpful tests include:
- cholecystography and cholangiography to visualise the gallbladder and biliary duct system
- percutaneous transhepatic cholangiography to visualise the portal venous system
- WBC count, haematocrit and haemoglobin, albumin, serum electrolyte and cholinesterase levels (all decreased)
- globulin, serum ammonia, prothrombin time (PT), total bilirubin, alkaline phosphatase, ALT, AST and LD levels (all increased).

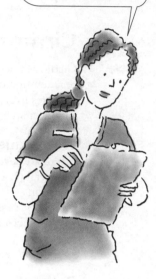

The signs and symptoms of cirrhosis are the same regardless of the cause.

How it's treated

Treatment for your patient with cirrhosis may include:
- high-calorie and moderate- to high-protein diet; restricted protein if hepatic encephalopathy develops, glucose in I.V. fluid regime
- sodium restricted to 200–500 mg/day; fluids to 1,000–1,500 ml/day
- possible enteral or parenteral feeding if the patient's condition continues to deteriorate
- drug therapy (requires special caution because the cirrhotic liver can't detoxify harmful substances efficiently; sedatives avoided or prescribed with great care)
- paracentesis and salt-poor albumin infusions to relieve ascites
- surgery (ligation of varices, splenectomy, oesophagogastric resection or liver transplantation).

What to do

- A patient with cirrhosis is generally admitted to the critical care unit because of a complication of cirrhosis, such as hepatic failure or bleeding oesophageal varices. (See *Managing bleeding from oesophageal varices*.)
- Monitor the patient's vital signs, oxygen saturation, cardiac rhythm and cardiopulmonary status.
- Observe the patient closely for signs of behavioural or personality changes. Report increasing stupor, lethargy, hallucinations or neuromuscular dysfunction. Watch for asterixis, a sign of developing hepatic encephalopathy.
- Assess the patient for fluid retention, weigh and measure their abdominal girth or intra-abdominal pressure and inspect their ankles and sacrum for dependent oedema.
- Accurately record the patient's intake and output.

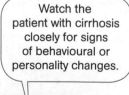

Watch the patient with cirrhosis closely for signs of behavioural or personality changes.

Managing bleeding from oesophageal varices

Oesophageal varices are dilated, tortuous veins in the submucosa of the lower oesophagus resulting from portal hypertension. Varices can go undetected and result in sudden and massive bleeding. Such varices commonly cause massive haematemesis, requiring emergency treatment to control haemorrhage and prevent hypovolaemic shock.

Managing bleeding

- Vasopressin infused into the superior mesenteric artery may stop bleeding temporarily. Vasopressin infused by I.V. drip diluted with dextrose 5% in water is less effective.
- Sclerotherapy is done by endoscopy to cause fibrosis and obliteration of the varices.

- A Minnesota or Sengstaken–Blakemore tube is used to control haemorrhage by applying pressure on the bleeding site.
- Iced saline lavage through the tube is used to control bleeding. Fresh blood and frozen plasma are given to replace clotting factors.
- Lactulose is administered to promote elimination of old blood from the GI tract and to combat excessive production and accumulation of ammonia.
- Surgical bypass procedures include portosystemic anastomosis, splenorenal shunt, portacaval shunt and mesocaval shunt.

Hepatic failure and encephalopathy

Hepatic failure is the possible end result of any liver disease. When the liver fails, a complex syndrome involving impairment of many organs and body functions ensues. Failure can be caused by hepatitis, cirrhosis, liver cancer or as part of multiorgan failure. (See *Viral hepatitis from A to E—plus G*, page 424.)

Ammonia coma

Hepatic encephalopathy, also called hepatic coma, is a neurological syndrome that develops as a manifestation of hepatic failure. It usually reflects ammonia intoxication of the brain.

What causes it

Hepatic encephalopathy is the result of increasing blood ammonia levels, such as from:
- improper shunting of blood from portal hypertension or from surgically created portosystemic shunts
- excessive protein intake
- sepsis
- excessive accumulation of nitrogenous body wastes (caused by constipation or GI bleeding)
- bacterial action on protein and urea to form ammonia.

Viral hepatitis from A to E—plus G

Use this table to compare the features of various types of viral hepatitis characterised to date. Other types are emerging.

Feature	Hepatitis A	Hepatitis B	Hepatitis C	Hepatitis D	Hepatitis E	Hepatitis G
Incubation	15–45 days	30–180 days	15–160 days	14–64 days	14–60 days	2–6 weeks
Onset	Acute	Insidious	Insidious	Acute	Acute	Presumed insidious
Age-group commonly affected	Children, young adults	Any age	More common in adults	Any age	Ages 20–40	Any age, primarily adults
Transmission	Faecal–oral, sexual (especially oral–anal contact), nonpercutaneous (sexual, maternal–neonatal), percutaneous (rare)	Blood-borne; parenteral route, sexual, maternal–neonatal; virus is shed in all body fluids	Blood-borne; parenteral route	Parenteral route; most people infected with hepatitis D are also infected with hepatitis B	Primarily faecal–oral	Blood-borne; similar to Hepatitis B and C
Severity	Mild	Commonly severe	Moderate	Can be severe and lead to fulminant hepatitis	Highly virulent with common progression to fulminant hepatitis and hepatic failure, especially in pregnant patients	Moderate
Prognosis	Generally good	Worsens with age and debility	Moderate	Fair, worsens in chronic cases; can lead to chronic hepatitis D and chronic liver disease	Good unless pregnant	Generally good; no current treatment recommendations
Progression to chronicity	None	Occasional	10–50% of cases	Occasional	None	Not known; no association with chronic liver disease

Pathophysiology

Hepatic encephalopathy—a set of CNS disorders—results when the liver can no longer detoxify the blood. Liver dysfunction and collateral vessels that shunt blood around the liver to the systemic circulation permit toxins absorbed from the GI tract to circulate freely to the brain.

Ammonia's role

Ammonia is one of the main toxins causing hepatic encephalopathy. Ammonia is a by-product of protein metabolism. The liver transforms ammonia to urea, which the kidneys excrete. When the liver fails to do this, ammonia levels increase and ammonia is delivered to the brain.

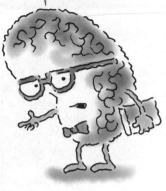

When the liver can't transform ammonia to urea, ammonia is delivered to the brain.

What to look for

Signs and symptoms vary, depending on the severity of neurological involvement. The disorder progresses through these four stages, with symptoms that can fluctuate from one stage to another:

 prodromal stage—slight personality changes (disorientation, forgetfulness and slurred speech) and a slight tremor

 impending stage—tremor progresses to asterixis (the hallmark of hepatic encephalopathy), characterised by quick irregular extensions and flexions of the wrists and fingers, lethargy, aberrant behaviour and apraxia

 stuporous stage—hyperventilation with stupor; noisy and abusive patient when stimulated

 comatose stage—includes hyperactive reflexes, upgoing plantars, coma and a musty, sweet breath odour.

What tests tell you

Tests that aid in diagnosing hepatic encephalopathy include:
- elevated liver function tests and PT
- increased serum albumin and decreased urea and blood glucose levels
- serum electrolytes that reveal hypokalaemia and hyponatraemia.

How it's treated

Treatment goals for the patient with hepatic failure are correcting the underlying cause and reducing blood ammonia levels. Treatment measures include:
- administration of antibiotics to destroy intestinal bacteria that breaks down protein into ammonia
- continuous aspiration of blood from the stomach
- limitation on dietary protein
- lactulose administration to reduce blood ammonia levels
- if hepatic encephalopathy is present neurological management must also be included (see Chapter 3).

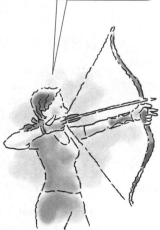

Aim for the treatment targets: correcting the underlying cause and reducing your patient's blood ammonia levels.

But wait, there's more

Other possible treatments include:
- potassium supplements
- haemodialysis to temporarily clear toxic blood
- exchange transfusions

- salt-poor albumin to maintain fluid and electrolyte balance
- shunt placement or paracentesis if ascites is a problem.

What to do

- Use ABCDE assessment. Monitor the patient's airway and respiratory status frequently, at least every 1–2 hours. Maintain a patent airway, and position the patient with the head of the bed elevated.
- Monitor the patient's oxygen saturation levels.
- Assess the patient's neurological status to establish a baseline, and report any changes. Reorient the patient as necessary.
- Monitor the patient's cardiac status and vital signs often, at least every hour.
- Assess the patient's haemodynamic parameters closely, at least every hour. Monitor for indications of fluid volume deficit or excess.
- Assess the patient's urinary output hourly. Notify the doctor if output is less than 0.5 ml/kg/hour.
- Measure the patient's abdominal girth or intra-abdominal pressure.
- Assess the patient for signs and symptoms of fluid excess, including peripheral oedema, jugular vein distention, tachypnoea and crackles that don't clear with coughing.
- Monitor blood results, such as renal function, liver enzymes, serum albumin, total protein and serum electrolytes.
- Monitor the patient's nutritional intake and maintain calorie count.
- Check finger-stick blood glucose levels every 4 hours or as ordered and assess for signs and symptoms of hyperglycaemia and hypoglycaemia.
- Institute bleeding precautions and monitor the patient for signs and symptoms of bleeding.
- Administer prescribed medications. Check with the doctor to adjust the dose of lactulose to allow for three to four semiformed stools per day.
- Assist with paracentesis, as indicated.
- Begin emergency treatment to control bleeding if variceal rupture occurs.
- Provide supportive care to the patient and their family.

Intra-abdominal hypertension

Intra-abdominal hypertension, the elevation of intra-abdominal pressure, commonly occurs in the critical care unit and affects medical patients just as often as it does trauma and surgical patients. If untreated, intra-abdominal hypertension can lead to abdominal compartment syndrome, a medical emergency that accounts for significant morbidity and mortality in critically ill patients.

Clear-cut measures

Intra-abdominal hypertension is defined as an elevation of intra-abdominal pressure of 12 mmHg or greater. The World Society on Abdominal

Compartment Syndrome has identified four grades of severity of intra-abdominal hypertension:

Grade I—IAP between 12 and 15 mmHg

Grade II—IAP between 16 and 20 mmHg

Grade III—IAP between 21 and 25 mmHg

Grade IV—IAP greater than 25 mmHg.

Organ breakdown

According to the World Society, abdominal compartment syndrome is organ dysfunction that occurs as the end-stage complication of untreated intra-abdominal hypertension. This complication affects the mesenteric, hepatic and intestinal arterial systems and can diminish blood flow to various intra-abdominal organs.

What causes it

Both intra-abdominal hypertension and abdominal compartment syndrome result from capillary endothelial damage and widespread interstitial oedema in the body, including the bowel and mesentery. Many medical and surgical patients requiring care in the critical care unit have these conditions. The incidence of intra-abdominal hypertension in high-risk critical care unit patients is 5–50%.

Common conditions

Intra-abdominal hypertension is especially prevalent in patients with systemic inflammatory response syndrome and sepsis. Other causes include:
- abdominal trauma
- GI haemorrhage
- pancreatitis
- pelvic fracture
- ruptured aortic aneurysm
- burns (large areas, full-thickness)
- shock
- aggressive fluid resuscitation
- cirrhosis
- peritonitis
- postabdominal surgery
- morbid obesity.

How it happens

Interstitial oedema in the bowel and mesentery as a result of capillary endothelial damage is the primary pathophysiological cause of intra-abdominal hypertension and abdominal compartment syndrome. Although

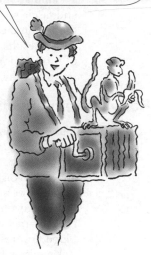

Abdominal compartment syndrome, the end-stage complication of untreated intra-abdominal hypertension, can diminish blood flow to various intra-abdominal organs.

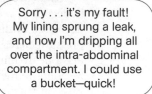

Sorry . . . it's my fault! My lining sprung a leak, and now I'm dripping all over the intra-abdominal compartment. I could use a bucket—quick!

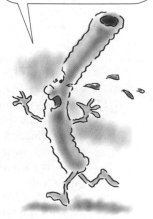

an initial event triggers the capillary damage, the release of proinflammatory cytokines in response to this insult also contributes to the widespread endothelial damage that occurs.

Leaks and stretching

As a result of 'leaky' capillaries, several litres of interstitial fluid can accumulate in the intra-abdominal compartment. The abdominal wall and fascia slowly stretch as this fluid accumulates. Overstretching of the abdominal tissues quickly leads to decreased abdominal compliance, which results in elevated intra-abdominal pressure. Sustained elevation of intra-abdominal pressure has significant adverse effects on organ perfusion throughout the body.

Body system effects

Pathophysiological changes associated with intra-abdominal hypertension and abdominal compartment syndrome produce these body system effects:

- *Gastrointestinal*—Elevated pressure in the abdominal cavity leads to abdominal distention and compression on the mesenteric, hepatic and intestinal vessels. Capillary blood flow within the abdomen becomes completely obstructed if the intra-abdominal pressure rises to the point that it equals that of the capillary bed (15–25 mmHg). Obstruction of capillary blood flow results in decreased venous flow, venous congestion, worsening ischaemia and, eventually, bowel necrosis. In addition, decreased portal blood flow results in visceral oedema within the portal system, further aggravating the rise in intra-abdominal pressure.
- *Cardiovascular*—Compression of the vena cava and portal vein results in decreased venous return to the heart (decreased preload), resulting in decreased cardiac output. Intrathoracic pressure rises as the intra-abdominal pressure increases, causing a reduction in cardiac compliance and severe diastolic dysfunction. Increased systemic afterload also occurs as the body responds to the drop in cardiac output by promoting vasoconstriction. This vasoconstriction, along with the low cardiac output, leads to further cardiac decompensation.
- *Pulmonary*—As intrathoracic pressure rises due to increased intra-abdominal pressure, the diaphragm is pushed upwards into the chest, resulting in respiratory compromise. In a mechanically ventilated patient to maintain an adequate tidal volume, peak pressures rise (increased pulmonary vascular resistance) as the ventilator drives air into the lungs. If these pressures continue to go unchecked, barotrauma can result quickly, leading to hypercapnia (elevated carbon dioxide) and hypoxia. Decreased cardiac output in combination with increased pulmonary vascular resistance can trigger the release of inflammatory mediators from the gut, resulting in pulmonary capillary damage, pulmonary interstitial oedema and a syndrome that closely mirrors acute respiratory distress syndrome.
- *Renal*—Direct pressure on the renal parenchyma (especially the renal capsule) and renal veins leads to oedema of the kidneys. At the same time,

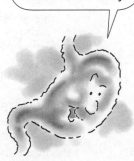

It's hard to believe that a little extra fluid in the gut can wreak so much havoc on the body.

decreased cardiac output and aortic compression compromise renal perfusion. Consequently, glomerular filtration decreases, leading to decreased urine output and possible renal insufficiency and failure.

- *Central nervous system*—Venous return to the chest is hampered by increased intrathoracic pressure caused by intra-abdominal hypertension. This decrease in venous return results in venous congestion of the arms and neck. Elevations in intracranial pressure occur as the congestion progresses up through the internal jugular vein into the cranial vault.

> Assess the abdomen for tenseness, tenderness, and increased girth.

What to look for

Intra-abdominal hypertension and abdominal compartment syndrome produce significant adverse systemic and haemodynamic effects. Assess the patient for these signs and symptoms:

- tense abdominal wall
- increased abdominal girth (round belly sign characterised by abdominal distention with increased ratio of anteroposterior-to-transverse diameter)
- abdominal tenderness
- shallow respirations
- oliguria or anuria
- tachycardia
- hypotension
- hypercapnia
- hypoxia
- decreased cardiac output and index
- increased central venous pressure (CVP)
- increased intra-abdominal pressure (via urinary bladder catheter).

What tests tell you

The gold standard for diagnosing intra-abdominal hypertension is measurement of the intra-abdominal pressure. (See *Measuring intra-abdominal pressure*, page 430.)

Off the gold standard

Other diagnostic findings include:
- elevated urea and creatinine.
- ABG levels that indicate hypoxia and hypercapnia.

How it's treated

Treatment goals include reducing intra-abdominal pressure and improving perfusion to the affected organs. Specific treatments may include:
- diuretics to reduce interstitial oedema
- possible fluid restriction
- I.V. albumin to maintain CVP between 8 and 12 mmHg
- inotropic support with vasopressors to improve cardiac output and tissue perfusion

Measuring intra-abdominal pressure

Intra-abdominal pressure can be measured either directly (via a peritoneal catheter) or indirectly (using an intraluminal bladder catheter). The indirect bladder technique is used most commonly and involves placing the patient in a supine position and instilling 50–100 ml of fluid into the bladder. It uses a pressure transducer or fluid manometer connected to the bladder catheter and the patient's urine as a transmitting medium. A pressure measurement is made from the catheter after it has been occluded distal to the transducer or air release port.

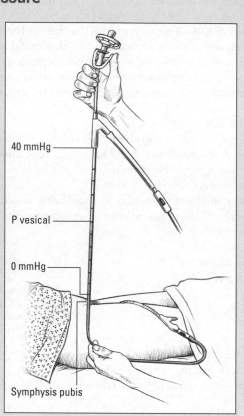

40 mmHg

P vesical

0 mmHg

Symphysis pubis

- continuous renal replacement therapy for fluid removal and management
- mechanical ventilation to maintain adequate gas exchange
- NG suctioning to remove excess air and fluid from intestinal lumen
- possible bowel purging using enemas or rectal tubes
- positioning to reduce vena cava compression (semirecumbent, tilted to left side)
- surgical decompression.

What to do
- Administer I.V. fluids to help minimise abdominal ischaemia.
- Administer oxygen to help maximise tissue perfusion.
- Be prepared to provide mechanical ventilation if the patient begins to experience respiratory distress.
- Administer sedation and analgesics to help decrease tissue oxygenation needs.
- Be prepared to assist with paracentesis.

> The key to success is reducing intra-abdominal pressure and improving perfusion to the affected organs.

- Monitor intra-abdominal pressures at least every 2 hours, or according to your unit's policy.
- Maintain NG suctioning to remove all air and fluid from the intestinal tract.
- If the patient needs surgical decompression, prepare the patient for surgery.
- Provide emotional support to the patient and their family.

Quick quiz

1. The stomach's major functions include all of the following actions except:

A. moving the gastric contents into the small intestine.
B. completing digestion.
C. serving as a temporary storage area for food.
D. breaking down food into chyme.

Answer: B. The stomach doesn't complete the digestion process.

2. Bowel sounds that are high-pitched and gurgling and occurring 10 times per minute are classified as:

A. hypoactive.
B. hyperactive.
C. dull.
D. normal.

Answer: D. Normal bowel sounds are high-pitched, gurgling and occur irregularly from 5 to 34 times per minute. Hypoactive sounds are heard infrequently. Hyperactive bowel sounds are loud, high-pitched and occur frequently.

3. During abdominal paracentesis, the aspirated fluid amount should be limited to:

A. 1,500–2,000 ml.
B. 2,000–3,000 ml.
C. 1,000–2,000 ml.
D. 1,000–1,500 ml.

Answer: A. Removing more than 1,500–2,000 ml of peritoneal fluid at one time may lead to hypovolaemic shock.

4. Signs and symptoms of bowel perforation usually include all of the following findings except:

A. abdominal pain.
B. pyrexia.
C. pruritis.
D. absent bowel sounds.

Answer: C. Pruritis is usually associated with cirrhosis of the liver caused by bile pigments irritating the skin.

5. Grade IV intra-abdominal hypertension measures:

A. between 12 and 15 mmHg.
B. between 16 and 20 mmHg.

C. between 21 and 25 mmHg.
D. greater than 25 mmHg.

Answer: D. The World Society of Abdominal Compartment Syndrome defines Grade IV intra-abdominal hypertension as above 25 mmHg.

Scoring

☆☆☆   If you answered all five questions correctly, you deserve a gourmet meal! Clearly, you've digested all the information in this chapter.

☆☆   If you answered four questions correctly, read up and try again! Your hunger for GI information makes it easy to swallow.

☆   If you answered fewer than four questions correctly, you may be fact-starved. Chew over the chapter and then take the test again.

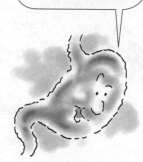

Now that you're full of GI knowledge, I'm passing you on to the renal system.

Just the facts

In this chapter, you'll learn:

♦ structure and function of the renal system
♦ assessment of the renal system
♦ diagnostic tests and treatments
♦ common renal disorders and related nursing care.

> The renal system is the body's water treatment plant; it collects waste products and expels them as urine.

Understanding the renal system

The renal system is the body's water treatment plant. The structures of the renal system include:

- kidneys
- ureters
- bladder
- urethra.

Kidney sitting

The kidneys are located on each side of the abdomen near the lower back. These compact organs contain a filtration system that processes about 180 L of fluid each day (120 ml/minute)—99% of this is reabsorbed leaving around 1–2 L of urine, which contains water and waste products. (See *A close look at a kidney*, page 434.)

It's all downhill from there

After it's produced by the kidneys, urine passes through the urinary system and is expelled from the body. The other structures of the system, extending downwards from the kidneys, include:

- ureters—two 40.5–45.5-cm muscular tubes that contract rhythmically (peristalsis) to transport urine from each kidney to the bladder

A close look at a kidney

Illustrated below is a kidney along with an enlargement of a nephron, the kidney's functional unit.

Kidney keys

Major structures of the kidney include:

- medulla—inner portion of the kidney, made up of renal pyramids and tubular structures
- renal artery—supplies blood to the kidney
- renal pyramid—channels output to the renal pelvis for excretion
- renal calyx—channels formed urine from the renal pyramids to the renal pelvis
- renal vein—about 99% of filtered blood is circulated through the renal vein back to the general circulation; the remaining 1%, which contains waste products, undergoes further processing in the kidney
- renal pelvis—after blood that contains waste products is processed in the kidney, the urine thus formed is channelled to the renal pelvis
- ureter—a tube that terminates in the urethra; urine enters the urethra for excretion
- cortex—outer layer of the kidney.

Note the nephron

The nephron is the functional and structural unit of the kidney. Each kidney contains about 1 million nephrons. Their two main activities are selective readsorption and secretion of ions and mechanical filtration of fluids, wastes, electrolytes and acids and bases. Components of the nephron include:

- glomerulus—a network of twisted capillaries that acts as a filter for the passage of protein-free and red blood cell-free filtrate to the proximal convoluted tubules
- Bowman's capsule—the structure that contains the glomerulus and acts as a filter for urine
- proximal convoluted tubule—the site of readsorption of glucose, amino acids, metabolites and electrolytes from filtrate; resorbed substances then return to the circulation
- loop of Henle—a U-shaped nephron tubule located in the medulla and extending from the proximal convoluted tubule to the distal convoluted tubule; the site for further concentration of filtrate through readsorption
- distal convoluted tubule—the site from which filtrate enters the collecting tubule
- collecting tubule—the structure that releases urine.

Kidney

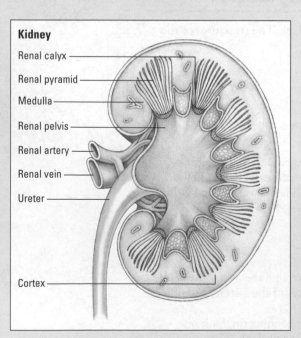

Renal calyx
Renal pyramid
Medulla
Renal pelvis
Renal artery
Renal vein
Ureter
Cortex

Nephron

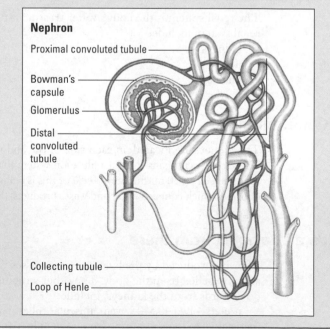

Proximal convoluted tubule
Bowman's capsule
Glomerulus
Distal convoluted tubule
Collecting tubule
Loop of Henle

- urinary bladder—a sac with muscular walls that collects and holds urine (300–500 ml) expelled from the ureters every few seconds
- urethra—a narrow passageway (surrounded by the prostate gland in men) from the bladder to the outside of the body through which urine is excreted.

That isn't all

The renal system is a major regulatory system as well. Its roles include:
- maintaining fluid and electrolyte balance
- maintaining acid–base balance
- detoxifying the blood and eliminating wastes
- regulating blood pressure
- aiding red blood cell (RBC) production.

I'm a major player in a major regulatory system. Doo-wah-doo, Daddio.

Fluid and electrolyte balance

The kidneys maintain fluid and electrolyte balance in the body by regulating the amount and makeup of the fluid inside and around the cells.

Exchange interchange

The kidneys maintain the volume and composition of extracellular and, to a lesser extent, intracellular fluid. They do so by continuously exchanging water and solutes across their cell membranes. The solutes include electrolytes, such as hydrogen, sodium, potassium, chloride, bicarbonate, sulphate and phosphate ions.

Hormones and osmoreceptors

Hormones partly control the kidneys' role in fluid balance by regulating the response of specialised sensory nerve endings (osmoreceptors) to changes in osmolality (the ionic concentration of a solution). Problems in hormone concentration can cause fluctuations in sodium and potassium concentrations that, in turn, may lead to hypertension.

The two hormones involved are:

Two hormones— ADH and aldosterone— are involved in fluid balance.

   antidiuretic hormone (ADH), produced by the pituitary gland

   aldosterone, produced by the adrenal cortex.

The ABCs of ADH

ADH changes the collecting tubules' permeability to water. Here's how:
- When ADH concentration in plasma is high, the tubules are most permeable to water. This condition creates a highly concentrated but small volume of urine.
- When ADH concentration is low, the tubules are less permeable to water. This situation creates a larger volume of less concentrated urine.

Age and ADH

As a person ages, tubular readsorption and renal concentrating ability decline because the size and number of functioning nephrons decrease.

All about aldosterone and sodium

Aldosterone regulates water readsorption by the distal tubules and changes urine concentration by increasing sodium readsorption. Here's how:
• A high plasma aldosterone concentration increases sodium and water readsorption by the tubules and decreases sodium and water excretion in the urine.
• A low plasma aldosterone concentration promotes sodium and water excretion.

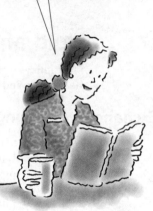

Aldosterone regulates water readsorption and changes urine concentration by increasing sodium readsorption.

Aldosterone and potassium

Aldosterone also helps control the secretion of potassium by the distal tubules. A high aldosterone concentration increases the excretion of potassium. Other factors that affect potassium secretion include:
• amount of potassium ingested
• number of hydrogen ions secreted
• potassium levels in the cells
• amount of sodium in the distal tubule
• glomerular filtration rate (GFR), which is the rate at which plasma is filtered as it flows through the glomerular capillary filtration membrane.

Going against the current

The kidneys concentrate urine through the countercurrent exchange system. In this system, fluid flows in opposite directions through parallel tubes, up and down parallel sides of the loops of Henle. A concentration gradient causes fluid exchange; the longer the loop, the greater the concentration gradient.

Acid–base balance

To regulate acid–base balance, the kidneys:
• secrete hydrogen ions
• resorb sodium and bicarbonate ions
• acidify phosphate salts
• produce ammonia.

Earning a PhD in pH balance

All of these regulating activities keep the blood at its normal pH of 7.35–7.45. Acidosis occurs when the pH falls below 7.35, and alkalosis occurs when the pH rises above 7.45.

Detoxification and waste elimination

The kidneys collect and eliminate wastes from the body in a three-step process:

glomerular filtration, in which the kidney's blood vessels, or glomeruli, filter blood flowing through them

tubular reabsorption, in which the tubules (minute canals that make up the kidney) reabsorb the filtered fluid

tubular secretion, in which the filtered substance is then released by the tubules.

Clear the way

Clearance is the complete removal of a substance from the blood. It's commonly described as the amount of blood that can be cleared in a specific time. For example, creatinine clearance is the volume of blood in millilitres that the kidneys can clear of creatinine in 1 minute.

Some substances are filtered out of the blood by the glomeruli. Dissolved substances that remain in the fluid may be resorbed by the renal tubular cells. (See *Understanding GFR*, page 438.)

Nephron compensation

In a patient whose kidneys have atrophied from disease, healthy nephrons (the filtering units of the kidney) enlarge to compensate. As nephron damage progresses, the enlargement no longer adequately compensates and the patient's GFR slows. (See *Age-related renal changes*, page 438.)

Tubular transport-ability

The amount of a substance that's resorbed or secreted depends on the substance's maximum tubular transport capacity, or the maximum amount of a substance that can be reabsorbed or secreted in 1 minute without saturating the renal system.

For example, in diabetes mellitus, excess glucose in the blood overwhelms the renal tubules and causes glucose to appear in the urine (glycosuria).

Blood pressure regulation

High blood pressure (hypertension) can damage blood vessels as well as cause hardening of the kidneys (nephrosclerosis), a leading cause of chronic renal failure.

Hypertension regulation

Hypertension can stem from renin—angiotensin hyperactivity (as well as from fluid and electrolyte imbalance). The kidneys aid blood pressure

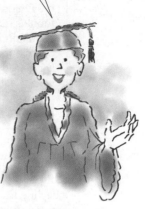

Normal blood pH has a narrow range. Acidosis occurs when pH falls below 7.35, and alkalosis occurs when pH rises above 7.45. PhDs need a different kind of grading system.

Understanding GFR

Glomerular filtration rate (GFR) is the rate at which the glomeruli filter blood. A normal GFR is about 120 ml/minute. GFR depends on:

- permeability of capillary walls
- vascular pressure
- filtration pressure.

GFR and clearance

Clearance is the complete removal of a substance from the blood. The most accurate way of estimating glomerular filtration is by using creatinine since it is filtered by the glomeruli but not resorbed by the tubules. Creatinine clearance has for many years been the way of estimating GFR. However, because creatinine levels are dependent on muscle mass, age, gender and race calculations of how well creatinine is cleared takes account of these. eGFR is the most recently advocated way of estimating GFR and though there are several ways of calculating this, the most common takes account of age, race and gender. Your laboratory should do this for you if given the variables.

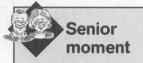

Senior moment

Age-related renal changes

By age 70, a person's blood urea levels increase by 21%. Other age-related changes that affect renal function include:

- diminished kidney size
- impaired renal clearance of drugs
- reduced bladder size and capacity
- decreased renal response to sodium intake.

regulation by producing and secreting the enzyme renin in response to reduced glomerular filtrate. Reduced glomerular filtrate is often a result of a decline in kidney perfusion. So the aim is to improve perfusion through increasing blood pressure. Renin, in turn, forms angiotensin I, which is converted into the more potent angiotensin II.

Pressure promotion

Angiotensin II increases low arterial blood pressure levels by:
- increasing peripheral vasoconstriction
- stimulating aldosterone secretion.

The increase in aldosterone promotes the readsorption of sodium and water to correct the fluid deficit and inadequate blood flow (renal ischaemia).

RBC production

Erythropoietin is a hormone that prompts the bone marrow to increase RBC production (erythropoiesis). The kidneys secrete erythropoietin when the oxygen supply to the kidneys drops or is chronically low (as in severe COPD for example). Chronic renal failure results in anaemia.

Vitamin D and calcium formation

The kidneys also produce active vitamin D and help regulate calcium balance and bone metabolism. Loss of renal function results in insufficient calcium levels (hypocalcaemia).

Simply put, the kidneys secrete renin, which forms angiotensin I, which is converted into angiotensin II.

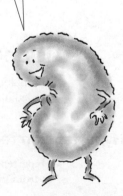

Renal assessment

Renal assessment and monitoring are major parts of critical care nursing and will usually take place regularly in the critically ill. The frequency depends on the severity of illness. It is important to think about a framework for assessment.

Being systematic

Assessment of the renal system includes knowing:
- History of the present complaint
- Health history
- Clinical assessment and monitoring
- Results and significance of diagnostic tests and investigations

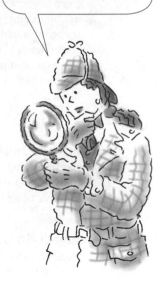

Collect clues from the patient's health history to find out about the cause and severity of their renal condition.

History of the present complaint

In essence you need to know why the patient has come into hospital and into critical care, to know any timescales and key events. In particular, find out an symptoms and how these relate to renal function.

Health history

Build your patient's health history by asking short, open-ended questions. Conduct the interview in several short sessions if you have to, depending on the severity of your patient's condition. Ask their family to provide information if your patient can't.

The health history includes information about the patient's current and previous illnesses and treatments as well as medication and family and lifestyle factors.

Current health status

Find out how the patient's symptoms developed and progressed. Ask how long they have had the problem, how it affects their daily routine and when and how it began. Ask about related signs and symptoms, such as nausea and vomiting. If your patient has any pain, ask about its location, radiation, intensity, duration and what precipitates or relieves it.

Previous health status

For clues about the patient's current condition, explore their past medical problems. Certain systemic diseases, such as diabetes mellitus, systemic lupus erythematosus, hypertension, sickle cell anaemia, Goodpasture's syndrome, acute glomerulonephritis and acute pyelonephritis may contribute to the development of acute renal failure.

Ask the patient whether they have a history of renal disease or have ever had a kidney or bladder tumour. Find out what treatments they received and the treatment outcomes. Ask about any traumatic injuries, surgery or conditions that required hospitalisation or any recent diagnostic test that involved the use of a contrast medium.

> I need to stay in shape. Many drugs are eliminated by the kidneys.

Drug check

Ask your patient if they're now taking any medications and what they are. Ask if they have any known allergies to foods or medications.

Many drugs are eliminated by the kidneys, so the patient with compromised kidney function, such as chronic renal failure, may need to avoid certain drugs or receive reduced dosages to prevent further renal problems. Drugs that may require a reduced dosage include angiotensin-converting enzyme inhibitors, ciprofloxacin, digoxin, histamine-2 receptor antagonists, penicillins, sulphonamides and low-molecular-weight heparins.

Examples of drugs that impose a risk of nephrotoxicity include aminoglycosides (such as gentamicin). In the acutely ill, shocked or elderly, drugs such as ACE inhibitors and NSAIDs may reduce renal perfusion. ACE inhibitors block the renin–angiotensin–aldosterone pathway described above as an important controller of blood pressure. A kidney that is underperfused or insulted by some other mechanism such as toxins or infection produces prostaglandins which cause vasodilation in the kidney and improve local blood flow. Since NSAIDs block prostaglandins the result is that yet another mechanism of improving renal perfusion is blocked.

Family history

Because some renal disorders are hereditary, ask the patient whether anyone in their family has a history of renal disease. Polycystic kidney disease is one example of an inherited disorder that can lead to renal failure.

Lifestyle patterns

Psychological and sociologic factors can affect the patient's health. To determine how such factors may have contributed to your patient's current problem, ask about their:
- home life
- stress level
- occupation.

> Environmental agents that could cause kidney problems might be found in the patient's home or workplace.

At work and play

Ask your patient about possible exposure at work or home to agents that may be nephrotoxic, such as cleaning products, pesticides, lead and mercury. Also ask about their alcohol, tobacco, caffeine and drug use, as well as their dietary habits, cultural practices that affect diet and dietary restrictions, such as a vegetarian or low-potassium diet.

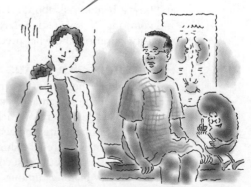

Clinical assessment and monitoring

Proceed in an orderly way with the physical examination of your patient's renal system. Use what skills you have and report any abnormal findings. (See *Interpreting renal findings*.)

Interpreting renal findings

After assessment is complete the findings may inform a diagnostic impression of the patient's condition. Check this table to find groupings of significant signs and symptoms, related findings you may discover during the health history and physical assessment and the possible cause indicated by a cluster of these findings.

Key signs and symptoms	Related findings		Possible cause
• Oliguria, possibly progressing to anuria • Haematuria or coffee-coloured urine • Smoky urine	• Poststreptococcal throat or skin infection • Systemic lupus erythematosus, vasculitis or scleroderma • Pregnancy	• Elevated blood pressure • Periorbital oedema progressing to dependent oedema • Ascites • Pleural effusion	Acute glomerulonephritis
• Oliguria • Dark, smoky urine • Anorexia and vomiting	• Crush injury or illness associated with shock such as sepsis • Muscle necrosis • Exposure to nephrotoxic agent such as lead • History of recently received contrast medium for radiological investigation.	• Recent aminoglycoside therapy • Oliguria progressing to anuria • Dyspnoea • Bibasilar crackles • Dependent oedema	Acute tubular necrosis
• Proteinuria, haematuria, vomiting and pruritus (patient may be asymptomatic until advanced disease stage)	• Primary renal disorder, such as membranoproliferative glomerulonephritis and focal segmental glomerulosclerosis	• Elevated blood pressure • Ascites and dependent oedema • Dyspnoea • Bibasilar crackles	Chronic glomerulonephritis
• Urinary frequency and urgency • Burning sensation on urination • Nocturia, cloudy haematuria and dysuria • Lower back or flank pain	• Female patient • Recurrent urinary tract infection • Recent chemotherapy or systemic antibiotic therapy	• Recent vigorous sexual activity • Suprapubic pain on palpation • Fever • Inflamed perineal area	Cystitis
• Severe radiating pain from costovertebral angle to flank and suprapubic region and from external genitalia • Nausea and vomiting • Haematuria	• Strenuous physical activity in hot environment • Previous renal calculi • Recent kidney infection	• Fever and chills • Poor skin turgor, concentrated urine and dry mucous membranes	Nephrolithiasis
• Abdominal or flank pain • Gross haematuria	• Youth (especially younger than age 7) • Congenital anomalies • Firm, smooth, palpable abdominal mass in enlarged abdomen	• Fever • Elevated blood pressure • Urine retention	Wilms' tumour

Inspection

In a normal adult, the abdomen is smooth, flat or scaphoid (concave), and symmetrical. Abdominal skin should be free from scars, lesions, bruises and discolouration.

Disclosing dysfunction Patients'

Abdomens should be inspected for gross enlargements or fullness by comparing the left and right sides, noting asymmetrical areas. Extremely prominent veins may accompany other vascular signs associated with renal dysfunction, such as hypertension.

Distention, skin tightness and glistening, and striae (streaks or linear scars caused by rapidly developing skin tension) may signal fluid retention.

Urethral meatus inspection

Urethral meatus inspection may reveal several abnormalities. In a male patient, a meatus deviating from the normal central location may represent a congenital defect. In any patient, inflammation and discharge may signal urethral infection. Ulceration usually indicates a sexually transmitted disease.

Assess fluid-volume status

Fluid-volume status should be assessed by observing for jugular vein distention and peripheral oedema, periorbital oedema and sacral oedema. The skin should be checked for turgor and mobility. Inspect the tongue and mucous membranes for moisture.

Skin turgor may be an unreliable sign of hydration in older people because of reduced subcutaneous tissue. Check turgor by pinching the subcutaneous tissue at the forehead or over the xiphoid process and watching for a quick return to baseline.

Calcium culprit

When your patient complains of muscle spasms and paraesthesia in their limbs, check for signs of calcium deficiency such as cramps and twitching muscles. The most accurate way of diagnosing hypocalcaemia is to measure serum calcium.

Diagnostic tests

Diagnostic tests commonly ordered for a patient with known or suspected renal disease may include blood studies, radiography, renal angiography, renal ultrasound and urine studies.

Blood studies

Blood studies used to diagnose and evaluate kidney function include:
- full blood count (FBC) to evaluate white blood cells, RBCs, haemoglobin (Hb) and haematocrit (Hct)
- blood urea testing
- electrolyte measurements to evaluate calcium, phosphorus, chloride, potassium and sodium levels
- serum creatinine, serum osmolality, serum protein, uric acid, creatinine clearance and urea clearance measurements. (See *Interpreting blood studies in renal disease*.)

Renal angiography

Renal angiography is used to visualise the arterial tree, capillaries and venous drainage of the kidneys. The test involves the use of a contrast medium injected under fluoroscopy into a catheter in the femoral artery or vein.

Interpreting blood studies in renal disease

Here's how you may interpret the results of blood studies used in diagnosing renal disease.

Full blood count

An increased white blood cell count may indicate urinary tract infection, peritonitis (in peritoneal dialysis patients) or kidney transplantation infection and rejection.

Red blood cell (RBC) count, haemoglobin level and haematocrit (Hct) decrease in a patient with chronic renal insufficiency resulting from decreased erythropoietin production by the kidneys. Hct also provides an index of fluid balance because it indicates the percentage of RBCs in the blood.

Blood urea

Increased blood urea levels may indicate glomerulonephritis, extensive pyogenic infection, oliguria (from mercuric chloride poisoning or posttraumatic renal insufficiency), tubular obstruction or other obstructive uropathies. Because nonrenal conditions can cause urea levels to increase, interpret urea levels in conjunction with serum creatinine levels.

Electrolytes

Because the kidneys regulate fluid and electrolyte balance, a critically ill patient with renal disease may experience significant serum electrolyte imbalances. The most commonly measured electrolytes are:

- *calcium and phosphorus*—calcium and phosphorus levels have an inverse relationship; when one increases, the other decreases. In renal failure, the kidneys aren't able to excrete phosphorus, resulting in hyperphosphataemia and hypocalcaemia.
- *chloride*—chloride levels relate inversely to bicarbonate levels, reflecting acid–base balance. In renal disease, elevated chloride levels suggest metabolic acidosis. Hyperchloraemia occurs in renal tubular necrosis, severe dehydration and complete renal shutdown. Hypochloraemia may occur with pyelonephritis.
- *potassium*—hyperkalaemia occurs with renal insufficiency or acidosis. In renal shutdown, potassium may rapidly increase to life-threatening levels. Hypokalaemia may reflect renal tubular disease and the inability to reabsorb potassium from the tubules.

(continued)

Interpreting blood studies in renal disease (continued)

- *sodium*—sodium helps the kidneys regulate body fluid. Renal disease may result in the loss of sodium through the kidneys, again because of the inability of the tubules to reabsorb sodium.

Serum creatinine

Serum creatinine level reflects the glomerular filtration rate (GFR). Renal damage is indicated more accurately by increases in serum creatinine than by urea levels.

Serum osmolality

An increase in serum osmolality (ion concentration in the blood) with a simultaneous decrease in urine osmolality indicates diminished distal tubule responsiveness to circulating antidiuretic hormone. This is because the distal tubules are where antidiuretic hormone usually causes reabsorbtion of water.

Serum proteins

Levels of the serum protein albumin may decline sharply from loss in the urine when the glomerular vessels are damaged and leaky during nephritis or nephrosis. This in turn causes oedema as fluid leaks out of the systemic blood vessels when there is insufficient albumin to hold it in the blood. Nephrosis may also cause total serum protein levels to decrease.

Uric acid

Because uric acid clears from the body by glomerular filtration and tubular secretion, elevated levels may indicate impaired renal function; below-normal levels may indicate defective tubular absorption.

Creatinine and GFR

Creatinine has traditionally been the way that renal function has been measured. A raised creatinine level indicates reduced renal function. Creatinine is filtered but not is monitored in CKD (chronic kidney disease). Laboratories usually calculate eGFR using the four-variable MDRD (modification of diet in renal disease) method. These are serum creatinine concentration, age, sex and ethnic origin (for African-Caribbean people only, eGFR multiplied by 1.21). The eGFR is reported in ml/min/1.73 m^2. This only gives an estimate of GFR and is not valid in the following: children, acute renal failure, pregnancy, oedematus states, muscle-wasting disease states, amputees and malnourished patients. The estimation is most reliable in the UK Caucasian individuals and may be less reliable in other ethnic groups. (See *interpreting eGFR*.)

Urea clearance

While urea clearance is a less reliable measurement of GFR than creatinine clearance, it still provides a measure of overall renal function. High urea clearance rates may indicate that urea is not being filtered in the glomerulus as in shock and hypotension. In this case it will be accompanied by a rise in creatinine. But it also rises as increased amounts of water are reabsorbed from the tubules in dehydration. Urea levels are also raised when the blood is concentrated—so urea can be an indicator of dehydration if is not accompanied by a corresponding rise in creatinine.

Interpreting eGFR

Stage of CKD	ml/min/1.73 m^2	Recommended frequency of monitoring
1—Normal GFR	>90	Annually
2—Mild impairment	60–89	Annually
3—Moderate impairment	30–59	6 monthly
4—Severe impairment	15–29	3 monthly
5—Established	<15	3 monthly

Angiography of arteries

Renal arteriography (angiography of the arteries) may reveal:
- abnormal renal blood flow
- hypervascular renal tumours
- renal cysts
- renal artery stenosis
- renal artery aneurysms and arteriovenous fistulas
- pyelonephritis
- renal abscesses or inflammatory masses
- renal infarction
- renal trauma.

> Renal arteriography may reveal disorders such as these.

Nursing considerations
- Explain the procedure to the patient and confirm that they aren't allergic to iodine or shellfish. A patient with these allergies may have an adverse reaction to the contrast medium. If they have a seafood or dye allergy, a pretest preparation kit with prednisolone and chlorpheniramine may be given.
- Preprocedure testing should include evaluation of renal function (serum creatinine and urea) and potential risk of bleeding (prothrombin time, partial thromboplastin time and platelet count). Notify the doctor if results are abnormal.
- Report adverse reactions, such as nausea, vomiting, dizziness, headache and urticaria.
- Depending on the patient's renal status, the doctor may order increased fluids after the procedure or an increased rate of I.V. fluid infusion to flush the contrast medium out of the patient's system.
- The doctor may also order *N*-acetylcysteine to help limit the damage done to the renal tissues by the contrast medium.
- After the procedure, check the patient's serum creatinine and urea levels to evaluate renal function (contrast media can cause acute renal failure).

Renal ultrasound

Renal ultrasound is used to visualise kidney size, shape and placement. Renal ultrasound may reveal:
- hydronephrosis
- tumours
- cysts
- abscess
- trauma.

Nursing considerations
- Explain the procedure to the patient.
- No pretest preparation is needed.
- The test may be done at the bedside if the patient is unstable.

Urine studies

Urine studies, such as urinalysis and urine osmolality, can indicate acute renal failure, renal trauma and other disorders. Urinalysis can indicate renal or systemic disorders, warranting further investigation. A random urine specimen is used, preferably the first-voided morning specimen. (See *What urinalysis findings mean.*)

What urinalysis findings mean

Test	Normal values or findings	Abnormal findings	Possible causes of abnormal findings
Colour and odour	• Straw colour	Clear to black	Dietary changes; use of certain drugs; metabolic, inflammatory, or infectious disease
	• Slightly aromatic odour	Fruity odour	Diabetes mellitus, starvation, dehydration
	• Clear appearance	Turbid appearance	Renal infection
Specific gravity	• Between 1.005 and 1.030, with slight variations from one specimen to the next	Below-normal specific gravity (dilute urine)	Diabetes insipidus, glomerulonephritis, pyelonephritis, acute renal failure, alkalosis
		Above-normal specific gravity (concentrated urine)	Dehydration, nephrosis
		Fixed specific gravity	Severe renal damage
pH	• Between 4.5 and 8.0	Alkaline pH (above 8.0)	Chronic renal disease, urinary tract infection (UTI), metabolic or respiratory alkalosis
		Acidic pH (below 4.5)	Renal tuberculosis, phenylketonuria, acidosis
Protein	• No protein	Proteinuria	Renal disease (such as glomerulosclerosis, acute or chronic glomerulonephritis, nephrolithiasis, polycystic kidney disease, and acute or chronic renal failure)
Ketones	• No ketones	Ketonuria	Diabetes mellitus, starvation, conditions causing acutely increased metabolic demands and decreased food intake (such as vomiting and diarrhoea)
Glucose	• No glucose	Glycosuria	Diabetes mellitus, hyperglycaemia
Red blood cells (RBCs)	• 0–3 RBCs per high-power field	Numerous RBCs	UTI, obstruction, inflammation, trauma, or tumour; glomerulonephritis; renal hypertension; lupus nephritis; renal tuberculosis; renal vein thrombosis; hydronephrosis; pyelonephritis; parasitic bladder infection; polyarteritis nodosa; haemorrhagic disorder
Epithelial cells	• Few epithelial cells	Excessive epithelial cells	Renal tubular degeneration, acute tubular necrosis
White blood cells (WBCs)	• 0–4 WBCs per high-power field	Numerous WBCs	Urinary tract inflammation, especially cystitis or pyelonephritis
		Numerous WBCs and WBC casts	Renal infection (such as acute pyelonephritis and glomerulonephritis, nephrotic syndrome, pyogenic infection, and lupus nephritis)

(continued)

What urinalysis findings mean (continued)

Test	Normal values or findings	Abnormal findings	Possible causes of abnormal findings
Casts	• No casts (except occasional hyaline casts)	Excessive casts	Renal disease
		Excessive hyaline casts	Renal parenchymal disease, inflammation, glomerular capillary membrane trauma
		Epithelial casts	Renal tubular damage, nephrosis, eclampsia, chronic lead intoxication
		Fatty, waxy casts	Nephrotic syndrome, chronic renal disease, diabetes mellitus
		RBC casts	Renal parenchymal disease (especially glomerulonephritis), renal infarction, subacute bacterial endocarditis, sickle cell anaemia, blood dyscrasias, malignant hypertension, collagen disease
Crystals	• Some crystals	Numerous calcium oxalate crystals	Hypercalcaemia
		Cystine crystals (cystinuria)	Inborn metabolic error
Yeast cells	• No yeast crystals	Yeast cells in sediment	External genitalia contamination, vaginitis, urethritis, prostatovesiculitis
Parasites	• No parasites	Parasites in sediment	External genitalia contamination
Creatinine clearance	• Males (age 20): 90 mg/minute/1.73 m^2 of body surface • Females (age 20): 84 ml/minute/1.73 m^2 of body surface • Older patients: normally decreased concentrations (by 6 ml/minute/decade)	Above-normal creatinine clearance	Little diagnostic significance
		Below-normal creatinine clearance	Reduced renal blood flow (associated with shock or renal artery obstruction), acute tubular necrosis, acute or chronic glomerulonephritis, advanced bilateral renal lesions (as in polycystic kidney disease, renal tuberculosis, and cancer), nephrosclerosis, heart failure, severe dehydration

Urine osmolality is used to evaluate the diluting and concentrating ability of the kidneys and varies greatly with diet and hydration status. The ability to concentrate urine is one of the first functions lost in renal failure.

Nursing considerations
• Before urinalysis, collect a random urine specimen from the indwelling urinary catheter or, preferably, the first-voided morning specimen. Send the specimen to the laboratory immediately.
• For urine osmolality testing, collect a random urine sample, preferably the first-voided morning specimen.

Treatments

Renal disorders can adversely affect virtually every body system in a critically ill patient and may be fatal without effective treatment. Drug therapy is a treatment option in some cases, and others require dialysis of some kind.

Drug therapy

Drug therapy for renal disorders includes such agents as diuretics, vasoactive drugs for increased blood pressure and renal perfusion, and sulphonate cation-exchange resins to correct hyperkalaemia. (See *Commonly used drugs for renal disorders*.)

Ideally, drug therapy should be effective without impairing renal function. Drugs excreted mainly by the kidneys may require dosage adjustments to prevent nephrotoxicity.

Commonly used drugs for renal disorders

Drugs	Indications	Adverse reactions	Practice pointers
Adrenergic agent			
Noradrenaline	To maintain systemic blood pressure in acute hypotensive states refractory to fluid resuscitation	Anxiety, dizziness, headache, bradycardia, cardiac arrhythmias, hypertension, tissue necrosis (associated with extravasation of peripheral I.V. infusion), increased blood glucose, peripheral vasoconstriction leading to ischaemic peripheries.	• Continuously monitor the patient's cardiac rhythm and blood pressure. • Correct hypovolaemia before starting the infusion. • Administer I.V. infusion with an infusion device to control flow. • Don't mix other drugs with the infusion or administer via the same I.V. port as another infusion. • Administer into a central vein.
Alkalinising agent			
Sodium bicarbonate	To correct metabolic acidosis in patients with renal failure	Metabolic alkalosis, hypernatraemia, local pain and irritation at the injection site, hypokalaemia.	• Use with caution in patients with heart failure or renal insufficiency and patients receiving corticosteroids. • Assess the patient's cardiopulmonary status. • Monitor the patient for metabolic alkalosis and electrolyte imbalance, especially hypocalcaemia and hypokalaemia. • Monitor the I.V. site for irritation and infiltration. (Extravasation may cause tissue damage and necrosis.)
Loop diuretics			
Bumetanide Furosemide Torasemide	To inhibit sodium reabsorption in the renal tubule, promote diuresis and manage oedema	Mild GI disturbances, hyperglycaemia, hypotension, headache, fluid and electrolyte imbalance (hypokalaemia, hypochloraemia and hyponatraemia), metabolic alkalosis, electrocardiogram (ECG) changes, tinnitus and deafness with large rapid doses.	• Monitor the patient for fluid and electrolyte imbalance. • Monitor the patient for cardiac arrhythmias, especially ventricular. • Avoid using in the patient with sulphonamide hypersensitivity. • Use is contraindicated in anuria. • Be aware that ototoxicity may result with rapid I.V. administration of high dosages. • Carefully monitor the patient's intake and output.

(continued)

Commonly used drugs for renal disorders (continued)

Drugs	Indications	Adverse reactions	Practice pointers
Polystyrene sulphonate resins			
Calcium Resonium	To correct hyperkalaemia associated with renal failure	Rectal ulceration with rectal administration, hypernatraemia, hypercalcaemia, hypomagnesaemia, gastric irritation, nausea and vomiting, constipation, diarrhoea.	• Monitor the patient for electrolyte imbalance. • Monitor the patient for ECG changes (flat, inverted T wave and prominent U wave) and ventricular arrhythmias. • For oral administration, mix resin with water or sorbitol–never orange juice because of high potassium content. • Monitor elderly patients for constipation and faecal impaction. • Use cautiously in patients who require sodium restriction, such as those with heart failure or hypertension, to prevent the risk of sodium overload.

Renal replacement therapies

A critically ill patient with a renal disorder may need blood purifying treatments to remove toxic waste and excess fluid from the body. These are collectively called RRT (renal replacement therapies). The same treatments may also be used in sepsis, metabolic acidosis and in some drug overdoses.

What's it all about?

RRT has several key components and mechanisms:
- Blood is withdrawn from the patient via a mechanical pump.
- Anticoagulant is usually added to the blood to prevent it coagulating whilst in the 'extracorporeal' (out of the body) circuit.
- Water and solutes are removed via a filter and collected in waste bags.
- Dialysate/substitute/replacement fluid is added to the circuit to facilitate the process of solute removal (dialysis) or to replace essential water volume and solutes that will have been unavoidably removed in the process of filtration (haemofiltration).
- The treated blood is returned to the patient.

All methods of RRT involve these but the physiological mechanisms and mechanics of the extracorporeal circuit differ to some extent. The key differences of importance are discussed below in order that you can understand how they relate to practice in your area.

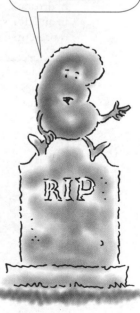

A renal disorder can affect every body system of a critically ill patient. It may be fatal without effective treatment.

Here comes the science . . .

There are several key concepts that explain how fluid and solutes move. This is essential knowledge prior to applying the science within RRT. These concepts are:

- diffusion
- ultrafiltration
- convection.

Diffusion describes the passive movement of *particles* (e.g. electrolytes in a solution) from an area of high-solute concentration to an area of low-solute concentration. The process is represented in the diagram below where particles are moving across a membrane.

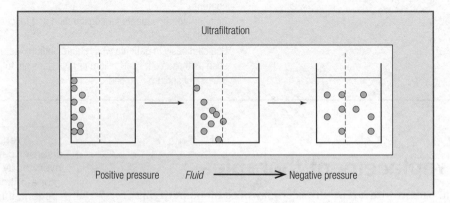

Ultrafiltration is the movement of fluid across a membrane driven by hydrostatic pressure. (Blood pressure and pressure applied by a roller pump in an RRT system are examples of hydrostatic pressure.) The process is represented in the diagram below.

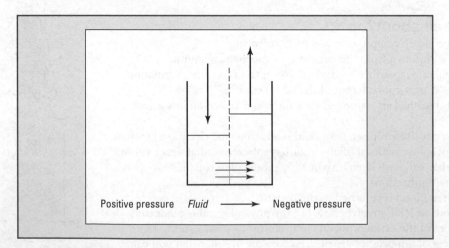

The pressure drives the fluid across the membrane. A positive pressure on one side will 'push' fluid through the membrane. A negative pressure on the other side will 'pull' fluid through the membrane. The positive and negative pressures produce a combined force called the *transmembrane pressure*— that is often measured and displayed on RRT machines in critical care.

Convection is the movement of solutes occurring with the flow of fluid across a semipermeable membrane. This is represented in the diagram below.

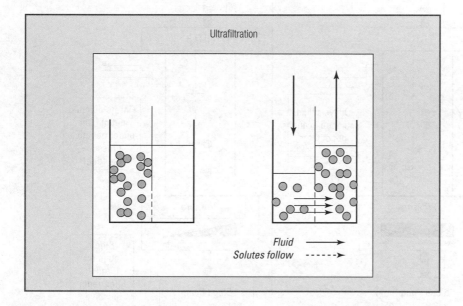

Whenever large volumes of fluid are drawn across a semipermeable membrane, substances dissolved in the fluid may be transported across the membrane, depending on their size. They are literally 'dragged' across the membrane and this has been referred to as 'solute drag'. This phenomenon can be likened to leaves being carried by wind; the harder the wind blows– the more leaves are transported.

Now let's apply the science

RRT is usually delivered by haemofiltration or dialysis in the critically ill. Haemodiafiltration combines haemofiltration and dialysis. The characteristics of these systems are presented in the diagram '*Dialysis and Haemofiltration compared*'.

Cellular components of blood (e.g. white and red bloods cells) and large protein molecules (e.g. albumin) will not pass through the filtration membrane used in RRT. However, many of the substances dissolved in

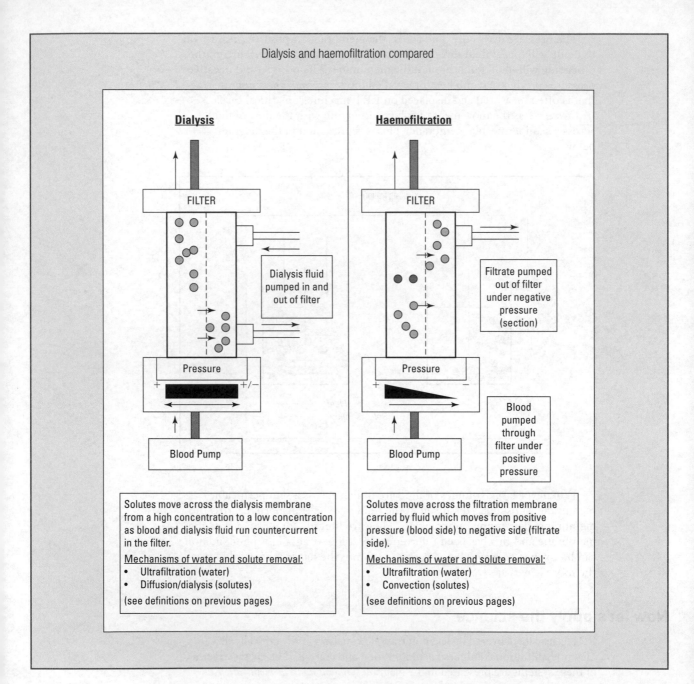

Dialysis and haemofiltration compared

Dialysis

FILTER

Dialysis fluid pumped in and out of filter

Pressure

+   +/−

Blood Pump

Solutes move across the dialysis membrane from a high concentration to a low concentration as blood and dialysis fluid run countercurrent in the filter.

Mechanisms of water and solute removal:
- Ultrafiltration (water)
- Diffusion/dialysis (solutes)

(see definitions on previous pages)

Haemofiltration

FILTER

Filtrate pumped out of filter under negative pressure (section)

Pressure

+   −

Blood pumped through filter under positive pressure

Solutes move across the filtration membrane carried by fluid which moves from positive pressure (blood side) to negative side (filtrate side).

Mechanisms of water and solute removal:
- Ultrafiltration (water)
- Convection (solutes)

(see definitions on previous pages)

What RRT removes from the blood	
Substances removed by RRT	*Substances not removed*
Water	White blood cells
Sodium	Red blood cells
Potassium	Platelets
Chloride	Proteins (albumin, fibrinogen)
Magnesium	
Calcium	
Phosphate	
Bicarbonate	
Hydrogen ions	
Glucose	
Urea	
Creatinine	
Endotoxins	
Drugs	

blood will pass through the membrane. (See *What RRT removes from the blood*.)

Haemofiltration (e.g. CVVH) uses high fluid flow rates causing significant *convection* and resultant rapid solute removal. It also uses highly permeable membranes.

Because dialysis does not use convection and instead relies on diffusion to cause solute movement—it is less effective at removing solutes. This is the reason that in the critically ill, where rapid biochemical/toxin abnormality correction is needed, haemofiltration is often the chosen method of renal replacement therapy in critical care.

One of the other advantages of the high convection in haemofiltration is that it allows the removal of soluble mediators of systemic inflammation that cause sepsis. These mediators are relatively 'heavy'. (One of the other methods of removal of sepsis mediators is through the binding of these to the filtration membrane.)

Understanding the effects of RRT on cellular and biochemical blood components puts the nurse in a position to be proactive—preventing complications, anticipating patients' needs and negotiating management plans with other clinical professionals. It is important to know when it is needed, when there may be contraindications or difficulties using RRT and when it might be stopped. (See *RRT—Indications, contraindications and termination of therapy*, page 454.)

RRT—Indications, contraindications and termination of therapy

Criteria for considering/initiating RRT

- Oliguria (urine output <200 ml/12 hours) with fluid overload/biochemical disorders.
- Anuria (urine output <50 ml/12 hours) with fluid overload/biochemical disorders.
- Azotaemia (urea >30 mmol/L).
- Symptoms of azotaemia: pericarditis, GI bleeding, encephalopathy, myopathy.
- Serum creatinine >400.
- Hyperkalaemia (K^+>6.5 mmol/L or rapidly rising).
- Severe dysnatraemia (Na^+>160 or <115 mmol/L).
- Severe metabolic acidaemia (pH<7.1).
- Drug toxicity with dialysable toxin.
- Severe sepsis.
- Multiorgan dysfunction syndrome.

Contraindications/difficulties

- Unethical to escalate treatment (e.g. in patient very unlikely to survive).
- Lack of vascular access.
- Haemodynamic instability (CVVH is the least haemodynamically compromising form of RRT because it is continuous whereas haemodialysis, for example, is often undertaken in rapid treatment episodes. Hypovolaemia should be addressed but in the face of serious effects of renal/metabolic disease—haemodynamic instability may not be a good reason for holding off with CVVH and it may even improve depending on the cause).

Criteria for weaning off RRT

- All criteria for initiating RRT are absent.
- Urine output averages 1 ml/kg over 24-hour period.
- Fluid balance can be kept approximately neutral with current urine output.
- There is a complication related to RRT.
- Biochemical abnormalities are resolved.

The RRT circuit

Knowing the key components of an RRT circuit should lead you to understand what equipment is needed to prepare for setting up, lining, priming and troubleshooting the circuit. However, you should refer to your specific local policy/protocol and recommended practice standards.

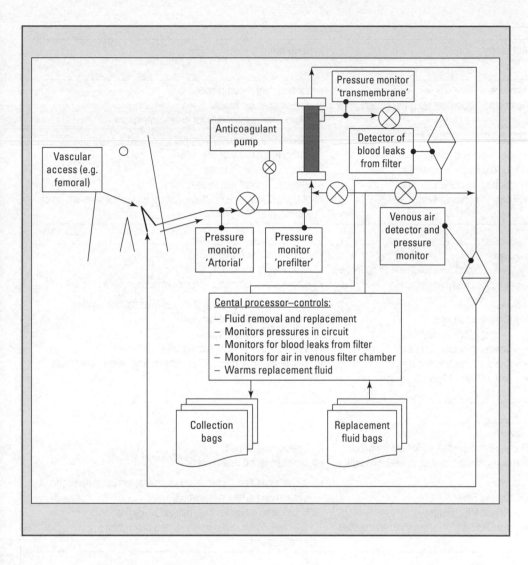

Common system alarms and circuit problems

Modern RRT machines have numerous alarms. These are all usually explained in the technical manual for each machine. Some alarms require prompt action since they indicate problems that compromise patient safety or the continuity of the circuit. The alarms requiring prompt action are presented in the following table.

Alarm	Aetiology	Management
Arterial/access pressure		
	Essence: Restricted blood flow from the patient	• Reduce blood pump speed • Check lines for kinks • Check vascular cannula for displacement/kink
	Causes: • Kinked blood lines • Kinked vascular cannula • Clotted vascular cannula • Cannula against vessel wall	• Change patient position if it is suspected that position is affecting patency of cannula • Flush vascular cannula • Reverse arterial and venous lines • If unresolvable, discontinue system and request re-sitting of cannula
Venous/return pressure		
	Essence: Restricted blood flow returning to patient via air detector chamber.	• Reduce blood pump speed • Check lines for kinks • Check vascular cannula for displacement/kink
	Causes: • Kinked blood lines • Kinked vascular cannula • Clotted vascular cannula • Cannula against vessel wall • Clot in filter at base of air detector chamber	• Change patient position if it is suspected that position is affecting patency of cannula • Flush vascular cannula • Reverse arterial and venous lines • If unresolvable, discontinue system and prime new circuit
Transmembrane pressure		
	Essence: Pressure required to suck fluid from blood through the filter membrane is increased.	• Check lines for kinks • Check coagulation • Increase blood pump speed
	Causes: • Clotted filter • Kinked filtrate line • Insufficient blood flow through the filter	• If sustained and incremental pressure increase, discontinue system and prime new circuit • If successive circuits clot, request re-evaluation of anticoagulation/consider increased predilution configuration
Blood leak		
	Essence: The filaments of the filter have ruptured and red blood cells are leaking through into the filtrate	• Check for blood (dip-stick) filtrate • Discontinue system and prime new circuit if blood leak is confirmed
	Other causes: • Occasionally this can be due to bubbles or other small artefacts in the blood leak detector chamber	

There are numerous other machine-specific errors that can occur—these will generate an error message and an error code will be displayed on the machine. The type of error and how to resolve it will be explained in the machine's manual. Examples of other problems related to RRT are presented in the following table.

RRT problems

Problem	Aetiology	Manifestations	Management
Hypotension			
	Increased ultrafiltration rate	Bleeding	Control amount of ultrafiltration
	Blood leak	Hypotension	Reconnect if disconnected
	Disconnection of lines		Control bleeding Raise patients legs Call Doctor Administer fluid as prescribed Stop system
Fluid and electrolyte changes			
	Too much/little removal of fluid	Changes in mentation ↓ or ↑ CVP, PCWP	Observe for changes in CVP or PCWP
	Inappropriate replacement of electrolytes	ECG changes	Observe for changes in vital signs
	Inappropriate replacement fluid	↓ or ↑ BP and HR abnormal electrolyte levels	Observe ECG for changes as a result of electrolyte abnormalities Monitor input and output values
Bleeding			
	System disconnection	Oozing from catheter insertion site or connections	Monitor clotting (APTT)
	Excessive anticoagulant dose	↓ Hb Faecal occult blood	Adjust anticoagulant
		Shock	Observe dressing on vascular access for blood loss
		↓ Consciousness	Observe for blood in filtrate (filter leak)
			Observe for signs of occult/internal bleeding
Access dislodgement or infection			
	Catheter/connections not secure Break in sterile technique Excessive patient movement	Bleeding from catheter Site or connections Inappropriate	Ensure as much of lines are visible Observe access site regularly Ensure that clamps are within easy reach at all times
		Flow/infusion Fever Inflammation at catheter site	Observe strict sterile technique when dressing vascular access, or manipulating lines

(continued)

RRT problems (continued)

Problem	Aetiology	Manifestations	Management
Temperature derangement			
	Cooling effect of giving large volumes of replacement fluid/ extracorporeal blood circulation	Clinical signs of hypothermia	Monitor temperature
		Low temperature readings on monitoring	Adjust replacement fluid heater
			Use patient warming systems
			Insulate extracorporeal circuit

There are several key things you can do to help minimise problems:
• Do not be afraid of the machine—it is a relatively simple circuit driven by pumps and monitored by pressure transducers and air detectors.
• Get to know your machine well and the circuit well—talk yourself through where each line comes from and goes to and what the function of each button and display is on your machine—refer to the technical manual/ local trainers whenever you are not sure.
• Gain experience at troubleshooting and problem solving—work with colleagues who are experienced with haemofiltration and your particular machine—do not hand problems over to others to solve—ask them to help you solve them.

Intravascular lines used in RRT

Dual lumen venous catheters are the most commonly used forms of vascular access for RRT used in the critically ill. Common sites for insertion are subclavian and femoral veins. Because of the prevalence of bacteria in the groin area, femoral lines are more likely to become infected. Other complications of these lines are presented in the following table.

Femoral access	Subclavian (and internal jugular) access
Complications include:	Complications include:
• Air or thrombo embolus	• Pneumothorax
• Vessel damage (including adjacent vessels)	• Air or thrombo embolus
	• Vessel damage
• Haemorrhage	• Haemorrhage
• Haematoma	• Haematoma
• Catheter misplacement	• Catheter misplacement
• Infection	• Infection
	• Cardiac arrhythmias and hypotension caused by guide wire on insertion

It is important that the nurse is aware of these complications and is vigilant in monitoring for them and promptly intervening when necessary. Lines should always be treated aseptically and should be dressed and flushed according to local policy/protocols and standards of practice.

RRT ABCs

Nursing considerations

• If the patient is undergoing RRT for the first time, explain its purpose and what to expect during treatment.
• Prime the haemofilter and tubing according to the manufacturer's instructions.
• Assist with catheter insertion, if necessary, using strict aseptic technique.
• Flush the catheters with a heparin flush solution to prevent clotting as prescribed.

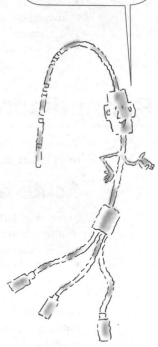

Flush the catheters with a heparin flush solution to prevent clotting.

Get dressed

• Apply transparent occlusive dressings to the insertion sites, and mark the dressings with the date and time.
• Before treatment, weigh the patient, take baseline vital signs and make sure all necessary laboratory studies have been done (usually electrolyte levels, clotting screen, FBC, urea and creatinine levels).
• Record the time the treatment begins, fluid balance figures, vital signs, weight, complications, medications given and the patient's tolerance of the procedure. Document patient assessment parameters when the treatment course has ended.
• Monitor the patient's vital signs and oxygen saturation.
• If the patient has haemodynamic monitoring in place, monitor and chart parameters especially as RRT is commenced.
• Be alert for indications of hypovolaemia (such as decreasing blood pressure and decreases in CVP) from too rapid removal of ultrafiltrate or hypervolaemia due to excessive fluid replacement with a decrease in ultrafiltrate.
• Provide continuous cardiac monitoring because arrhythmias can occur with electrolyte imbalances.
• Monitor the patient's weight and vital signs frequently.

Colour is key

• Inspect the ultrafiltrate during the procedure. It should remain clear yellow, with no gross blood.
• Pink-tinged or bloody ultrafiltrate may signal a membrane leak in the haemofilter, which permits bacterial contamination and loss of RBCs. With a CVVH system, look for the blood leak detector to signal this. If a leak occurs, notify the doctor so the haemofilter can be replaced.

- Assess the leg used for vascular access (if femoral line is in place) for signs of obstructed blood flow, such as coolness, pallor and weak pulse. Check the groin area on the affected side for signs of haematoma. Ask the patient if they have pain at the insertion sites.
- Obtain serum electrolyte levels every 4–6 hours or as requested; anticipate adjustments in replacement fluid or dialysate based on the results.
- Check filtrate volumes each hour, record fluid intake and total output and calculate fluid balance against the target prescribed.
- Check haemofilter programme against the prescription.
- Monitor and record system pressures and pump speed and record according to local policy.
- Infuse heparin in low doses, or epoprostenol, as prescribed, into an infusion port on the arterial side of the setup to prevent blood clotting during haemofiltration.
- Measure APTT (activated partial thromboplastin times) or ACT (activated clotting time) and titrate heparin according to local protocol. When epoprostenol is used, check clotting screen at least once per shift.
- Inspect the site dressing for infection and bleeding.

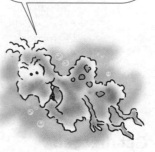

I'm in! A membrane leak in the haemofilter could permit bacterial contamination.

Renal disorders

The most common renal disorders seen in critical care units include acute renal failure and acute tubular necrosis.

Acute renal failure

Acute renal failure is the sudden interruption of renal function resulting from:
- obstruction
- reduced circulation
- renal parenchymal disease.

Acute renal failure is sometimes reversible, but if it's left untreated, permanent damage can lead to chronic renal failure. As a critical care nurse, you play a vital role in assessing and treating patients with acute renal failure.

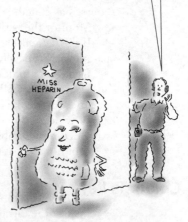

Five minutes to curtain call, Miss Heparin.

What causes it

Acute renal failure may be classified as prerenal, intrarenal or postrenal. Each type has different causes. (See *Causes of acute renal failure*, page 461.)

How it happens

Each classification of acute renal failure–prerenal, intrarenal and postrenal–has its own pathophysiology:

- *Prerenal failure* results from conditions that diminish blood flow to the kidneys (hypoperfusion). Examples include hypovolaemia, hypotension, vasoconstriction or inadequate cardiac output. One condition, prerenal azotaemia (excess nitrogenous waste products, such as urea and creatinine, in the blood), accounts for 40–80% of all cases of acute renal failure. Azotemia occurs as a response to renal hypoperfusion. Typically, it can be rapidly reversed by restoring renal blood flow and glomerular filtration.
- *Intrarenal failure*, also called *intrinsic* or *parenchymal* renal failure, results from damage to the filtering structures of the kidneys, usually from acute tubular necrosis, a disorder that causes cell death such as hypoperfusion, or from nephrotoxic substances, such as certain antibiotics or radiological dyes.
- *Postrenal failure* results from bilateral obstruction of urine outflow, as in prostatic hyperplasia or bladder outlet obstruction.

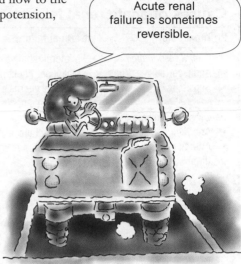

Acute renal failure is sometimes reversible.

Causes of acute renal failure

Acute renal failure is classified as prerenal, intrarenal or postrenal. All conditions that lead to prerenal failure impair blood flow to the kidneys (renal perfusion), resulting in a decreased glomerular filtration rate and increased tubular reabsorption of sodium and water. Intrarenal failure results from damage to the kidneys. Postrenal failure results from obstructed urine flow. The causes of each type of acute renal failure are listed here.

Prerenal failure	Intrarenal failure	Postrenal failure
Cardiovascular disorders	*Acute tubular necrosis*	*Bladder obstruction*
• Arrhythmias	• Ischaemic damage to renal parenchyma from unrecognised or poorly treated prerenal failure	• Anticholinergic drugs
• Cardiac tamponade		• Autonomic nerve dysfunction
• Cardiogenic shock	• Nephrotoxins, including analgesics; antibiotics such as gentamicin; heavy metals such as lead; radiographic contrast media; and organic solvents	• Infection
• Heart failure		• Tumour
• Myocardial infarction		
	• Obstetric complications, such as eclampsia, postpartum renal failure, septic abortion and uterine haemorrhage	*Urethral obstruction*
Hypovolaemia		• Blood clots
• Burns	• Myoglobin release, such as crush injury, myopathy, sepsis and transfusion reaction	• Calculi
• Dehydration		• Oedema or inflammation
• Diuretic overuse		• Necrotic renal papillae
• Haemorrhage	*Other parenchymal disorders*	• Retroperitoneal fibrosis or haemorrhage
• Hypovolaemic shock	• Acute glomerulonephritis	• Surgery (accidental ligation)
• Trauma	• Acute interstitial nephritis	• Tumour
	• Acute pyelonephritis	• Uric acid crystals

(continued)

Causes of acute renal failure (continued)

Prerenal failure	Intrarenal failure	Postrenal failure
Peripheral vasodilation • Antihypertensive drugs • Sepsis *Renovascular obstruction* • Arterial embolism • Arterial or venous thrombosis • Tumour *Severe vasoconstriction* • Disseminated intravascular coagulation • Eclampsia • Malignant hypertension • Vasculitis	• Bilateral renal vein thrombosis • Malignant nephrosclerosis • Papillary necrosis • Periarteritis nodosa (inflammatory disease of the arteries) • Renal myeloma • Sickle cell disease • Systemic lupus erythematosus • Vasculitis	*Ureteral obstruction* • Prostatic hyperplasia or tumour • Strictures • Blocked urinary catheter

Going through phases

With treatment, the patient passes through three distinct phases:

1. oliguric (decreased urine output)

2. diuretic (increased urine output)

3. recovery.

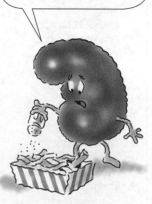

I just heard that after damage occurs, I may not be able to conserve sodium!

Output down

Oliguria is a decreased urine output (less than 400 ml/24 hours). Prerenal oliguria results from decreased blood flow to the kidney. Before damage occurs, the kidney responds to decreased blood flow by conserving sodium and water. Once damage occurs, the kidney's ability to conserve sodium is impaired. Untreated prerenal oliguria may lead to acute tubular necrosis.

During this phase, urea and creatinine rise. Hypervolaemia also occurs, causing oedema, weight gain and elevated blood pressure.

Output up

The diuretic phase is marked by urine output that can range from normal (1–2 L/day) to as great as 4–5 L/day. High urine volume has two causes, including:
- the kidney's inability to conserve sodium and water
- osmotic diuresis produced by high urea levels.

During the diuretic phase, which lasts several days to 1 week, urea and creatinine levels slowly increase and hypovolaemia and weight loss result. These conditions can lead to deficits of potassium, sodium and water that can be deadly if left untreated. If the cause of the diuresis is corrected, azotaemia gradually disappears and the patient improves greatly—leading to the recovery stage.

On the road to recovery...

The recovery phase is reached when urea and creatinine levels return to normal and urine output is between 1 and 2 L/day.

It gets complicated...

Primary damage to the renal tubules or blood vessels results in kidney failure (intrarenal failure). The causes of intrarenal failure are classified as nephrotoxic, inflammatory, or ischaemic.

Irreparable damage

When nephrotoxicity or inflammation causes the damage, the delicate layer under the epithelium (basement membrane) becomes irreparably damaged, commonly proceeding to chronic renal failure.

Severe or prolonged lack of blood flow (ischaemia) may lead to renal damage (ischaemic parenchymal injury) and excess nitrogen in the blood (intrinsic renal azotaemia).

A change in blood pressure and volume signals prerenal failure.

What to look for

The signs and symptoms of prerenal failure depend on the cause. If the underlying problem is a decrease in blood pressure and volume, the patient may have:
- oliguria
- tachycardia
- hypotension
- dry mucous membranes
- flat jugular veins
- lethargy progressing to coma
- decreased cardiac output and cool, clammy skin in a patient with heart failure.

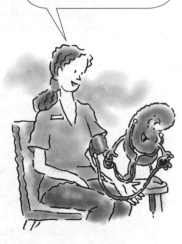

Negative progress

As renal failure progresses, the patient may show signs and symptoms of uraemia, including:
• confusion or drowsiness
• GI symptoms, including ulceration and bleeding, paralytic ileus and hiccups
• fluid in the lungs
• infection.

About 5% of all hospitalised patients develop acute renal failure. The condition is usually reversible with treatment; however, if it isn't treated, it may progress to end-stage renal disease, excess urea in the blood (prerenal azotaemia or uraemia) and death.

What tests tell you

These tests are used to diagnose acute renal failure:
• Blood studies reveal elevated urea, creatinine and potassium levels and decreased blood pH, bicarbonate, Hct and Hb levels.
• Urine studies show casts, cellular debris, decreased specific gravity and, in glomerular diseases, proteinuria and urine osmolality close to serum osmolality. Urine sodium <20 mEq/L if oliguria results from decreased perfusion and sodium >40 mEq/L if it results from an intrarenal problem.
• Arterial blood gas analysis reveals decreased pH and bicarbonate levels, indicating metabolic acidosis.
• Creatinine clearance testing is used to measure the GFR and estimate the number of remaining functioning nephrons.
• Electrocardiogram (ECG) shows tall, peaked T waves, a widening QRS complex and disappearing P waves if increased blood potassium (hyperkalaemia) is present.
• Other studies used to determine the cause of renal failure include kidney ultrasonography, plain films of the abdomen, KUB radiography, excretory urography, renal scan, retrograde pyelography, computed tomography scan and nephrotomography.

How it's treated

Supportive measures include nutritional modifications. In chronic renal failure, reducing dietary protein may be advised in order to reduce the end products of protein breakdown—urea and creatinine. This may in turn prevent or reduce the need for RRT such as intermittent dialysis. However, in renal failure associated with acute and critical illness things are often more complex. In patients such as those with sepsis or who have undergone surgery, reducing protein intake would not be advised as it would reduce tissue healing and immunity. Other nutritional considerations will include reducing potassium, phosphate and sodium intake to minimise derangements in blood levels. Supplemental vitamins, restricted fluids and meticulous electrolyte monitoring are also important elements of supportive care.

Send in the drugs

Drug therapy for acute renal failure may include:
• sodium bicarbonate for treatment of metabolic acidosis and to reduce potassium in hyperkalaemia
• to reduce potassium, hypertonic glucose and insulin infusions administered I.V., polystyrene sulphanate resins (Calcium Resonium) by mouth or by enema, as well as salbutamol
• calcium chloride is used to antagonise the toxic effects of hyperkalaemia at the myocardial cell membrane
• diuretics to manage hypervolaemia and facilitate potassium loss
• fluid replacement to correct hypovolaemia.

Overload overview

Even with treatment, an elderly patient is susceptible to volume overload, possibly precipitating acute pulmonary oedema, hypertensive crisis, hyperkalaemia and infection.

If hyperkalaemia can't be reduced with drugs, acute therapy may include dialysis or haemofiltration. To control uraemic symptoms, haemodialysis or peritoneal dialysis may be necessary.

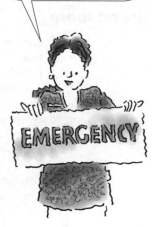

Calcium gluconate may be given in an emergency to protect the heart in hyperkalaemia.

What to do

• If the patient is to receive a diuretic, be sure to obtain a urine sample for urine studies before giving the diuretic because these drugs can alter urine results.
• Measure and record the patient's intake and output hourly, including wound drainage, NG tube output and diarrhoea. Insert a urinary catheter if indicated. Assess skin turgor; evidence of peripheral, sacral or periorbital oedema; and degree of pitting, if any. Monitor the patient's daily weight for trends.
• Check urine specific gravity and osmolality, as ordered. With prerenal failure, urine specific gravity is typically greater than 1.020 and urine osmolality is increased up to 500 mOsm; with intrarenal failure, specific gravity is typically less than 1.010 and osmolality is approximately 350 mOsm.
• Anticipate the commencement of haemodynamic monitoring to assess the patient's haemodynamic status. Monitor and chart parameters according to the method of haemodynamic monitoring used.
• Assess Hb levels and Hct and replace blood components, as prescribed.

Whole lotta blood

• Don't use whole blood to transfuse the patient if they're prone to heart failure and can't tolerate extra fluid volume. Packed RBCs deliver the necessary blood components without added volume.

• Assess the patient's cardiopulmonary status, including breath sounds. Monitor their cardiac rhythm. Report any shortness of breath, crackles and tachycardia.

• Monitor the patient's level of consciousness at least 2 hourly, or more often if indicated.

• Maintain electrolytes within normal range. Strictly monitor the patient's potassium levels, especially during emergency treatment to reduce potassium levels. Avoid administering drugs containing potassium.

• Watch the patient for symptoms of hyperkalaemia (malaise, anorexia, paraesthesia or muscle weakness) and ECG changes (tall, peaked T waves; widening QRS complex; and disappearing P waves), and report them to medical staff immediately.

• Provide a high-calorie, low-potassium, low-sodium diet, with vitamin supplements. Give anorexic patients small, frequent meals.

• Use sterile technique when performing procedures because a critically ill patient with renal failure is highly susceptible to infection.

• Encourage coughing and deep breathing and perform passive limb exercises to reduce complications of bed rest.

Dry no more

• Provide mouth care frequently because mucous membranes become dry.

• Assess the patient for signs and symptoms of GI bleeding. Administer drugs to reduce gastric acid and risk of peptic ulcer.

• Use appropriate safety measures, such as side rails or assistance with ambulation, because the patient with central nervous system involvement may be dizzy or confused. Institute bleeding precautions to minimise the patient's risk of bleeding.

• Provide appropriate care to a patient receiving RRT. Provide emotional support to the patient and their family and explain diagnostic tests, treatments and procedures. Caring for the patient with renal failure requires the involvement of a multidisciplinary team.

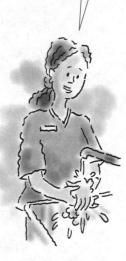

Use sterile technique when performing procedures on a critically ill patient with renal failure. They're at high risk for infection.

Acute tubular necrosis

Acute tubular necrosis causes 75% of all cases of acute renal failure. This disorder destroys the tubular segment of the nephron, causing renal failure and uraemia (excess by-products of protein metabolism in the blood). Because acute tubular necrosis is fatal in 40–70% of cases, prevention, prompt recognition and intervention by the critical care nurse are vital.

What causes it

Acute tubular necrosis may follow two types of kidney injury:

• *Ischaemic* injury, the most common cause, interrupts blood flow to the kidneys. The longer the blood flow is interrupted, the worse the kidney damage.

• *Nephrotoxic* injury usually affects debilitated patients, such as the critically ill and those who have undergone extensive surgery.

Blood disruption

In ischaemic injury, blood flow to the kidneys may be disrupted by:
- circulatory collapse
- severe hypotension
- trauma
- haemorrhage
- dehydration
- cardiogenic or septic shock
- surgery
- anaesthetics
- transfusion reactions.

Toxic talk

Nephrotoxic injury can result from:
- ingesting or inhaling toxic chemicals, such as carbon tetrachloride, and heavy metals
- a hypersensitivity reaction of the kidneys to such substances as antibiotics and radiographic contrast agents.

Cause and effect

Some specific causes of acute tubular necrosis and their effects include:
- a diseased tubular epithelium that allows glomerular filtrate to leak through the membranes and be reabsorbed into the blood
- obstructed urine flow from the collection of damaged cells, RBCs and other cellular debris in the tubules
- ischaemic injury to glomerular epithelial cells, causing cellular collapse and poor glomerular capillary permeability
- ischaemic injury to the vascular endothelium, eventually causing cellular swelling and tubular obstruction.

How it happens

Deep or shallow lesions may occur in acute tubular necrosis.

Lesion lesson

With ischaemic injury, necrosis creates deep lesions, destroying the tubular epithelium and basement membrane (the delicate layer underlying the epithelium). Ischaemic injury causes patches of necrosis in the tubules. Ischaemia can also cause lesions in the connective tissue of the kidney.

With nephrotoxic injury, necrosis occurs only in the epithelium of the tubules, leaving the basement membrane of the nephrons intact. This type of damage may be reversible. (See *A close look at acute tubular necrosis*, page 468.)

Nephrotoxic injury can result from ingesting or inhaling toxic chemicals.

RENAL WASTE INC.

A close look at acute tubular necrosis

In acute tubular necrosis caused by ischaemia, patches of necrosis occur, usually in the straight portions of the proximal tubules.

In areas without lesions, tubules are usually dilated. In acute tubular necrosis caused by nephrotoxicity, the tubules have a more uniform appearance.

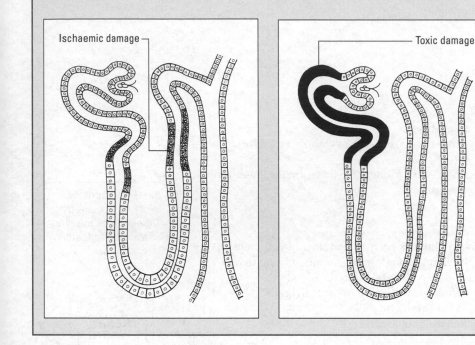

Ischaemic damage

Toxic damage

> Common complications of acute tubular necrosis include infections, GI haemorrhage and hypercalcaemia.

Toll-taking

Toxicity takes a toll on renal structures. Nephrotoxic agents can injure tubular cells by:
- direct cellular toxic effects
- coagulation and destruction (lysis) of RBCs
- oxygen deprivation (hypoxia)
- crystal formation of solutes.

Getting complicated

There are several common complications of acute tubular necrosis:
- Infections (frequently septicaemia) complicate up to 70% of all cases and are the leading cause of death.
- GI haemorrhage, fluid and electrolyte imbalance and cardiovascular dysfunction may occur during the acute or recovery phase.

- Neurological complications are common in elderly patients and occur occasionally in younger patients.
- Excess blood calcium (hypercalcaemia) may occur during the recovery phase.

What to look for

Early-stage acute tubular necrosis may be hard to spot because the patient's primary disease may obscure the signs and symptoms. The first recognisable sign may be decreased urine output, usually less than 400 ml/24 hours.

Difficult to detect

Acute tubular necrosis is difficult to detect in its early stages, so look closely at members of high-risk populations, such as elderly patients or those with diabetes, and be alert for subtle signs and symptoms during your nursing assessments.

Other signs and symptoms depend on the severity of systemic involvement and may include:
- bleeding abnormalities
- vomiting of blood
- dry skin and mucous membranes
- lethargy
- confusion
- agitation
- oedema
- fluid and electrolyte imbalances
- muscle weakness with hyperkalaemia
- cardiac arrhythmias.

Mortality can be as high as 70%, depending on complications from underlying diseases. The patient with a nonoliguric form of acute tubular necrosis has a better prognosis.

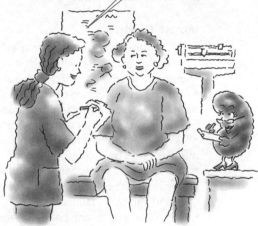

Acute tubular necrosis is difficult to detect in its early stages, so look closely at patients who are members of high-risk groups, such as elderly people.

What tests tell you

Acute tubular necrosis is difficult to diagnose except in advanced stages. The following tests are commonly performed:
- Urinalysis shows dilute urine, low osmolality, high sodium levels and urine sediment containing RBCs and casts.
- Blood studies reveal high urea and creatinine levels, low serum protein levels, anaemia, platelet adherence defects, metabolic acidosis and hyperkalaemia.
- ECG may show arrhythmias from electrolyte imbalances and, with hyperkalaemia, a widening QRS complex, disappearing P waves and tall, peaked T waves.

How it's treated

The patient with acute tubular necrosis requires vigorous supportive measures during the acute phase until normal kidney function is restored. Therapy may include:

- diuretics and fluids to flush tubules of cellular casts and debris and to replace lost fluids (initially)
- adrenergic drugs such as noradrenalin to improve renal blood flow in hypotensive states
- emergency I.V. infusion of 50% glucose, regular insulin and sodium bicarbonate in case of hyperkalaemia
- polystyrene sulphonates (Calcium Resonium) given by mouth or by enema to reduce potassium levels.

All this talk about vigorous treatment has tired me out!

Furthermore

Treatment for the patient with acute tubular necrosis may also include:
- daily replacement of projected and calculated fluid losses
- transfusion of packed RBCs for anaemia
- nonnephrotoxic antibiotics for infection
- renal replacement therapy to prevent severe fluid and electrolyte imbalance and uraemia.

What to do

- Take steps to maintain the patient's fluid balance. Accurately record intake and output, including wound drainage, NG tube output and RRT balances. Weigh the patient daily if facilities are available.
- Assist with insertion of a central venous or with establishing haemodynamic monitoring to monitor fluid status. Monitor and chart haemodynamic parameters as indicated.
- Watch the patient for fluid overload, a common complication when infusing large fluid volumes.
- Monitor Hb levels and Hct, and administer blood products, as prescribed. Use fresh packed cells instead of whole blood to prevent fluid overload and heart failure.
- Maintain electrolyte balance. Monitor laboratory results and report imbalances.
- Monitor the patient's vital signs, oxygen saturation, cardiac rhythm and cardiopulmonary status. Treat hypotension immediately to avoid renal ischaemia. Monitor vital signs closely. Fever and chills may signal the onset of an infection, which is the leading cause of death in acute tubular necrosis. (See *Temperature regulation in elderly patients*, page 471.)
- Check for potassium content in prescribed drugs (for example, potassium penicillin). Provide dietary restriction of foods containing sodium and potassium, such as bananas, orange juice and baked potatoes.
- Provide adequate calories and essential amino acids while restricting potassium and phosphate. Total parenteral nutrition may be indicated for a critically ill and debilitated or catabolic patient.
- Use aseptic technique, especially when handling catheters, because the critically ill or debilitated patient is vulnerable to infection.
- Administer sodium bicarbonate, as prescribed, for acidosis or assist with dialysis in severe cases.

Watch out for fluid overload! It's a common complication when infusing large fluid volumes.

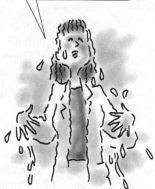

• Provide the patient with reassurance and emotional support. Encourage them and their family to verbalise their concerns. Fully explain each procedure.
• To prevent acute tubular necrosis, make sure the patient is well hydrated before surgery or after x-rays requiring use of a contrast medium. Administer N-acetylcysteine as prescribed to the high-risk critically ill patient before and during these procedures. Administer nephrotoxic drugs cautiously and avoid using contrast dyes in the high-risk patient.

Quick quiz

1. The kidneys secrete erythropoietin when:
  A. oxygen supply in tissue decreases.
  B. calcium levels are insufficient.
  C. vitamin D becomes inactive.
  D. pH level drops below 7.35.

Answer: A. The kidneys secrete erythropoietin when the oxygen supply in tissue decreases.

2. In dialysis, particles move through a semipermeable membrane from an area of high-solute concentration to an area of low-solute concentration in a process called:
  A. diffusion.
  B. active transport.
  C. permission.
  D. osmosis.

Answer: A. Diffusion is the movement of particles through a semipermeable membrane from an area of high-solute concentration to an area of low-solute concentration. In dialysis, waste products and excess electrolytes in the blood cross through the semipermeable membrane of a dialysis filter through diffusion.

3. Prerenal failure results from:
  A. bilateral obstruction of urine outflow.
  B. conditions that diminish blood flow to the kidneys.
  C. damage to the kidneys.
  D. ischaemic damage to renal parenchyma.

Answer: B. Prerenal failure is caused by any condition that reduces blood flow to the kidneys, such as hypotension, hypovolaemia, vasoconstriction and inadequate cardiac output.

4. Acute tubular necrosis following ischaemic renal injury may be due to:
  A. fluid-volume overload.
  B. nephrotoxic drugs.
  C. a hypersensitivity reaction to radiographic contrast agents.
  D. severe hypotension.

Answer: D. Acute tubular necrosis may follow ischaemic or nephrotoxic injury to the kidney. Ischaemic injury may be caused by severe hypotension as well as circulatory collapse, trauma, haemorrhage, dehydration, surgery, transfusion reactions and cardiogenic or septic shock.

Scoring

☆☆☆ If you answered all four questions correctly, take a dip in a kidney-shaped pool. Your information-filtering system is intact.

☆☆ If you answered three questions correctly, try to reabsorb what you've read. With a little concentration, you can detoxify your thinking and restore balance through work and play regulation.

☆ If you answered fewer than three questions correctly, don't expel yourself. Reread the chapter to flush out the facts and then take the test again.

Just the facts

In this chapter, you'll learn:

♦ structure and function of the endocrine system

♦ assessment of the endocrine system

♦ diagnostic tests and treatments for critically ill patients

♦ endocrine system disorders and related nursing care.

Understanding the endocrine system

The endocrine system regulates and integrates the body's metabolic activities and maintains internal homeostasis. It has three major components:

1 glands, which are specialised organs that secrete hormones and chemical transmitters into the bloodstream to regulate body functions

2 hormones, which are chemical substances secreted by glands in response to stimulation from the nervous system and other sites

3 receptors, which are protein molecules that trigger specific physiological changes in target cells in response to hormonal stimulation.

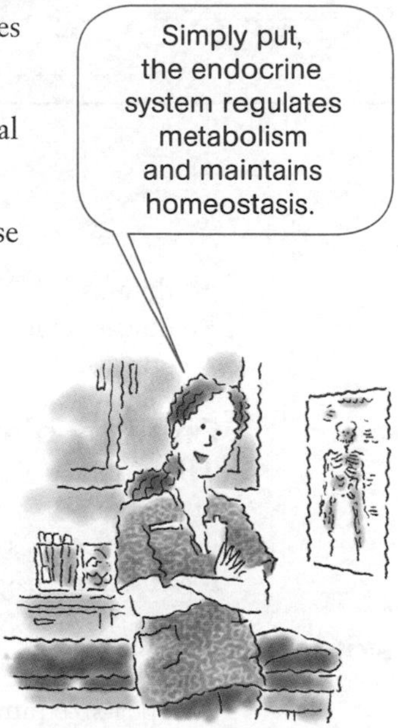

Glands

The major glands of the endocrine system are the:
- pituitary gland
- thyroid gland
- parathyroid glands
- adrenal glands
- pancreas

> Simply put, the endocrine system regulates metabolism and maintains homeostasis.

Endocrine gland sites

The illustration below shows the location of the major endocrine glands (except the gonads).

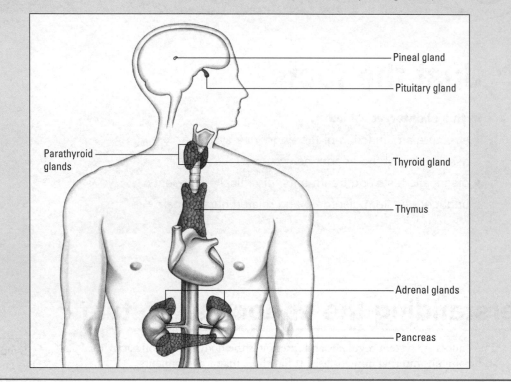

Pineal gland

Pituitary gland

Parathyroid glands

Thyroid gland

Thymus

Adrenal glands

Pancreas

- thymus
- pineal gland
- gonads. (See *Endocrine gland sites*.)

Pituitary gland

The pituitary gland rests in a depression in the sphenoid bone at the base of the brain. It's connected by the infundibulum to the hypothalamus, from which it receives chemical and nervous stimulation. (*See Understanding the hypothalamus,* page 475.)

Powerful pea

The pea-size pituitary gland has two regions, or lobes: posterior and anterior. The posterior pituitary lobe stores and releases oxytocin and antidiuretic

Understanding the hypothalamus

The hypothalamus integrates the endocrine and autonomic nervous systems. It controls some endocrine gland functions through neural and hormonal stimulation.

Pathways to the posterior pituitary

Neural pathways connect the hypothalamus to the posterior pituitary gland. These neurones stimulate the posterior pituitary gland to secrete two effector hormones—antidiuretic hormone (ADH) and oxytocin—which are stored in the posterior pituitary.

When ADH is secreted, the body retains water. Oxytocin stimulates uterine contractions during labour and milk secretion in lactating women.

Inhibition and stimulation

The hypothalamus produces many other inhibiting and stimulating hormones and other factors that regulate functions of the anterior pituitary.

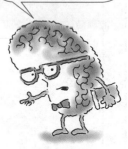

The hypothalamus integrates the endocrine and autonomic nervous systems.

hormone, which are produced by the hypothalamus. The larger anterior pituitary lobe produces at least six hormones:

 growth hormone (GH)

thyroid-stimulating hormone (TSH)

corticotrophin

follicle-stimulating hormone (FSH)

leuteinising hormone (LH)

 prolactin.

Thyroid gland

The thyroid gland is directly beneath the larynx and partly in front of the trachea. It has two lobes—one on either side of the trachea—connected by a strip of tissue called the isthmus, which gives the gland a butterfly shape. (See *A close look at the thyroid gland*, page 476.)

Metabolism master

The thyroid gland regulates the body's metabolism and produces three hormones:

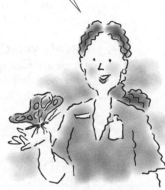

The thyroid gland is shaped like a butterfly.... I'm sure it isn't as colourful though.

A close look at the thyroid gland

This illustration shows the structure and location of the thyroid gland.

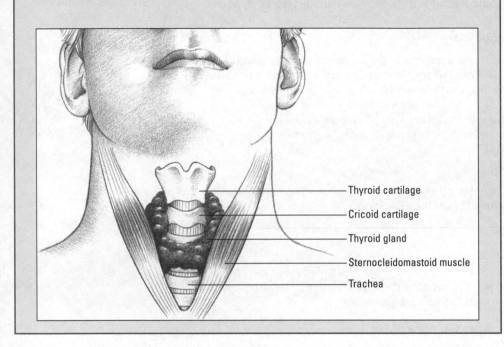

- Thyroid cartilage
- Cricoid cartilage
- Thyroid gland
- Sternocleidomastoid muscle
- Trachea

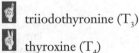 triiodothyronine (T_3)

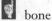 thyroxine (T_4)

 calcitonin.

T_3 and T_4 work together to regulate cellular metabolism. Calcitonin maintains blood calcium levels by inhibiting calcium release from bone.

Parathyroid glands

There are four parathyroid glands, one in each corner of the thyroid gland. Together, they produce parathyroid hormone (PTH) or parathormone, which maintains the body's calcium levels by travelling to three target tissue types, including:

 bone

GI tissue

renal tissue.

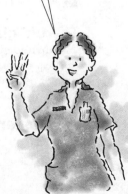

Three thyroid hormones regulate metabolism and blood calcium levels: T_3, T_4, and calcitonin.

Adrenal glands

There are two adrenal glands, one above each kidney. Each adrenal gland has an inner layer (the medulla) and an outer layer (the cortex).

Innie

The adrenal medulla produces catecholamines and is considered a neuroendocrine structure because catecholamines play an important role in the autonomic nervous system.

Outie

The adrenal cortex is the larger, outer layer and has three zones, or cell layers:

🖐 zona glomerulosa, the outermost zone, which produces mineralocorticoids, primarily aldosterone

✌ zona fasciculata, the middle and largest zone, which produces the glucocorticoids cortisol (hydrocortisone), cortisone, and corticosterone, and small amounts of the sex hormones androgen and oestrogen

✌ zona reticularis, the innermost zone, which produces mainly glucocorticoids and some sex hormones.

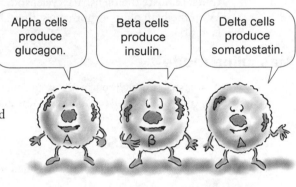

Alpha cells produce glucagon.

Beta cells produce insulin.

Delta cells produce somatostatin.

Pancreas

The pancreas has endocrine and exocrine functions. It's located behind the stomach, extending to the spleen and within the duodenal curve.

Visit the islets of Langerhans

The islets of Langerhans, which perform the endocrine function of the pancreas, contain alpha, beta, and delta cells. Alpha cells produce glucagon; beta cells, insulin; and delta cells, somatostatin.

Thymus

The thymus is located below the sternum and contains lymphatic tissue. This gland produces hormones (thymosin and thymopoietin), but its major role is related to the immune system: it produces T cells, which are involved in cell-mediated immunity.

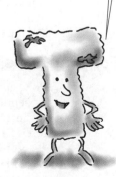

The thymus produces T cells, which are involved in cell-mediated immunity.

Pineal gland

The tiny pineal gland lies at the back of the third ventricle of the brain. It produces the hormone melatonin, which regulates a person's sleep-wake cycles and plays a role in mood regulation and the female reproductive cycle.

Gonads

The gonads include the:
- ovaries (in females)
- testes (in males).

Feminine function

The ovaries promote the development and maintenance of female sex-related traits, regulate the menstrual cycle, and maintain the uterus for pregnancy. With the help of other hormones, they also prepare the mammary glands for lactation.

Masculine mode

The testes produce spermatozoa and the male sex hormone testosterone. Testosterone stimulates and maintains male sex-related traits.

Hormones

Hormones can be structurally classified into three types:

📖 amines

📖 polypeptides

📖 steroids.

Amenable amines

Amines are derived from tyrosine, an essential amino acid found in most proteins. They include the thyroid hormones (T_3 and T_4) and the catecholamines (adrenaline, noradrenaline, and dopamine).

Poly want a peptide?

Polypeptides are protein compounds made of many amino acids connected by peptide bonds. They include:
- anterior pituitary hormones (somatotrophin [GH], TSH, corticotrophin, FSH, LH, melanocyte-stimulating hormone, and prolactin)
- posterior pituitary hormones (antidiuretic hormone [ADH] and oxytocin)
- PTH
- pancreatic hormones (insulin and glucagon).

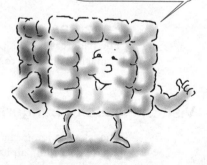

Amines are derived from tyrosine, an essential amino acid found in most proteins.

Senior moments

Endocrine changes with ageing

A common endocrine change in older adults is a decreased ability to tolerate stress.

Age matters

When stress stimulates an older person's pancreas, the blood glucose concentration increases more and remains elevated longer than in a younger adult. Such diminished glucose tolerance is a normal part of ageing. Keep this in mind when evaluating an older person for diabetes.

If coma develops

Older adults rarely become ketoacidotic, even with extremely elevated blood glucose levels. When coma develops, it's usually from hyperosmolar hyperglycaemic nonketotic syndrome, which can be triggered by acute illness or surgery in older adults.

Other changes

Other normal variations in endocrine function include a decreased cortisol secretion rate and decline in serum aldosterone levels. Changes in endocrine function during menopause vary from woman to woman, but normally oestrogen levels diminish and follicle-stimulating hormone production increases. In men, testosterone levels may decrease.

Steroidal secretions

Steroids, derived from cholesterol, include:
• adrenocortical hormones (aldosterone and cortisol) secreted by the adrenal cortex
• sex hormones (oestrogen and progesterone in females and testosterone in males) secreted by the gonads.

Hormone release and transport

All hormone release results from endocrine gland stimulation, but release patterns vary greatly. For example:
• Corticotrophin (secreted by the anterior pituitary lobe) and cortisol (secreted by the adrenal cortex) are released in irregular spurts in response to body rhythm cycles, with levels peaking in the early morning.
• Secretion of PTH (by the parathyroid gland) and prolactin (by the anterior pituitary) occurs fairly evenly throughout the day.
• Secretion of insulin by the pancreas has both steady and sporadic release patterns. (See *Endocrine changes with aging*)

Hormone function

When a hormone reaches its target site, it binds to a specific receptor on the cell membrane or in the cell:

- Polypeptides and some amines bind to membrane receptor sites.
- Smaller, more lipid-soluble steroids and thyroid hormones diffuse through cell membranes and bind to intracellular receptors.

Right on target!

After binding to the receptor, each hormone produces a unique physiological change, depending on the target site and the hormone's action at that site. A particular hormone may produce different effects at different target sites.

Hormonal regulation

Hormonal regulation is a complex feedback mechanism involving hormones, the central nervous system and blood chemicals and metabolites that maintain the body's delicate equilibrium by regulating hormone synthesis and secretion. (Feedback is information sent to endocrine glands that signals the need for changes in hormone levels, either increasing or decreasing hormone production and release.) (See *The feedback loop*, page 481.)

Heart and hormones

The heart has a role in endocrine function. In the walls of the atria, there are cells that produce atrial natriuretic hormone (ANH), also referred to as *atrial natriuretic peptide*. The atria secrete ANH in response to increased atrial wall stretching due to increased blood pressure or blood volume. ANH causes increased renal excretion of sodium and water, thus reducing blood volume and blood pressure.

In summary

The endocrine system acts throughout the body, some of the activity is vital but the remainder can cause serious illness or aggravate other conditions if it is not functioning normally.

> When a hormone reaches its target site, it binds to a receptor on the cell membrane or in the cell.

> ANH reduces blood volume and pressure by increasing sodium and water excretion by the kidneys.

The feedback loop

This diagram depicts the negative feedback mechanism that regulates the endocrine system.

From simple . . .

Simple feedback occurs when the level of one substance regulates the secretion of hormones (simple loop). For example, a low blood calcium level stimulates the parathyroid gland to release parathyroid hormone (PTH). PTH, in turn, promotes resorption of calcium. A high blood calcium level inhibits PTH secretion.

. . . to complex

When the hypothalamus receives negative feedback from target glands, the mechanism is more complicated (complex loop). *Complex feedback* occurs through an axis established between the hypothalamus, pituitary gland and target organ. For example, secretion of corticotrophin-releasing hormone from the hypothalamus stimulates release of corticotrophin by the pituitary, which, in turn, stimulates cortisol secretion by the adrenal gland (the target organ). A rise in blood cortisol levels inhibits corticotrophin secretion by decreasing corticotrophin-releasing hormone.

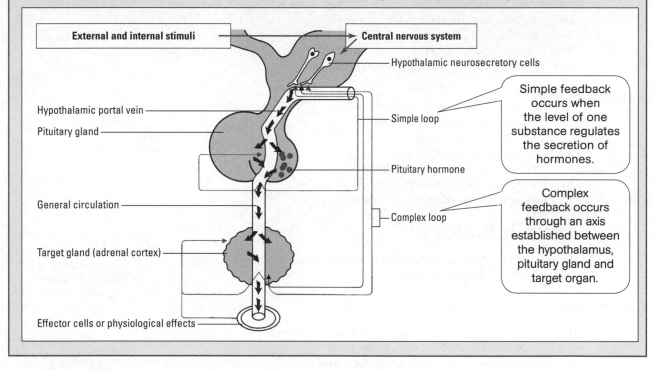

Endocrine system assessment

To assess the patient's endocrine system, take an accurate health history and conduct a thorough physical examination. When an acutely ill patient with an endocrine disorder arrives in the critical care unit, the information you obtain from the health history, physical examination and diagnostic tests is used to

treat and stabilise the patient. After the patient is stable, you may obtain additional data. You are trying to answer the following questions:
- Is there an acute endocrine problem?
- Is there an underlying chronic endocrine condition?
- Is there a potential for endocrine deterioration?

To carry out a complete assessment, it is useful to adopt a structured approach:
- History of the present complaint
- Health history
- Clinical assessment and monitoring
- Results and significance of diagnostic tests and investigations.

History of the present complaint

Because the endocrine system interacts with all other body systems, conduct a complete body systems review. Ask the patient/relatives to describe the chief complaint. Common complaints associated with endocrine disorders include fatigue, weakness, weight changes, mental status changes, polyuria, polydipsia and abnormalities of sexual maturity and function.

Ask questions

Be sure to ask the patient/relatives the following questions:
- How is the patient feeling?
- Why did they come to hospital?
- What has happened over the past 24–48 hours?
- How different are they to their usual state of health?
- How long has the patient been unwell?

Health history

Ask the patient/relatives about overall patterns of health and illness, paying attention to the details they provide.

Ask questions

Be sure to ask the patient/relatives the following questions:
- Have you noticed any changes to the skin?
- Does bruising happen more easily than it used to?
- Have you noticed any change in the amount or distribution of body hair?
- Do the eyes burn or feel gritty when closed?
- How good is the sense of smell?

Previous health status

Ask about the patient's medical history. You may identify insidious and vague symptoms of endocrine dysfunction if the patient has had a skull fracture, surgery, complications of surgery or brain infection, such as meningitis or encephalitis.

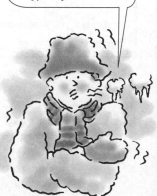

Intolerance of cold may indicate hypothyroidism . . .

Family history

Ask about the patient's family history because some endocrine disorders, such as diabetes mellitus and thyroid disease, are inherited or have strong familial tendencies.

Lifestyle patterns

Ask the patient about temperature intolerance, which may indicate certain thyroid disorders. For example, intolerance of cold may indicate hypothyroidism and intolerance of warmth, hyperthyroidism.

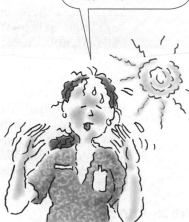

. . . and intolerance of heat may indicate hyperthyroidism.

Clinical assessment and monitoring

A total body evaluation and neurological assessment is usually included in the physical examination because the hypothalamus plays an important role in regulating endocrine function. An ABCDE assessment should be used treating any critical abnormalities as they are found. When the patient is stable a more detailed assessment can be done.

Permissive condition

If the patient's condition permits, begin by measuring height and weight. Measure blood pressure with the patient lying, sitting and standing. Compare the findings with normal expected values and the patient's baseline measurements, if available.

Exposure

Systematically inspect the patient's overall appearance and examine all areas of the body.

Outward appearance

Evaluate general body development, including posture, body build, proportionality of body parts and distribution of body fat.

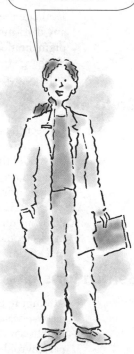

Inspect the patient's outward appearance from head to toe.

Skin deep

Assess the patient's overall skin colour and inspect the skin and mucous membranes for lesions or areas of increased, decreased or absent pigmentation. As you do so, be sure to consider racial and ethnic variations. In a dark-skinned patient, colour variations are best assessed in the sclera, conjunctiva, mouth, nail beds and palms. Next, assess the patient's skin texture and hydration.

Hairy topic

Inspect the hair for amount, distribution, condition and texture. Observe scalp and body hair for abnormal patterns of growth or hair loss. Remember to consider normal racial-, ethnic- and sex-related differences in hair growth and texture.

Nail it

Next, check the patient's fingernails for cracking, peeling, separation from the nail bed (onycholysis) or clubbing; observe the toenails for fungal infection, ingrown nails, discolouration, length and thickness.

Face it

Assess the patient's face for overall colour and the presence of erythematous areas, especially in the cheeks. Note facial expression. Is it pained and anxious, dull and flat, or alert and interested? Note the shape and symmetry of the eyes and look for eyeball protrusion, incomplete eyelid closure or periorbital oedema. Have the patient extend their tongue, and inspect it for colour, size, lesions, positioning and tremors or unusual movements.

Neck check

While standing in front of the patient, examine the neck first with it—held straight, then slightly extended. Check for neck symmetry and midline positioning and for symmetry of the trachea.

Chest check

Evaluate the overall size, shape and symmetry of the patient's chest, noting any deformities. In females, assess the breasts for size, shape, symmetry, pigmentation (especially on the nipples and in skin creases) and nipple discharge (galactorrhoea). In males, observe for bilateral or unilateral breast enlargement (gynaecomastia) and nipple discharge.

Go to extremes

Inspect the patient's extremities. Check the arms and hands for tremors. To do so, have the patient hold both arms outstretched in front with the palms down and fingers separated. Note any muscle wasting, especially in the upper arms. Have the patient grasp your hands to assess the strength and symmetry of their grip.

Next, inspect the legs for muscle development, symmetry, colour and hair distribution. Examine the feet for size and note lesions, corns, calluses or marks from socks or shoes. Inspect the toes and the spaces between them for maceration and fissures.

Search for signs

Attempt to elicit Chvostek's sign and Trousseau's sign if you suspect a patient has hypocalcaemia (low serum calcium levels) related to deficient or ineffective PTH secretion from hypoparathyroidism or surgical removal of the parathyroid glands.

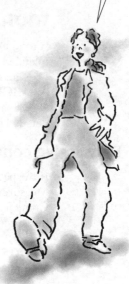

Examine the patient's feet for size and other characteristics.

To elicit Chvostek's sign, tap the facial nerve in front of the ear with a finger; if the facial muscles contract towards the ear, the test is positive for hypocalcaemia.

To elicit Trousseau's sign, place a blood pressure cuff on the arm and inflate it above the patient's systolic pressure. In a positive test, the patient exhibits carpal spasm (ventral contraction of the thumb and digits) within 3 minutes.

Results and significance of diagnostic tests and investigations

Various tests are used to suggest, confirm or rule out an endocrine disorder. Some test results also identify a dysfunction as hyperfunction or hypofunction or indicate whether a problem is primary, secondary or functional. (See *Common endocrine laboratory studies*, pages 486–488.) Endocrine function is tested through direct and indirect testing and imaging studies.

Direct and indirect testing

Direct and indirect testing measure hormone levels or substances controlled by hormones. When test results are borderline, provocative testing may be done (For example attempting to stimulate an underactive gland or suppress an overactive gland to measure reaction depending on the suspected disorder).

Direct testing

The most common method, direct testing, is used to measure hormone levels in the blood or urine. Accurate measurement requires special techniques because the body contains only minute amounts of hormones.

Methods of direct testing used to measure hormone levels in the blood and urine are:
- immunoradiometric assays (IRMAs)
- radioimmunoassay (RIA)
- 24-hour urine testing.

Indirect testing

Indirect testing is used to measure the substance controlled by a hormone–not the hormone itself. For example, glucose measurements are used to evaluate insulin levels and calcium measurements are used to assess PTH activity. Although RIAs measure these substances directly, indirect testing is easier and less costly.

Not so fast

Glucose levels obtained indirectly accurately reflect insulin's effectiveness. Even so, various factors that affect calcium may alter PTH levels and, thus, result in indirect testing.

Common endocrine laboratory studies

When a patient exhibits signs and symptoms of an endocrine disorder, laboratory studies provide valuable clues to the possible cause, as shown in the table below. (*Note:* Keep in mind that abnormal findings may stem from a problem unrelated to the endocrine system.) Remember that values differ among laboratories; check the normal range for the specific laboratory.

Test and purpose	Normal findings	Abnormal findings	Possible causes of abnormal findings
Blood tests			
Calcium Used to detect bone and parathyroid disorders	2.12–2.65 mmol/L	Above-normal level	Parathyroid tumours, hyperparathyroidism
		Below-normal level	Hypoparathyroidism
Cortisol Used to evaluate adrenocortical function	*8 a.m.*: 280 to 700 nmol/L *4 p.m.*: 140 to 280 nmol/L (Usually, the 4 p.m. level is half the 8 a.m. level.)	Above-normal level	Cushing's disease, Cushing's syndrome
		Below-normal level	Addison's disease
Glucose tolerance test, oral Used to detect diabetes mellitus and hypoglycaemia	11.1 mmol/L within 1 hour of oral glucose test dose; returns to fasting levels or lower within 3 hours	Above-normal level	Cushing's disease, phaeochromocytoma, diabetes mellitus
		Below-normal level	Addison's disease, hypothyroidism, hypopituitarism, hypoglycaemia
Glycosylated haemoglobin Used to monitor the degree of glucose control in diabetes mellitus over 3 months	<6% of total haemoglobin — good control	Above-normal level	Uncontrolled diabetes mellitus
Gonadotrophin (follicle-stimulating hormone [FSH], luteinising hormone [LH]) Used to distinguish a primary gonadal problem from pituitary insufficiency	*Males* FSH: 2–8 U/L *Females–dependent on phase of menstrual cycle*	Above-normal level	Primary gonadal failure
		Below-normal level	Pituitary insufficiency
Growth hormone (GH) radioimmunoassay Used to evaluate GH oversecretion	<20 mU/L	Above-normal level	Pituitary or hypothalamic tumour; diabetes mellitus
		Below-normal level	Pituitary infarction

(continued)

Common endocrine laboratory studies (continued)

Test and purpose	Normal findings	Abnormal findings	Possible causes of abnormal findings
Blood tests (continued)			
Insulin-induced hypoglycaemia Used to detect hypopituitarism	GH increase two to three times greater than baseline	Below-normal level of GH	Hypopituitarism
Parathyroid hormone Used to evaluate parathyroid function	<0.1–0.73 mcg/L	Above-normal level	Hyperparathyroidism
		Below-normal level	Hypoparathyroidism
Phosphate Used to detect parathyroid disorders and renal failure	0.8–1.45 mmol/L	Above-normal level	Hypoparathyroidism, renal failure, diabetic ketoacidosis
		Below-normal level	Hyperparathyroidism
Thyroid-stimulating hormone Used to detect primary hypothyroidism	0.5–5.7 mU/L	Above-normal level	Hypothyroidism, thyroid cancer
		Below-normal level	Hyperthyroidism
Thyroxine (T$_4$) radioimmunoassay Used to evaluate thyroid function and monitor iodine or antithyroid therapy	70–140 nmol/L	Above-normal level	Hyperthyroidism
		Below-normal level	Hypothyroidism
Triiodothyronine (T$_3$) radioimmunoassay Used to detect hyperthyroidism if T$_4$ levels are normal	1.2–3 nmol/L	Above-normal level	Hyperthyroidism
		Below-normal level	Hypothyroidism
Urine studies			
Cortisol Used to measure free cortisol to evaluate adrenocortical function	<280 nmol/24 hour	Above-normal level	Cushing's disease
Catecholamine **Used to assess adrenal medulla function** Adrenaline Noradrenaline	0–144 nmol/24 hours 0–560 nmol/24 hours	Above-normal level Above-normal level	Phaeochromocytoma
17-Hydroxycorticosteroid Used to evaluate adrenal function	*Males:* 4–14 mg/24 hours *Females:* 2–12 mg/24 hours	Above-normal level	Cushing's syndrome, pituitary tumour
		Below-normal level	Hypopituitarism, Addison's disease

(continued)

Common endocrine laboratory studies (continued)

Test and purpose	Normal findings	Abnormal findings	Possible causes of abnormal findings
Urine studies (continued)			
17-Ketosteroid Used to evaluate adrenocortical and gonadal function	*Males:* 8–20 mg/24 hours *Females:* 6–12 mg/24 hours	Above-normal level	Congenital adrenal hyperplasia
		Below-normal level	Adrenal insufficiency

For example, abnormal protein levels can lead to seemingly abnormal calcium levels because nearly half of calcium binds to plasma proteins. Therefore, other possibilities must be ruled out before assuming that an abnormal calcium level reflects a PTH imbalance.

Nursing considerations

For indirect testing, hormone measurement may include serum or urine collection. Ensure appropriate organisation and explanation to the patient/relatives:
• Accurate testing may require several blood samples taken at different times of the day because physiological factors—such as stress, diet, episodic secretions and body rhythms—can change circulating hormone levels.
• Urine is collected for 24 hours using the appropriate collection device. If a specimen is accidentally discarded, the collection must be restarted.

Imaging studies

X-rays

Routine x-rays are used to evaluate how an endocrine dysfunction affects body tissues, although they don't reveal endocrine glands. For example, a bone x-ray, routinely ordered for a suspected parathyroid disorder, can show the effects of a calcium imbalance.

Nursing considerations
• Explain the procedure to the patient.
• Radiographic studies require no special pre- or posttest care.

CT scan and MRI

CT scan and MRI are used to assess an endocrine gland by providing high-resolution, tomographic, three-dimensional (3D) images of the gland's structure, and may be used to identify tumours.

Nursing considerations

- Explain the procedure to the patient.
- Confirm that the patient isn't allergic to iodine or shellfish. A patient with such allergies may have an adverse reaction to the contrast medium. If the patient has an allergy, a pretest allergy preparation may be given.
- If contrast medium is ordered, explain that it's injected into an existing I.V. cannula or a new cannula may be inserted.
- Preprocedure testing should include evaluation of renal function (serum creatinine and urea levels) because the contrast medium can cause acute renal failure.
- After the procedure, encourage oral fluid intake to flush the contrast medium out of the patient's body, or increased I.V. fluids may be prescribed.

Nuclear medicine studies

Nuclear medicine studies include radioactive iodine uptake (RAIU) test and radionuclide thyroid imaging.

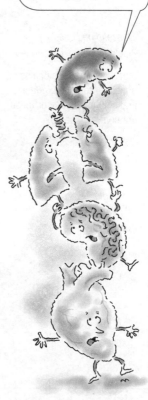

Endocrine dysfunction can affect all body systems.

Treatments

Endocrine dysfunction can affect all body systems and, if not corrected, can be life-threatening. Treatment of an acutely ill patient with an endocrine disorder is a complex process that may include drug therapy, nonsurgical and surgical treatments.

Drug therapy

Drugs are commonly used to treat endocrine disorders, such as adrenal crisis, diabetic ketoacidosis (DKA), myxoedema coma and thyrotoxic crisis. Some drug therapies commonly used to treat critical care patients with acute endocrine disorders include:
- insulin therapy
- antithyroid medications
- antihypertensives
- inotropes
- thyroid replacement medications
- corticosteroids
- antidiuretic hormone. (See *Common endocrine medications*, pages 490–492.)

Common endocrine medications

Drugs	Indications	Adverse reactions	Practice pointers
Sulphonylureas			
Glibenclamide Gliclazide	• Type 2 diabetes	• Agranulocytosis • Dizziness • Hypoglycaemia • Nausea • Thrombocytopaenia • Rash	• Check for signs and symptoms of hypoglycaemia and hyperglycaemia. • Monitor blood glucose levels. An increased risk as longer acting.
Biguanides Metformin	• Type 2 diabetes	• Diarrhoea • Flatulence • Headache • Lactic acidosis • Nausea and vomiting	• Give drug with meals. • Assess renal function. • Monitor for lactic acidosis, especially in patients with renal insufficiency. • Be aware that contrast dye may increase risk of lactic acidosis. Stop metformin 48 hours before procedure using contrast dye.
Thiazolidinediones Pioglitazone Rosiglitazone (not recommended unless unable to tolerate biguanide and sulphonylureas or these are contraindicated)	• Type 2 diabetes	• Oedema • Headache • Hypoglycaemia (rare if used as a single agent) • Myalgia • Pharyngitis • Upper respiratory infection • Weight gain	• Monitor liver function studies. • Don't use in patients with active liver disease. • Use cautiously in patients with oedema or heart failure.
Alpha glucosidase inhibitors Acarbose	• Type 2 diabetes	• Abdominal pain • Diarrhoea • Flatulence	• Acarbose alone doesn't cause hypoglycaemia; however, when given with a sulphonylurea or insulin, it may increase the hypoglycaemic potential of the sulphonylurea. If hypoglycaemia occurs, treat with glucose (dextrose) rather than sucrose or starch because acarbose blocks uptake of these.

(continued)

Common endocrine medications (continued)

Drugs	Indications	Adverse reactions	Practice pointers
Insulins			
Short-acting: Actrapid Intermediate-acting: Isophane Insulin Long-acting: Insulin glargine	• All types of diabetes	• Hypoglycaemia • Weight gain	• Monitor for hypoglycaemia. • Monitor blood glucose levels. • Educate the patient about the symptoms and treatment of hypoglycaemia and hyperglycaemia. • For critically ill patients Actrapid insulin by continuous I.V. infusion, titrated to blood sugars.
Antithyroid medications			
Thyroid hormone antagonist Propylthiouracil	• Hyperthyroidism	• Arthralgia • Diarrhoea • Drowsiness • Nausea and vomiting • Headache • Loss of taste perception • Myxoedema coma • Systemic lupus erythematosus–like syndrome • Vertigo • Agranulocytosis • Leucopenia • Hepatotoxicity	• Use cautiously with anticoagulants because bleeding risk is increased. • Instruct the patient to report any signs of bleeding. • Monitor the effects of cardiac medications after hyperthyroidism is corrected; cardiac medication dosages may need to be decreased. • Be aware that frequent thyroid tests may be necessary initially to adjust dosing. • Educate the patient about symptoms of hypothyroidism (myxoedema coma).
Thyroid replacement medications			
Thyroid hormone Levothyroxine	• Hypothyroidism	• Hypertension • Insomnia • Intolerance to heat • Menstrual irregularities • Nervousness • Tachycardia • Thyrotoxicosis • Weight loss • Tremor	• Instruct the patient to avoid aluminium-and magnesium-containing antacids, which decrease thyroxine absorption. • Be aware that requirements for antidiabetic medications may change with treatment. • Instruct patient to take medications in the early morning on an empty stomach.

(continued)

Common endocrine medications (continued)

Drugs	Indications	Adverse reactions	Practice pointers
Thyroid replacement medications (continued)			
			• Keep in mind that frequent thyroid tests may be necessary initially to adjust dosing. • Monitor for toxicity. • Teach the patient about symptoms of toxicity (thyrotoxicosis symptoms). • Use cautiously in elderly patients and in those with renal impairment or cardiovascular disorders. • Monitor for cardiac arrhythmias such as tachycardia.
Corticosteroids			
Glucocorticoid			
Hydrocortisone	• Acute adrenal crisis	• Cataracts • Delirium and hallucinations • Diabetes mellitus • Hirsutism • Hypertension • Increased appetite • Insomnia • Muscle wasting • Peptic ulcer • Seizures • Delayed wound healing	• Avoid abrupt cessation because the adrenal gland is suppressed during steroid use. • Be aware that drug-induced diabetes can result. • Use cautiously if the patient is on concomitant anticoagulant therapy. Prothrombin time results may differ after steroids are initiated. • Use cautiously if potassium-depleting diuretics are used. Steroids can worsen hypokalaemia. • Keep in mind that initial signs of infection may be masked due to the drug's antiinflammatory effects. • Administer with food or milk to avoid GI distress. • Monitor blood pressure, weight, glucose and electrolyte levels.

Nonsurgical treatments

Fluid management and electrolyte replacement is an important aspect of treating many endocrine disorders including disorders of the pancreas, adrenal and pituitary glands. Cooling blankets and ice may be used to treat patients with hyperthermia due to an increased hypermetabolic state in thyrotoxic crisis.

Surgery

In the critical care unit, you may care for patients requiring thyroidectomy (full or partial) or who have been admitted with bleeding or airway complications following thyroidectomy. Because of the position of the thyroid gland and its proximity to the airway, monitoring and maintaining the airway are vital. Make sure emergency equipment is readily available and contact the doctor if you have any concerns.

Endocrine system disorders

Some common endocrine disorders you may encounter in the critical care environment are presented here alphabetically. You will see that some disorders result from either an excess or a deficiency in a particular hormone. Those encountered are acute adrenal crisis (Addison's disease), diabetes inspidus, diabetes mellitus, DKA, hyperglycaemic hyperosmolar nonketotic coma (HONK), myxoedema coma, syndrome of inappropriate antidiuretic hormone (SIADH) and thyroid storm.

Addison's disease

Addison's disease, also called adrenal *hypofunction or adrenal insufficiency*, occurs in two forms: primary and secondary. This relatively uncommon disorder occurs in people of all ages and both sexes. Either primary or secondary Addison's disease can progress to adrenal crisis.

Acute adrenal crisis, also called Addisonian crisis, is a deficiency of mineralocorticoids and glucocorticoids that requires immediate treatment. (See *Understanding adrenal crisis*, page 494.)

What causes it

Causes of Addison's disease are classified according to whether they result in primary or secondary hypofunction.

Who's on first?

In primary hypofunction, the cause lies with the adrenal glands when approximately 90% of the gland is destroyed, apparently through an autoimmune process.

Understanding adrenal crisis

Adrenal crisis (acute adrenal insufficiency) is the most serious complication of Addison's disease. It may occur gradually or suddenly.

Who's at risk

This potentially lethal condition usually develops in patients who:

- don't respond to hormone replacement therapy
- undergo extreme stress without adequate glucocorticoid replacement (often undiagnosed patients)
- abruptly stop hormone therapy

- undergo trauma
- undergo bilateral adrenalectomy
- develop adrenal gland thrombosis after a severe infection (Waterhouse–Friderichsen syndrome).

What happens

In adrenal crisis, destruction of the adrenal cortex leads to a rapid decline in the steroid hormones cortisol and aldosterone. This directly affects the liver, stomach and kidneys. The flowchart below depicts what happens in adrenal crisis.

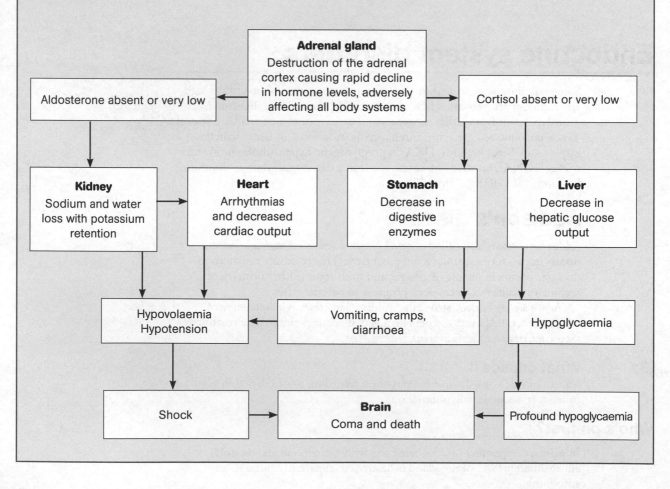

Other causes of primary hypofunction include:
- tuberculosis
- bilateral adrenalectomy
- haemorrhage into the adrenal glands
- tumours (benign or malignant)
- infections.

What's on second?

In secondary hypofunction, the causes include:
- pituitary gland (decreased function)
- abrupt steroid withdrawal due to adrenal atrophy from long-term therapy (which suppresses corticotrophin secretion by the pituitary)
- removal of a corticotrophin-secreting tumour.

Pathophysiology

Addison's disease is characterised by decreased secretion of the adrenal hormones glucocorticoids (cortisol and aldosterone), mineralocorticoids and androgens. Addisonian crisis can occur with severe stress, such as illness, surgery, sepsis, trauma and abrupt discontinuation of steroid therapy. If the cause of the Addison's disease can be removed the condition will not be permanent.

Release the aldosterone!

Normally aldosterone release occurs in response to hypovolaemia as the body attempts to maintain vascular volume. Aldosterone causes the renal tubules to reabsorb sodium. As sodium is reabsorbed, water naturally follows and is reabsorbed. Vascular volume and pressure increase. Cortisol release causes an increase in glucose production as the body attempts to supply the body with this fuel.

Emergency!

In acute Addisonian crisis, both hormones are suddenly depleted. Here's what happens:

First, blood pressure drops, due to vascular collapse. Standard vasopressor therapy is difficult to regulate because the response to catecholamines by the patient is unpredictable.

Second, blood glucose plummets and coma and death ensue if immediate treatment isn't available.

What to look for

Typical clinical features of Addison's disease include:
- profound hypotension
- dehydration

- profound weakness and fatigue
- nausea and vomiting
- hypoglycaemia
- neurological changes
- hyperkalaemia
- hyponatraemia.

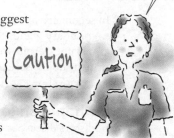

With acute Addisonian crisis, coma and death ensue without immediate treatment.

What tests tell you

In a patient with typical Addisonian symptoms, findings that strongly suggest acute adrenal insufficiency include:
- decreased plasma cortisol
- decreased serum sodium and fasting blood glucose
- increased corticotrophin
- increased serum potassium
- increased serum urea
- various radiological tests identifying adrenal gland size such as x-rays showing adrenal calcification.

How it's treated

Treatment for the patient with adrenal crisis is prompt I.V. bolus administration of 100 mg of hydrocortisone, followed by hydrocortisone as an I.V. infusion until the patient's condition stabilises.

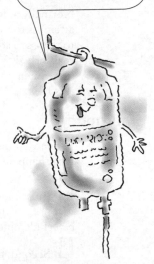

Treatment of adrenal crisis begins with prompt I.V. hydrocortisone administration.

Furthermore…

Further treatment includes:
- aggressive fluid replacement with up to 5 L I.V. saline and glucose solutions
- vasopressors (if the patient doesn't respond to the initial treatment), such as adrenaline or noradrenaline, titrated to the patient's blood pressure
- blood glucose management with I.V. dextrose solution
- use of corticosteroid (hydrocortisone) replacement when the patient's condition is stable.

What to do

- Explain all procedures and tests to the patient and their family.
- Monitor the patient's vital signs and oxygen saturation closely. Assist with insertion of a central venous catheter as indicated for fluid status evaluation. Assess haemodynamic parameters and monitor for shock.
- Assess the patient's respiratory status and auscultate breath sounds for crackles, which may indicate fluid overload.
- Monitor cardiac rhythm and assess for possible arrhythmias secondary to electrolyte imbalance (evidenced by tall, tented T waves and widening QRS complex associated with hyperkalaemia).
- Monitor the patient's intake and output, fluid replacement therapy and weight if possible.

- Monitor the patient's blood glucose levels and administer I.V. glucose if necessary.
- Monitor electrolytes for sodium and potassium imbalances, including hyponatraemia and hyperkalaemia during crisis.
- Monitor renal function studies and laboratory test results, including haemoglobin and haematocrit, serum electrolyte and blood glucose levels.
- Monitor the patient's NG tube in case of vomiting.
- Institute emergency measures if needed, such as mechanical ventilation in case of respiratory failure.
- Maintain a quiet environment.
- Maintain standard infection control measures.

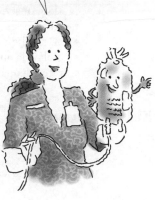

Monitor the patient's blood glucose levels and administer I.V. glucose if necessary

Diabetes insipidus

Diabetes insipidus is a water metabolism disorder caused by deficiency of ADH. ADH is also called vasopressin. The absence of ADH allows filtered water to be excreted in the urine instead of being reabsorbed. Diabetes insipidus causes excessive urination and excessive thirst and fluid intake.

What causes it

Possible causes of diabetes insipidus include:
- pituitary tumour
- hypothalamic tumour
- cranial trauma (basilar skull fracture)
- cranial surgery
- stroke
- certain medications (lithium, phenytoin and alcohol)
- rare genetic form of an X-linked recessive trait
- other idiopathic, nephrogenic or neurogenic causes.

Pathophysiology

Diabetes insipidus is a syndrome resulting from a lack of ADH secretion. ADH is a hormone released by the posterior pituitary in response to increased serum osmolality. It controls the body's ability to retain water.

Three forms

There are three forms of diabetes insipidus:

 neurogenic

 nephrogenic

 psychogenic.

Some nerve!

Neurogenic or central diabetes insipidus is caused by inadequate synthesis or release of ADH. It occurs when an organic lesion of the hypothalamus or posterior pituitary partially or completely blocks ADH synthesis, transport or release. Causes of such organic lesions include brain tumours, hypophysectomy, aneurysms, thrombosis, infection and raised intracranial pressure.

The onset of neurogenic diabetes insipidus is acute and involves:
- progressive loss of nerve tissue and increased diuresis
- normal diuresis
- polyuria and polydipsia due to permanent loss of the ability to secrete adequate ADH.

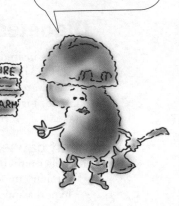

Oh no! Nephrogenic diabetes insipidus is caused by inadequate renal response to ADH.

Kidney cause

Nephrogenic diabetes insipidus is caused by inadequate renal response to ADH. It's caused by such conditions as pyelonephritis, polycystic disease and intrinsic renal disease.

Fluid overflow

Psychogenic diabetes insipidus is caused by extremely large fluid intake, which may be idiopathic or related to psychosis or sarcoidosis. The polydipsia and resultant polyuria wash out ADH more quickly than it can be replaced.

Chronic polyuria can overwhelm the renal medullary concentration gradient, rendering patients partially or totally unable to concentrate urine. Regardless of the cause, insufficient ADH causes the immediate excretion of large volumes of dilute urine and consequent plasma hyperosmolality.

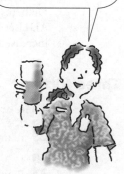

Most signs and symptoms of diabetes insipidus are related to fluid intake and output.

What to look for

Your assessment findings in a patient with diabetes insipidus may include:
- abrupt onset of increased urine output (polyuria), sometimes producing 4–16 L of dilute urine per day
- extreme thirst (polydipsia) leading to fluid intake of 5–20 L/day
- weight loss
- dizziness, weakness
- nocturia leading to sleep disturbance and fatigue
- signs of dehydration, such as fever and dry skin and mucous membranes
- hypotension and tachycardia
- risks of thromboembolism
- change in LOC.

What tests tell you

Diagnostic test findings may include:
- urinalysis showing almost colourless urine with low urine osmolality (50–200 mOsm/kg)
- increased serum osmolality (greater than 300 mOsm/kg), very concentrated blood
- decreased urine specific gravity (less than 1.005), very dilute urine
- serum sodium greater than 147 mmol/L
- dehydration test or water deprivation test to identify vasopressin deficiency, which differentiates nephrogenic from pituitary effects.

How it's treated

Until the cause of diabetes insipidus is identified and eliminated, vasopressin or a vasopressin stimulant is given to control fluid balance and prevent dehydration. Treatment measures include:
- hypotonic I.V. solution administration (1 ml for every 1 ml of urine output) to replace free water lost in urine
- medications (subcutaneous [S.C.] or I.M. vasopressin aqueous preparations; S.C., I.V. or nasal spray desmopressin acetate [DDAVP] to maintain volume
- thiazide diuretics for patients with nephrogenic diabetes insipidus
- transphenoidal hypophysectomy for patients with pituitary tumours.

What to do

- Vasopressin administration can cause hypertension, angina and MI due to the vasoconstrictive effects of the drug. Monitor the patient's cardiac status closely, including vital signs, cardiac rhythm and haemodynamic parameters.
- Monitor urine output and urine specific gravity.
- Monitor other output sources such as drainage tubes.
- Monitor daily weights, serum laboratory test results and skin turgor.
- Assess the patient's LOC.
- Assess the patient receiving vasopressin for signs of water intoxication, including drowsiness, headache, light-headedness, seizure or coma. Notify the doctor immediately if any occur.

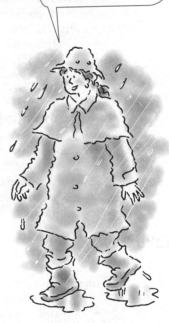

Treatment measures for the patient with diabetes insipidus include controlling fluid balance and preventing dehydration.

Diabetes mellitus

Diabetes mellitus is a chronic disease of absolute or relative insulin deficiency or resistance. It's characterised by disturbances in carbohydrate, protein or fat metabolism.

Diabetes is the leading cause of blindness in adults. It's also a major risk factor for myocardial infarction (MI), stroke, renal failure and peripheral vascular disease.

What causes it

Diabetes is classified as type 1 or type 2.

Virus or environment

One cause of type 1 diabetes is thought to be an autoimmune process that's triggered by a virus or environmental factor. However, the cause of the idiopathic form isn't known; patients with this form exhibit no evidence of an autoimmune process.

Lifestyle and heredity

The cause of type 2 diabetes is thought to be beta cell exhaustion due to lifestyle habits and hereditary factors. Risk factors thought to contribute to the development of type 2 diabetes include:
- increased weight
- family history
- Black or Hispanic ethnicity
- history of gestational diabetes during pregnancy
- advanced age

> Lifestyle habits and hereditary factors such as these can cause type 2 diabetes.

Pathophysiology

When a person is genetically susceptible to type 1 diabetes, a triggering event, possibly a viral infection, causes production of autoantibodies against the beta cells of the pancreas. The resultant destruction of the beta cells leads to a decline and ultimate absence of insulin secretion. After more than 90% of the beta cells are destroyed, hyperglycaemia, enhanced lipolysis (decomposition of fat) and protein catabolism result.

Take 2

Genetic factors are significant in type 2 diabetes. Obesity and a sedentary lifestyle accelerate its onset. Type 2 diabetes is a chronic disease caused by one or more dysfunctions, including:
- impaired insulin secretion
- inappropriate hepatic glucose production
- peripheral insulin receptor insensitivity.

Compliance or resistance

Patients with type 1 diabetes require insulin to prevent death. Type 2 diabetes is sometimes called an insulin-resistant disease. In this type of diabetes, beta cells secrete higher and higher levels of insulin to move glucose into the cell and, over time, the cells become exhausted.

What to look for

Patients with type 1 diabetes usually report rapid muscle wasting and loss of subcutaneous fat, they tend to present from 10–20 years old. With type 2 diabetes, symptoms are generally vague, long-standing and develop gradually, they tend to present in the 50 years plus age group. Although increasing obesity and poor diet is causing increasing numbers to present with type 2 diabetes at a younger age.

Similar signs and symptoms

Signs and symptoms of hyperglycaemia reported by patients with type 1 or type 2 diabetes include:
- excessive urination (polyuria)
- excessive thirst (polydipsia)
- excessive eating (polyphagia)
- weight loss
- fatigue
- weakness
- vision changes
- frequent skin infections
- dry, itchy skin
- vaginal infections or discomfort.

What tests tell you

Test results that define diabetes when they occur on two separate occasions include:
- fasting serum glucose level greater than 7.8 mmol/L
- 2-hour oral glucose tolerance test greater than 11.1 mmol/L with 75-g carbohydrate load
- nonfasting draw of serum glucose greater than 11.1 mmol/L at any time of the day.

Other results

Other diagnostic tests used to assess and manage diabetes include urinalysis (showing the presence of ketones) and an HbA1c or glycosylated haemoglobin test, which reflects serum glucose levels over a 3-month period.

When glucose enters the blood, it binds with haemoglobin. The HbA1c test is used to measure the percent of glucose bound to haemoglobin. People without diabetes average 4–6% glucose. For people with diabetes, the goal is to achieve 6% glucose or less. The closer the result is to the normal range, the lower the likelihood of developing complications in the long run.

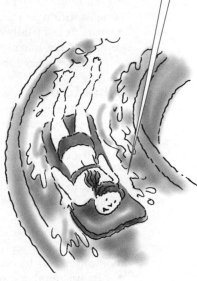

When glucose enters the blood, it binds with haemoglobin.

How it's treated

The goal of effective treatment for patients with all types of diabetes is to optimise blood glucose control and decrease complications.

Type 1 treatment

Treatment for patients with type 1 diabetes includes:
- insulin replacement
- meal planning
- exercise
- pancreas transplantation.

Type 2 treatment

Treatment for patients with type 2 diabetes includes:
- in the early stages diet modification may be enough to control blood glucose levels
- oral antidiabetic drugs to stimulate endogenous insulin production, increase insulin sensitivity in cells, suppress hepatic gluconeogenesis and delay GI carbohydrate absorption
- insulin therapy if control isn't achieved with oral agents.

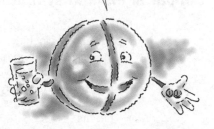

If type 2 diabetes isn't controllable with oral antidiabetic drugs, insulin therapy is used.

Types 1 and 2 treatment

Treatment for patients with either type 1 or type 2 diabetes includes:
- careful monitoring of blood glucose levels
- individualised meal planning designed to meet nutritional needs, control blood glucose and lipid levels and reach and maintain appropriate body weight
- weight reduction (for an obese patient with type 2 diabetes) or high caloric allotment depending on the growth stage and activity level (for patients with type 1 diabetes)
- patient and family education about the disease process, possible complications, nutritional management, exercise regimen, blood glucose self-monitoring and insulin or oral medications.

What to do

In the critical care unit, you may care for patients who have a history of diabetes but are admitted to the unit because of surgery or another medical condition. Some medical conditions, such as stroke or renal failure, result from diabetic effects on the cardiovascular or renal systems.
- Monitor blood glucose levels and assess for acute complications of diabetic therapy, especially DKA and hypoglycaemia (blood glucose less than 3 mmol/L); signs and symptoms include tachycardia, pallor, diaphoresis, weakness, vagueness, slow cerebration, dizziness, irritability, seizure and coma. Some medications, such as beta-adrenergic blockers, can mask the symptoms of a hypoglycaemic reaction, so more frequent blood glucose monitoring may be necessary.
- Treatment in case of a hypoglycaemic reaction is glucose. If the patient is able to swallow, provide oral glucose or a sucrose-containing drink. If the patient can't drink, give a bolus of 25 g of 50% dextrose. Obtain blood glucose measurements before administering glucose to confirm the diagnosis.

Document blood glucose levels after treatment as well as the patient's response to treatment.

• Assess for diabetic effects on the cardiovascular system, such as stroke, acute coronary syndromes, peripheral vascular impairment and peripheral neuropathy. Assess cardiovascular and neurovascular status and fluid balance and monitor for cardiac arrhythmias.

• More frequent blood glucose monitoring and insulin dose adjustments may be necessary during periods of physiological stress, such as acute illness and surgery, because blood glucose levels increase as a result of elevated stress hormones (such as adrenaline and cortisol).

Many patients who are not suffering from diabetes mellitus may require insulin therapy while critically ill to maintain blood glucose levels within the normal range. In fact there has been research to suggest that maintaining blood glucose levels within the range 4.5–6 mmol/L improves survival for critically ill patients.

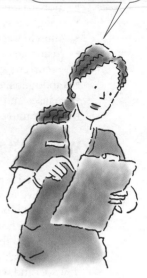

Patients in critical care units may have diabetes but are usually there because of surgery or another medical condition.

Diabetic ketoacidosis

DKA is an acute complication of hyperglycaemic crisis in patients with diabetes mellitus. It's a life-threatening complication that's most common in patients with type 1 diabetes and is sometimes the first evidence of the disease.

What causes it

DKA may result from:
• infection
• illness
• surgery
• stress
• insufficient or absent insulin.

Pathophysiology

In DKA, production and release of glucose into the blood is increased or uptake of glucose by the cells is decreased.

What happens?

In the absence of endogenous insulin, the body breaks down fats for energy. In the process, fatty acids develop too rapidly and are converted into ketones, resulting in severe metabolic acidosis.

Acidosis also affects potassium levels. For every 0.1 change in pH, there's a reciprocal 0.6 change in potassium. As acidosis worsens, blood glucose levels increase and hyperkalaemia worsens. The cycle continues until coma and death occur.

As with diabetes, the liver responds to the lack of fuel (glucose) in cells by converting glycogen into glucose for release into the bloodstream. Excess glucose molecules in the blood trigger osmosis and fluid shifts occur.

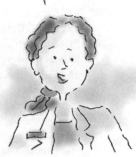

Monitor blood glucose more often and adjust the insulin dose if necessary when the patient is under stress.

What to look for

The patient may have a rapid onset of confusion appearing inebriated, which progresses to drowsiness, stupor and coma. Other assessment findings include:

- severe dehydration
- rapid and deep breathing (Kussmaul's respirations)
- fruity breath odour due to ketones
- polyuria, polydipsia and polyphagia
- weight loss
- muscle wasting
- vision changes
- recurrent infections
- abdominal cramps
- nausea and vomiting
- leg cramps.

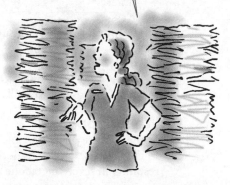

When glucose is lacking, I convert glycogen into glucose for release into the bloodstream.

What tests tell you

Findings used to diagnose DKA include:

- elevated serum glucose of 11–45 mmol/L
- positive urine ketones
- arterial blood gas (ABG) analysis that reveals metabolic acidosis
- initially, normal potassium or hyperkalaemia, depending on the level of acidosis, and then hypokalaemia
- electrocardiogram (ECG) changes related to hyperkalaemia (tall, tented T waves and widened QRS complex); later, with hypokalaemia, flattened T wave and presence of U wave
- elevated serum osmolality, showing evidence of dehydration.

There's a stack of findings used to diagnose DKA.

How it's treated

Treatment goals for the patient with DKA include rehydration, control of glucose levels and restoration of electrolyte and acid–base balance. If the patient is comatose, airway support and mechanical ventilation may be indicated.

What to do

- Correct dehydration first, using nondextrose-based I.V. fluids to prevent hypovolaemic shock.
- Administer I.V. insulin therapy and fluid and electrolyte replacements based on laboratory test results. The aim is to reduce blood glucose steadily and consistently.
- Monitor blood glucose levels. As blood glucose level nears 15 mmol/L, give dextrose-based I.V. fluid to prevent hypoglycaemia. Blood glucose should be checked every 30 minutes. Blood glucose levels must be reduced gradually to prevent cerebral fluid shifting and subsequent cerebral oedema.

• Monitor potassium levels. As blood glucose level normalises, add potassium as ordered to I.V. fluid to prevent hypokalaemia.
• Monitor ABG levels. Bicarbonate is rarely required, as blood glucose level normalises, acidosis is corrected.
• Assess the patient's GCS and ability to maintain a patent airway. Monitor respiratory status, including breath sounds and oxygen saturation. Monitor cardiac rhythm for arrhythmias that may result from electrolyte imbalance.
• Monitor the patient's vital signs because changes reflect hydration status.
• Monitor blood glucose and serum electrolyte levels, especially potassium levels and ABG results.
• Administer I.V. fluid replacement initially with 1–2 L normal saline. When the patient's blood glucose levels reach 15 mmol/L, anticipate the addition of glucose to the fluid replacement to prevent hypoglycaemia.
• Consider the cause of the DKA and treat accordingly.
• When the patient is stable, consult the diabetes team to assist with patient teaching.

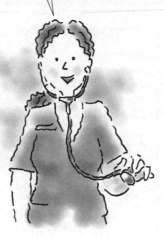

Monitor the patient's vital signs because changes reflect hydration status.

Hyperglycaemic hyperosmolar nonketotic syndrome

HONK is an acute hyperglycaemic crisis accompanied by hyperosmolality and severe dehydration without ketoacidosis. If not treated properly, it can cause coma or death.

HONK is most common in patients with type 2 diabetes (usually middle-aged or older) and is often their first presentation. It can occur in anyone whose insulin tolerance is stressed and in patients who have undergone certain therapeutic procedures, such as peritoneal dialysis, haemodialysis or total parenteral nutrition.

What causes it
Causes of HONK include illness, infection and stress.

Pathophysiology
With HONK in patients with type 2 diabetes, glucose production and release into the blood is increased or glucose uptake by the cells is decreased. When the cells don't receive fuel (glucose), the liver responds by converting glycogen into glucose for release into the bloodstream. When all excess glucose molecules remain in the blood, osmosis causes fluid shifts. The cycle continues until fluid shifts in the brain causing intracellular dehydration which results in coma and death.

What to look for

The onset of HONK is usually gradual and may not be noticed by the patient. The manifestations of HONK are similar to those of DKA, but there are differences. (See *Comparing HONK and DKA*.)

Comparing HONK and DKA

Hyperglycaemic hyperosmolar nonketotic syndrome (HONK) and diabetic ketoacidosis (DKA) are both acute complications of diabetes mellitus. They share some similarities, but are two distinct conditions. Use this flowchart to determine which condition your patient has.

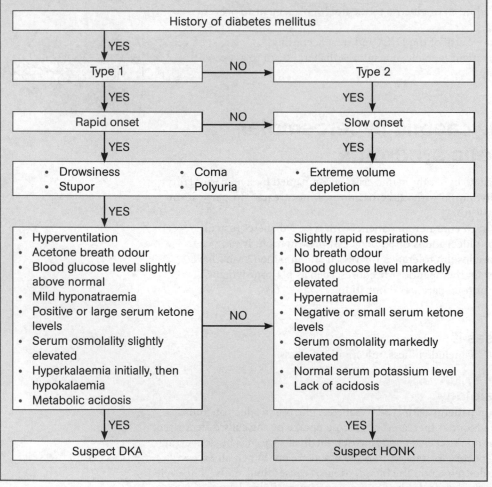

History of diabetes mellitus

↓ YES

| Type 1 | → NO → | Type 2 |

↓ YES (Type 1)   ↓ YES (Type 2)

| Rapid onset | → NO → | Slow onset |

↓ YES   ↓ YES

| • Drowsiness   • Coma | • Extreme volume |
| • Stupor   • Polyuria | depletion |

↓ YES

(DKA features)	→ NO →	**(HONK features)**
• Hyperventilation	• Slightly rapid respirations
• Acetone breath odour	• No breath odour
• Blood glucose level slightly above normal	• Blood glucose level markedly elevated
• Mild hyponatraemia	• Hypernatraemia
• Positive or large serum ketone levels	• Negative or small serum ketone levels
• Serum osmolality slightly elevated	• Serum osmolality markedly elevated
• Hyperkalaemia initially, then hypokalaemia	• Normal serum potassium level
• Metabolic acidosis	• Lack of acidosis

↓ YES   ↓ YES

| Suspect DKA | | Suspect HONK |

Making progress

As HONK progresses, assessment findings may include:
- severe dehydration
- hypotension and tachycardia
- diaphoresis
- tachypnoea
- polyuria, polydipsia and polyphagia
- vision changes
- rapid onset of lethargy
- stupor and coma
- neurological changes.

> As HONK progresses, your assessment may turn up these findings.

What tests tell you

These findings may be helpful in diagnosing HONK:
- Serum glucose level is elevated, sometimes greater than 40 mmol/L.
- Ketones are absent, so there's no acidosis and urine ketone results are negative.
- Urine glucose levels are positive.
- Serum osmolality is increased.
- Serum sodium levels are elevated and serum potassium level is usually normal.
- ABG results are usually normal, without evidence of acidosis.

How it's treated

Treatment for patients with HONK is focused on correcting fluid volume deficits and electrolyte imbalances and addressing the underlying cause:
- I.V. fluids are given to correct dehydration. Administer isotonic or half-normal saline as prescribed to prevent rapid fluid and sodium shifts which may cause cerebral oedema. When the patient's blood glucose level approaches 15 mmol/L, add dextrose to the fluid to prevent hypoglycaemia.
- I.V. insulin and electrolyte replacement therapy are delivered.
- Blood glucose levels are monitored. As blood glucose levels normalise, so do sodium levels.

What to do

- Assess the patient's GCS and ability to maintain a patent airway. Monitor respiratory status and oxygen saturation.
- Monitor the patient's vital signs. Changes reflect the patient's hydration status.
- Monitor the patient's blood glucose and serum electrolyte levels.
- Administer regular insulin I.V. as ordered, by continuous infusion, and titrate the dosage based on the patient's blood glucose levels.
- Remember, the patient with HONK has severely elevated glucose levels, but less insulin is usually needed (compared with that required by patients

with DKA) to reduce the glucose level because the patient typically secretes some insulin and may be sensitive to additional doses.
• Provide patient and family education to foster prevention of future episodes.

Myxoedema coma

Myxoedema coma is a life-threatening disorder that progresses from hypothyroidism.

What causes it
Causes of hypothyroidism include:
• pituitary failure to produce TSH
• hypothalamic failure
• chronic autoimmune thyroiditis (Hashimoto's disease)
• amyloidosis and sarcoidosis
• inability to synthesise hormones
• use of antithyroid hormones
• postthyroidectomy effects
• postradiation therapy effects.

Pathophysiology
There are two classifications of hypothyroidism: primary and secondary. Primary hypothyroidism originates as a disorder of the thyroid gland. Secondary hypothyroidism is caused by a failure to stimulate normal thyroid function or an inability to synthesise thyroid hormones due to an iodine deficiency (usually dietary) or use of antithyroid medications.

A myx of causes

Myxoedema coma can result from either primary or secondary hypothyroidism and progresses slowly and gradually. It's usually precipitated by infection, exposure to cold or sedative use. Cellular metabolism decreases to a fatal level if the patient with myxoedema coma is left untreated.

What to look for
The progression to myxoedema coma is usually gradual but may develop abruptly if stress aggravates severe or prolonged hypothyroidism. It can happen in critically ill patients with a history of hypothyroidism.

Inspect and assess

Periorbital oedema, dry flaky skin, thick brittle nails and sacral or peripheral oedema may be present in the patient with myxoedema coma. In addition, look for changes in the patient's overall appearance and behaviour, including:
• decreased mental ability (slight mental slowing to severe obtundation)
• thick and dry tongue
• hoarseness
• slow and slurred speech.

> Myxoedema coma is a life-threatening form of hypothyroidism.

What else?

Assessment findings also include:
- progressive stupor
- significantly depressed respirations and adventitious breath sounds
- hypoglycaemia
- hyponatraemia
- hypotension and bradycardia
- severe hypothermia without shivering.

What tests tell you

The following test findings are used to diagnose myxoedema coma:
- Serum levels of T_3 and T_4 are decreased.
- Serum levels of TSH are increased.
- Low serum levels of thyroid hormones.
- Radioisotope scanning of thyroid tissue is used to identify ectopic thyroid tissue.
- A CT scan, MRI or skull x-ray may disclose an underlying cause, such as pituitary or hypothalamic lesions.
- Chest x-ray may show pleural effusion.

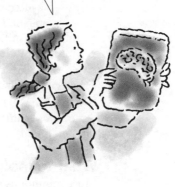

In myxoedema coma, a CT scan, MRI or skull x-ray may disclose an underlying cause, such as pituitary or hypothalamic lesions.

How it's treated

Rapid treatment may be necessary for patients in myxoedema coma, including:
- administration of I.V. hydrocortisone and I.V. levothyroxine (a thyroid agent)
- possible ventilatory support if the patient is comatose
- I.V. fluid replacement
- warming devices
- maintenance thyroid replacement.

What to do

- Assess the patient's GCS and ability to maintain a patent airway.
- Monitor the patient's respiratory status, adequacy of ventilation and oxygen saturation and ABG levels. Administer supplemental oxygen as ordered and anticipate the need for intubation and mechanical ventilation.
- Monitor vital signs and cardiac arrhythmias.
- Monitor temperature closely until the patient is stable, and institute warming measures such as applying a warming blanket.
- Administer medications as ordered. Sedatives are contraindicated.
- Administer I.V. fluids as ordered and monitor fluid balance status, serum electrolytes and blood glucose levels.
- Assess for possible sources of infection—such as blood, sputum and urine—and provide meticulous skin care.

Syndrome of inappropriate antidiuretic hormone

SIADH is a relatively common complication of surgery or critical illness.

What causes it

The most common cause of SIADH is oat-cell lung cancer, which secretes ADH or a vasopressor-like substance that the body responds to as if ADH were secreted.

Many other possibilities

Other causes include:
- neoplasms (pancreatic, brain and prostatic tumours; Hodgkin's disease; and thymoma)
- brain abscess
- stroke
- Guillain–Barré syndrome
- pulmonary disorders
- adverse effects of medications (glibenclamide, tolbutamide, vincristine, cyclophosphamide, haloperidol, carbamazepine, morphine and thiazides)
- adrenal insufficiency
- anterior pituitary insufficiency.

Pathophysiology

In SIADH, ADH is secreted excessively and the body responds by retaining water. Fluid shifts within compartments cause decreased serum osmolality (diluted blood).

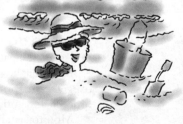

In SIADH, excessive ADH is secreted and the body responds by retaining water.

What to look for

Most commonly, a patient with SIADH complains of anorexia, nausea and vomiting. Despite these symptoms, the patient may report weight gain. Assessment findings also may include:
- thirst
- neurological changes—such as lethargy, headache and emotional and behavioural changes—and sluggish deep tendon reflexes
- tachycardia associated with increased fluid volume
- hyponatraemia.

What tests tell you

Diagnostic test results may indicate:
- decreased serum osmolality (less than 280 mOsm/kg)
- increased urine sodium
- decreased serum sodium level
- elevated serum ADH level.

How it's treated
Treatment is based on the underlying cause and the patient's symptoms.

First thing first

Treatment begins with restricting fluid intake to 500–1,000 ml/day. Other measures include administration of I.V. normal saline. Haemofiltration may be considered for patients with severe hyponatraemia. A loop diuretic may also be ordered to reduce the risk of heart failure.

What to do
• Assess the patient's neurological, cardiac and respiratory status.
• Implement seizure and safety precautions if the patient's serum sodium levels are dangerously low. Monitor serum electrolyte levels.
• Monitor the patient's vital signs, oxygen saturation and cardiac rhythm for potential arrhythmias.
• Administer medications and I.V. fluids as ordered. If hypertonic sodium chloride is ordered, monitor for fluid overload and administer diuretics as ordered.
• Monitor the patient's intake and output and weight.
• Enforce fluid restrictions and explain to the patient and their family why this is necessary.

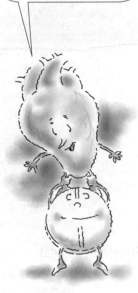

Help me, please! The patient may need a loop diuretic to reduce the risk of heart failure.

Thyroid storm

Thyroid storm, also called thyrotoxic crisis, is a life-threatening emergency in a patient with hyperthyroidism. Thyroid storm may be the initial symptom in a patient with hyperthyroidism that hasn't been diagnosed.

What causes it
The onset of thyroid storm is almost always abrupt and evoked by a stressful event, such as trauma, surgery or infection.

Not-so-common causes

Other, less common causes include:
• metastatic carcinoma of the thyroid
• pituitary tumour secreting TSH
• DKA.

Pathophysiology
Thyroid storm develops when there's a surge of thyroid hormones. Hyperthyroidism can result from genetic and immunological factors.

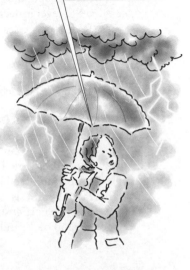

Thyroid storm is a life-threatening emergency in a patient with hyperthyroidism.

Grave's is grave

Grave's disease—the most common form of hyperthyroidism—is an autoimmune process in which the body makes an antibody similar to TSH and the thyroid responds to it. Overproduction of T_3 and T_4 increases adrenergic activity and severe hypermetabolism results. This can rapidly lead to cardiac, sympathetic nervous system, and GI collapse.

What to look for

A patient in thyroid storm initially shows marked tachycardia, vomiting and stupor. Other findings may include:
- irritability and restlessness
- vision disturbances such as diplopia
- tremor
- weakness
- heat intolerance
- angina
- shortness of breath
- cough
- swollen extremities.

Raise the flag

On palpation, an enlarged thyroid may be felt. Any change in LOC and increasing temperature in a patient with hyperthyroidism should raise red flags. Fever, typically above 38°C, begins insidiously and rises rapidly to a lethal level. Without treatment, the patient may experience vascular collapse, hypotension, coma and death.

What tests tell you

The following diagnostic test findings may indicate impending thyroid storm:
- Serum T_3 and T_4 levels are elevated.
- TSH level is decreased.
- Radioisotope scanning shows increased uptake.
- CT scan or MRI may disclose an underlying cause such as pituitary lesion.
- 12-lead ECG may show atrial fibrillation or supraventricular tachycardia.

How it's treated

Immediate treatment for a patient with thyroid storm is necessary to prevent death and includes:
- beta-adrenergic blockers to block adrenergic effects
- propylthiouracil and carbimazole to block thyroid hormone synthesis
- possible corticosteroid administration to block conversion of T_3 and T_4

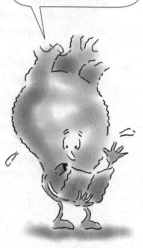

Without treatment, thyroid storm can lead to vascular collapse, hypotension, coma and death.

Monitor ECG readings because increased adrenergic activity can produce arrhythmias.

- avoidance of aspirin because salicylates block binding of T₃ and T₄
- cooling measures; icepacks, fans, cooling blankets, paracetamol.

What to do

- Assess the patient's GCS and cardiopulmonary status.
- Monitor the patient's vital signs and core body temperature and institute cooling measures.
- Monitor ECG readings. Increased adrenergic activity may produce arrhythmias.
- Monitor the patient for signs of heart failure.
- Monitor I.V. fluids and fluid and electrolyte balance.
- Monitor the patient for high blood glucose levels. Excessive thyroid activity can lead to glycogenolysis.
- Provide a quiet environment.

Quick quiz

1.   Pituitary hormones are controlled by the:
    A.   hypothalamus.
    B.   midbrain.
    C.   adrenal glands.
    D.   target organs.

Answer: A. The hypothalamus receives, integrates and directs hormone secretion.

2.   Which dysfunction should you address first in a patient with DKA?
    A.   Acidosis
    B.   Hyperkalaemia
    C.   Hyperglycaemia
    D.   Hypovolaemia

Answer: D. Hypovolaemia may be severe and should be addressed first, followed by hyperglycaemia, and then hyperkalaemia. Acidosis is corrected by correcting the other imbalances.

3.   Which of the following is an appropriate treatment measure for a patient with Addisonian crisis?
    A.   I.V. fluid replacement
    B.   I.V. corticosteroids
    C.   Blood glucose management
    D.   All of the above

Answer: D. All of the therapies indicated are first-line treatment measures during Addisonian crisis.

4.   The patient is experiencing thyroid storm. Which of the following drugs is contraindicated?
    A.   I.V. beta-adrenergic blockers
    B.   Aspirin

    C. Propylthiouracil
    D. Corticosteroids

Answer: B. Aspirin is contraindicated in patients with thyroid storm because it blocks the binding of T_3 and T_4.

5. Which of the following signs is seen in patients with diabetes insipidus?
    A. Decreased urine output
    B. Increased serum osmolality
    C. Increased urine osmolality
    D. Decreased blood glucose

Answer: B. Urine output increases with diabetes insipidus; therefore, serum osmolality is increased.

Scoring

✰✰✰   If you answered all five questions correctly, give yourself a gland! Your endocrine energy is practically radioactive.

✰✰   If you answered four questions correctly, don't worry about your target cells. Your knowledge receptors are still uptaking information.

✰   If you answered fewer than four questions correctly, quit the hemming and hormoning and review the chapter.

9 Haematological and immune systems

Just the facts

In this chapter, you'll learn:

♦ structure and function of the haematological and immune systems

♦ assessment of the haematological and immune systems

♦ diagnostic tests and treatments for critically ill patients

♦ haematological and immune system disorders and related nursing care.

Understanding the haematological and immune systems

The haematological system consists of the blood and bone marrow. The immune system consists of specialised cells, tissues and organs found throughout the body.

Transport and delivery

Functions of the haematological system include:
* transporting blood cells and immunity-related cells, hormones and gases throughout the body
* delivering oxygen and nutrients to all body tissues
* removing wastes collected from cells and tissues.

Defence! Defence!

The immune system defends the body against invasion by harmful organisms and chemical toxins. The blood plays an important part in this protective system.

> Cells of the haematological and immune systems originate in the same place and travel together.

Kin systems

The haematological and immune systems are distinct, yet closely related. Their cells share a common origin in the bone marrow, and the immune system uses the bloodstream to transport defensive components to the site of invasion.

Haematological system

The haematological system consists of various formed elements, or blood cells, suspended in a fluid called plasma.

Formed elements in the blood include:
* red blood cells (RBCs), or erythrocytes
* platelets
* white blood cells (WBCs), or leucocytes.

RBCs and platelets function entirely within blood vessels. WBCs act mainly in the tissues outside the blood vessels.

Red blood cells

RBCs transport oxygen and carbon dioxide to and from body tissues. They contain haemoglobin (Hb), the oxygen-carrying molecule that gives blood its red colour. The RBC surface carries antigens (substances that trigger immune responses), which determine a person's blood group, or blood type.

Days of their lives

RBCs have an average life span of 120 days. Bone marrow releases RBCs into circulation in an immature form as reticulocytes. The reticulocytes mature into RBCs in about 1 day. The spleen sequesters, or isolates, old, worn-out RBCs, removing them from circulation.

The rate of reticulocyte release usually equals the rate of old RBC removal. When RBC depletion occurs (for example, with haemorrhage), the bone marrow increases reticulocyte production to maintain the normal RBC count.

Platelets

Platelets are small, colourless, disk-shaped cytoplasmic fragments split from cells in bone marrow called *megakaryocytes*.

Sticky stabilisers

In the peripheral blood, the sticky platelets contribute to blood clotting in three ways:

They congregate at an injury site in a larger vessel and close the wound so a clot can form.

They release substances that stabilise the clot. For example, they release serotonin, which reduces blood flow by vasoconstriction, and thromboplastin, an enzyme essential to clotting.

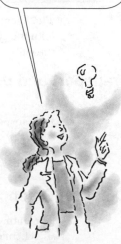

The rate of reticulocyte release equals the rate of RBC removal. That makes sense!

White blood cells

Five types of WBCs participate in the body's defence and immune systems. They are:

- neutrophils
- eosinophils
- basophils
- monocytes
- lymphocytes.

The WBCs are classified as either granulocytes or agranulocytes.

Granulocytes

Granulocytes are polymorphonuclear leucocytes. Each contains a single multilobular nucleus and granules in the cytoplasm. Each type of granulocyte exhibits different properties and each is activated by different stimuli. The granulocytes include:

- neutrophils
- eosinophils
- basophils.

> A granulocyte contains a single multilobed nucleus and granules.

Neutrophils engulf, ingest and digest

The most abundant granulocytes—the neutrophils—account for 47–77% of circulating WBCs. Neutrophils are phagocytic, meaning they engulf, ingest and digest foreign materials. They leave the bloodstream by passing through the capillary walls into the tissues (a process called *diapedesis*), then migrate to accumulate at infection sites.

Replacement bands

Worn-out neutrophils form the main component of pus. Bone marrow produces their replacements, which are immature neutrophils called bands. In response to infection, bone marrow produces many immature cells and releases them into circulation, elevating the band count.

Ingestion by eosinophils

Eosinophils account for 0.3–7% of circulating WBCs. Eosinophils migrate from the bloodstream by diapedesis (passage through the walls of capillaries) in response to an allergic reaction. Eosinophils accumulate in loose connective tissue, where they're involved in ingesting antigen—antibody complexes.

Basophils secrete histamine

The least common granulocyte—basophils—usually make up fewer than 2% of circulating WBCs. They possess little or no phagocytic ability. The basophils' cytoplasmic granules secrete histamine, bradykinin and heparin in response to certain inflammatory and immune stimuli. This increases vascular permeability and eases fluid passage from capillaries into body tissues.

Agranulocytes

Agranulocytes have nuclei without lobes and lack specific cytoplasmic granules. They include:

- monocytes
- lymphocytes

Monstrous monocytes

Monocytes, the largest WBCs, constitute only 0.6–9.6% of WBCs in circulation. Like neutrophils, monocytes enlarge and mature, becoming macrophages, or histiocytes. As macrophages, monocytes may roam freely through the body when stimulated by inflammation. Usually, they remain immobile, populating most organs and tissues.

Defence against infection

Monocytes are part of the reticuloendothelial system, which defends the body against infection and disposes of cell breakdown products. Macrophages concentrate in structures that filter large amounts of body fluid, such as the liver, spleen and lymph nodes, where they defend against invading organisms.

Macrophages are efficient phagocytes (cells that ingest microorganisms, cellular debris such as worn out neutrophils and necrotic tissue). When mobilized at an infection site, they phagocytise cellular remnants and promote wound healing.

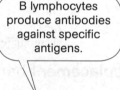

T lymphocytes attack infected cells directly.

B lymphocytes produce antibodies against specific antigens.

Lymphocytes: Least but not last

Lymphocytes, the smallest and the second most numerous (16.2–43%) of the WBCs, originate from stem cells in the bone marrow. There are two types of lymphocytes:

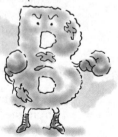

T lymphocytes, which attack infected cells directly

B lymphocytes, which produce molecules called *antibodies* that attack specific antigens.

Blood clots

Haemostasis (blood clotting) is the complex process by which platelets, plasma and coagulation factors interact to control bleeding.

Extrinsic coagulation cascade

When a blood vessel ruptures, local vasoconstriction (decrease in the calibre of blood vessels) and platelet clumping (aggregation) at the injury site initially prevent haemorrhage. This initial activation of the coagulation system, called the *extrinsic cascade*, requires the release of tissue thromboplastin from the damaged cells.

Intrinsic clotting cascade

Formation of a more stable clot requires initiation of the complex clotting mechanisms known as the *intrinsic cascade system*. This clotting system is activated by a protein called *factor XII*, which is one of 13 substances necessary for coagulation and derived from plasma and tissue.

The final result of the intrinsic and extrinsic cascade is a fibrin clot, an accumulation of a fibrous, insoluble protein at the injury site. (See *Understanding clotting*, page 520.)

Blood groups

A person's blood is one of four blood types: A, B, AB and O.

A is for antigen...

In type A blood, A antigens appear on RBCs. Type B blood contains B antigens. Type AB blood contains both antigens. Type O blood has neither antigen.

Testing, testing: A, B, AB, O

Testing for the presence of A and B antigens on RBCs is the most important system for classifying blood. Plasma may contain antibodies that interact with these antigens, causing the cells to agglutinate, or combine into a mass. Plasma can't contain antibodies to its own cell antigen or it would destroy itself. For example, type A blood has A antigens but no A antibodies; however, it does have B antibodies.

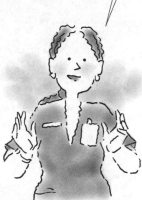

Plasma can't contain antibodies to its own cell antigen or it would destroy itself.

Cross-matching for compatibility

Precise blood-typing and cross-matching (mixing and observing for agglutination of donor cells) are essential, especially before blood transfusions. A donor's blood must be compatible with a recipient's or the result can be fatal. The following blood groups are compatible:
• type A with type A or O
• type B with type B or O
• type AB with type A, B, AB or O
• type O with type O only. (See *Compatible blood types*, page 521.)

Factor in Rhesus

Rh typing is used to determine whether a substance, called an *Rh factor*, is present or absent in a person's blood. Of the eight types of Rh antigens, only C, D and E are common. The presence or absence of the D antigen determines whether a person has Rh-positive or Rh-negative blood.

Blood typically is Rh-positive, meaning it contains Rh D antigen. Blood without the Rh D antigen is Rh-negative. Anti-Rh antibodies occur only in a person who has become sensitised to the Rh factor.

Understanding clotting

When a blood vessel is severed or injured, clotting begins within minutes to stop blood loss. Coagulation factors are essential to normal blood clotting. Absent, decreased or excess coagulation factors can cause a clotting abnormality. Coagulation factors are commonly designated by Roman numerals.

Two pathways to clotting

Clotting is initiated through two different pathways, the intrinsic pathway or the extrinsic pathway. The intrinsic pathway is activated when plasma comes in contact with damaged vessel surfaces. The extrinsic pathway is activated when tissue thromboplastin, a substance released by damaged endothelial cells, comes in contact with one of the clotting factors.

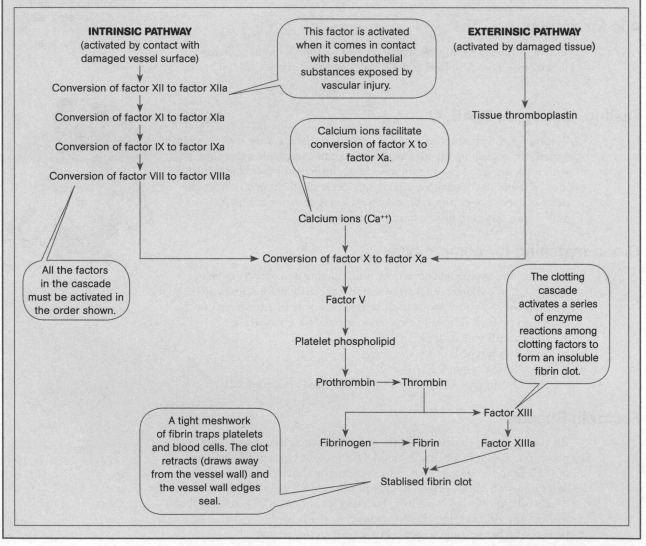

(Text continues on page 521)

Liver failure

The liver performs more than 100 separate functions in the body. When it fails, a complex syndrome involving the impairment of many different organs and body functions ensues. The only cure for liver failure is liver transplantation.

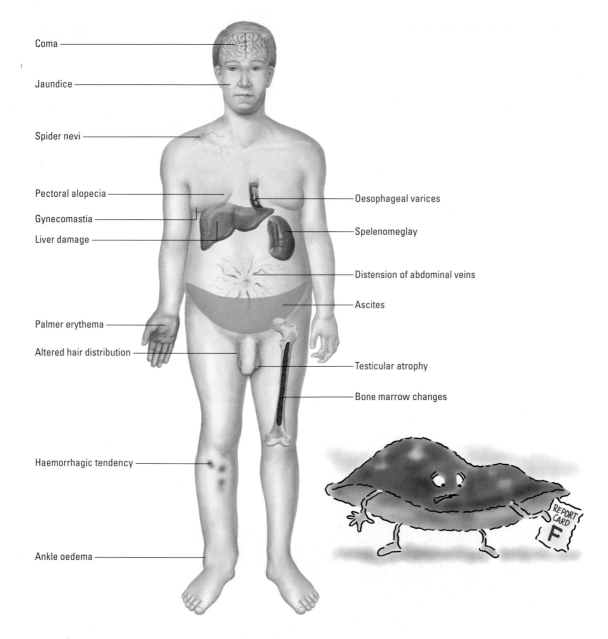

Coma

Jaundice

Spider nevi

Pectoral alopecia

Gynecomastia

Liver damage

Palmer erythema

Altered hair distribution

Haemorrhagic tendency

Ankle oedema

Oesophageal varices

Spelenomeglay

Distension of abdominal veins

Ascites

Testicular atrophy

Bone marrow changes

REPORT CARD F

Anaphylaxis

Anaphylaxis is an acute, potentially life-threatening immediate hypersensitivity reaction marked by rapidly progressive urticaria and respiratory distress. A severe reaction may precipitate vascular collapse, leading to systemic shock and, sometimes, death.

Anaphylaxis requires previous sensitisation or exposure to the specific antigen, resulting in immunoglobulin (Ig)E production by plasma cells in the lymph nodes and enhancement by helper T cells. IgE antibodies then bind to membrane receptors on mast cells in connective tissue and basophils in the blood.

1. Response to antigen

IgM and IgG recognise and bind to the antigen. The patient has no signs or symptoms.

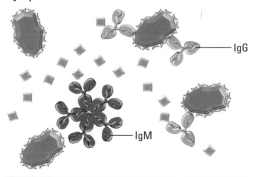

IgG

IgM

■ Complement cascade

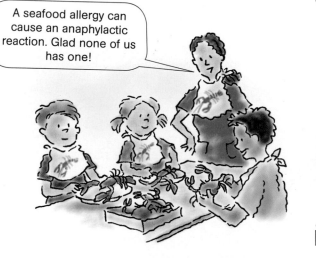

A seafood allergy can cause an anaphylactic reaction. Glad none of us has one!

2. Release of chemical mediators

Activated IgE on basophils promotes the release of mediators: histamine, serotonin and leukotrienes. The patient develops nasal congestion, itchy and watery eyes, flushing, weakness and anxiety.

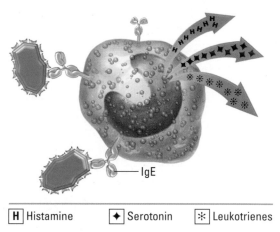

IgE

| H Histamine | ◆ Serotonin | ✳ Leukotrienes |

3. Intensified response

Mast cells release more histamine and eosinophil chemotactic factor of anaphylaxis (ECF-A), which create venule-weakening lesions. Signs and symptoms appear; swelling and wheals.

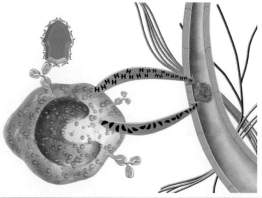

| ▶ ECF-A | H Histamine |

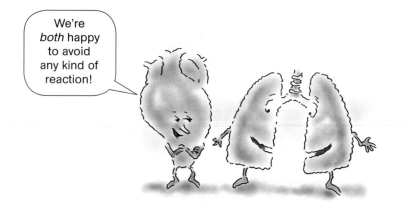

5. Deterioration

Meanwhile, mediators increase vascular permeability, causing fluid to leak from the vessels. Shock, confusion, tachycardia and hypotension signal vascular collapse.

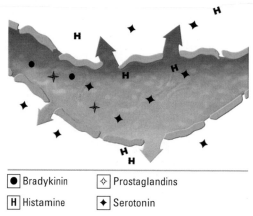

● Bradykinin	◇ Prostaglandins
H Histamine	✦ Serotonin

4. Respiratory distress

In the lungs, histamine causes endothelial cell destruction and fluid to leak into alveoli. The patient develops changes in level of consciousness, respiratory distress and, possibly, seizures.

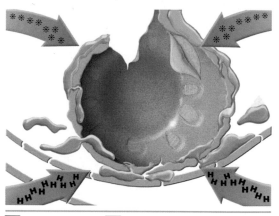

✳ Leukotrienes	H Histamine

6. Failure of compensatory mechanisms

Endothelial cell damage causes basophils and mast cells to release heparin and mediator-neutralising substances. However, anaphylaxis is now irreversible. Haemorrhage, disseminated intravascular coagulation and cardiac arrest can occur.

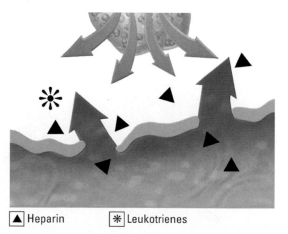

▲ Heparin	✳ Leukotrienes

Renovascular hypertension

Renovascular hypertension is a rise in systemic blood pressure resulting from stenosis of the major renal arteries or their branches or from intrarenal atherosclerosis. The narrowing or sclerosis may be partial or complete, and the resulting blood pressure elevation may be benign or malignant. Approximately 5–10% of patients with high blood pressure display renovascular hypertension.

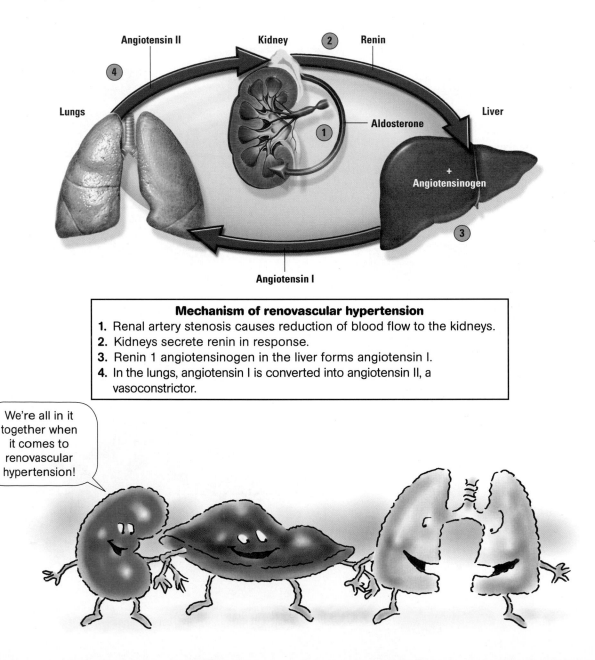

Mechanism of renovascular hypertension

1. Renal artery stenosis causes reduction of blood flow to the kidneys.
2. Kidneys secrete renin in response.
3. Renin 1 angiotensinogen in the liver forms angiotensin I.
4. In the lungs, angiotensin I is converted into angiotensin II, a vasoconstrictor.

We're all in it together when it comes to renovascular hypertension!

Compatible blood types

Precise blood-typing and cross-matching can prevent the transfusion of incompatible blood, which can be fatal. Usually, typing the recipient's blood and cross-matching it with available donor blood takes less than 1 hour.

Matchmaking

Agglutinogen (an antigen in red blood cells [RBCs]) and agglutinin (an antibody in plasma) distinguish the four ABO blood groups. This table depicts ABO compatibility from the perspectives of recipients and donors.

Blood group	Antibodies in plasma	Compatible RBCs	Compatible plasma
Recipient			
0	Anti-A and anti-B	0	0, A, B, AB
A	Anti-B	A, 0	A, AB
B	Anti-A	B, 0	B, AB
AB	Neither anti-A nor anti-B	AB, A, B, 0	AB
Donor			
0	Anti-A and anti-B	0, A, B, AB	0
A	Anti-B	A, AB	A, 0
B	Anti-A	B, AB	B, 0
AB	Neither anti-A nor anti-B	AB	AB, A, B, 0

Anti-Rh antibodies can only appear in the blood of an Rh-negative person after introduction of Rh-positive RBCs into the bloodstream such as from transfusion of Rh-positive blood. An Rh-negative female who carries an Rh-positive foetus may also acquire anti-Rh antibodies from exposure to Rh-positive blood during pregnancy and especially during labour and delivery.

A person with Rh-negative blood should only receive a transfusion with Rh-negative blood. Repeated transfusions of Rh-positive blood to an Rh-negative patient puts the patient at risk for haemolysis and agglutination. (See Chapter 10 for more information about blood transfusions and adverse reactions.)

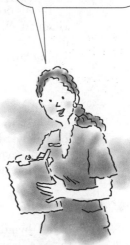

Anti-Rh antibodies occur in an Rh-negative person after Rh-positive RBCs are introduced into the bloodstream.

Immune system

The organs and tissues of the immune system are involved with the growth, development and dissemination of lymphocytes. (See *Organs and tissues of the immune system*, page 523.)

Immunity divided by 3

The immune system has three major divisions:

 central lymphoid organs and tissues

peripheral lymphoid organs and tissues

accessory lymphoid organs and tissues.

Central lymphoid organs and tissues
The bone marrow and thymus play roles in developing B cells and T cells, which are the two major types of lymphocytes.

Bone marrow
The bone marrow contains stem cells, which are multipotential, meaning they may develop into several different cell types. The immune system and blood cells develop from stem cells in a process called *haematopoiesis*.

Stemming from stem cells

Soon after differentiation from the stem cells, some of the cells become part of the immune system and sources of lymphocytes; others develop into phagocytes, which ingest microorganisms and cellular debris.

To B or to be T

The lymphocytes further differentiate into either B cells (which mature in the bone marrow) or T cells (which travel to the thymus and mature). B cells and T cells are distributed throughout the lymphoid organs, especially the lymph nodes and spleen.

B cells don't attack pathogens themselves but instead produce antibodies, which attack pathogens or direct other cells, such as phagocytes, to attack them. This response is regulated by T cells and their products, lymphokines, which determine the immunoglobulin class a B cell will manufacture.

Thymus
In a foetus or an infant, the thymus is a two-lobed mass of lymphoid tissue located over the base of the heart in the mediastinum. The thymus forms T lymphocytes for several months after birth and gradually atrophies until only a remnant persists in adults.

Teaching T cells

In the thymus, T cells undergo a process called *T-cell education*, in which the cells 'learn' to recognise other cells from the same body (self cells) and

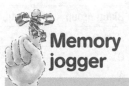

Memory jogger

To help you remember where lymphocytes mature, remember:

B cells mature in the **B**one marrow

T cells mature in the **T**hymus.

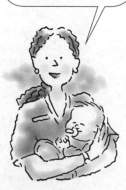

The thymus forms T lymphocytes until several months after birth and then gradually atrophies.

Organs and tissues of the immune system

The immune system includes cells that circulate in the bloodstream as well as organs and tissues in which lymphocytes predominate. This illustration depicts the central, peripheral and accessory lymphoid organs and tissue.

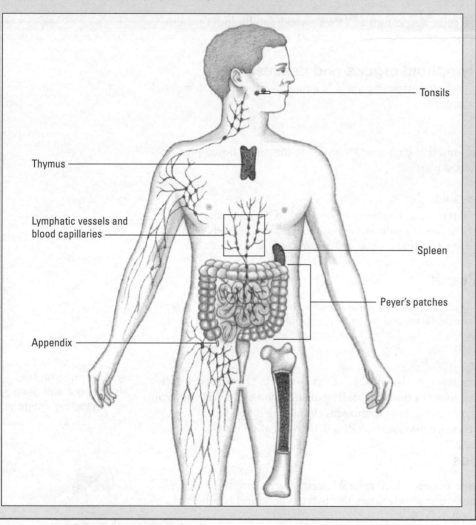

Tonsils

Thymus

Lymphatic vessels and blood capillaries

Spleen

Peyer's patches

Appendix

distinguish them from all other cells (nonself cells). There are five types of T cells with specific functions:

memory cells, which are sensitised cells that remain dormant until second exposure to an antigen

lymphokine-producing cells, which are involved in delayed hypersensitivity reactions cytotoxic T cells, which direct destruction of an antigen or the cells carrying the antigen

helper T cells, also known as *T4 cells*, which facilitate the humoral and cell-mediated responses

suppressor T cells, also known as *T8 cells*, which inhibit humoral and cell-mediated responses.

Peripheral lymphoid organs and tissues

The peripheral lymphoid structures include lymph and the lymphatic vessels, lymph nodes and spleen.

Lymph

Lymph is a clear fluid that bathes body tissues. It contains a liquid portion that resembles blood plasma.

Lymphatic vessels

The lymphatic vessels form a network of thin-walled channels that drain lymph from body tissues. Lymph seeps into the lymphatic vessels through their thin walls. (See *Lymphatic vessels and lymph nodes*, page 525.)

Fluid enters but can't exit

Lymphatic capillaries are located throughout most of the body. They're wider than blood capillaries and permit interstitial fluid to flow into them but not out.

Lymph nodes

Lymph nodes are small, oval-shaped structures along the lymphatic vessels. They're most abundant in the head, neck, axillae, abdomen, pelvis and groin. Lymph nodes remove and destroy antigens circulating in the blood and lymph because they are filled with WBCs that engulf and destroy.

From vessels to nodes

Afferent lymphatic vessels, which resemble veins, carry lymph into the lymph nodes; the lymph slowly filters through the node and is collected into efferent lymphatic vessels.

Node-to-node

Lymph usually travels through more than one lymph node because numerous nodes line the lymphatic vessels that drain a region. For example, axillary nodes filter drainage from the arms and femoral nodes filter drainage from the legs. This prevents organisms that enter peripheral areas from entering central areas.

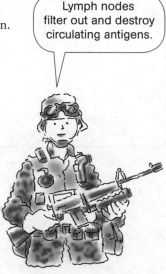

Lymph nodes filter out and destroy circulating antigens.

Lymphatic vessels and lymph nodes

The primary lymphatic vessels and structures of a lymph node are depicted below.

Into the nodes

Afferent lymphatic vessels carry lymph into the subcapsular sinus (or cavity) of the lymph node. From there, lymph flows through cortical sinuses and smaller radial medullary sinuses.

Phagocytic cells in the deep cortex and medullary sinuses attack antigens in lymph. Antigens may also be trapped in the follicles of the superficial cortex.

Back into the vessels

Cleansed lymph leaves the node through efferent lymphatic vessels at the hilum (a depression at the exit or entrance of the node). The efferent vessels drain into lymph node chains that, in turn, empty into large lymph vessels, or trunks, that drain into the subclavian vein of the vascular system.

Lymphatic vessels and capillaries

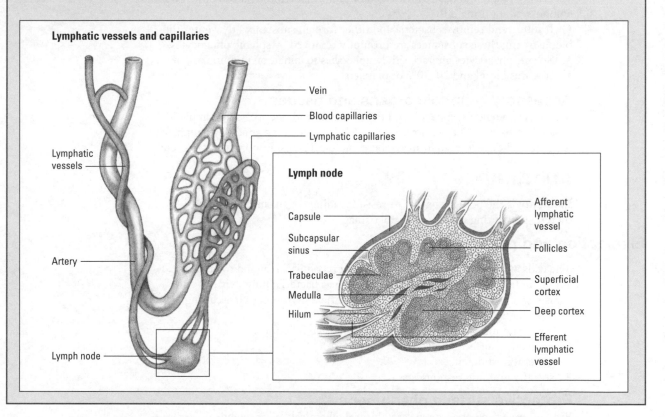

Spleen

A person's spleen is in the left upper abdominal quadrant beneath the diaphragm. This dark red, oval structure is about the size of a fist. Bands of connective tissue from the dense fibrous capsule surrounding the spleen extend into the spleen's interior.

Red, white and blood-filled

The interior spleen, called the splenic pulp, contains white and red pulp:
• White pulp contains compact masses of lymphocytes surrounding branches of the splenic artery.
• Red pulp is a network of blood-filled sinusoids supported by a framework of reticular fibres and mononuclear phagocytes, along with some lymphocytes, plasma cells and monocytes.

Splenic work

The spleen has several functions:
• Its phagocytes engulf and break down worn-out RBCs, causing the release of Hb, which then breaks down into its components. These phagocytes also selectively retain and destroy damaged or abnormal RBCs and cells with large amounts of abnormal Hb.
• It filters and removes bacteria and other foreign substances that enter the bloodstream; these substances are promptly removed by splenic phagocytes.
• Splenic phagocytes interact with lymphocytes to initiate an immune response.
• It stores blood and 20–30% of platelets.

Accessory lymphoid organs and tissues

The tonsils, adenoids, appendix and Peyer's patches are the accessory lymphoid organs and tissues. They remove foreign debris in much the same way lymph nodes do. They're located in areas where microbial access is more likely to occur.

Immunity

Immunity is the body's capacity to resist invading organisms and toxins, thereby preventing tissue and organ damage.

Elimination and preservation

The cells and organs of the immune system recognise, respond to, and eliminate foreign substances (antigens), such as bacteria, fungi, viruses and parasites. They also preserve the body's internal environment by scavenging dead or damaged cells.

The immune system has three basic defensive functions:
• protective surface phenomena
• general host defences
• specific immune responses.

Protective surface phenomena

Protective surface phenomena are physical, chemical and mechanical barriers that prevent organisms from entering the body. Such phenomena include organs, structures and processes of many body systems:
• integumentary (skin, tissues and mucous membranes)
• respiratory
• GI
• genitourinary.

Skin-deep defences

Intact and healing skin and mucous membranes physically defend against microbial invasion by preventing attachment of microorganisms. Skin desquamation (normal cell turnover) and low pH further impede bacterial colonisation.

Antibacterial substances, such as the enzyme lysozyme (in tears, saliva and nasal secretions) chemically protect seromucous surfaces, such as the conjunctiva of the eye and oral mucous membranes.

Defensive breathing

In the respiratory system, turbulent airflow through the nostrils and nasal hairs filters foreign materials. Nasal secretions contain an immunoglobulin that discourages microbe adherence, and the mucous layer lining the respiratory tract is continually sloughed off and replaced. Coughing and sneezing aid removal of bacteria and excess secretions.

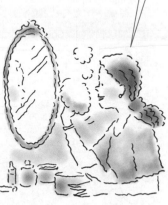

The skin and mucous membranes prevent microbial invasions.

GI system GIs

Bacteria that enter the GI system are mechanically removed through salivation, swallowing, peristalsis, defecation and vomiting when required. The low pH of gastric secretions is bactericidal, making the stomach virtually free from live bacteria. In addition, resident bacteria in the intestines prevent colonisation by other microorganisms, protecting the rest of the GI system through a process called *colonisation resistance*.

Urinary sterility

The urinary system is sterile except for the distal end of the urethra and the urinary meatus. Urine flow, low urine pH, immunoglobulin, and the bactericidal effects of prostatic fluid impede bacterial colonisation. A series of sphincters also inhibits upward bacterial migration into the urinary tract.

Says here, 'Resident bacteria in the intestines protect the GI system through a process called *colonisation resistance*'.

General host defences

When an antigen does penetrate the skin or mucous membrane, the immune system launches a nonspecific cellular response to identify and remove the invader.

First response

The first nonspecific response against an antigen, the inflammatory response, involves vascular and cellular changes that eliminate dead tissue, microorganisms, toxins and inert foreign matter. (See *Understanding inflammation*, page 528.)

Next effect

Phagocytosis occurs after inflammation or during chronic infection. In this nonspecific response, neutrophils and macrophages engulf, digest and dispose of the antigen.

Understanding inflammation

The inflammatory response to an antigen involves vascular and cellular changes that eliminate dead tissue, microorganisms, toxins, and inert foreign matter. This nonspecific immune response aids tissue repair in a stepwise fashion.

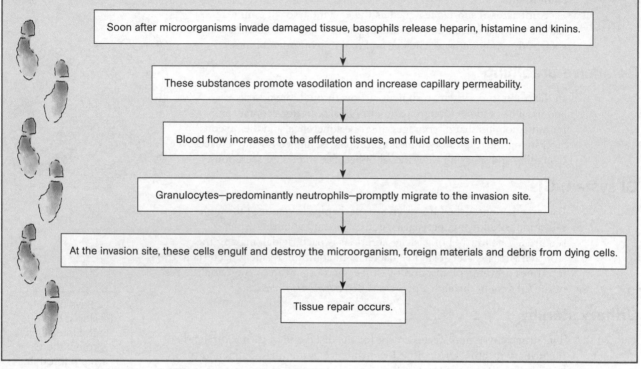

Soon after microorganisms invade damaged tissue, basophils release heparin, histamine and kinins.

↓

These substances promote vasodilation and increase capillary permeability.

↓

Blood flow increases to the affected tissues, and fluid collects in them.

↓

Granulocytes—predominantly neutrophils—promptly migrate to the invasion site.

↓

At the invasion site, these cells engulf and destroy the microorganism, foreign materials and debris from dying cells.

↓

Tissue repair occurs.

Specific immune responses

All foreign substances elicit the same general host defences. In addition, particular microorganisms or molecules activate specific immune responses produced by lymphocytes (B cells and T cells) and can initially involve specialised sets of immune cells. Such specific responses are classified as either:
- humoral immunity, or
- cell-mediated immunity.

Humoral immunity

In humoral immunity, an invading antigen causes B cells to divide and differentiate into plasma cells. Each plasma cell then produces and secretes a large amount of antigen-specific immunoglobulin into the bloodstream.

Each of the five types of immunoglobulins (IgA, IgD, IgE, IgG and IgM) has a specific function:
- IgA, IgG and IgM guard against viral and bacterial invasion.
- IgD is an antigen receptor of B cells.
- IgE causes an allergic response.

Defence depends on the antigen

Depending on the antigen, immunoglobulins work in one of several ways:
- They can disable certain bacteria by linking with toxins that the bacteria produce; these immunoglobulins are called *antitoxins*.
- They can coat bacteria, making them targets for scavenging by phagocytosis.
- Most commonly, they link to antigens, causing the immune system to produce and circulate enzymes called *complements*.

Telling time lag

After an initial exposure to an antigen, a time lag occurs during which little or no antibody can be detected in the body. During this time, the B cell recognizes the antigen, and the antigen–antibody complex forms. The complex has several functions:
- A macrophage processes the antigen and presents it to antigen-specific B cells.
- The antibody activates the complement system, causing an enzymatic cascade that destroys the antigen.
- The activated complement system, which bridges humoral and cell-mediated immunity, attracts phagocytic neutrophils and macrophages to the antigen site.

Complement system

The complement system consists of about 25 enzymes that complement the work of antibodies by aiding phagocytosis or destroying bacteria (by puncturing their cell membranes).

Cascading complements

Complement proteins travel in the bloodstream in an inactive form. When the first complement substance is triggered by an antibody interlocked with an antigen, it sets in motion a ripple effect. As each component is activated in turn, it acts on the next component in a controlled sequence called the *complement cascade*.

Attack complex

The complement cascade leads to formation of the membrane attack complex, which enters the membrane of a target cell and creates a channel through which fluids and molecules flow in and out. The target cell then swells and eventually bursts.

Complementary effects

Effects of the complement cascade also include:
- the inflammatory response (resulting from release of the contents of mast cells and basophils)
- stimulation and attraction of neutrophils (which participate in phagocytosis)
- coating of target cells by C3b (an inactivated fragment of the complement protein C3), making them attractive to phagocytes.

The complement cascade causes a ripple effect.

Cell-mediated immunity

Cell-mediated immunity protects the body against bacterial, viral and fungal infections and provides resistance against transplanted cells and tumour cells.

T cells destroy and survey

In cell-mediated immunity, a macrophage processes the antigen, which is then presented to T cells. Some T cells become sensitised and destroy the antigen; others release lymphokines, which activate macrophages that destroy the antigen. Sensitised T cells then travel through the blood and lymphatic systems, providing ongoing surveillance for specific antigens.

Haematological and immune systems assessment

Many signs and symptoms of haematological disorders are nonspecific and difficult to assess. Others are more specific; use these to focus on possible disorders. Assess the haematological system if the patient reports any of these specific signs or symptoms, including:

- abnormal bleeding
- bone and joint pain
- exertional dyspnoea
- ecchymoses
- fatigue and weakness
- fever
- lymphadenopathy
- petechiae
- shortness of breath
- chills
- night sweats.

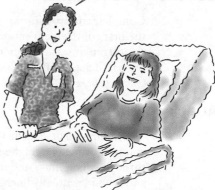

If the patient reports the specific signs or symptoms discussed here, assess for haematological disorders.

Immune challenges

Accurately assessing a patient's immune system can likewise challenge your skills. Immune disorders sometimes produce characteristic signs—such as butterfly rash in systemic lupus erythematosus (SLE)—but they usually cause vague symptoms, such as fatigue or dyspnoea, which initially seem related to other body systems. For this reason, assess the immune system whenever a patient reports such symptoms as:

- malaise
- fatigue
- frequent or recurrent infections
- slow wound healing.

If the critically ill patient requires immediate stabilising treatment always use an ABCDE approach, otherwise begin with a thorough assessment adopting this structured approach:
- History of the present complaint
- Health history and medication
- Clinical assessment and monitoring
- Results and significance of diagnostic tests and investigations

Health history

History of the present complaint
Ask the patient/relatives how long the patient has had the problem, when it began and how suddenly or gradually. What are the main symptoms? What is causing the most concern?

Next, determine the location and character of the problem and precipitating conditions. Ask if anything makes the problem better or worse. Also ask about other signs and symptoms that occur at the same time as the primary ones.

Health history and medication
Examine the patient's medical history for additional clues to their present condition. Look for information about allergies, immunisations, previously diagnosed illnesses (childhood and adult), past hospitalisations and surgeries and current medications, both prescription and over-the-counter.

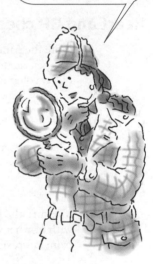

Examine the patient's medical history to find clues about their present condition.

Look back
Look at the patient's history for information about past disorders (such as acute leukaemia, Hodgkin's disease, sarcoma and rheumatoid arthritis) that required aggressive immunosuppressant or radiation therapies. Such treatment can diminish blood cell production. Has the patient received any blood products? If so, note when and how often blood product transfusions were used to assess the patient's risk of harbouring a blood-borne infection.

Family history
Some haematological disorders are inherited. Ask about deceased family members; note their ages at death and causes. Note any inheritable haematological disorders.

Lifestyle patterns
The patient may be reluctant to discuss certain habits or lifestyles. Take steps to develop trust between you and the patient to increase cooperation. Inquire about alcohol intake, diet, sexual habits and possible drug abuse, all of which can impair haematological or immune function.

Work and service
Make sure you gather a comprehensive occupational history. Exposure to certain hazardous substances can cause bone marrow dysfunction, especially leukaemia.

Clinical assessment and monitoring

Because haematological and immune disorders can involve almost every body system, perform a complete physical examination.

Assessing vital signs

Vital signs can provide important clues about the patient's haematological and immune system health.

Thermomeasurement

Take the patient's temperature. Frequent fevers can indicate a poorly functioning immune system. Subnormal temperatures usually accompany gram-negative infections.

Heart and BP checks

Note the patient's heart rate. The heart may pump harder or faster to compensate for a decreased oxygen supply resulting from anaemia or decreased blood volume from bleeding. This problem can cause tachycardia, palpitations or arrhythmias. Measure the patient's blood pressure observing for hypotension.

O₂ inquiry

Check the patient's breathing. If they're having difficulty meeting the body's oxygen needs, they may have pronounced tachypnoea.

Size up

Measure the patient's height and weight if possible. Compare the findings with normal values for the patient's bone structure. Weight loss may result from anorexia or other GI problems related to immune disorders.

Haematological inspection

Next, concentrate on areas most relevant to a haematological disorder, including the:
- skin
- mucous membranes
- fingernails
- eyes
- lymph nodes
- liver and spleen.

Skin-deep assessment

The patient's skin colour directly reflects body fluid composition. Observe for pallor, cyanosis or jaundice. Check for erythema and plethora (ruddy colour), which appear with local inflammation and polycythaemia, respectively. Assess the mucous membranes for jaundice, bleeding, redness, swelling or ulceration.

> Because haematologic and immune disorders can involve almost every body system, perform a complete physical examination.

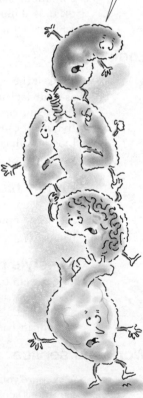

Examine skin, nails and eyes

If you suspect a blood-clotting abnormality, check the patient's skin for purpuric lesions, which may vary in size and usually result from thrombocytopaenia. Also, inspect for abnormalities, such as telangiectases (dilated capillary blood vessels), and note their locations. Check the patient's skin for dryness and coarseness, which may indicate iron deficiency anaemia.

Note abnormalities in the patient's nails. Longitudinal striations can indicate anaemia. Spoon-shaped nails characterise iron deficiency anaemia. Nail clubbing indicates chronic tissue hypoxia, which can result from such haematological disorders as anaemia.

Inspect the patient's eyes for jaundice, which may occur from excessive haemolysis. Retinal haemorrhages and exudates suggest severe anaemia and thrombocytopaenia.

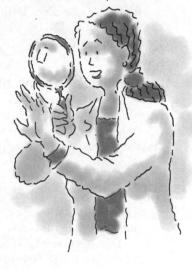

Abnormalities in the patient's nails, such as longitudinal striations, spoon shape and clubbing, can result from anaemia.

Abdominal assessment

Inspect the patient's abdominal area for enlargement, distention and asymmetry, possibly indicating a tumour. Hepatomegaly and splenomegaly may result from:
- congestion caused by cell overproduction, as in polycythaemia or leukaemia
- excessive cell destruction, as in haemolytic anaemia.

Immune system inspection

An immune disorder can affect the skin and nails as described earlier. It can also affect the mouth and nose, so assess the nasal cavity for mucous membrane ulceration, which may indicate SLE.

Inspect the oral mucosa. White patches scattered throughout the mouth may indicate candidiasis, and lacy white plaques on the buccal mucosa may be associated with acquired immunodeficiency syndrome (AIDS). Such lesions can occur in a patient with an immunosuppressive disorder or one who receives chemotherapy.

LOC signs

Evaluate the patient's level of consciousness (LOC). Neurological effects may provide clues to an underlying disease. A patient with SLE may experience altered mentation, depression or psychosis. Calculate GCS and evaluate mental status.

Eyes, fingers, toes, ears and nose

Observe the patient's eyelids for signs of infection or inflammation. Assess the fundus of the eye; haemorrhage or infiltration may indicate vasculitis.

Assess the patient's peripheral circulation for Raynaud's phenomenon (intermittent arteriolar vasospasm of the fingers or toes and sometimes of the ears and nose). This phenomenon may be caused by SLE or scleroderma.

Urinary system inspection

Because immune dysfunction can affect the urinary system, obtain a urine specimen and evaluate its colour, clarity and odour. Cloudy, offensive smelling urine may result from a urinary tract infection.

Inspect the urinary meatus. In a patient with WBC deficiency or immunodeficiency, the external genitalia may be focal points for inflammation, which is commonly accompanied by discharge or bleeding related to infection.

Look for lumps

Inspect the lymph node areas (see *Palpating the lymph nodes*, page 535) where the patient reports swollen glands or lumps for colour abnormalities and visible lymph node enlargement. Then inspect all other nodal regions. Proceed from head to toe to avoid missing any region. Normally, lymph nodes can't be seen. Visibly enlarged nodes suggest a current or previous inflammation. Nodes covered with red-streaked skin suggest acute lymphadenitis.

Auscultating the abdomen

With the patient lying down, auscultate the abdomen before palpation and percussion to avoid altering bowel sounds. Listen for a loud, high-pitched, tinkling sound, which heralds the early stages of intestinal obstruction. Lymphoma is a haematological cause of such obstruction.

Consider the liver

The medical staff will examine the liver and spleen, to determine size, and possibly detect tumours.

Doctors percuss all four abdominal quadrants to determine liver and spleen size and to detect tumours.

Cell-packing problem

As lymph nodes are palpated you may discover sternal tenderness. This problem occurs with cell packing in the marrow from anaemia, leukaemia and immunoproliferative disorders.

Liver and spleen palpation

Accurate liver palpation is difficult and can depend on the patient's size and comfort level and possible fluid accumulation. The spleen is palpated to detect tenderness and confirm splenomegaly. The spleen must be enlarged about three times normal size to be palpable.

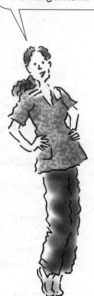

Look from head to toe for lumps or visible lymph node enlargement.

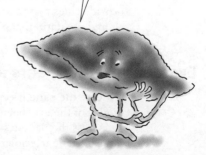

Remember, palpate tender areas last. I'm a sensitive fellow, you know.

Palpating the lymph nodes

When assessing a patient for signs of an immune disorder, the superficial lymph nodes of the head and neck and of the axillary, epitrochlear, inguinal and popliteal areas should be palpated, using the pads of index and middle fingers. Always palpate gently, beginning with light pressure and gradually increasing the pressure.

Head and neck nodes

Head and neck nodes are best palpated with the patient sitting.

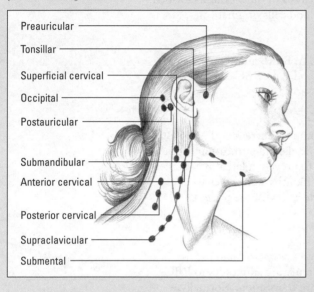

Preauricular
Tonsillar
Superficial cervical
Occipital
Postauricular
Submandibular
Anterior cervical
Posterior cervical
Supraclavicular
Submental

Inguinal and popliteal nodes

Palpate the inguinal and popliteal nodes with the patient lying in a supine position. Palpate the popliteal nodes with the patient sitting or standing.

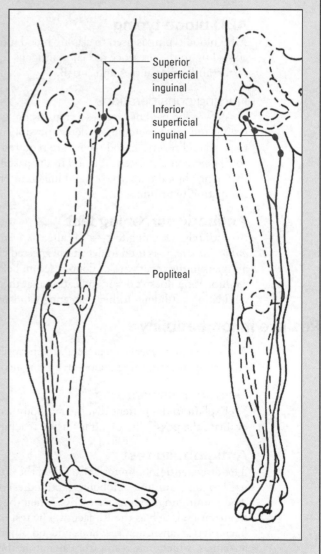

Superior superficial inguinal
Inferior superficial inguinal
Popliteal

Results and significance of diagnostic tests and investigations

Various tests may be ordered to diagnose haematological and immune disorders.

Haematological system tests

Haematological diagnostic tests allow direct analysis of the blood, its formed elements (cells) and the bone marrow, where blood cells originate.

ABO blood typing

ABO blood typing is used to classify blood into A, B, AB and O groups according to the presence of major antigens A and B on RBC surfaces and serum antibodies anti-A and anti-B.

Nursing considerations
• Before the patient receives a transfusion, compare current and past ABO typing and cross-matching to detect possible mistaken identification. Both forward and reverse blood typing are required to prevent a lethal reaction.
• If a patient has received blood in the past 3 months, antibodies to this donor blood may develop and linger, interfering with the patient's compatibility testing.

Antibody screening test

An antibody screening test—also called *an indirect Coombs' test* and *indirect antiglobulin test*—is used to detect unexpected circulating antibodies to RBC antigens in the recipient's or donor's serum before transfusion. Normally, agglutination doesn't occur, indicating that the patient's serum contains no circulating antibodies (other than anti-A and anti-B).

Positive incompatibility

A positive result reveals the presence of unexpected circulating antibodies to RBC antigens, indicating donor—recipient incompatibility.

Nursing considerations
• Explain to the patient that the antibody screening test is used to evaluate the possibility of a transfusion reaction.

Antiglobulin test

The direct antiglobulin test, also called the *direct Coombs' test*, is used to detect immunoglobulins (antibodies) on RBC surfaces. These immunoglobulins coat RBCs when they become sensitised to an antigen such as the Rh factor. The test is used to investigate haemolytic transfusion reactions and aid differential diagnosis of anaemias, which may result from an autoimmune reaction or a drug's adverse effect.

Hold it! Withhold medications that can induce autoimmune haemolytic anaemia.

Nursing considerations
• As ordered, withhold medications that can induce autoimmune haemolytic anaemia, e.g. high-dose penicillin, paracetamol, quinine, levodopa.

Cross-matching
Cross-matching is used to establish the compatibility or incompatibility of donor and recipient blood and is the final check for such compatibility.

Always necessary, except . . .
Blood is always cross-matched before transfusion, except in extreme emergencies. Because a complete cross-match may take 45 minutes to 2 hours, an incomplete (10-minute) cross-match may be acceptable in emergencies. Meanwhile, transfusion can begin with limited amounts of group O negative packed RBCs. It is important to recognise that O negative blood is only available in small amounts so should only be used when absolutely necessary, e.g. massive uncontrolled haemorrhage in an obviously shocked patient. When an emergency transfusion is necessary, proceed with special awareness of the complications that may arise because of incomplete typing and cross-matching. (See Chapter 10 for more information about transfusion reactions).

Nursing considerations
• If more than 48 hours have elapsed since a previous transfusion, previously cross-matched donor blood must be cross-matched with a new recipient serum sample to detect newly acquired incompatibilities before transfusion.
• If the recipient hasn't received a transfusion, donor blood need not be cross-matched again for 72 hours.
• If the patient is scheduled for surgery and has received blood during the previous 3 months, their blood must be cross-matched again to detect recently acquired incompatibilities.

Rh blood typing
The Rh system is used to classify blood according to the presence or absence of antigen D on RBC surfaces. Rh blood typing is used to determine if donors and recipients are compatible before transfusions and to learn whether the patient needs an Anti D immunoglobulin injection.

Nursing considerations
• Before the patient receives a transfusion, the Rh factor must be checked along with ABO typing.

Haematocrit
Haematocrit (HCT) test results indicate the percentage of RBCs in whole blood samples. Although normal HCT varies widely, it's roughly three times the person's Hb level and amounts to:
• in men, 42–52%
• in women, 36–48%
• in children, 30–42%.
  Below-normal HCT suggests anaemia or haemodilution; above-normal, polycythaemia or haemoconcentration due to fluid loss.

Nursing considerations
- Explain the purpose of blood tests to the patient.
- Notify the doctor of significant findings and administer blood products, fluid or diuretics as prescribed based on test results.

Haemoglobin level (total Hb)
Hb—the main component of RBCs—contains *haem*, a complex molecule of iron and porphyrin that gives blood its colour, and globin, a simple protein.

O_2 delivery

Hb delivers oxygen from the lungs to the cells and buffers carbon dioxide formed during metabolic activity. A below-normal Hb level may result from anaemia, recent haemorrhage or fluid retention causing haemodilution; an above-normal Hb level may result from haemoconcentration due to polycythaemia or dehydration. An Hb of <7 g/dl is the usual trigger for transfusion in critically ill patients unless obvious coronary ischaemia or bleeding exist. This level is used because above this the side effects of transfusion outweigh the benefits.

Nursing considerations
- Explain the purpose of blood tests to the patient.
- Notify the doctor of significant findings and administer blood products as prescribed based on test results. Remember that there is time delay in both Hb dropping and rising. After bleeding or transfusion it can take around 2 hours for the Hb result to change.

RBC count
RBC count—also known as *erythrocyte count*—indicates the number of RBCs in whole blood. A depressed RBC count may indicate anaemia, fluid overload, recent haemorrhage or leukaemia; an elevated count, dehydration, polycythaemia or acute poisoning.

Nursing considerations
- Explain the purpose of RBC tests to the patient.
- Notify the doctor of significant findings and administer blood products as prescribed based on test results.

Coagulation screening tests
Coagulation screening tests are used to detect bleeding disorders and specific coagulation defects. They inform titration of anticoagulants and determine the risk of bleeding especially prior to invasive procedures, e.g. surgery and central line insertion.

Nursing considerations
- Explain the test to the patient.
- Allow no more than 4 hours between blood sampling and coagulation testing. Allow only 2 hours between blood centrifugation and coagulation testing because once centrifuged, RBCs lose their buffering effect on the plasma.

• Avoid using haemolysed plasma, which may decrease clotting times. Send blood sample to the laboratory immediately after it's collected to preserve its labile factors.

Activated partial thromboplastin time

Activated partial thromboplastin time (APTT) is used to evaluate all intrinsic pathway clotting factors (except factors VII and XIII) by measuring the time needed for a fibrin clot to form after calcium and phospholipid emulsion is added to a plasma sample. APTT is commonly used to monitor heparin therapy.

Normal time

Normally, a fibrin clot forms 25–36 seconds after reagent is added. Prolonged times may mean that the plasma sample contains plasma clotting factor deficiencies, heparin, fibrin split products or circulating anticoagulants that act as antibodies to clotting factors.

Nursing considerations
• Explain to the patient receiving heparin therapy that this test may be repeated at regular intervals to assess their response to treatment.
• Notify the doctor of test results and adjust the heparin infusion dosage as ordered.
• For a patient on anticoagulant therapy, additional pressure may be needed at the venepuncture site to control bleeding.

D-dimer

D-dimer testing is used to help diagnose disseminated intravascular coagulation (DIC) by confirming the presence of fibrin split products. Fibrin split products are pieces of clot that enter the circulation after the clot has been broken down. DIC is a process that continually builds and breaks down clots, until all the clotting factors in the body have been depleted. As more clots break down, the D-dimer rises.

Nursing considerations
• Explain the purpose of the test to the patient.
• If the patient is being tested for coagulopathies, apply additional pressure to the venepuncture site to prevent haematoma formation.

Platelet count

Platelet count is used to evaluate platelet (thrombocyte) production, which is necessary for blood clotting. Accurate counts are essential for monitoring chemotherapy and radiation therapy and for assessing the severity of thrombocytosis (abnormally increased platelet count) or thrombocytopaenia.

Count down

A normal platelet count varies from 150 to 400 $\times 10^9$ per L. A platelet count below 50 can result in spontaneous bleeding; a count below 5 usually indicates potential

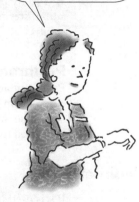

Normally, a fibrin clot forms 25–36 seconds after reagent is added. Anything longer can be a problem.

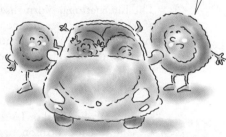

HCT test results indicate the percentage of RBCs in whole blood samples.

for massive haemorrhage. A decreased platelet count may result from autoimmune processes, some drugs (such as heparin which may lead to heparin-induced thrombocytopaenia [HIT]), infection or platelets may be lost during renal replacement therapy by adhering to the filter.

Count up

An increased platelet count may result from haemorrhage, infectious disorders, cancer, iron deficiency anaemia, surgery, pregnancy, splenectomy or an inflammatory disorder. It is regularly seen in critically ill patients as they mount a response to the insult on their body.

Nursing considerations
• Explain the purpose of platelet tests to the patient.
• Notify the doctor of significant findings and administer blood products as prescribed based on test results.

Prothrombin time and INR
Prothrombin time (PT) is the time required for a fibrin clot to form in a citrated plasma sample after calcium ion and tissue thromboplastin (factor III) are added. The result is compared to the fibrin clotting time in a control plasma sample.

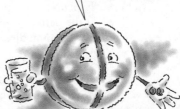

Not so fast... nobody gets by unless they're on the list and their I.D. checks out.

Indirect test

PT is used to indirectly measure prothrombin and is an excellent screening method for evaluating prothrombin, fibrinogen and extrinsic coagulation factors V, VII and X. It's the test of choice for monitoring oral anticoagulant therapy (e.g. warfarin). In a patient receiving an oral anticoagulant, PT usually remains between one and one-half and three times the normal control value.

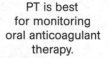

PT is best for monitoring oral anticoagulant therapy.

INR standards

The International Normalised Ratio (INR) system is the best means of standardising measurement of PT to monitor oral anticoagulant therapy. Normal INR for those receiving warfarin therapy is two to three times the control. Increased INR values may indicate:
• DIC
• cirrhosis
• vitamin K deficiency
• uncontrolled oral or I.V. anticoagulation
• salicylate intoxication

- massive blood transfusion
- inadequate reversal of intraoperative anticoagulation, for example in vascular and cardiac surgery.

Nursing considerations
- Explain to a patient receiving oral anticoagulant therapy that this test may be repeated at regular intervals to assess their response to treatment.
- For a patient on anticoagulant therapy, additional pressure may be needed at the venepuncture site to control bleeding.
- Notify the doctor of test results; oral anticoagulant therapy dosage adjustments are based on test results.

Biopsy

Biopsies involve removing small samples of tissue for testing.

Bone marrow aspiration and needle biopsy
In aspiration biopsy, a fluid specimen containing bone marrow cells in suspension is collected. Bone marrow aspiration is an important test for evaluating the blood's formed elements.

Needle biopsy is done to remove a marrow core containing cells but no fluid. The best possible marrow specimens are obtained by using both methods.

Aspire to biopsy

Because most haematopoiesis takes place in bone marrow, histology and haematological bone marrow examination yields valuable diagnostic information about blood disorders. Bone marrow aspiration and needle biopsy are used to obtain material for that examination.

Bone marrow biopsy is used to diagnose aplastic, hypoplastic and vitamin B_{12} deficiency anaemias; granulomas; leukaemias; lymphomas; myelofibrosis; and thrombocytopaenia. It's also used to evaluate chemotherapy effectiveness and to monitor myelosuppression.

Nursing considerations
- Describe the procedure and answer the patient's questions. Confirm any medication allergies or past history of hypersensitivity to local anaesthetics. Inform the patient that a local anaesthetic is used but that they may feel pressure during the biopsy.
- Tell them the test takes 5–10 minutes and test results are usually available in 1 day.
- Tell the patient which bone is to be used for the biopsy. (See *Bone marrow aspiration and biopsy sites*, page 542.)
- Explain to the patient that they may receive I.V. sedation before the procedure.

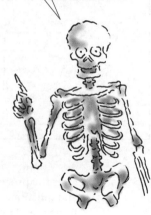

Bone marrow examination yields valuable information about blood disorders.

Bone marrow aspiration and biopsy sites

The drawings below depict the most common sites for bone marrow aspiration and biopsy. These sites are used because the involved bone structures are relatively accessible and rich in marrow cavities.

Posterior superior iliac crest

The posterior superior iliac crest is the preferred site for aspiration and biopsy because no vital organs or vessels are nearby. The patient lies in a prone or lateral position. The needle is inserted several centimetres lateral to the iliosacral junction and directed downwards and towards the anterior inferior spine or entered a few centimetres below the crest at a right angle to the surface of the bone.

Spinous process

The spinous process is preferred if multiple punctures are necessary or if marrow is absent at other sites. The patient sits on the edge of the bed, leaning over the bedside stand. The spinous process of the third or fourth lumbar vertebrae is selected, the needle is inserted at the crest or slightly to one side, and advanced in the direction of the bone plane.

Sternum

The sternum involves the greatest risk but provides the best access. The patient is in a supine position with a small pillow beneath their shoulders to elevate their chest and lower their head. The doctor secures the needle guard 3–4 mm from the tip of the needle to avoid accidentally puncturing the heart or a major vessel. Then they insert the needle at the midline of the sternum at the second intercostal space.

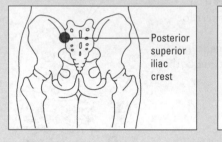

Posterior superior iliac crest

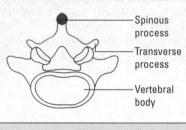

Spinous process

Transverse process

Vertebral body

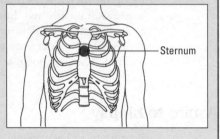

Sternum

• Monitor vital signs, oxygen saturation and cardiac rhythm during and after the procedure. After the procedure, check the biopsy site for bleeding and inflammation. Monitor for these signs of bleeding or infection: rapid heart rate, low blood pressure or fever.

• Change the dressing over the biopsy site every 24 hours to reduce the risk of infection.

Immune system tests

The doctor may order various tests to evaluate the patient's immune response. Commonly ordered studies include cellular tests, such as T- and B-lymphocyte assays, to detect immunomediated disease.

T- and B-lymphocyte surface marker assays

Surface marker assays are used to identify the specific cells involved in the immune response and to examine the balance between the regulatory activities of several interacting cell types, notably T-helper and T-suppressor cells.

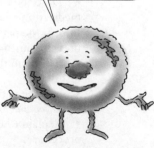

Surface marker assays are used to analyse both normal and malignant cells.

The test involves use of highly specific monoclonal antibodies to define levels of lymphocyte differentiation and to analyse both normal and malignant cells. This information is used to assess immunocompetence in chronic infections, evaluate immunodeficiencies and classify lymphocytic leukaemia, lymphoma and immunodeficiency disease and AIDS.

Nursing considerations
- Explain the test to the patient.
- Send the sample to the laboratory immediately; don't refrigerate or freeze it.

Treatments

Treatments for patients with haematological and immune disorders may include drug therapy and transfusion therapy.

Drug therapy

Haematological drugs include anticoagulants, blood derivatives, iron supplements, vitamin B_{12} supplements, erythropoietin and heparin and warfarin antagonists. (See *Common haematological medications*, pages 544–545.)

For patients with some immune disorders, drugs are the primary treatment. For example, following oxygen and fluids, adrenaline is the drug of choice for correcting an anaphylactic reaction. For patients with other disorders, drugs are prescribed to treat associated symptoms. (See *Drug therapy in immune disorders*, pages 546–547.)

Corticosteroid potentials

Corticosteroids (e.g. hydrocortisone) are adrenocortical hormones used to treat patients with immune-mediated disorders because of their potent anti-inflammatory and immunosuppressant effects.

Corticosteroids stabilise the vascular membrane, blocking tissue infiltration by neutrophils and monocytes and thus inhibiting inflammation. They also affect T cells in the bone marrow, causing leukopaenia. However, because these drugs aren't cytotoxic, lymphocyte concentration can quickly return to normal within 24 hours after they're withdrawn.

Corticosteroid cautions

Steroids should be used cautiously in patients with GI ulceration, renal disease, hypertension, diabetes mellitus and psychotic tendencies. On discontinuation they must be gradually reduced.

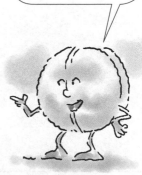

Corticosteroids aren't cytotoxic, so lymphocytes can quickly return to normal afterwards.

Common haematological medications

Haematologic drugs include those to boost red blood cell production which help arrest anaemia; anticoagulants, which impede clotting; haemostatics, which arrest blood flow or reduce capillary bleeding; blood derivatives, which replace blood loss from disease or surgical procedures. This chart outlines common haemolytic drugs, their indications and adverse effects, and practice considerations.

Drugs	Indications	Adverse effects	Practice pointers
Anticoagulants			
Heparin Low-molecular-weight heparins (Dalteparin Sodium, Enoxaparin Sodium, Tinzaparin Sodium)	• Prevention of pulmonary embolism and deep vein thrombosis (DVT) after hip- or knee-replacement surgery • Continuous I.V. or subcut therapy for DVT, myocardial infarction (MI), pulmonary embolism, instead of warfarin therapy during acute illnes	Haemorrhage, thrombocytopaenia, chills, fever, pruritis, urticaria, anaphylactoid reactions	• Never administer I.M. • Don't massage the site after subcutaneous injection. Rotate injection sites, keeping a record of sites used. • Monitor platelet count and for signs of bleeding. • Check I.V. infusions regularly for underdosing and overdosing. • Measure APTT. Anticoagulation is present when APTT values are 1.5–2 times control values for heparin. Clotting times remain unchanged in low-molecular-weight heparin use. • Reversed by protamine.
Warfarin	• Treatment of pulmonary embolism • Prevention and treatment of DVT, MI, rheumatic heart disease with heart valve damage, atrial arrhythmias	Anorexia, nausea, vomiting, haematuria, haemorrhage, jaundice, urticaria, fever, headache, rash	• Prothrombin time (PT) determinations measured as International Normalised Ratio (INR) are essential for proper controls; maintain INR 1.5–3 times. • Give drug at the same time daily. • Regularly inspect for bleeding gums, bruises, petechiae, nosebleeds, melaena, haematuria and haematemesis. • In critical illness vastly abnormal INR may be seen. Vitamin K is used to treat this. • The long-acting nature of warfarin makes it unsuitable for use in acute illness.

(continued)

Common haematological medications (continued)

Drugs	Indications	Adverse effects	Practice pointers
Blood derivatives			
Human albumin solution 4.5% Human albumin solution 20%	• Hypovolaemic shock • Hypoproteinaemia	Vascular overload after rapid infusion, hypotension, nausea, vomiting, dyspnoea, pulmonary oedema, chills, fever	• Don't give more than 250 g in 48 hours. • Watch for haemorrhage or shock if used after surgery or injury. • Watch for signs of vascular overload (heart failure or pulmonary oedema). • Don't use cloudy solutions or those with sediment. • Monitor blood pressure; reduce infusion rate if hypotension occurs. • Watch for signs of vascular overload (heart failure or pulmonary oedema). • Monitor intake and output; watch for decreased urine output.
Anaemia treatment			
Ferrous sulphate Erythropoietin	• Iron deficiency • hypoplastic, haemolytic and renal anaemias, Jehovah's witnesses	Nausea, epigastric pain, vomiting, constipation, black stools, diarrhoea, anorexia Hypertension, headache, thrombosis, rarely red cell aplasia	• Dilute liquid in orange juice or water, not milk or antacids. • GI upset is related to dosage; give the drug between meals. • Monitor blood pressure, platelets and Hb.
Heparin antagonist			
Protamine	• Heparin overdose	Bradycardia, circulatory collapse, nausea, vomiting, pulmonary oedema, acute pulmonary hypertension, anaphylaxis	• Use cautiously to avoid clotting. • Give slowly to reduce adverse effects. • Watch for spontaneous bleeding.

Transfusion therapy

Transfusion procedures allow administration of a wide range of blood products, such as RBCs, which can revive oxygen-starved tissues; leucocytes, which can combat infections beyond the reach of antibiotics; and clotting factors, plasma and platelets, which can help patients with clotting disorders live virtually normal lives.

Drug therapy in immune disorders

The practitioner may order drug therapy to suppress a patient's immune response. Immune serum studies may be ordered after specific antigens are identified. Immunosuppressants may be used to combat tissue rejection or relieve inflammation. Antiviral agents, which include nucleoside reverse transcriptase inhibitors, protease inhibitors and nonnucleoside reverse transcriptase inhibitors, are used to correct human immunodeficiency virus (HIV) infections. Use this table to find information necessary to administer these drugs.

Drugs	Indications	Adverse effects	Practice pointers
Nucleoside reverse transcriptase inhibitors			
Lamivudine	• Treatment of HIV infection in combination with other antivirals	Headache, fatigue, dizziness, insomnia, neutropaenia, thrombocytopaenia, cough, fever, chills, malaise, nausea	• Monitor serum amylase levels. Stop drug if clinical signs and symptoms suggest pancreatitis. • Give with another antiviral. Not indicated for use alone.
Stavudine	• Treatment of HIV-infected patients who have received prolonged zidovudine therapy	Peripheral neuropathy, headache, malaise, insomnia, anxiety, dizziness, chest pain, abdominal pain, diarrhoea, nausea, anorexia, weight loss, neutropenia, thrombocytopaenia, anaemia, rash, hepatotoxicity, chills, fever, pancreatitis	• May be taken with or without food. • Teach patient signs and symptoms of peripheral neuropathy, which is the major dose-limiting effect. It may not resolve after drug is discontinued. • Monitor liver function tests.
Zidovudine, AZT	• Symptom-producing HIV infection	Headache, seizures, paresthesia, somnolence, anorexia, nausea, vomiting, diarrhoea, constipation, severe bone marrow suppression (resulting in anaemia), rash, myalgia, fever, increased liver enzymes	• Use cautiously in patients with severe bone marrow depression. • Monitor blood studies every 2 weeks to detect anaemia or granulocytopaenia.
Protease inhibitors			
Saquinavir	• Treatment of advanced HIV infection in combination with other antivirals	Headache, dizziness, chest pain, pancreatitis, pancytopaenia, thrombocytopaenia, portal hypertension, hyperglycaemia, cough, rash	• Watch for adipogenic adverse effects (redistribution of body fat, peripheral wasting and breast enlargement). • Use cautiously in patients with liver impairment.

(continued)

Drug therapy in immune disorders (continued)

Drugs	Indications	Adverse effects	Practice pointers
Protease inhibitors (continued)			
Indinavir	• HIV infection	Headache, abdominal pain, nausea, acute renal failure, haemolytic anaemia, neutropenia, hepatic failure, hyperglycaemia, back pain, insomnia, dizziness, malaise	• Instruct patient to drink at least six glasses of water per day. • Give the drug on an empty stomach. • Monitor blood glucose levels.
Ritonavir	• HIV infection	Generalized tonic–clonic seizure, pancreatitis, thrombocytopaenia, leukopaenia, hepatitis, diabetes mellitus, hypersensitivity reaction, rash, myalgia, anorexia, abdominal pain, constipation, diarrhoea, nausea, vomiting	• Monitor liver functions studies and blood glucose levels. • Administer with food.
Nonnucleoside reverse transcriptase inhibitors			
Nevirapine	• Prevention of maternal–foetal transmission of HIV • Adjunct therapy for HIV infection	Headache, fever, nausea, diarrhoea, abdominal pain, hepatitis, hepatotoxicity, Stevens–Johnson syndrome, severe hypersensitivity reaction	• Monitor patient for and immediately report blistering rash.
Immune serums			
Hepatitis B immune globulin (H-BIG) I.V. immunoglobulin	• Hepatitis B exposure, needle stick injury • Hypogammaglobulina emia, idiopathic thrombocytopaenic purpura, post bone marrow transplant, Kawasaki syndrome, Guillain–Barré syndrome	Urticaria, pain and tenderness at injection site, anaphylaxis, angioedema Headache, faintness, nausea, vomiting, hip pain, chest pain, chest tightness, dyspnoea Allergic reaction, rarely thromboembolic events	• Obtain a history of allergies. • Inject into the anterolateral aspect of thigh or deltoid area. • Use cautiously in patients with a history of cardiovascular disease of thrombotic episodes. • Use is closely monitored owing to restricted availability and cost.
Immunosuppressants			
Cyclosporine	Prophylaxis of organ rejection in kidney, liver, bone marrow and heart transplants, treatment of psoriasis and rheumatoid arthritis	Tremor, headache, seizures, confusion, hypertension, nephrotoxicity, leukopaenia, thrombocytopaenia, hepatotoxicity, flushing, acne, infections, increased low-density lipoproteins, anaphylaxis	• Give dose once daily in the morning at the same time each day. • Oral preparations may be taken with meals if drug causes nausea.

Common procedures include blood transfusions and clotting factor replacement. Owing to the risks involved (hypersensitivity and allergic reactions, transmission of infection and thrombosis), a trigger Hb of 7 g/dl has been recommended when considering transfusion of packed red blood cells. Exceptions to this would be patients who are actively bleeding or have signs of cardiac ischaemia. (See Chapter 10 for more information about adverse reactions to transfusions.)

Factor replacement

I.V. infusion of deficient clotting elements is a major part of treatment for patients with coagulation disorders. Factor replacement typically corrects clotting factor deficiencies, thereby stopping or preventing haemorrhage.

Products depend on disorders

Various blood products are used, depending on the specific disorder being treated and dosage will usually be advised by a haematologist:
* Fresh frozen plasma (FFP) is used to treat clotting disorders with unknown causes, clotting factor deficiencies resulting from hepatic disease or blood dilution, consumed clotting factors secondary to DIC and deficiencies of clotting factors for which no specific replacement product exists.
* Cryoprecipitate is used to treat von Willebrand's disease, fibrinogen deficiencies and factor XIII deficiencies.
* Factor VIII (antihaemophiliac factor) concentrate serves as the long-term treatment of choice for patients with haemophilia A.
* Prothrombin complex is given to correct haemophilia B, severe liver disease and acquired deficiencies for the factors it contains (II, VII, IX and X).

Nursing considerations when administering blood products
* Explain the procedure to the patient and assemble equipment. Ensuring good I.V. access.
* Verify the prescription.
* Obtain the blood product from the blood bank or pharmacy.
* Identify the patient. Ask another registered health care professional (nurse or doctor) to double-check the patient's name, date of birth, medical record number and ABO and Rh status (as well as other compatibility factors). This information should be compared with the identification label on the blood product's bag.
* Check the expiration date, and inspect the product for cloudiness or turbidity.
* Infusion of all blood products must commence within 30 minutes of leaving a blood fridge to reduce infection and should always be completed within 6 hours. Platelets should be agitated once defrosted then infused immediately to prevent aggregation.
* Administer platelets and packed cells using a blood component drip administration set; don't use a microaggregate filter or platelets and red blood cells will not be infused.
* Monitor the patient's vital signs before, during and after transfusion.
* During and after administration, monitor for signs of anaphylaxis and other allergic reactions (rash, loin pain, pyrexia, rigours, tachycardia, hypotension) and fluid overload.

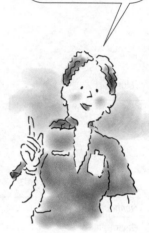

Good news! Transfusion can revive oxygen-starved tissues, combat infections and aid patients with haemophilia.

Administer fresh frozen plasma within 4 hours because it doesn't contain preservatives.

- Monitor for bleeding, increased pain or swelling at the transfusion site and fever.
- Never add anything to blood products or piggyback anything on to the I.V. line.
- Complete all relevant documentation ensuring transfusion records are traceable.

Haematological and immune system disorders

Haematological and immune system disorders commonly seen in the critical care environment include acute leukaemia, anaemias, anaphylaxis, autoimmune disorders, clotting disorders, DIC, human immunodeficiency virus (HIV) infection and idiopathic thrombocytopaenic purpura.

Acute leukaemia

Leukaemia is a group of malignant disorders characterised by abnormal proliferation and maturation of lymphocytes and nonlymphocytic cells leading to suppression of normal cells. It's classified as acute or chronic:
- Acute lymphoblastic leukaemia (ALL) involves abnormal growth of lymphoblasts. It accounts for 80% of all childhood leukaemias.
- Acute myelogenous leukaemia (AML) involves rapid accumulation of myeloblasts. It's one of the most common leukaemias in adults.
- Chronic myeloid leukaemia (CML) is characterised by myeloproliferation in bone marrow. It's common in middle age but may occur in any age group.
- Chronic lymphatic leukaemia (CLL) is characterised by an increase in well-differentiated lymphocytes in the bone marrow and peripheral blood. It's most common in elderly people.

Age is no object

Acute leukaemia ranks 20th as the cause of cancer-related deaths among people of all age groups. Without treatment, acute leukaemia invariably leads to death, usually because of complications. With treatment, the prognosis varies.

What causes it
The cause of acute leukaemia isn't known. Risk factors seem to include some combination of viruses, genetic and immunological factors, and exposure to radiation and certain chemicals.

How it happens
Malignant WBC precursors (blasts) proliferate in bone marrow or lymph tissue and accumulate in peripheral blood, bone marrow and body tissues.

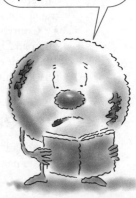

Says here, 'Without treatment, acute leukaemia is deadly. With treatment, the prognosis varies'.

What to look for

Typical clinical features include sudden onset of high fever, night sweats, abnormal bleeding (such as nosebleeds, gingival bleeding, purpura, ecchymoses, and petechiae), easy bruising after minor trauma, and prolonged menses indicating bone marrow failure.

Nonspecific signs and symptoms include low-grade fever, night sweats, pallor and weakness that may persist for days or months before other symptoms appear.

What tests tell you

• Bone marrow aspiration typically shows a proliferation of immature WBCs and is used to confirm the diagnosis.
• Full blood count (FBC) and clotting screen shows anaemia, thrombocytopaenia and neutropenia.
• Differential leukocyte count is used to determine cell type.

How it's treated

Systemic chemotherapy is used to eradicate leukaemic cells and induce remission. Chemotherapy varies with the specific disorder. Bone marrow transplants are also an option.

What to do when a patient with acute leukaemia is admitted to critical care

• Preventing infection is vital for the patient with acute leukaemia. Strict infection control measures must be carried out and protective isolation in cases of neutropenia. Observations must be monitored closely for early signs of infection (fever, chills, tachycardia and tachypnoea). Patients with a temperature over 38.3°C and decreased WBC counts should have thorough infection screening (sputum, urine and blood cultures) and receive antibiotic therapy promptly.
• Avoid taking rectal temperatures, giving rectal suppositories, doing digital examinations and employ measures to prevent constipation to reduce risks of bacterial translocation.
• Avoid mechanical ventilation, using invasive lines, indwelling catheters and giving I.M. injections to reduce risks of infection transmission.
• Control mouth ulceration by checking the patient's mouth often and by providing frequent mouth care.
• Provide psychological support by establishing a trusting relationship to promote communication.

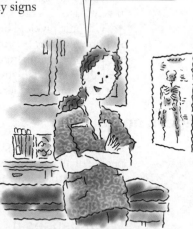

Preventing infection is an important part of care for the patient with acute leukaemia.

Anaemia

Anaemia is present when the Hb level is below the normal range expected for the patient. Relative anaemia is seen commonly within critical care units owing to blood loss in patients, excessive blood sampling, poor nutrition and critical illness, reducing RBC production and haemodilution.

Questions to ask

It is useful to know the reason for the anaemia so that the cause as well as the blood result may be treated. Sometimes this will be obvious but in other cases more difficult to work out. Asking the following questions will help:
- How long has the patient been anaemic?
- How quickly has the Hb dropped?
- What associated conditions does the patient have which may account for the anaemia?
- Is blood loss suspected?
- Is inability to generate Hb the cause?
- Is there evidence of haemolysis (in urine, raised bilirubin, splenomegaly)?

What to look for

When searching for blood loss; abdominal distension, wound leakage, drain output, NG output or vomit, melaena or fresh blood per rectum and hidden bleeding around fracture sites or into the pleural cavity and peritoneum must be considered.

Typical clinical features of anaemia include pale or yellow tinged skin, shortness of breath, cardiac ischaemia, fatigue, tachycardia and hypotension that only responds transiently to fluid boluses.

What tests tell you
- Hb level to measure the severity of anaemia.
- Haematocrit to measure the concentration of RBC to plasma.
- Folate and ferritin levels for diagnosis of iron deficiency anaemia.
- B_{12} levels for diagnosis of iron deficiency anaemia or pernicious anaemia.
- Electrophoresis to distinguish Hb variants (sickle cell).

How it's treated

When the Hb is below 7 g/dl a blood transfusion is required. If the patient has an objection to this, e.g. Jehovah's witness, medication to boost the Hb level may be administered. In cases of pernicious anaemia B_{12} in the form of hydroxocobalamin I.M. is required. In haemolytic anaemia the treatment depends on the cause but splenectomy may be required. In sickle cell crisis priorities of treatment are oxygen, I.V. fluids, analgesia and blood transfusion.

Anaphylaxis

Anaphylaxis is an exaggerated hypersensitivity reaction to a previously encountered antigen. A severe reaction may precipitate vascular collapse, leading to systemic shock and sometimes death.

What causes it

Causes of anaphylaxis include:
- exposure to sensitising drugs (such as antibiotics, vaccines, allergen extracts, enzymes, hormones, local anaesthetics, salicylates, polysaccharides and antineoplastics)
- exposure to diagnostic chemicals (including radiographic contrast media containing iodine)
- foods (nuts, eggs, shellfish)
- sulphites
- insect venom (bee and wasp stings)
- latex.

How it happens

An anaphylactic reaction requires previous sensitisation or exposure to the specific antigen. This sensitisation causes production of specific IgE antibodies by plasma cells. IgE antibodies then bind to membrane receptors or mast cells and basophils.

Take two

Upon re-exposure, the antigens bind to adjacent IgE antibodies or cross-linked IgE receptors, activating a series of reactions that triggers the release of powerful chemical mediators (histamine) from mast cell stores. IgG or IgM enters into the reaction and activates the release of complement fractions.

At the same time, two other chemical mediators, bradykinin and leukotrienes, induce vascular collapse by causing certain smooth muscles to contract and increasing vascular permeability. This collapse leads to decreased peripheral resistance to plasma leakage from the circulation to extravascular tissues. Hypotension ensues, leading to hypovolaemic shock and cardiac dysfunction.

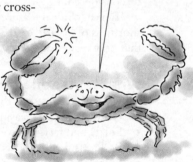

Re-exposure to a specific antigen (such as foods like me!) triggers the release of histamine.

What to look for

An anaphylactic reaction usually produces sudden distress within seconds or minutes after exposure to an allergen. (A delayed or persistent reaction may occur up to 24 hours later.)

Signs and symptoms from head to toe

Initial signs and symptoms include a feeling of impending doom or fright, weakness, sweating, sneezing, pruritus, urticaria and angioedema. Cardiovascular signs include hypotension, shock and arrhythmias. Respiratory signs and symptoms include nasal mucosal oedema, profuse watery rhinorrhoea, nasal congestion, sudden sneezing attacks, hoarseness, stridor and dyspnoea. GI and genitourinary signs and symptoms include severe stomach cramps, nausea, diarrhoea, urinary urgency, and incontinence.

What tests tell you

Anaphylaxis can be diagnosed by the rapid onset of severe respiratory or cardiovascular reactions after exposure to an allergen.

How it's treated

Anaphylaxis is always an emergency, remove the antigen if possible, call for help, give 100% oxygen and I.V. fluids and perform an ABCDE assessment. Prepare adrenaline 0.5 mg for I.M. injection. Adrenaline should be given if there are any signs of respiratory or cardiovascular compromise. If cardiac arrest occurs initiate cardiopulmonary resuscitation.

What to do

Use an ABCDE approach:
*   Maintain airway patency using head tilt and chin lift. Observe for early signs of laryngeal oedema (stridor, hoarseness and dyspnoea), which may necessitate endotracheal (ET) intubation, cricothyrotomy or a tracheostomy.
*   Give 100% oxygen via mask or ventilator. Auscultate for air entry and wheeze. Administer salbutamol or adrenaline nebulisers as prescribed.
*   Maintain circulatory volume with fluid boluses. I.V. crystalloids 500 ml infused as rapidly as possible as prescribed. Watch for hypotension and shock. Stabilise the patient's blood pressure with I.V. vasopressors, such as noradrenaline. Monitor the patient's observations, cardiac rhythm, oxygen saturation and urine output as a response index.
*   Monitor LOC using AVPU or GCS scoring and position patient accordingly to protect airway and maintain safety.
*   Examine patient from head to toe for rashes and other abnormalities.
    After initial emergency measures, administer other medications as ordered, such as I.V. hydrocortisone and chlorphenamine. Follow up must involve good documentation and information to the patient, relatives and health care team in order to prevent recurrence. Blood testing to confirm anaphylactic reaction is carried out over the next 24 hours.

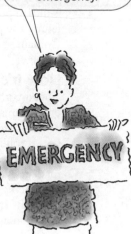

Rapid onset of severe respiratory or cardiovascular reactions are telltale signs of anaphylaxis. It's always an emergency.

Autoimmune disorders

Autoimmune disorders are caused by the breakdown of immunoregulation allowing the immune system to become autoaggressive. Cellular and tissue damage occur because cellular and blood components of the inflammatory response are activated. Autoimmune disease can be an acute self-limiting intermittent disorder or a chronic perpetuating one. It might have an identified trigger, such as infection, trauma or pregnancy, which is followed 10–21 days later by the inflammatory disorder.

Immunological diseases

Goodpasture's syndrome is caused by antiglomerular membrane antibodies. Patients present with renal failure and pulmonary haemorrhage. Early diagnosis and intensive plasma exchange may be required to reduce mortality. Patients with anuric renal failure rarely regain renal function.

Acetylcholine receptor autoantibodies cause myasthenia gravis. Respiratory failure and aspiration lead to critical care admission. Drug treatment with pyridostigmine and supportive ventilation until the crisis resolves may be required. Patients with the immune complex disease SLE causing renal failure, cerebritis and pneumonitis may be treated in critical care with plasma exchange. Guillain–Barré is an acute self-limiting disease causing demyelinating neuropathy. There is evidence that the demyelination is due to postinfectious autoimmunity. If it causes respiratory compromise or failure the patient will be admitted to critical care. (More information about Guillain–Barré can be found in Chapter 3.)

How it's treated

Therapy in acute and chronic autoimmune disease aims to minimise irreparable organ damage and support patients during the acute illness. It can include:
- nonspecific therapy to suppress effector mechanisms, e.g. corticosteroids, nonsteroidal antiinflammatory drugs and antiplatelet therapy
- therapy to reduce circulating levels of toxic factor antibodies and mediators of inflammation, e.g. plasma exchange
- specific or broad spectrum immunosuppressive agents to suppress or block the immune response, e.g. corticosteroids and cytotoxic agents
- mechanical ventilation to support respiratory function
- renal replacement therapy, e.g. continuous veno-venous haemofiltration (CVVH) or dialysis to support renal function.

Clotting disorders

A variety of clotting disorders are seen in patients in critical care units. DIC is probably the most severe of these and is detailed separately below. A variety of factors may cause an inability of the blood to clot and all may result in life-threatening haemorrhage.

What causes it

Conditions that can prevent blood clotting include:
- absence, inability to produce or loss of clotting factors
- anticoagulant overdose
- abnormal reactions to anticoagulants.

Congenital clotting defects

Congenital clotting defects like Haemophilia and Christmas disease are caused by a single factor defect so replacement of this factor either prophylactically or in cases of emergency is usually enough to enable blood clotting. Von Willebrand's disease, the commonest hereditary haemostatic disorder, cryoprecipitate and FFP are used, and desmopressin given prior to procedures to induce a haemostatic state by release of factor VIII and von Willebrand factor.

Acquired clotting defects

Acquired haemostatic disorders are more common in critical care. Massive blood transfusion means that a loss and dilution of coagulation factors can occur. Coagulation tests should be done and FFP and platelets infused as advised by the haematologist. The liver produces nearly all factors involved in coagulation so bleeding associated with liver disease is difficult to manage. Vitamin K, FFP and cryoprecipitate may be used but last for only a short time so must be repeated if there is continued bleeding or risk of bleeding.

Anticoagulant and antiplatelet associated clotting defects

Oral anticoagulants, e.g. warfarin, cause a deficiency of vitamin K dependent clotting factors and can be reversed by giving vitamin K. Heparin acts on several sites of the clotting pathway and effects are commonly measured by APTT. It can be immediately reversed with protamine sulphate, approximately 1 mg of protamine will neutralise 100 U of heparin. HIT may be seen after 7–10 days of heparin therapy when an immune reaction causes platelets to aggregate. Blood tests will demonstrate this reaction. The risk of HIT is reduced with low-molecular-weight heparins or if therapy is kept short. Antiplatelet drugs are widely used prophylactically for arterial disease and many of the nonsteroidal antiinflammatory are also platelet-inhibitory. Aspirin has an irreversible effect on platelet function lasting around 10 days and is one of the commonest causes of post-op bleeding.

Disseminated intravascular coagulation

DIC is a grave coagulopathy that accelerates clotting, causing small blood vessel occlusion, organ necrosis, depletion of circulating clotting factors and platelets and activation of the fibrinolytic system.

These processes in turn can provoke severe haemorrhage. Clotting in the microcirculation usually affects the kidneys and extremities, but may occur in the brain, lungs, pituitary and adrenal glands and GI mucosa.

What causes it

Conditions that can cause DIC include:
- infection
- obstetric complications
- neoplastic disease
- disorders that produce necrosis, such as extensive burns, trauma, brain tissue destruction, transplant rejection and hepatic necrosis
- heat stroke
- shock
- severe venous thrombosis
- cirrhosis

DIC can be caused by brain tissue destruction? I don't like the sound of that!

- fat embolism
- incompatible blood transfusion
- cardiac arrest
- surgery necessitating cardiopulmonary bypass
- poisonous snakebite.

How it happens
Regardless of how DIC begins, the typical accelerated clotting causes generalised activation of prothrombin and a consequent excess of thrombin.

Clotting and coagulating
Excess thrombin converts fibrinogen into fibrin, producing fibrin clots in the microcirculation. This process consumes large amounts of coagulation factors, causing hypoprothrombinaemia, thrombocytopaenia and deficiencies in factors V and VIII.

Circulating thrombin activates the fibrinolytic system, which lyses fibrin clots into fibrin degradation products. Haemorrhage may be the result of the anticoagulant activity of fibrin degradation products as well as depletion of plasma coagulation factors.

What to look for
Abnormal bleeding without a history of serious haemorrhagic disorder can signal DIC.

Blood out of place
Principal signs of such bleeding include cutaneous oozing, petechiae, ecchymoses, haematomas, bleeding from sites of surgical or invasive procedures and bleeding from the GI tract.

Other signs and symptoms
Related or possible signs and symptoms include dyspnoea, oliguria, seizures, coma, shock, failure of major organ systems and severe muscle, back and abdominal pain.

What tests tell you
Laboratory findings supporting a tentative diagnosis include:
- decreased platelets
- decreased fibrinogen level
- increased fibrin degradation products
- prolonged PT
- prolonged APTT
- decreased urine output (less than 30 ml/hour), elevated urea and creatinine.

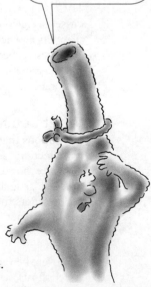

Look for evidence of unusual bleeding, such as cutaneous oozing, petechiae, ecchymoses, haematomas and bleeding from surgical sites, invasive procedures or even the GI tract.

How it's treated

Effective treatment for patients with DIC requires prompt recognition and adequate attention to the underlying disorder. Treatment may be generally supportive or highly specific.

If the patient isn't actively bleeding, supportive care alone may reverse DIC. However, active bleeding may require administration of blood, FFP, cryoprecipitate, platelets or packed RBCs to support haemostasis. (See *Understanding DIC and its treatment*, page 558.)

What to do

- Monitor the patient's cardiac, respiratory and neurological status closely. There is a high risk of stroke.
- Assess the patient for signs of haemorrhage and hypovolaemic shock. Observe the patient's skin colour and check peripheral circulation and capillary refill. Inspect skin and mucous membranes for signs of bleeding.
- Check all I.V. and venepuncture sites often. Apply pressure to injection sites for at least 15 minutes.
- Administer supplemental oxygen as indicated. Monitor oxygen saturation and blood gas results, assess for hypoxaemia, and anticipate the need for ET intubation and mechanical ventilation.
- Keep the patient as quiet and comfortable as possible to minimise oxygen demands. Place the patient in 45 degrees head elevation, as tolerated, to maximise chest expansion.
- Monitor the patient's blood results and administer blood and clotting products as prescribed.
- Monitor the patient's intake and output hourly, especially when administering blood products. Watch for transfusion reactions and signs of fluid overload.
- Assess the patient for potential complications of DIC, including pulmonary emboli due to accelerated clotting, neurological compromise from stroke or bleeding, renal failure from acute tubular necrosis or multiple organ failure.
- Provide emotional support to the patient and their family.

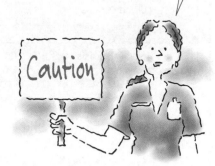

Assess the patient with DIC for signs of haemorrhage and hypovolaemic shock.

HIV infection

HIV infection is characterised by progressive decline of immune function that, if left untreated, results in susceptibility to opportunistic infections and malignancies. The most profound state of immunodeficiency caused by HIV is AIDS.

AIDS is defined as a confirmed presence of HIV infection and a CD4+ T cell (helper T) count less than 200 per μl, or presence of HIV with an opportunistic infection. (See *Conditions associated with AIDS*, page 559.)

What causes it

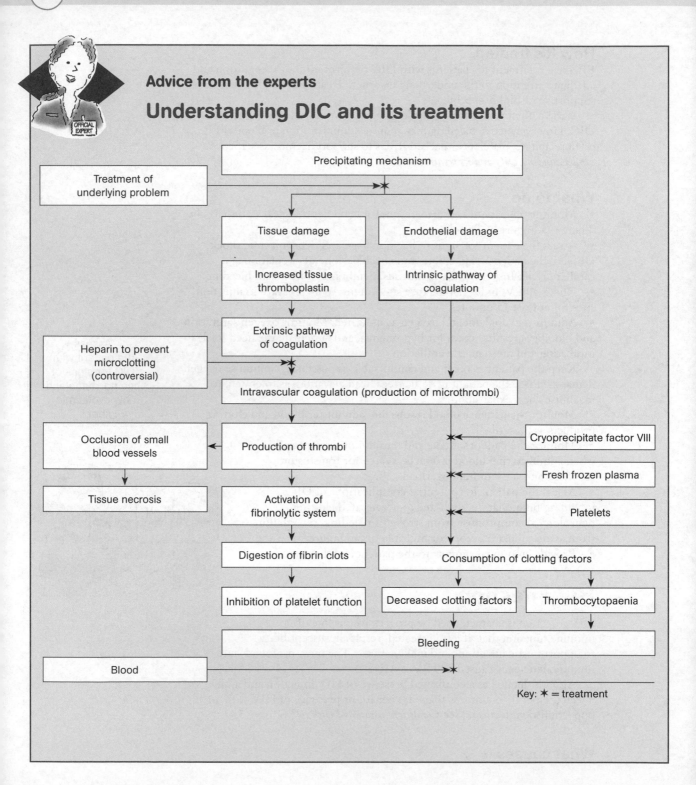

Advice from the experts

Understanding DIC and its treatment

Precipitating mechanism

Treatment of underlying problem

Tissue damage

Endothelial damage

Increased tissue thromboplastin

Intrinsic pathway of coagulation

Extrinsic pathway of coagulation

Heparin to prevent microclotting (controversial)

Intravascular coagulation (production of microthrombi)

Occlusion of small blood vessels

Production of thrombi

Cryoprecipitate factor VIII

Tissue necrosis

Fresh frozen plasma

Activation of fibrinolytic system

Platelets

Digestion of fibrin clots

Consumption of clotting factors

Inhibition of platelet function

Decreased clotting factors

Thrombocytopaenia

Bleeding

Blood

Key: ✳ = treatment

The retrovirus HIV causes AIDS. This virus appears in body fluids, such as blood and semen. Modes of transmission include:

- sexual contact, especially with trauma to the rectal or vaginal mucosa, in patients from any age group (see *HIV in elderly patients*, page 560)
- transfusion of contaminated blood or blood products
- use of contaminated needles
- perinatal transmission from mother to foetus.

How it happens

For patients with AIDS, the number of CD4$^+$ T cells declines, mainly because HIV selectively binds with and destroys them. A substance called *gp 120* binds HIV to CD4$^+$ T-cell receptor sites.

Enter HIV

After binding to a target cell, HIV enters the cell and sheds its envelope. How the virus enters the cell isn't known. After HIV enters the cell, the enzyme reverse transcriptase transcribes the genomic ribonucleic acid into deoxyribonucleic acid

---

Conditions associated with AIDS

The Centre for Disease Control and Prevention (CDC) USA lists diseases associated with acquired immunodeficiency syndrome (AIDS) under three categories with category C being the most advanced stage of the illness.

Category A

- Persistent generalised lymph node enlargement
- Acute primary human immunodeficiency virus (HIV) infection with accompanying illness
- HIV infection without symptoms

Category B

- Bacillary angiomatosis
- Oropharyngeal or persistent vulvovaginal candidiasis
- Fever or diarrhoea lasting longer than 1 month
- Idiopathic thrombocytopaenic purpura
- Pelvic inflammatory disease, especially with a tubulo-ovarian abscess
- Peripheral neuropathy
- Cervical dysplasia
- Oral leukoplakia (hairy)

- Herpes zoster, with at least two different episodes or involving more than one dermatone
- Listeriosis

Category C

- Candidiasis of the bronchi, trachea, lungs or oesophagus
- Invasive cervical cancer
- Disseminated or extrapulmonary coccidioidomycosis
- Extrapulmonary cryptococcosis
- Chronic interstitial cryptosporidiosis
- Cytomegalovirus (CMV) disease affecting organs other than the liver, spleen or lymph nodes
- CMV retinitis with vision loss
- Encephalopathy related to HIV
- Herpes simplex infection with chronic ulcers or herpetic bronchitis, pneumonitis or oesophagitis

- Disseminated or extrapulmonary histoplasmosis
- Chronic intestinal isosporiasis
- Kaposi's sarcoma
- Burkitt's lymphoma
- Immunoblastic lymphoma
- Primary brain lymphoma
- Disseminated or extrapulmonary *Mycobacterium avium-intracellulare* complex or *M. kansasii*
- Pulmonary or extrapulmonary *M. tuberculosis*
- Disseminated or extrapulmonary infection with any other species of *Mycobacterium*
- *Pneumocystis carinii* pneumonia
- Recurrent pneumonia
- Progressive multifocal leukoencephalopathy
- Recurrent *Salmonella* septicaemia
- Toxoplasmosis of the brain
- Wasting syndrome caused by HIV

(DNA). Afterwards, during cell division, a virus-encoded enzyme integrates the DNA into the host genome. At this point, HIV's replication cycle may be suspended until the infected CD4+ T cell is activated.

Critical destruction

Because CD4+ T cells are critically important in the immune response, destruction of even part of their population can cause immunodeficiencies. These immunodeficiencies leave the patient vulnerable to the potentially fatal opportunistic infections and cancers characteristic of AIDS.

What to look for

Signs and symptoms of AIDS vary widely; nonspecific ones include:
* fatigue
* afternoon fevers
* night sweats
* weight loss
* diarrhoea
* cough.

That's all 'til later

Patients may be otherwise asymptomatic until the abrupt onset of complications, such as opportunistic infection and HIV encephalopathy (dementia) marked by confusion, apathy and paranoia. (See *Opportunistic infections in AIDS*, page 561.)

What tests tell you

* The most widely used test determines the presence of antibodies for HIV. If the results are positive, the test is repeated. If the results are still positive, the findings are confirmed by another method, usually the Western blot or an immunofluorescence assay.
* Direct testing is more reliable because it detects HIV itself. Direct testing includes antigen testing, HIV cultures, nucleic acid probes of peripheral blood lymphocytes and polymerase chain reaction tests.
* CD4+ T-cell and CD8+ T-cell subset counts are used to evaluate the severity of immunosuppression and response to treatment.

How it's treated

Although no cure has yet been found, signs and symptoms can be managed with treatment. Primary therapy for HIV infection includes three different types of antiretrovirals used in combination:
* protease inhibitors
* nucleoside reverse transcriptase inhibitors
* nonnucleoside reverse transcriptase inhibitors.

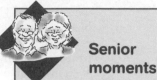

Senior moments

HIV in elderly patients

HIV infection occurs predominantly in young people (in most cases ages 25–55). However, incidence is rapidly increasing in people ages 50 and older. This group may not have benefited from HIV-prevention messages, which are commonly targeted at younger people. Make sure you take a sexual history from older patients or inquire about their sexual activity, which may aid in diagnosing the disease.

HIV is picky. It selectively binds with and destroys helper T cells, causing immunodeficiencies.

Opportunistic infections in AIDS

The chart below lists microbial forms and specific organisms that cause opportunistic infections in patients with acquired immunodeficiency syndrome (AIDS).

Microbiological agent	Organism	Infection
Protozoa	*Pneumocystis carinii*	Pneumocystosis
	Cryptosporidium	Cryptosporidiosis
	Toxoplasma gondii	Toxoplasmosis
	Histoplasma	Histoplasmosis
Fungi	*Candida albicans*	Candidiasis
	Cryptococcus neoformans	Cryptococcosis
Viruses	Herpes	Herpes simplex 1 and 2
	Cytomegalovirus (CMV)	CMV retinitis
Bacteria	*Mycobacterium tuberculosis*	Tuberculosis
	Mycobacterium avium	*M. avium* complex

Note: Other opportunistic conditions include Kaposi's sarcoma, wasting syndrome and AIDS dementia complex.

The most widely used test determines the presence of antibodies for HIV, but direct testing is more reliable because it detects HIV itself.

Other options

Other potential therapies include:
• immunomodulatory drugs designed to boost the weakened immune system
• antiinfective and antineoplastic drugs to combat opportunistic infections and associated cancers.

What to do

• Adhere to standard precautions and anticipate the need for protective isolation. Keep invasive lines to a minimum owing to high risks of infection.
• Assess the patient's cardiopulmonary status—including breath sounds, vital signs, oxygen saturation and cardiac rhythm.
• Report any cough, sore throat or adventitious sounds that may indicate respiratory infection such as pneumonia. Administer supplemental oxygen as indicated. Anticipate the need for ET intubation and mechanical ventilation if the patient's respiratory status deteriorates.
• Monitor the patient for pyrexia, noting its pattern. Watch for signs and symptoms of infection, such as skin breakdown, cough, sore throat and diarrhoea and send samples for culture as indicated.

- Assess the patient for tender, swollen lymph nodes and check blood results.
- Assess for pain and administer analgesia as prescribed according to needs.
- Provide comprehensive mouth care and regular oral assessment.
- Monitor the patient's nutritional status providing supplements as indicated. Although parenteral nutrition may be needed for adequate caloric intake, it should be avoided owing to high risks of infection.
- For the patient with Kaposi's sarcoma, monitor the progression of lesions and provide meticulous skin care.
- An AIDS diagnosis is profoundly distressing because of the social impact and the discouraging prognosis. Offer support to the patient, friends and family.

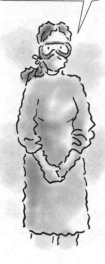

Adhere to standard precautions and anticipate the need for protective isolation.

Idiopathic thrombocytopaenic purpura

Idiopathic thrombocytopaenic purpura (ITP) results from immunological platelet destruction. It may be acute (postviral thrombocytopaenia) or chronic (Werlhof's disease, pupura haemorrhagica, essential thrombocytopaenia and autoimmune thrombocytopaenia).

Acute ITP usually affects children. Chronic ITP mainly affects adults younger than age 50, especially women ages 20–40.

What causes it

Acute ITP usually follows a viral infection, such as rubella or chickenpox. Chronic ITP seldom follows infection and is associated with immunologic disorders, such as SLE, or is linked to drug reactions.

How it happens

The platelet membrane is coated with IgG or another antibody and then these sensitised platelets are destroyed. Their destruction is brought about by the reticuloendothelial system of the liver and spleen.

What to look for

Signs and symptoms of ITP include:
- petechiae
- ecchymoses
- mucosal bleeding from the mouth, nose or GI tract
- purpuric lesions in vital organs (such as the lungs, kidneys or brain) that may be fatal.

What tests tell you

- A platelet count less than 20×10^9 per L and prolonged bleeding time suggest ITP.
- Platelets may be abnormal in size and morphologic appearance.
- Anaemia may be present.
- Bone marrow studies show an abundance of megakaryocytes and a shortened circulating platelet survival time.

How it's treated

Corticosteroids promote capillary integrity, but are only temporarily effective in chronic ITP. Alternative therapy includes:

- immunosuppression
- high-dose I.V. gamma globulin
- splenectomy for which the patient may require blood, blood products and vitamin K delivery.

What to do

- Monitor the patient's cardiopulmonary status and assess for signs of bleeding. Monitor laboratory results and administer immunoglobulin as ordered.
- Closely monitor patients receiving immunosuppressants for signs of bone marrow depression, infection, mucositis, GI tract ulceration and severe diarrhoea or vomiting.

Quick quiz

1. The spleen must be enlarged about how many times normal size to be palpable?

- A. One
- B. Two
- C. Three
- D. Four

Answer: C. To detect an enlarged spleen on palpation, it must be about three times its normal size.

2. Which is the preferred site for a bone marrow biopsy?

- A. Sternum
- B. Spinous process
- C. Posterior superior iliac crest
- D. Anterior superior iliac crest

Answer: C. The posterior superior iliac crest is the preferred site because no vital organs or vessels are nearby.

3. The first drug of choice for a patient experiencing anaphylaxis is:

- A. adrenaline.
- B. aminophylline.
- C. hydrocortisonedopamine.
- D. chlorphenamine.

Answer: A. Adrenaline provides physiological reversal of the immediate symptoms, such as laryngeal oedema, bronchospasm and hypotension.

4. Which blood result may be an indication of DIC?

- A. Increased platelets
- B. Increased fibrinogen levels
- C. Decreased fibrin degradation products
- D. Decreased fibrinogen levels

> We're next! Read on to learn about multisystem issues.

Answer: D. Decreased fibrinogen levels in the absence of haemorrhage support a diagnosis of DIC. Reduced platelets, increased fibrin degradation products and prolonged clotting times also support this diagnosis.

Scoring

☆☆☆   If you answered all four questions correctly, go and have some fun! You're already a bloody genius, mate!

☆☆   If you answered three questions correctly, don't despair. No one is immune to an occasional information mismatch.

☆   If you answered fewer than three correctly, your oxygen levels may need a boost. Take a break, have a platelet of something nutritious, and get back into circulation as soon as possible.

Just the facts

In this chapter, you'll learn:

♦ types of multisystem disorders
♦ indications for blood and fluid replacement
♦ treatments specific to multisystem issues
♦ nursing care of the patient with multisystem issues.

A look at multisystem issues

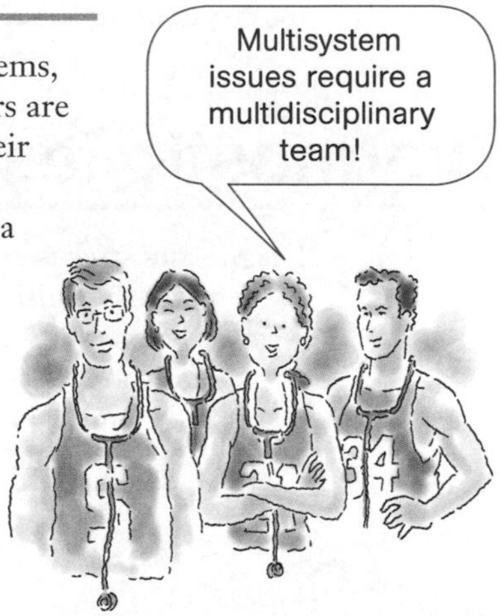

Some disorders are so severe that they have effects across multiple systems, for example sepsis, burns or trauma. Whilst other multisystem disorders are not severe they are common to all critically ill patients regardless of their initial problem, for example, fluid and electrolyte disorders.

Prompt, efficient and organised care of multisystem issues requires a multidisciplinary team approach. Typically, assessment, treatment and care of multisystem issues occur simultaneously.

> Multisystem issues require a multidisciplinary team!

Assessment

Rapid assessment followed by appropriate interventions influence the outcome of the patient with multisystem issues. General assessment measures should be paired with more rapid focused and directed assessment techniques that are specific to the patient's condition.

History lesson

Begin your assessment by obtaining the patient's history, including:
• chief complaint
• present and previous illnesses and surgery

- current medications, prescribed and over-the-counter
- family and social history.

If the patient is unstable, you may need to wait until they have stabilised to obtain a complete health history or ask the family, consult the general practitioner and review any case notes from previous hospital admissions.

Is it life-threatening?

Assess the patient for life-threatening problems (such as respiratory distress in the burn victim), and initiate emergency measures such as cardiopulmonary resuscitation (CPR) as appropriate.

Use an ABCDE approach in your 'primary survey' of the patient. Treat problems you find with A-Airway before you move onto B-Breathing. Then treat problems with B-Breathing before moving onto C-Circulation. Use this assess-treat-move-on approach through D-Disability (neurological disability) and E-Exposure as well. Your treatment interventions may be basic but they may be life-saving. Simple airway manoeuvres and adjuncts, oxygen and I.V. fluid bolus preparation may save lives and valuable time until a suitably experienced doctor attends.

The once-over

Your physical examination of the patient includes assessment of all body systems, with particular attention to the body systems involved in the multisystem disorder.

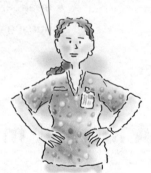

Always assess for life-threatening problems first, and initiate emergency measures as needed.

Diagnostic tests

Diagnostics studies are performed to help determine the cause or extent of the patient's multisystem issues. Tests may include laboratory studies (such as haematology, coagulation, biochemistry, urine studies and cultures of blood or body fluids), radiographic studies, electrocardiography, computed tomography (CT) scans, magnetic resonance imaging (MRI), ultrasonography, nuclear medicine scans and interventional radiological studies.

Treatment

Treating multisystem issues is a challenge. At times, the causative factors in a patient's deteriorating condition may not be known. As more organ systems are affected, care becomes more complex. Supportive measures are a crucial part of treatment; they include drug therapy, blood transfusion and fluid replacement.

Drug therapy

Drug therapy for multisystem issues varies depending on the patient's underlying condition. For example, antibiotics may be used to treat severe sepsis/septic shock or multiple traumas. Vasopressors may be used to treat various types of shock. Corticosteroids and immunosuppressants are used to treat graft-versus-host disease (GVHD). (See *Drug therapy for multisystem disorders*.)

Drug therapy for multisystem disorders

Use the chart below as a guide to drug therapy appropriate for multisystem disorders.

Drugs	Indications	Adverse reactions	Practice pointers
Corticosteroids			
Dexamethasone Hydrocortisone Prednisolone	• Inflammatory conditions • Immunosuppression • Graft-versus-host disease	• Euphoria • Insomnia • Acute delirium • Heart failure or arrhythmias • Thromboembolism • Gastric ulceration • Pancreatitis • Acute adrenal insufficiency	• Use cautiously in patients with myocardial infarction, hypertension, renal disease or GI ulcer. • Sudden withdrawal after prolonged use may be fatal. • Administer oral drug with milk or food. • Monitor serum electrolytes and blood glucose levels at onset of therapy.
Vasopressors			
Noradrenaline	• Hypotension • Sepsis/septic shock	• Restlessness and anxiety • Dizziness, headache • Bradycardia or tachycardia • Palpitations • Cardiac arrhythmias • Hypertension and hypertensive crisis • Stroke and cerebral haemorrhage • Angina • Gangrene of extremities in high doses	• Use a central venous catheter for administration. Use a continuous infusion pump to regulate infusion flow rate. • When discontinuing, taper dosage slowly to evaluate stability of blood pressure.
Immunosuppressants			
Cyclosporine	• Prophylaxis of organ rejection	• GI disturbances, anorexia, nausea and vomiting • Hepatic dysfunction • Renal dysfunction • Electrolyte imbalance • Hypoglycaemia	• Monitor the patient for signs of nephrotoxicity, hepatic dysfunction, hyperkalaemia and hypokalaemia. • Monitor blood glucose level regularly.

(continued)

Drug therapy for multisystem disorders (continued)

Drugs	Indications	Adverse reactions	Practice pointers
Antibiotics			
Cefuroxime Metronidazole	• Serious infections of the lower respiratory and urinary tracts • Intra-abdominal, bone and joint, skin and gynaecological infections • Bacteraemia • Sepsis	• Leucopenia • Serum sickness • Anaphylaxis • Phlebitis or thrombophlebitis • Diarrhoea • Thrombocytopaenia • Pseudomembranous colitis	• Obtain a specimen for culture and sensitivity tests before giving first dose.
Other			
Activated protein C Drotrecogin alfa (activated)	• Severe sepsis associated with organ failure	• Bleeding • Stroke	• Don't administer to a patient with an epidural catheter in place. • Don't use concurrently with heparin.

Blood transfusion

Blood transfusions treat decreased haemoglobin (Hb) level and haematocrit (Hct). A whole blood transfusion replenishes the volume and oxygen-carrying capacity of the circulatory system by increasing the mass of circulating red blood cells (RBCs). Because of the risk of circulatory overload, whole blood transfusions are rarely used, except in cases of severe haemorrhage.

Packing it in

Packed RBCs, a blood component from which 80% of the plasma has been removed, are transfused to restore the circulatory system's oxygen-carrying capacity. Packed RBCs are used when the patient has a normal blood volume to avoid possible fluid and circulatory overload. (See *Transfusing blood and blood components,* page 569.)

Washed for patient protection

Washed packed RBCs, commonly used for patients previously sensitised to transfusions, are rinsed with a special solution that removes white blood cells (WBCs) and platelets, thus decreasing the chance of transfusion reaction.

Transfusing blood and blood components

Blood component	Indications	ABO and Rh compatibility	Nursing considerations
Packed red blood cells (RBCs)			
Like whole blood but with most of the plasma removed	• Symptomatic chronic anaemia • Prevention of morbidity from anaemia in patients at greatest risk for tissue hypoxia • Active bleeding with signs and symptoms of hypovolaemia • Preoperative haemoglobin < 9 g/dl, with possibility of major blood loss • Sickle cell disease (red cell exchange)	• ABO compatibility: Type A receives type A or O, type B receives type B or O, type AB receives type AB or O, type O receives type O • Rh match necessary	• Use a blood administration set to infuse blood within 4 hours. • Administer only with normal saline solution. • Keep in mind that an RBC transfusion isn't appropriate for anaemias treatable by nutritional or drug therapies.
Platelets			
Platelet sediment from whole blood	• Bleeding due to critically decreased circulating platelet counts or functionally abnormal platelets • Prevention of bleeding due to thrombocytopaenia • Platelet count <50,000 per µl before surgery or a major invasive procedure	• ABO identical when possible • Rh-negative recipients should receive Rh-negative platelets when possible	• Use a filtered component drip administration set to infuse. • Keep in mind that platelets shouldn't be used to treat autoimmune thrombocytopaenia or thrombocytopaenic purpura unless patient has a life-threatening haemorrhage.
Fresh frozen plasma (FFP)			
Uncoagulated plasma separated from RBCs and rich in clotting factors	• Bleeding • Coagulation factor deficiencies • Warfarin reversal • Thrombotic thrombocytopaenic purpura	• ABO compatibility required • Rh match not required	• Use a blood administration set to infuse rapidly. • Monitor patient for signs and symptoms of hypocalcaemia because the citric acid in FFP may bind to calcium. • Remember that FFP must be infused within 24 hours of being thawed.
Cryoprecipitate			
Insoluble plasma portion of FFP containing fibrinogen, Factor VIII:c, Factor VIII:vWF, Factor XIII and fibronectin	• Bleeding associated with hypofibrinogenaemia or dysfibrinogenaemia • Significant factor XIII deficiency (prophylactic or treatment)	• ABO compatibility preferred but not necessary • Rh match not required	• Use a blood administration set to infuse. • Keep in mind that cryoprecipitate must be administered within 6 hours of thawing. • Be aware that patients with haemophilia A or von Willebrand's disease should only be treated with cryoprecipitate when appropriate factor VIII concentrates aren't available.

(continued)

Transfusing blood and blood components (continued)

Blood component	Indications	ABO and Rh compatibility	Nursing considerations
Factor VIII concentrate			
Recombinant, genetically engineered product; derivative obtained from plasma	• Haemophilia A • von Willebrand's disease	• Not required	• Administer by I.V. injection using a filter needle or use the administration set supplied by the manufacturer.
Albumin 5% (buffered saline); albumin 20% (salt poor)			
A small plasma protein prepared by fractionating pooled plasma	• Volume loss due to burns, trauma, surgery or infection • Hypoproteinaemia (with or without oedema)	• Not required	• Use the administration set supplied by the manufacturer and set rate based on patient condition and response. • Administer cautiously in cardiac and pulmonary disease because heart failure may result from volume overload.
Immune globulin			
Processed human plasma from multiple donors that contains 95% immunoglobulin (Ig) G, <2.5% IgA and a fraction of IgM	• Primary immune deficiencies • Secondary immune deficiencies • Kawasaki syndrome • Idiopathic thrombocytopaenic purpura • Neurological disorders (Guillain–Barré syndrome, dermatomyositis, myasthenia gravis)	• Not required	• Reconstitute the lyophilised powder with normal saline solution injection, 5% dextrose or sterile water. • Administer at the minimal concentration available and at the slowest practical rate.

Self-supplier

In some cases, the patient may receive their own blood during a transfusion, called *autotransfusion* or *autologous transfusion*. In this process, the patient's own blood is collected, filtrated and reinfused. With the concern over acquired immunodeficiency syndrome and other blood-borne diseases, the use of autologous transfusion is currently on the rise.

Autologous transfusion may be indicated for:
• elective surgery (where the patient donates blood over an extended period of time before surgery)
• nonelective surgery (where the patient's blood is withdrawn immediately before surgery)
• perioperative and emergency blood salvage during and after thoracic or cardiovascular surgery and hip, knee or liver resection
• perioperative and emergency blood salvage for traumatic injury of the lungs, liver, chest wall, heart, pulmonary vessels, spleen, kidneys, inferior vena cava and iliac, portal or subclavian veins.

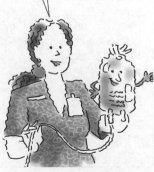

With the concern over blood-borne diseases, the use of autologous transfusion is on the rise.

How low is too low?

Published evidence suggests that liberal transfusion of blood in the critically ill can increase mortality. A randomised multicentre trial found that critically ill patients who were not transfused until their Hb dropped below 7 g/dl, and had a target Hb of 7–9 g/dl, had a greater chance of survival than those who were transfused according to a more liberal strategy. The hospital mortality in the restrictive transfusion group was 22.2 versus 28.1 in the liberal transfusion group ($p = 0.05$).

Source: Hebert, P.C., Wells, G., Blajchman, M.A., et al. A multicenter randomised controlled trial of transfusion requirements in critical care. *New England Journal of Medicine.* 340: 409–417, 1999.

Refuse to transfuse?

In some cases, a patient may refuse a blood transfusion. For example, a Jehovah's Witness may refuse a transfusion because of their religious beliefs. A competent adult has the right to refuse treatment. You may be able to use other treatment options if the patient refuses the blood transfusion, such as using blood-conservation strategies during surgery or providing erythropoietin iron and folic acid supplements preoperatively and postoperatively. Using available alternative treatments supports the patient's right of self-determination and honours the patient's wishes.

What to do
- Obtain the prescription and check whether it has been signed.
- Notify the doctor if the patient refuses the blood transfusion or if family members tell you that their religious beliefs may mean that if they were able they would refuse (in an unconscious patient).
- Obtain baseline vital signs and start an I.V. line if one isn't already started. Use a 20G or larger-diameter catheter.

Double-check identity

- Identify the patient by asking them their name and date of birth if they are able to respond. Also check their identification bracelet details against the cross-match report and then with the unit of blood before transfusion. Double-check all this with a colleague. Follow local policy for blood administration.
- Obtain the patient's vital signs after the first 15 minutes and then every 30 minutes (or according to the facility's policy) for the remainder of transfusion therapy.
- If administering platelets or fresh frozen plasma, administer each unit immediately after obtaining it.
- Use a blood transfusion administration set. When administering multiple units of blood under pressure, use a blood warmer to avoid hypothermia. Do not mix blood with other infusions.
- Remember to always replace the administration set if more than 1 hour elapses between transfusions.

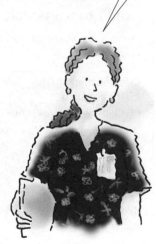

A patient may refuse a transfusion because of religious beliefs.

Rapid replacement

- For rapid blood replacement, use a pressure bag or rapid transfusion device if necessary. Be aware that excessive pressure may develop, leading to broken blood vessels and extravasation with haematoma if administered peripherally, and haemolysis of the infusing RBCs.
- Obtain follow-up laboratory tests as requested to determine the effectiveness of therapy.
- Record the date and time of the transfusion (time started and completed); the type and amount of transfusion product; the type and gauge of the catheter used for infusion; the patient's vital signs before, during and after transfusion; a verification check of all identification data (including the nurses' names verifying the information); and the patient's response.
- Document the patient's transfusion reaction and the treatment (if any) required. (See *Guide to transfusion reactions*.)

Guide to transfusion reactions

There are a range of transfusion reactions that you may see in practice; here's a guide to the key things you should know.

Classification of life-threatening reactions	Key things to know
Acute haemolytic transfusion reactions	- Most commonly due to ABO mismatches. Causes DIC and acute renal failure. - Begins after a few millilitres of blood have been transfused. - Treatment is aimed at maintaining blood pressure and renal perfusion. - Infusion of ABO incompatible blood or plasma almost always arises from sampling, clerical or administration errors—therefore prevention is by good checking and documentation procedures.
Acute bacterial contamination	- Blood is a good culture medium for bacteria. Contamination can occur at any point, from donation to delivery and is associated with severe and often fatal septicaemia if transfused into the patient. Skin flora (i.e. Staphylococcus aureus/epidermis) can contaminate the unit at donation or may be introduced to the patient with venous cannulation prior to, or during, transfusion. - Usually begins during first 100 ml of transfusion. - Treatment involves treatment of the sepsis with fluids, antibiotics and vasopressors. - Can be a particular problem with platelets which are stored at room temperature.
Acute anaphylaxis	- Patients who are IgA deficient may produce anti-IgA which can cause severe cardiovascular collapse if they are transfused components containing IgA (i.e. FFP, cryoprecipitate, platelets and I.V. immunoglobulin). - Reactions are usually seen 1–45 minutes post commencing the infusion. - Treatment involves airway management, adrenaline by slow I.V. injection, fluid boluses and chlorpheniramine. - Prevention involves using washed red cells and platelets or using IgA-deficient donor blood.

(continued)

Guide to transfusion reactions (continued)

Classification of life-threatening reactions	Key things to know
Acute fluid overload	• Patients with chronic anaemic and/or cardiac/renal insufficiency may experience acute fluid overload if blood products are transfused too quickly, with diuretic cover. • In patients who have previously and/or are deemed at risk of acute fluid overload, transfusion should be prescribed over a longer administration period (2–3 hours), with diuretic cover. • At risk renal patients or those with renal dysfunction may need to be transfused on haemodialysis.
Transfusion-related acute lung injury (TRALI)	• Often underreported condition linked to acute respiratory distress syndrome. May be life-threatening. • TRALI is most frequently seen within 1–2 hours of the start of a transfusion, but can be delayed for up to 6 hours. • Clinical presentation following transfusion involves respiratory distress, cough, fever and marked hypoxia with diffused bilateral infiltrates on chest x-ray. Treatment includes management as for ARDS.
Classification of non-life-threatening reactions	
Febrile nonhaemolytic transfusion reaction	• Common and can be distressing for patients, but not life-threatening. • Often associated with fever and rigours during red cell and/or platelet infusion. • Febrile nonhaemolytic reactions are due to antileucocyte antibodies. • Note: it is very important to distinguish a febrile nonhaemolytic reaction from a more serious haemolytic or infective crisis.
Allergic reactions	• These can be troublesome to patients, but not life-threatening. • Usually present as urticaria and itching within minutes of commencing a transfusion. However, reactions should respond to oral/I.V. chlorpheniramine.

Fluid replacement

Fluid replacement is a vital part of treating multisystem illnesses. To maintain the patient's health, the fluid and electrolyte balance in the intracellular and extracellular spaces needs to remain relatively constant. Whenever a person experiences an illness or a condition that prevents normal fluid intake or causes excessive fluid loss, I.V. fluid replacement may be necessary.

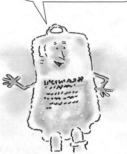

I provide immediate and predictable therapeutic effects!

So predictable

I.V. therapy provides the patient with life-sustaining fluids, electrolytes and medications and offers the advantage of immediate and predictable therapeutic effects. Solutions used for I.V. fluid replacement fall into the broad categories of crystalloids and colloids. (See *Understanding electrolytes*, page 574.)

Easy flowing

Crystalloids are solutions with small molecules that flow easily from the bloodstream into cells and tissues. Crystalloids can be divided into three

Understanding electrolytes

Electrolytes help regulate water distribution, govern acid–base balance, facilitate muscle contraction and transmit nerve impulses. They also contribute to energy generation and blood clotting. The lists here summarise what the body's major electrolytes do. Check the illustration below to see how electrolytes are distributed in and around the cell.

Potassium (K)

- Main intracellular fluid (ICF) cation
- Regulates cell excitability
- Permeates cell membranes, thereby affecting the cell's electrical status
- Helps to control ICF osmolality and, consequently, ICF osmotic pressure

Magnesium (Mg)

- A leading ICF cation
- Contributes to many enzymatic and metabolic processes, particularly protein synthesis
- Modifies nerve impulse transmission and skeletal muscle response (unbalanced Mg concentrations dramatically affect neuromuscular processes)

Phosphorus (P)

- Main ICF anion
- Promotes energy storage and carbohydrate, protein and fat metabolism
- Acts as a hydrogen buffer

Sodium (Na)

- Main extracellular fluid (ECF) cation
- Helps govern normal ECF osmolality (a shift in Na concentrations triggers a fluid volume change to restore normal solute and water ratios)
- Helps maintain acid–base balance
- Activates nerve and muscle cells
- Influences water distribution (with chloride)

Chloride (Cl)

- Main ECF anion
- Helps maintain normal ECF osmolality
- Affects body pH
- Plays a vital role in maintaining acid–base balance; combines with hydrogen ions to produce hydrochloric acid

Calcium (Ca)

- A major cation in teeth and bones; found in fairly equal concentrations in ICF and ECF

- Also found in cell membranes, where it helps cells adhere to one another and maintain their shape
- Acts as an enzyme activator within cells (muscles must have Ca to contract)
- Aids coagulation
- Affects cell membranes' permeability and firing level

Bicarbonate (HCO$_3^-$)

- Present in ECF
- Primary function is regulating acid–base balance

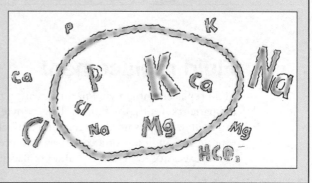

categories according to how much osmotic force they exert, in other words its osmolality.

- *Isotonic crystalloids* contain about the same concentration of osmotically active particles as extracellular fluid, so fluid doesn't shift between the extracellular and intracellular areas.

- *Hypotonic crystalloids* are less concentrated than extracellular fluid so they move from the bloodstream into the cell, causing the cell to swell.
- *Hypertonic crystalloids* are more highly concentrated than extracellular fluid, so fluid is pulled into the bloodstream from the cell, causing the cell to shrink. (See *A look at I.V. solutions*, pages 575–578.)

A look at I.V. solutions

This chart shows examples of commonly used I.V. fluids and includes some of the clinical uses and special consideration associated with their use.

	Osmolarity (mOsm/L)	Indications and incompatibilities	Precautions, comments, contraindications
Normal saline		**Indications**	
(0.9% Sodium chloride) Sodium 152 mmol/L Chloride 152 mmol/L pH 5	308 Relatively isotonic	• Replaces ECF losses by expanding the intravascular space when chloride loss is greater than sodium. • Corrects hyponatraemia. • Replaces sodium losses. • Corrects hypovolaemia. • Corrects mild metabolic acidosis. • Corrects metabolic alkalosis when fluid depletion exists because the chloride ions cause a decrease in bicarbonate ions. • Only infusate compatible with blood; used to initiate and follow blood transfusions. • Diluent for medications. • Used as an irrigant for intravascular devices (flush). — maintains patency. **Incompatibilities** • Amphotericin B • Chlordiazepoxide hydrochloride • Diazepam • Fat emulsions • Mannitol • Methylprednisolone sodium • Phenytoin sodium • Amiodarone	• Accurately monitor fluid balance. • Can cause intravascular overload. • Can cause hypokalaemia because saline promotes potassium excretion. • Can cause hypernatraemia. • Can induce hyperchloraemic acidosis due to loss of bicarbonate ions. • Can cause sodium retention during the intraoperative and early postoperative periods. • Does not provide free water. • Does not provide calories. • Use with caution in patients with decreased renal function. • Use with caution in patients with heart failure. • Use with caution in the elderly. • Contraindicated in oedema with sodium retention. • Causes excess sodium retention when used with glucocorticoids (steroids).

(continued)

A look at I.V. solutions (continued)

	Osmolarity (mOsm/L)	Indications and incompatibilities	Precautions, comments, contraindications
Dextrose saline		**Indications**	

(Sodium chloride 0.18% + glucose 4%) Sodium 32 mmol/L Chloride 32 mmol/L 150 kcal/L pH 4	266 Relatively isotonic	• Rehydration by replenishment of salt and water.
		• Fluid replacement for burns.
		• Supply calories.
		• Reduce nitrogen depletion.
		• As a maintenance infusion.
		
		Incompatibilities
		
		• Amphotericin B
		• Ampicillin sodium
		• Diazepam
		• Erythromycin lactobinate
		• Mannitol
		• Phenytoin
		• Warfarin sodium
		• Whole blood
		• Amiodarone
			To prevent circulatory overload, use with caution in patients with:
			• Congestive heart failure
			• Pulmonary oedema
			• Oedema with sodium retention
			• Patents undergoing corticosteroid therapy
			• Urinary obstruction
			  - Maintain strict fluid balance.
			  - Contraindicated in patients with diabetic coma.
			  - May falsely elevate laboratory urea reports.
			  - Once renal function is assured, electrolytes must be supplemented to prevent hypokalaemia.

Dextrose 5% (in water) 'D_5W'		**Indications**	
Anhydrous glucose 50 g/L 200 kcal/L pH 4.5	252 Relatively isotonic	• Hydration: replaces water losses in dehydration. • Provides free water for the excretion of solutes • Provides calories • Diluent for medications. **Incompatibilities** • Ampicillin sodium (after 2 hours) • Diazepam • Erythromycin lactobinate (after 6 hours) • Fat emulsions • Phenytoin sodium • Sodium bicarbonate • Warfarin Sodium • Whole blood • Vitamin B_{12}	• D_5W is isotonic in the container. Once infused the dextrose is rapidly metabolised and the infusion becomes hypotonic. • Do not administer to patients with increased intracranial pressure because it will cause oedema. • Use with caution in patients with systemic inflammatory response syndrome (e.g. sepsis and pancreatitis) and ARDS as D_5W may result in increased interstitial (and pulmonary) oedema. • Does not contain electrolytes. • Because of excess ADH secretions, as a stress response to surgery, use cautiously in the early postoperative period to prevent water intoxication.

(continued)

A look at I.V. solutions (continued)

	Osmolarity (mOsm/L)	Indications and incompatibilities	Precautions, comments, contraindications
Hartmann's solution		*Indications*	
Potassium 5 mmol/L Sodium 132 mmol/L Calcium 2 mmol/L Chloride 112 mmol/L Bicarbonate (as lactate) 30 mmol/L pH 6.5	281 Isotonic	• Used for dehydration in all types of dehydration. • Restores fluid volume deficit especially in postoperative losses. • Replaces fluid lost as a result of burns. • Treats mild metabolic acidosis associated with renal insufficiency because lactate is converted into bicarbonate. *Incompatibilities* • Amphotericin B • Ampicillin sodium • Cephradine • Diazepam • Erythromycin lactobinate • Methylprednisolone sodium • Oxytetracycline • Phenytoin sodium • Potassium phosphate • Sodium bicarbonate • Thiopentone • Warfarin • Whole Blood	• Risk of fluid overload • Risk of hypernatraemia • Risk of heart failure in the elderly
Sodium bicarbonate 8.4%		*Indications*	

NaHCO$_3$ 999.6 mmol/L
pH 7.75
	1,000	• Alkalinising agent for temporary treatment of severe metabolic acidosis.
		• Increases plasma bicarbonate and buffers excess hydrogen ions.
		• Dosage corresponds to degree of acidosis according to pH, HCO$_3$/BXS and electrolytes.
		• Treats hyperkalaemia.
		• Treatment for barbiturate, salicylate and tricyclic overdose
		
		Incompatibilities
		
		• Numerous infusion and drug interactions—consult pharmacist/medication datasheet.
			Contraindicated with:
			• respiratory acidosis
			• alkalosis
			• oedema
			• hypertension
			• hypocalcaemia
			• hypochloraemia
			• impaired renal function
			  - Use with extreme caution in patients with sodium retention.
			  - Use with extreme caution in patients on corticosteroids.
			  - Excessive or rapid administration can result in intracranial haemorrhage.
			  - Extravasation can result in severe tissue damage.
			  - Flush I.V. line before and after infusion.

(continued)

A look at I.V. solutions (continued)

	Osmolarity (mOsm/L)	Indications and incompatibilities	Precautions, comments, contraindications
Mannitol 20%		Indications	
	1,098	• Osmotic diuretic. • Reduces intraoccular, intracranial and intraspinal pressures by raising plasma osmolality and causing fluids in these areas to diffuse back into the plasma and intravascular space. • Promotes excretion of toxic substances. • Promotes diuresis during oliguric phase of acute renal failure. Incompatibilities • Blood • Imipenim	• Contraindicated in anuria. • Contraindicated in severely dehydrated patients. • Use with extreme caution in patients with congestive heart failure or pulmonary oedema. • Strict fluid balance needed every 30–60 minutes. • Haemodynamic monitoring. • Monitor electrolytes and urea. • Assess for signs of dehydration.
Hetastarch 6% in 0.9% NaCl		Indications	
Na 154 mmol/L Cl 154 mmol/L pH 5.5	308 Relatively isotonic	• Used in shock due to sepsis, acute haemorrhage or burns. • Similar to human albumin in colloid properties Incompatibilities • Ampicillin • Cefotaxime • Cefuroxime • Gentamycin • Phenytoin • Ranitidine • Theophylline • Tobramycin	• Haemodilution effect may worsen coagulation problems. • Contraindicated in congestive heart failure and renal failure. • Maintain strict fluid balance. • Monitor CVP and other haemodynamic monitoring to assess for circulatory overload.

Water movers

Hypertonic solutions called *colloids* may be used to increase blood volume. Colloids have molecules that will not cross a semipermeable membrane and which attract water. A normal physiological example is the protein albumin found in the blood. Colloids draw water from the interstitial space into the vasculature. Examples of colloid solutions that are given to correct hypovolaemia include 4.5% human albumin solution, starch containing fluids (e.g. hetastarch—see *A look at I.V. solutions*, pages 575–578), gelatine containing solutions and dextran.

The effects of colloids last between hours and several days if the lining of the capillaries is normal (i.e. not leaky due to systemic inflammation as in sepsis). The patient needs to be closely monitored during a colloid infusion for increased blood pressure, dyspnoea and bounding pulse, which are signs of hypervolaemia.

What to do

• Check the I.V. prescription for completeness and accuracy. A complete prescription should specify the amount and type of solution, specific additives and their concentrations and the rate and duration of the infusion.
• Keep in mind the size, age and history of the patient when giving I.V. fluids to prevent fluid overload.
• Change the site, dressing and tubing according to local policy. Solutions should be changed at least every 24 hours.
• Monitor the I.V. site for signs of complications, such as infiltration, phlebitis or thrombophlebitis, infection and extravasation.
• Monitor the patient for signs of complications of I.V. therapy, such as an allergic reaction, air embolism and fluid overload.
• Monitor intake and output. Notify the doctor if the patient's urine output falls below 0.5 ml/kg/hour—as a general rule 30 ml/hour is the minimum you should expect in most patients.
• Monitor the patient for potential fluid and electrolyte disturbances and check serum electrolyte values. (See *Interpreting serum electrolyte test results*.)
• Documentation for a patient receiving an I.V. infusion should include the date, time and type of catheter/cannula inserted, the site of insertion and its appearance, the type and amount of fluid infused, the patient's tolerance and response to therapy.

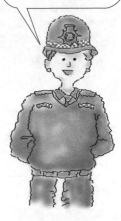

Thermal burns are the most common type of burn. They may result from fires, scalding accidents and sometimes abuse.

Interpreting serum electrolyte test results

Use the quick-reference chart below to interpret serum electrolyte test results for adult patients.

Electrolyte	Results	Implications	Common causes
Serum sodium	135–145 mmol/L	Normal	—
	<135 mmol/L	Hyponatraemia	Syndrome of inappropriate antidiuretic hormone
	>145 mmol/L	Hypernatraemia	Diabetes insipidus
Serum potassium	3.5–5 mmol/L	Normal	—
	<3.5 mmol/L	Hypokalaemia	Diarrhoea
	>5 mmol/L	Hyperkalaemia	Burns and renal failure

(continued)

Interpreting serum electrolyte test results (continued)

Electrolyte	Results	Implications	Common causes
Total serum calcium	2.0–2.5 mmol/L	Normal	—
	<2.0 mmol/L	Hypocalcaemia	Acute pancreatitis
	>2.5 mmol/L	Hypercalcaemia	Hyperparathyroidism
Ionised calcium	1.1–1.4 mmol/L	Normal	—
	<1.1 mg/dl	Hypocalcaemia	Massive transfusion
	>1.4 mg/dl	Hypercalcaemia	Acidosis

NB: Calcium is significantly albumin bound. Therefore, if albumin is low the total calcium will appear low. In this case it is most useful to look at ionised (unbound calcium) or corrected calcium – where the laboratories will correct for the low albumin. Corrected calcium should be in the normal calcium range as above.

Electrolyte	Results	Implications	Common causes
Serum phosphates	0.8–1.4 mmol/L	Normal	—
	<0.8 mmol/L	Hypophosphataemia	Diabetic ketoacidosis
	>1.4 mmol/L	Hyperphosphataemia	Renal insufficiency
Serum magnesium	0.7–1.0 mmol/L	Normal	—
	<0.7 mmol/L	Hypomagnesaemia	Malnutrition
	>1.0 mmol/L	Hypermagnesaemia	Renal failure
Serum chloride	98–108 mmol/L	Normal	—
	<98 mmol/L	Hypochloraemia	Prolonged vomiting
	>108 mmol/L	Hyperchloraemia	Hypernatraemia

Multisystem disorders

Multisystem disorders include burns, hypothermia, hypovolaemic shock, multiple organ dysfunction syndrome (MODS), severe sepsis/septic shock and trauma.

Burns

Burns are tissue injuries that result from contact with thermal, chemical or electrical sources or from friction or exposure to the sun. They can cause cellular skin damage and a systemic response, including inflammation that leads to altered body function. A major burn affects every body system and organ, usually requiring painful treatment and a long period of rehabilitation.

What causes it

Thermal burns, the most common burn type, typically result from:
- residential fires
- road traffic accidents

- playing with matches
- improper handling of fireworks
- scalding accidents and kitchen accidents
- abuse (in children or elderly people)
- clothes that have caught on fire.

Scorching brews

Chemical burns result from contact, ingestion, inhalation or injection of acids, alkalis or vesicants (blistering agents).

It's electric

Electrical burns usually result from contact with faulty electrical wiring and cords or high-voltage power lines.

Rubbing or sunning the wrong way

Friction or abrasion burns occur when the skin rubs harshly against a coarse surface. Sunburn results from excessive exposure to sunlight.

How it happens

Specific pathophysiological events depend on the cause and classification of the burn. (See *Visualising burn depth*.) The injuring agent denatures cellular proteins. Some cells die because of traumatic or ischaemic necrosis. Loss

Visualising burn depth

The most widely used system of classifying burn depth and severity categorises them by degree. However, it's important to remember that most burns involve tissue damage of multiple degrees and thicknesses. This illustration may help you to visualise burn damage at the various degrees.

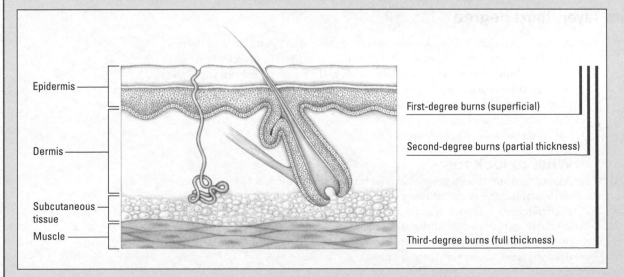

Epidermis

Dermis

Subcutaneous tissue

Muscle

First-degree burns (superficial)

Second-degree burns (partial thickness)

Third-degree burns (full thickness)

of collagen cross-linking also occurs with denaturation, creating abnormal osmotic and hydrostatic pressure gradients that cause intravascular fluid to move into interstitial spaces. Cellular injury triggers the release of mediators of inflammation, contributing to local and, in the case of major burns, systemic increases in capillary permeability.

For your epidermis only

A *first-degree burn* causes localised injury or destruction to the skin's epidermis by direct contact (such as a chemical spill) or indirect contact (such as sunlight). The barrier function of the skin remains intact. This type of burn isn't life-threatening.

Barrier-breaking blisters

A *second-degree superficial partial-thickness burn* involves destruction to the epidermis and some dermis. Thin-walled, fluid-filled blisters develop within a few minutes of the injury. As these blisters break, the nerve endings become exposed to the air. Because pain and tactile responses remain intact, subsequent treatments are painful. The barrier function of the skin is lost.

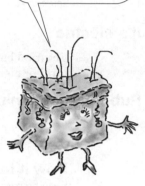

Yowza! Those second-degree deep partial-thickness burns involve blisters and oedema!

Deep into the dermis

A *second-degree deep partial-thickness burn* involves the epidermis and dermis. The patient develops blisters and experiences mild-to-moderate oedema and pain. The hair follicles remain intact, so the hair will regrow. Compared with a second-degree superficial partial-thickness burn, there's less pain sensation with this burn because the sensory neurons have undergone extensive destruction; however, because the barrier function of the skin is lost, sensitivity to pain remains in some areas around the burn.

Third layer, third degree

A *third-degree (full-thickness) burn* extends through the epidermis and dermis and into the subcutaneous tissue layer. It may also involve muscle, bone and interstitial tissues. Within hours, fluids and protein shift from capillary to interstitial spaces, causing oedema. A person's body has an immediate immunological response to a third-degree burn, making burn wound sepsis a potential threat. Finally, an increase in calorie demand after a third-degree burn increases the patient's metabolic rate.

What to look for

Assessment provides a general idea of burn severity. First, it is important to determine the depth of tissue damage. A partial-thickness burn damages the epidermis and part of the dermis; a full-thickness burn also affects subcutaneous tissue. Traditionally, burns were gauged by degree. Today, however, most assessment findings use degrees and depth of tissue damage to describe a burn, as previously discussed.

Tracking burn traits

Signs and symptoms depend on the type of burn and may include:
- localised pain and erythema, usually without blisters in the first 24 hours (first-degree burn)
- chills, headache, localised oedema and nausea and vomiting (more severe first-degree burn)
- thin-walled, fluid-filled blisters appearing within minutes of the injury, with mild-to-moderate oedema and pain (second-degree superficial partial-thickness burn)
- white, waxy appearance to damaged area (second-degree deep partial-thickness burn)
- white, brown or black leathery tissue and visible thrombosed vessels due to destruction of skin elasticity (dorsum of hand, most common site of thrombosed veins), without blisters (third-degree burn)
- silver-coloured, raised or charred area, usually at the site of electrical contact (electrical burn).

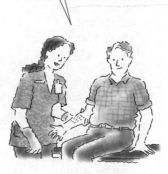

Assessment of the burn will give you an idea of the degree and depth of the tissue damage.

Configure this!

Inspection also reveals the location and extent of the burn. Note the burn's configuration. If the patient has a circumferential burn on an extremity, they run the risk of oedema occluding the circulation in that extremity. If they have burns on their neck, they may suffer airway obstruction; burns on the chest can lead to restricted respiratory excursion.

More to it than just skin

Inspect the patient for other injuries that may complicate recovery such as signs of pulmonary damage from smoke inhalation, including singed nasal hairs, mucosal burns, voice changes, coughing, wheezing, soot in the mouth or nose and darkened sputum.

Check a burn victim for pulmonary damage and smoke inhalation. These factors may complicate recovery.

What tests tell you

An assessment method that can be used to determine the size of a burn is the Rule of Nines chart, which determines the percentage of body surface area (BSA) covered by the burn. (See *Estimating the extent of a burn*, page 584.)

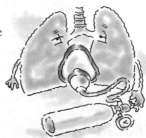

A matter of class

Burns may be classified into three categories: major, moderate and minor.
Major burns include:
- third-degree burns on more than 10% of BSA
- second-degree burns on more than 25% of BSA
- burns on hands, face, feet or genitalia
- burns complicated by fractures or respiratory damage
- electrical burns

Estimating the extent of a burn

You can estimate the extent of an adult patient's burn by using the Rule of Nines. This method quantifies body surface areas in multiples of nine, thus the name. To use this method, mentally transfer the burns on your patient to the body charts shown here. Add the corresponding percentages for each body section burned. You can use the total—a rough estimate of burn extent—to calculate fluid replacement needs.

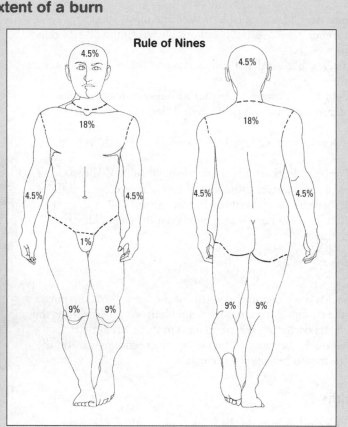

Rule of Nines

- burns in poor-risk patients.
  Moderate burns include:
- third-degree burns on 2–10% of BSA
- second-degree burns on 15–25% of BSA.
  Minor burns include:
- third-degree burns on less than 2% of BSA
- second-degree burns on less than 15% of BSA.

Back in the lab

Here are some additional diagnostic test results regarding burns:
- Arterial blood gas (ABG) levels may be normal in the early stages but may reveal hypoxaemia and metabolic acidosis later.
- Carboxyhaemoglobin level may reveal the extent of smoke inhalation due to the presence of carbon monoxide.

• Full blood count (FBC) may reveal a decreased Hb (due to haemolysis), increased haematocrit (secondary to haemoconcentration) and leucocytosis (resulting from a systemic inflammatory response or the possible development of sepsis).
• Electrolyte levels may show hyponatraemia (from massive fluid shifting) and hyperkalaemia (from fluid shifting and cell lysis). Other laboratory tests may reveal elevated urea levels (secondary to fluid loss or increased protein breakdown) and decreased total protein and albumin (resulting from plasma proteins leaking into the interstitial spaces).
• Creatine kinase (CK) and myoglobin levels may be elevated. Keep in mind that CK and myoglobin are helpful indicators of muscle damage. Therefore, the higher the CK or myoglobin level, the more extensive the muscle damage. The presence of myoglobin in urine may lead to acute tubular necrosis.

How it's treated
Initial burn treatments are based on the type of burn and may include:
• removing the source of the burn and any items that retain heat, such as clothing and jewellery
• maintaining an open airway; assessing airway, breathing and circulation (ABCs)
• administering supplemental humidified oxygen
• controlling active bleeding
• covering partial-thickness burns that are over 30% of BSA or full-thickness burns that are over 5% of BSA with a clean, dry, sterile sheet or drape (because of the drastic reduction in body temperature, don't cover large burns with saline-soaked dressings)
• fluid replacement (see *A closer look at fluid replacement*, page 586)
• antimicrobial therapy (for all patients with major burns)
• pain medication as needed
• antiinflammatory medications
• laboratory tests, such as FBC, urea and electrolytes, glucose and serum creatinine levels; ABG analysis; typing and cross-matching; urinalysis for myoglobinuria and haemoglobinuria
• close monitoring of intake and output and vital signs
• surgical intervention, including skin grafts and more thorough surgical debridement for major burns
• tetanus prophylaxis as ordered
• nutritional therapy.

What to do
• Immediately assess the patient's ABCs. Institute emergency resuscitative measures as necessary. Monitor arterial oxygen saturation and serial ABG values and anticipate the need for endotracheal (ET) intubation and mechanical ventilation should the patient's respiratory status deteriorate, especially with facial or neck burns.

A closer look at fluid replacement

Fluid replacement is essential for the patient with burns because of the massive fluid shifts that occur. However, extreme caution is needed because of the risk of fluid overload.

How much?

Numerous formulas may be used to determine the amount of fluid replacement to be administered during the first 24 hours after a burn injury. Typically, these formulas use body weight and the percentage of body surface area (BSA) burned. One of the most common formulas used is the Parkland formula shown here:

Fluid requirements
= Total BSA burned % × wt (kg) × 4 ml

Over how long?

Typically, one-half of the calculated amount is administered during the first 8 hours following the injury. (Note that the time of injury—not the time of the patient's arrival in the emergency department—is used as the initial start time of the 8-hour duration.) The remaining one-half of the amount is then administered over the next 16 hours.

What fluids?

During the first 24 hours, crystalloid solutions are commonly used because capillary permeability is greatly increased, allowing proteins to leak into the interstitial tissues. After the first 24 hours, colloid solutions can be included. Giving colloids before the initial 24-hour period would supply additional protein that could leak into the interstitial tissue.

Too much or too little?

During fluid replacement, always be alert for indications of overload and hypovolaemia. Signs and symptoms of heart failure and pulmonary oedema suggest overload. Assessment findings of circulatory shock suggest hypovolaemia.

Listen to the lungs

- Auscultate breath sounds for crackles, rhonchi or stridor. Observe for signs of laryngeal oedema or tracheal obstruction, including laboured breathing, severe hoarseness and dyspnoea.
- Administer supplemental humidified oxygen as prescribed.
- Perform oropharyngeal or tracheal suctioning as indicated by the patient's inability to clear their airway or evidence of abnormal breath sounds.
- Monitor the patient's cardiac and respiratory status closely, at least every 15 minutes, or more frequently, depending on their condition. Also monitor the patient for cardiac arrhythmias. Assess their level of consciousness (LOC) for changes, such as increasing confusion, restlessness or decreased responsiveness. (See *Electrical burn care*, page 587.)
- If the patient has a chemical burn, irrigate the wound with copious amounts of water or normal saline solution. If the chemical entered the patient's eyes, remove contact lenses if necessary and flush the eyes with large amounts of water or normal saline solution for at least 30 minutes. Have the patient close their eyes and cover them with a dry, sterile dressing. Note the type of chemical that caused the burn and any noxious fumes. If necessary, refer the patient for an ophthalmic examination.

Advice from the experts

Electrical burn care

Keep these tips in mind when caring for a patient with an electrical burn:
- Be alert for ventricular fibrillation as well as cardiac and respiratory arrest caused by the electrical shock; begin cardiopulmonary resuscitation immediately.
- Get an estimate of the voltage that caused the injury.
- Tissue damage from an electrical burn is difficult to assess because internal destruction along the conduction pathway usually is greater than the surface burn would indicate.
- An electrical burn that ignites the patient's clothes may also cause thermal burns.

- Place the patient in asemirecumbent position to maximise chest expansion. Keep them as quiet and comfortable as possible to minimise oxygen demands.
- Prepare the patient for an emergency escharotomy of the chest and neck for deep burns or circumferential injuries, if necessary, to promote lung expansion and decrease pulmonary compromise.
- Administer rapid fluid replacement therapy as prescribed, using a large-bore peripheral catheter or central venous catheter as indicated.

Shocking results

- Monitor the patient's vital signs and haemodynamic parameters for changes indicating hypovolaemic shock or evidence of fluid overload and pulmonary oedema.
- Assess the patient's intake and output every hour; insert a urinary catheter as to ensure accurate urine measurement.
- Assess the patient's level of pain, including nonverbal indicators, and administer analgesics such as morphine, as prescribed. Avoid I.M. injections because tissue damage associated with the burn injury may impair absorption of the drug when given I.M.
- Keep the patient calm, provide periods of uninterrupted rest between procedures, and use nonpharmacological pain relief measures as appropriate.
- Obtain daily weights and monitor intake, including daily calorie counts. Provide a high-calorie, high-protein diet. Assess the patient's abdomen for distention and presence of bowel sounds. Administer enteral and parenteral feedings as prescribed.
- Administer histamine-2 receptor antagonists or proton pump inhibitors, as prescribed, to reduce the risk of gastric ulcer formation.
- Assess the patient for signs and symptoms of infection, including fever, elevated WBC count, elevated CRP and changes in burn wound appearance

or drainage. Obtain a wound culture, and administer antipyretic and antimicrobial agents as prescribed.
- Administer tetanus prophylaxis, if indicated.
- Perform burn wound care as prescribed by burn specialist, wound care specialist or surgeons. Prepare the patient for possible grafting as indicated.
- Assess the neurovascular status of the injured area, including pulses, reflexes, paraesthesia, colour and temperature of the injured area at least every 2–4 hours, or more frequently, if indicated.
- Assist with splinting, positioning, compression therapy and exercise to the burned area as indicated. Maintain the burned area in a neutral position to prevent contractures and minimise deformity.
- Explain all procedures to the patient before performing them. Encourage them to actively participate in their care as much as possible, and provide opportunities for them to voice their concerns, especially about their altered body image.

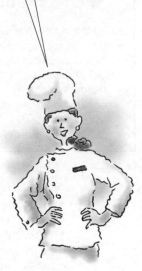

A burn patient needs a high-calorie, high-protein diet.

Hypothermia

Hypothermia is defined as a core body temperature below 35°C. It may be classified as mild (32–35°C), moderate (30–32°C) or severe (25–30°C). Severe hypothermia can be fatal as it is associated with life-threatening cardiac arrhythmias.

What causes it

Hypothermia commonly results from near drowning in cold water, prolonged exposure to cold temperatures, disease or debility that alters homeostasis and the administration of large amounts of cold intravenous fluids, blood or blood products.

Likely candidates

The risk of serious cold injury, especially hypothermia, increases with youth, old age, lack of insulating body fat, wet or inadequate clothing, drug abuse, cardiac disease, smoking, fatigue, malnutrition and depletion of caloric reserves and excessive alcohol intake.

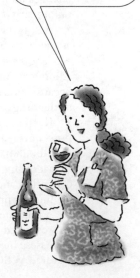

Excessive alcohol intake can increase the risk of hypothermia.

How it happens

In hypothermia, metabolic changes slow the functions of most major organ systems, resulting in decreased renal blood flow and decreased glomerular filtration. Vital organs are physiologically affected. Severe hypothermia results in depression of cerebral blood flow, diminished oxygen requirements, reduced cardiac output and decreased arterial pressure.

What to look for

Obtaining the history of a patient with a cold injury should reveal:
- cause of hypothermia
- temperature to which the patient was exposed
- length of exposure.

Temperature dependent

Assessment findings in a patient with hypothermia vary with the patient's body temperature:
- Mild hypothermia includes severe shivering, slurred speech and amnesia.
- Moderate hypothermia includes unresponsiveness, peripheral cyanosis and muscle rigidity. If the patient was improperly rewarmed, they may show signs of shock.
- Severe hypothermia includes absence of palpable pulses, dilated pupils and rigour mortis–like state. In addition, ventricular fibrillation and a loss of deep tendon reflexes commonly occur.

What tests tell you
- Doppler studies help determine pulses and the extent of frostbite after thawing.

How it's treated
Treatment for hypothermia consists of supportive measures and specific rewarming techniques, including:
- passive rewarming (the patient rewarms on their own)
- active external rewarming with heating blankets, warm ambient temperatures and heated objects such as water bottles
- active core rewarming with heated I.V. fluids, irrigation of urinary catheter and via NG tube with warm fluids, extracorporeal rewarming, haemodialysis and heated humidifiers.

Cardiac concerns

Arrhythmias that develop usually convert into normal sinus rhythm with rewarming. If the patient has no pulse or respirations, CPR is needed until rewarming raises the core temperature to at least 32°C.

Measure dependent on monitoring

The administration of oxygen, ET intubation, controlled ventilation, I.V. fluids and treatment for metabolic acidosis depend on test results and careful patient monitoring.

What to do
- Assess ABCs. Initiate CPR as appropriate. Keep in mind that hypothermia helps protect the brain from anoxia, which normally accompanies prolonged cardiopulmonary arrest. Therefore, even if the patient has been unresponsive for a long time, CPR may resuscitate them, especially after a cold-water near drowning.
- Assist with rewarming techniques as necessary.
- During rewarming, provide supportive measures as prescribed, including mechanical ventilation and heated, humidified oxygen therapy

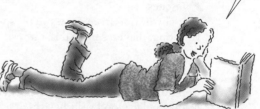

Here's a warm thought: hypothermia helps protect the brain from anoxia, so even if the patient has been unresponsive for a long time, CPR may resuscitate them.

to maintain tissue oxygenation, and I.V. fluids that have been warmed to correct hypotension and maintain urine output.

• Continuously monitor the patient's core body temperature and other vital signs during and after initial rewarming. Continuously monitor their cardiac status, including continuous cardiac monitoring for evidence of arrhythmias.

• If using active warming discontinue the warming when the core body temperature is within 0.6–1.1°C of the desired temperature. The patient's temperature will continue to rise even after devices are turned off.

• If the patient has been hypothermic for longer than 45–60 minutes, administer additional fluids as prescribed to compensate for the expansion of the vascular space that occurs during vasodilation in rewarming. Monitor the patient's heart rate and haemodynamic parameters closely to evaluate fluid needs and response to treatment.

• Monitor the patient's hourly urine output, fluid balance and serum electrolyte levels, especially potassium. Be alert for signs and symptoms of hyperkalaemia. If hyperkalaemia occurs, administer drugs to reduce potassium as prescribed. These may include calcium chloride, sodium bicarbonate, glucose and insulin as ordered. Anticipate the need for sodium polystyrene sulphonate enemas. If their potassium levels are extremely elevated, prepare the patient for dialysis or haemofiltration.

Hypovolaemic shock

Hypovolaemic shock occurs because of acute blood or other fluid losses. A loss of between 15% and 30% (750–1,500 ml) of circulating volume without sufficient blood or fluid replacement will cause hypovolaemic shock, leading to irreversible damage to organs and systems if not treated.

What causes it

Massive volume loss may result from:

• GI bleeding, internal or external haemorrhage or any condition that reduces circulating intravascular volume or other body fluids

• sepsis
• burns
• intestinal obstruction
• peritonitis
• acute pancreatitis
• ascites

• dehydration from excessive perspiration, severe diarrhoea or protracted vomiting, diabetes insipidus, diuresis or inadequate fluid intake.

How it happens

Potentially life-threatening, hypovolaemic shock stems from reduced intravascular blood volume, which leads to decreased cardiac output and inadequate tissue perfusion. The subsequent tissue anoxia prompts a shift in cellular metabolism from aerobic to anaerobic pathways. This results in an accumulation of lactic acid, which produces metabolic acidosis.

The road to shockville

When compensatory mechanisms fail, hypovolaemic shock occurs in this sequence:

 decreased intravascular fluid volume

diminished venous return, which reduces preload and decreases stroke volume

reduced cardiac output

decreased mean arterial pressure

impaired tissue perfusion

 decreased oxygen and nutrient delivery to cells

multisystem organ failure.

What to look for
The specific signs and symptoms exhibited by the patient depend on the amount of fluid loss. (See *Estimating fluid loss*.)

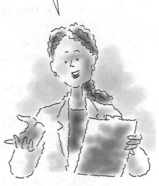

In many cases, the patient's history will reveal the cause of reduced blood volume—such as GI haemorrhage, trauma or severe diarrhoea, and vomiting—and guide your assessment.

Estimating fluid loss

The following assessment parameters indicate the severity of intravascular volume loss.

<750 ml (<15%)	750–1,500 ml (15–30%)	1,500–2,000 ml (30–40%)	>2,000 ml (>40%)
Signs and symptoms include:	Signs and symptoms include:	Signs and symptoms include:	Signs and symptoms include:
• Heart rate: slightly elevated/normal (<100) • Blood pressure: normal • Pulse pressure: normal • CRT: normal (<2 seconds) • RR: 14–20 • Urine output >30 ml/hour • Mental status: normal/alert	• Heart rate: elevated >100 • Blood pressure: normal systolic but elevated diastolic • Pulse pressure: narrowed • CRT: normal (>2 seconds) • RR: 20–30 • Urine output 20–30 ml/hour • Mental status: anxious	• Heart rate: elevated >120 • Blood pressure: reduced systolic and diastolic • Pulse pressure: narrowed • CRT: normal (>2 seconds) • RR: 30–40 • Urine output 5–15 ml/hour • Mental status: anxious and confused	• Heart rate: elevated >140 • Blood pressure: significantly reduced • Pulse pressure: significantly narrowed • CRT: undetectable • RR: >35 • Urine output anuria • Mental status: confusion/lethargy/unconsciousness

Oh where oh where has the blood volume gone?

Typically, the patient's history includes conditions that reduce blood volume, such as GI haemorrhage, trauma and severe diarrhoea and vomiting.

Assessment should proceed through an ABCDE approach initially. Findings from clinical assessment may include:

- pale skin
- decreased sensorium
- rapid, shallow respirations
- urine output below 30 ml/hour (or more accurately 0.5 ml/kg/hour)
- rapid, thready peripheral pulses
- cold skin with a capillary refill time (CRT) >2 seconds (often much longer)
- mean arterial pressure below 60 mmHg and a narrowing pulse pressure
- decreased CVP, right atrial pressure, PAWP and cardiac output.

What tests tell you

No single diagnostic test confirms hypovolaemic shock, but these test results help to support the diagnosis:

- low Hct
- decreased Hb level
- decreased RBC and platelet counts
- elevated serum potassium, sodium, lactate, creatinine and urea
- increased urine specific gravity (greater than 1.020) and urine osmolality
- decreased pH and partial pressure of arterial oxygen and increased partial pressure of arterial carbon dioxide ($PaCO_2$)
- gastroscopy, x-rays, aspiration of gastric contents through a nasogastric tube and tests for occult blood
- coagulation studies for coagulopathy from disseminated intravascular coagulation (DIC).

How it's treated

Emergency treatment relies on prompt and adequate fluid and blood replacement to restore intravascular volume and to raise blood pressure and maintain it above 80 mmHg. Rapid infusion of colloid plasma expanders, normal saline or Hartmann's solution may expand volume adequately. In the case of hypovolaemia from blood loss this may be followed by blood transfusion.

Treatment may also include oxygen administration, control of bleeding, inotrope or vasopressor infusions and surgery, if appropriate.

What to do

Assess the patient for the extent of fluid loss and begin fluid replacement as prescribed. Obtain a type and cross-match for blood component therapy if bleeding is suspected.

> Fluid and blood replacement is crucial to restoring intravascular volume and raising blood pressure in patients with hypovolaemic shock.

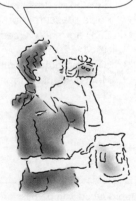

ABCs and ABGs

- Assess ABCs. If the patient experiences cardiac or respiratory arrest, start CPR.
- Administer supplemental oxygen as prescribed. Monitor oxygen saturation and ABGs for evidence of hypoxaemia and acidosis from elevated lactate. Anticipate the need for ET intubation and mechanical ventilation should the patient's respiratory status deteriorate. Place the patient with head of bed elevated to 45 degrees, if tolerated, to maximise chest expansion. Keep the patient as quiet and comfortable as possible to minimise oxygen demands.
- Monitor vital signs, neurological status and cardiac rhythm continuously for changes such as cardiac arrhythmias or myocardial ischaemia. Observe skin colour and check capillary refill. (See *When blood pressure drops*.)
- Monitor haemodynamic parameters, including CVP, PAWP and cardiac output, frequently—as often as every 15 minutes—to evaluate the patient's status and response to treatment.
- Monitor fluid intake and output closely. Insert a urinary catheter and assess urine output hourly. If bleeding from the GI tract is suspected as the cause, check all stools, emesis and gastric drainage for occult blood. If urine output falls below 30 ml/hour in an adult (or 1/2 ml/kg/hour), expect to increase the I.V. fluid infusion rate, but watch for signs of fluid overload such as elevated CVP and difficulty breathing with falling oxygen saturations. Notify the doctor if urine output doesn't increase.
- Administer blood and blood products as prescribed; monitor serial Hb values and Hct to evaluate effects of treatment.
- Administer dobutamine and/or noradrenaline as prescribed to increase renal perfusion.
- Watch for signs of impending coagulopathy (such as petechiae, bruising and bleeding or oozing from gums or venepuncture sites) and report them immediately.
- Provide emotional support and reassurance appropriately in the wake of massive fluid losses.
- Prepare the patient for surgery as appropriate.

Multiple organ dysfunction syndrome

MODS is a condition that occurs when two or more organs or organ systems are unable to function in their role of maintaining homeostasis. Intervention is necessary to support and maintain organ function. MODS isn't an illness itself; rather, it's a manifestation of another progressive underlying condition.

What causes it

MODS develops when widespread systemic inflammation, a condition known as systemic inflammatory response syndrome (SIRS), overtaxes a patient's compensatory mechanisms. SIRS can be triggered by infection, ischaemia, trauma, burns, reperfusion injury or multisystem injury. If allowed to progress, SIRS can lead to organ inflammation and ultimately, MODS.

Take charge!

When blood pressure drops

A drop below 80 mmHg in systolic blood pressure usually signals inadequate cardiac output from reduced intravascular volume. Such a drop usually results in inadequate coronary artery blood flow, cardiac ischaemia, arrhythmias and other complications of low cardiac output. If the patient's systolic blood pressure drops below 80 mmHg and their pulse is thready, increase the oxygen flow rate and notify the doctor immediately.

MODS isn't an illness itself. It's a manifestation of another underlying condition.

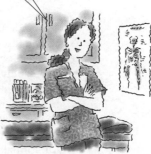

How it happens

MODS is classified as primary or secondary:
• Primary MODS involves organ or organ system failure that's caused by a direct injury (such as trauma, aspiration or near drowning) or a primary disorder (such as pneumonia or pulmonary embolism). Primary MODS commonly involves the lungs. Patients typically develop acute respiratory distress syndrome (ARDS), which progresses to encephalopathy and coagulopathy. As the syndrome continues, other organ systems are affected.
• Secondary MODS involves organ or organ system failure that's due to sepsis. Typically the infection source isn't associated with the lungs. The most common infection sources include intra-abdominal sepsis, extensive blood loss, pancreatitis or major vascular injuries. ARDS develops sooner and progressive involvement of other organs and organ systems occurs more rapidly than in primary MODS.

What to look for

The assessment findings associated with MODS typically reveal an acutely ill patient with signs and symptoms associated with SIRS. Early findings may include:
• fever (temperature usually greater than 38.3°C)
• tachycardia
• narrowed pulse pressure
• tachypnoea
• decreased pulmonary artery pressure (PAP), PAWP and CVP, and increased cardiac output.

As time goes by

As SIRS progresses, findings reflect impaired perfusion of the tissues and organs, such as:
• decreased LOC
• respiratory depression
• diminished bowel sounds
• jaundice
• oliguria or anuria
• increased PAP and PAWP and decreased cardiac output.

What tests tell you

No single test confirms MODS, and test results depend on the cause, such as trauma, aspiration, pulmonary embolism or sepsis:
• ABG analysis may reveal hypoxaemia with respiratory acidosis or metabolic acidosis.
• FBC may reveal decreased Hb level and Hct as well as leucocytosis
• X-rays may reveal fractures, a cervical spine injury, pulmonary infiltrates or abnormal air or fluid in the chest or abdominal organs.

Additional tests that may be performed include MRI, a CT scan and angiography.

How it's treated

Treatment focuses on supporting respiratory and circulatory function as a priority, and includes:

- mechanical ventilation and supplemental oxygen
- haemodynamic monitoring
- fluid infusion (crystalloids and colloids)
- vasopressors
- measuring fluid intake and output
- serial laboratory tests
- dialysis or haemofiltration
- antimicrobial agents.

What to do

- Keep in mind that nursing care for the patient with MODS is primarily supportive.
- Maintain the patient's airway and breathing with the use of mechanical ventilation and supplemental oxygen.
- Monitor vital signs, oxygen saturation, haemodynamic parameters and cardiac rhythm for arrhythmias.
- Administer I.V. fluids as prescribed.
- Monitor laboratory results.
- Monitor fluid intake and output.
- Administer medications as prescribed.
- Provide emotional support to the patient and family; explain diagnostic tests and treatments.

> Treatment for MODS focuses on supporting respiratory and circulatory function.

Sepsis, severe sepsis and septic shock

Up to 135,000 deaths occur from sepsis in Europe each year and this is set to rise even further in the future: 30–50% of patients who develop severe sepsis die within 1 month of the onset. Early recognition of sepsis and early intervention have been shown to significantly improve chances of survival so you need to be sure you know how to recognise sepsis and that you know what to do to increase chances of survival.

So what is sepsis?

SIRS occurs when there is a widespread inflammatory reaction to a major insult. The response involves release of inflammatory mediators such as tumour necrosis factor (TNF) or interleukin-1. Triggers might include major burns, trauma, pancreatitis or poisoning. However, when SIRS occurs in response to an infection of microorganisms this is sepsis.

How to identify infection

Health care staff should be constantly alert for signs and symptoms of infection. Evidence or suspicion of infection combined with SIRS means that your patient has sepsis so be alert for:
- fever >38.3°C
- rigours
- purulent discharge or sputum
- cellulitis, especially at the site of wounds, drains or invasive devices
- consolidation on chest x-ray
- elevated WBC
- elevated CRP.

How to identify SIRS

Remember that SIRS can have noninfective causes, but if there is evidence or suspicion of infection (see above) and the patient has two or more of the following SIRS criteria, sepsis is present:
- Hyperthermia > 38.3°C or hypothermia < 36°C
- WBC > 12,000 per μl or WBC < 4,000 per μl
- Tachycardia > 90 per minute
- Tachypnoea > 20 per minute
- Acutely altered mental status
- Glucose > 6.6 mmol/L

Who is at risk of sepsis?

Many things increase the risk of developing sepsis but you should be especially vigilant if your patient has any of the following:
- Injuries, wounds, trauma, burns
- Compromised immune system (e.g. severe illness, chemotherapy, transplants and AIDS)
- Pre-existing chronic conditions (e.g. COPD, heart failure, diabetes, pancreatitis and malignancy)
- Intravenous drug use or alcohol dependency
  Some patients with infections will have relatively mild systemic reactions, whilst other will have much more exaggerated reactions even despite treatment. This is thought to be because there are genetic factors that affect the inflammatory response in the presence of a major infection.

Differentiating sepsis from severe sepsis and septic shock

Many people will have experienced infections such as a virus causing fever and other markers of SIRS. This is the type of self-limiting illness we'll all experience throughout life. However, critical illness occurs when the inflammatory reaction is severe and begins to cause organ dysfunction and circulatory shock.

Severe sepsis exists when there is infection, SIRS and when organ dysfunction is present. Routine assessment and investigations allow assessment of organ dysfunction. Septic shock exists when there is hypotension despite intravenous fluid resuscitation. This is because of profound vasodilatation and loss of fluid through leaky capillary beds. Sepsis begins with a warm dilated phase but progresses to a cold decompensated phase as fluid is lost from circulation and organs begin to fail.

What tests tell you

Here are some of the markers of organ dysfunction to be alert for:
- SBP < 90 mmHg or decrease > 40 from baseline
- Arterial lactate > 4 mmol/L
- Urine < 0.5 ml/kg/hour for 2 hours or creatinine > 177 mmol/L
- Bilirubin > 34 mmol/L
- Platelets < 100×10^9 per L
- INR > 1.5 or APTT > 60 seconds
- Bilateral pulmonary infiltrates requiring supplemental oxygen to maintain SpO_2 > 90%

How it's treated initially

Rapid location and treatment of the underlying sepsis is essential to treating septic shock. The initial treatment should be achieved within the first hour of signs and symptoms. It is best to use a structured approach and a standardised protocol (See *Initial treatment of septic shock*.) This includes:

A Ensure patent airway
B Give oxygen – aim for SaO_2 > 94%
C Give a fluid challenge 500–1,000 ml Saline or Hartmann's (Colloid equivalent 300–500 ml) repeat based on *response* and *tolerance* up to 20 ml/kg.

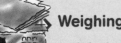

Weighing the evidence

Initial treatment of septic shock

Many hospitals are initiating standardised order sets for the treatment of different conditions. A recent study looked at the use of a standardised treatment protocol for patients with septic shock. A total of 120 patients were studied, 60 of whom were treated with the standardised treatment protocol, and the other 60 without the protocol. The patients with the standardised treatment received more appropriate fluid resuscitation and antimicrobial drugs, used less vasopressors, had a shorter hospital stay and experienced a lower 28-day mortality rate.

Source: Micek, S.T., et al. Before-after study of a standardized hospital order set for the management of septic shock, *Critical Care Medicine* 34(11): 2707–13, November 2006.

- Aim for mean BP > 65 mmHg
- If fluid challenges fail to achieve mean BP > 65/adequate organ perfusion—vasopressors or inotropes may be needed
- Measure arterial lactate (>2 = abnormal, >4 = septic shock/poor tissue perfusion)
- Catheterise and measure urine output hourly

D Continuous reassessment of consciousness/mental status

E Look for sources of sepsis, e.g. purulent sputum, wound drainage, cellulitis, infected indwelling lines and catheters and remove these immediately if they are suspected sources of sepsis. Send the tips for culture and draw blood culture samples from arterial or central venous catheters left *in situ*.

Other priorities include:

- Good I.V. access (>1 cannula—attempts may be more successful after initial fluid resuscitation). Ideally a central venous catheter should be inserted as part of the next stage of management.
- Take blood cultures immediately by venesection—taking care not to contaminate the sample.
- Broad spectrum antibiotics within 1 hour of developing signs and symptoms if severe sepsis/septic shock. (Seek microbiologist advice and review as soon as culture results are available.)
- Plasma glucose.
- ABGs, U&E, FBC, LFT and clotting.
- Reduce hyperthermia.
- Ensure observations are repeated at least hourly.

What next?

Once the immediate measures have been initiated to resuscitate the patient within the first hour the work isn't done. Those with severe sepsis and septic shock will need ongoing organ support and continuous monitoring. Here's what to do next:

- Commence continuous cardiac monitoring and be alert for cardiac arrhythmias.
- Monitor oxygen saturations continuously and be alert for falling levels.
- Be ready to assist with intubation and commencement of mechanical ventilation. A preventative lung strategy might be adopted where peak airway pressures are kept below 30 cmH$_2$O and tidal volumes of 6 ml/kg are used since these have been associated with better outcomes in patients with ARDS—common sequelae of severe sepsis.
- Assist with insertion of arterial and central venous catheters, as well as commencing haemodynamic monitoring according to your unit's method for measuring cardiac output/cardiac index (CO/CI) and systemic vascular resistance (SVR).
- Commence and titrate vasopressors and/or inotropes as prescribed to achieve explicit physiological goals. Aim for mean arterial blood pressure of > 65 mmHg.

- Measure central venous oxygen saturations (ScvO$_2$). The target should be >70%—give inotropes and/or blood transfusion as prescribed to achieve this goal. The central venous oxygen saturation indicates the balance of oxygen delivery and consumption—too low and not enough oxygen is being delivered. A high value (e.g. 80%) indicates that cardiac output may be too high due to low SVR. Vasopressors are usually used to tighten-up the peripheral circulation and increase blood pressure whilst returning the cardiac output to more normal levels.
- Give steroids as prescribed for those patients who are hypotensive despite adequate fluid resuscitation and high-dose vasopressors.
- Monitor intake and output closely and notify the doctor if urine output falls below 0.5 ml/kg/hour. Acute renal failure is a common sequelae of severe sepsis. Anticipate the need for RRT—high volume fluid exchanges may be used to rapidly correct pH and other biochemical abnormalities as well as clearing cytokines released as part of the sepsis process.
- Keep in mind that the patient's temperature is usually elevated in the early stages of septic shock and that they commonly experience shaking chills. As the shock progresses, the temperature typically drops and the patient experiences diaphoresis.
- Allow for frequent rest periods to minimise the patient's oxygen demands.
- Institute infection control precautions; use strict aseptic technique for all invasive procedures.
- Provide nutritional support therapy.
- Monitor laboratory test results, especially coagulation studies and hepatic enzyme levels, for changes indicative of DIC and hepatic failure, respectively.
- Provide emotional support to the patient and their family.
- Prepare the patient for surgery as appropriate.

Trauma

Trauma is a physical injury or wound that's inflicted by an external or violent act. Trauma may be intentional or unintentional. Multiple traumas involve injuries to more than one body area or organ and are the leading cause of death in persons younger than age 45.

What's your type?

The type of trauma determines the extent of injury:
- blunt trauma—leaves the body intact
- penetrating trauma—disrupts the body surface
- perforating trauma—leaves entrance and exit wounds as an object passes through the body.

What causes it

Trauma may be caused by weapons, road traffic accidents, physical confrontation, falls or any other unnatural occurrence to the body.

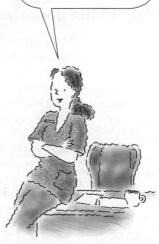

To put it bluntly, trauma may be considered blunt, penetrating or perforating, depending on the extent of the injury.

How it happens

Traumatic wounds include:

- abrasion—the skin is scraped, with partial loss of the skin surface
- laceration—the skin is torn, causing jagged, irregular edges; the severity of laceration depends on its size, depth and location
- puncture wound—when a pointed object, such as a knife or glass fragment, penetrates the skin
- traumatic amputation—part of the body (a limb or part of a limb) is removed.

What to look for

Assessment findings will vary according to the type and extent of trauma. A conscious patient with multiple injuries may be able to help focus the assessment on areas that need immediate attention, such as difficulty breathing or neurological symptoms.

Primary assessment

During the primary assessment the patient is assessed for life-threatening problems involving their airway, breathing, circulation, disability and exposure (ABCDEs). (See *Primary assessment of the trauma patient*, page 601.)

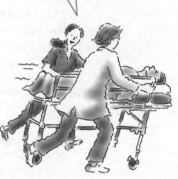

During an emergency, there's not much time for gathering health history. Focus on the most essential information, and fill in the details later, when the patient is stabilised.

Sport some life support

Monitor cardiac rhythm, initiate CPR and administer drugs and electrical defibrillation (defibrillation and synchronised cardioversion) as appropriate for cardiac arrhythmias.

Secondary assessment

After completing the primary assessment and treating life-threatening conditions, a secondary assessment is performed. This includes taking history and performing a more in-depth physical examination.

Skip to the important stuff...

During an emergency, there isn't time to obtain all of the patient's regular history. There needs to be a focus on the most important information, including:

- signs and symptoms related to the present condition
- allergies to drugs, foods, latex or environmental factors
- medication history, including prescription and over-the-counter medications, herbs and supplements
- past medical history
- last meal
- events leading to the injury or condition.

...then fill in the blanks

When the patient's condition is stabilised, fill in the other components of the normal health history. Remember to include history of blood transfusions and tetanus immunisation if the patient has an open wound.

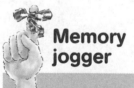

Memory jogger

To help remember what information to obtain during assessment of the trauma patient, use the acronym

SAMPLE:

Signs and symptoms

Allergies

Medications

Past medical history

Last meal

Events leading to injury.

Primary assessment of the trauma patient

This chart shows what to look for (ABCDEs) and what to do during the trauma patient's primary assessment.

Parameter	Assessment	Interventions
A = Airway	• Airway patency	• Position the patient. • To open the airway, make sure that the neck is midline and stabilised and then perform the jaw-thrust manoeuvere.
B = Breathing	• Respirations (rate, depth, effort) • Breath sounds • Chest wall movement and chest injury • Position of trachea (midline or deviation)	• Administer 15 L oxygen via a reservoir mask if breathing adequately or by bag-valve-mask if not. • Use airway adjuncts (such as oral or nasal airways) and prepare for endotracheal intubation or cricothyroidotomy if needed. • Suction as needed. • Remove foreign bodies that may obstruct breathing. • Anticipate and assist with treatment of life-threatening conditions (pneumothorax, tension pneumothorax).
C = Circulation	• Pulse and blood pressure • Bleeding or haemorrhage • Capillary refill, colour of skin and mucous membranes • Cardiac rhythm	• Administer cardiopulmonary resuscitation, medications, and prepare for defibrillation or synchronised cardioversion as necessary. • Control haemorrhaging with direct pressure. • Establish I.V. access and fluid resuscitation (colloids, crystalloids or blood). • Anticipate and assist in treating life-threatening conditions such as cardiac tamponade.
D = Disability	• Neurological assessment, including level of consciousness, pupils and motor and sensory function, presence and severity of pain	• Institute cervical spine immobilisation until x-rays confirm the absence of cervical spine injury. • Monitor and preserve airway • Administer and titrate analgesia as prescribed
E = Exposure and environment	• Injuries and environmental exposure (extreme cold or heat)	• Institute appropriate therapy (warming therapy for hypothermia or cooling therapy for hyperthermia).

Illicit or otherwise

Question the patient about alcohol and drug use. Patients in substance withdrawal may exhibit behavioural changes and be more difficult to manage. Determine the frequency of substance use to assess whether the patient may experience withdrawal postoperatively.

In the know from head to toe

During the secondary assessment a rapid head-to-toe examination may be performed that concentrates on areas relating to the patient's chief complaint rather than a body-systems examination because it's quicker. The head-to-toe examination includes assessing the patient's general appearance and vital signs, head and neck, chest and back, abdomen, perineal area and extremities.

All systems go

When the patient is stable, a body-system examination should be performed. A thorough assessment helps systematically identify and correct problems and establishes a baseline for future comparison.

What tests tell you

The diagnostic tests performed are based on the body system affected by the trauma. For example, a patient with a blunt chest injury would require a chest x-ray to detect rib and sternal fractures, pneumothorax, flail chest, pulmonary contusion and a lacerated or ruptured aorta. Angiography studies would also be performed with suspected aortic laceration or rupture. Diagnostic tests for a patient with head trauma may include a CT scan, cervical spine x-rays, skull x-rays or an angiogram.

Here are some other diagnostic tests that may be performed on the patient with multiple trauma:
• ABG analysis is used to evaluate respiratory status and determine acidotic and alkalotic states.
• FBC indicates the amount of blood loss.
• Coagulation studies are used to evaluate clotting ability.
• U&Es may indicate the presence of electrolyte imbalances or renal dysfunction.

How it's treated

Trauma care basics include:
• triage
• assessing and maintaining ABCs
• protecting the cervical spine
• assessing the LOC
• preparing the patient for transport and possible surgery.

Taking type into consideration

Management of traumatic wounds usually depends on the specific type of wound and degree of contamination. Treatment may include:

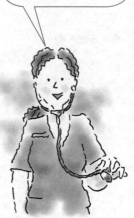

A head-to-toe examination may be performed when assessing a patient with multiple traumas because it's quicker than a body-systems examination.

- controlling bleeding, usually by applying firm, direct pressure and elevating the extremity
- cleaning the wound
- administering analgesic medication
- administering antibiotic therapy
- surgery.

Additional treatment is based on the body system that's affected by the trauma and the extent of injury. For example, treatment of a blunt chest injury may include maintaining a patent airway, providing adequate ventilation, maintaining fluid and electrolyte balance and inserting an intercostal drain for pneumothorax, hemothorax or tension pneumothorax.

What to do

- Assess ABCs and initiate emergency measures if necessary; administer supplemental oxygen as needed.
- Immobilise the head and neck with an immobilisation device, sandbags, backboard and tape. Assist with cervical spine x-rays.
- Monitor vital signs and note significant changes.
- Monitor oxygen saturation and cardiac rhythm for arrhythmias.
- Assess neurological status, including LOC and pupillary and motor response.
- Obtain blood studies, including type and cross-match.
- Insert/assist with insertion of two large-bore I.V. cannulas. For shocked or haemorrhaging patients infuse normal saline, Hartmann's solution or colloid initially.
- Quickly and carefully assess for multiple injuries.
- Assess wounds and provide wound care as appropriate. Cover open wounds and control bleeding by applying pressure and elevating extremities.
- Assess for increased abdominal distention and increased diameter of extremities.
- Administer blood products as prescribed.
- Monitor for signs of hypovolaemic shock.
- Provide analgesic medication, as appropriate.
- Provide reassurance to the patient and their family.
- Explain diagnostic tests and treatments.

Quick quiz

1. To replace clotting factors expand plasma volume and you would expect to give:

    A.   albumin.
    B.   fresh frozen plasma (FFP).
    C.   whole blood.
    D.   packed RBCs.

Answer: B. FFP is the product of choice for replacing clotting factors.

2. Hypertonic solutions cause fluids to move from the:
   A. interstitial space to the intracellular space.
   B. intracellular space to the extracellular space.
   C. extracellular space to the intracellular space.
   D. intracellular space to the interstitial space.

Answer: B. Because of their increased osmolality, hypertonic solutions draw fluids out of the cells and into the extracellular space.

3. Your patient has second- and third-degree burn injuries to their anterior chest, anterior abdomen and entire right arm. Using the Rule of Nines, the percent of total BSA involved can be estimated at:
   A. 18%.
   B. 27%.
   C. 45%.
   D. 50%.

Answer: B. The anterior chest and abdomen constitute 18% of the BSA, and the entire right arm is 9%, for a total of 27%.

4. What is the first step you should take for a patient with hypovolaemic shock?
   A. Assess for dehydration.
   B. Administer I.V. fluids.
   C. Insert a urinary catheter.
   D. Obtain blood for an FBC.

Answer: B. Hypovolaemic shock is an emergency that requires rapid infusion of I.V. fluids.

5. Signs of septic shock include:
   A. clear, watery sputum.
   B. severe hypertension.
   C. hypotension.
   D. increased urine output.

Answer: C. Hypotension despite I.V. fluids is a sign of septic shock when it is accompanied by evidence or suspicion of infection and two or more SIRS criteria.

Scoring

☆☆☆ If you answered all five questions correctly, way to go! You are multitalented when it comes to multisystem issues.

☆☆ If you answered four questions correctly, good work! This last quick quiz must not have been too traumatic for you.

☆ If you answered fewer than four questions correctly, don't go into shock. You can always review the chapter again.

Appendices and index

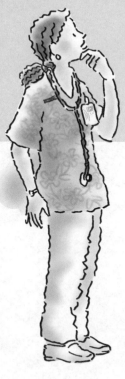

Web resources for critical care nursing

British Association of Critical Care Nurses
www.BACCN.org.uk

British Blood Transfusion Services
www.bbts.org.uk

British National Formulary
www.BNF.org/bnf

British Pain Society
www.britishpainsociety.org

British Thoracic Society
www.brit-thoracic.org.uk

Cardiac Nursing
www.cardiacnursing.co.uk

Delirium (ICU delirium)
www.icudelirium.co.uk

Department of Health
www.DH.gov.uk

Health talk on-line (patients' stories of critical illness)
www.healthtalkonline.org

Intensive care after care network (i-canuk)
www.i-canuk.com

Intensive care national audit and research centre (ICNARC)
www.icnarc.org

Intensive care society
www.ics.ac.uk

National outreach forum
www.norf.org.uk

The renal association
www.renal.org

Resuscitation Council (UK)
www.Resus.org.uk

Glossary

acid–base balance: mechanism by which the body's acids and bases are kept in balance

acidosis: condition resulting from the accumulation of acid or the loss of base

advance directive: document used as a guideline for life-sustaining medical care of a patient with an advanced disease or disability, who's no longer able to indicate his own wishes

afterload: resistance that the left ventricle must work against to pump blood through the aorta

agranulocyte: leucocyte (white blood cell) not made up of granules or grains; includes lymphocytes, monocytes and plasma cells

aldosterone: adrenocortical hormone that regulates sodium, potassium and fluid balance

alkalosis: condition resulting from the accumulation of base or the loss of acid

allergen: substance that induces an allergy or a hypersensitivity reaction

anaphylaxis: severe allergic reaction to a foreign substance

aneurysm: sac formed by the dilation of the wall of an artery, a vein or the heart

anoxia: absence of oxygen in the tissues

antibody: immunoglobulin molecule that reacts only with the specific antigen that induced its formation in the lymph system

antidiuretic hormone: hormone made by the hypothalamus and released by the pituitary gland that decreases the production of urine by increasing the reabsorption of water by the renal tubules

antigen: foreign substance, such as bacteria or toxins, that induces antibody formation

aphasia: language disorder characterised by difficulty expressing or comprehending speech

arrhythmia: disturbance of the normal cardiac rhythm from the abnormal origin, discharge or conduction of electrical impulses

ataxia: uncoordinated actions when voluntary muscle movements are attempted

atrial kick: amount of blood pumped into the ventricles as a result of atrial contraction;

contributes approximately 30% of total cardiac output

autologous transfusion (autotransfusion): reinfusion of the patient's own blood or blood components

automaticity: ability of a cardiac cell to initiate an impulse on its own

borborygmus: loud, gurgling, splashing sounds caused by gas passing through the intestine; normally heard over the large intestine

bruit: abnormal sound heard over peripheral vessels that indicates turbulent blood flow

capture: successful pacing of the heart, represented on the electrocardiogram tracing by a pacemaker spike followed by a P wave or QRS complex

cardiac cycle: the period from the beginning of one heartbeat to the beginning of the next; includes two phases, systole and diastole

cardiac output: amount of blood ejected from the left ventricle per minute; normal value is 4–8 L/minute

cardioversion: restoration of normal rhythm by electric shock or drug therapy

cerebral oedema: increase in the brain's fluid content; may result from correcting hypernatraemia too rapidly

Chvostek's sign: abnormal spasm of facial muscles that may indicate hypocalcaemia or tetany; tested by lightly tapping the facial nerve (upper cheek, below the zygomatic bone)

colloid: large molecule, such as albumin, that normally doesn't cross the capillary membrane

complement system: major mediator of inflammatory response; a functionally related system made up of 20 proteins circulating as functionally inactive molecules

conduction: transmission of electrical impulses through the myocardium

conductivity: ability of one cardiac cell to transmit an electrical impulse to another cell

contractility: ability of a cardiac cell to contract after receiving an impulse

care pathway: documentation tool used in managed care and case management in which a time line is defined for the patient's condition and for the achievement of expected outcomes; used by caregivers to determine where the patient should be in his progress towards optimal health

crystalloid: solute, such as sodium or glucose, that crosses the capillary membrane in solution

cytotoxic: destructive to cells

deep tendon reflex: involuntary muscle contraction in response to a sudden stretch that can be elicited by a hammer or finger tap on a tendon at its insertion

defibrillation: termination of ventricular fibrillation by electrical shock

dehydration: condition in which the loss of water from cells causes them to shrink

demyelination: destruction of a nerve's myelin sheath, which interferes with normal nerve conduction

depolarisation: response of a myocardial cell to an electrical impulse that causes movement of ions across the cell membrane, which triggers myocardial contraction

diastole: phase of the cardiac cycle when both atria (atrial diastole) or both ventricles (ventricular diastole) are at rest and filling with blood

diplopia: double vision

distal: farthest away

dysarthria: speech defect commonly related to a motor deficit of the tongue or speech muscles

dysphagia: difficulty swallowing

enhanced automaticity: condition in which pacemaker cells increase the firing rate above their inherent rate

excitability: ability of a cardiac cell to respond to an electrical stimulus

extravasation: leakage of intravascular fluid into surrounding tissue; can be caused by such medications as chemotherapeutic drugs, dopamine and calcium solutions that produce blistering and, eventually, tissue necrosis

granulocyte: any cell containing granules, especially a granular leucocyte (white blood cell)

haematopoiesis: production of red blood cells in the bone marrow

homeostasis: dynamic, steady state of internal balance in the body

hormone: chemical substance produced in the body that has a specific regulatory effect on the activity of specific cells or organs

host defence system: elaborate network of safeguards that protects the body from infectious organisms and other harmful invaders

hypervolaemia: excess of fluid and solutes in extracellular fluid; can be caused by increased fluid intake, fluid shifts in the body or renal failure

hypotonic: solution that has fewer solutes than another solution

hypovolaemia: condition marked by the loss of fluid and solutes from extracellular fluid that, if left untreated, can progress to hypovolaemic shock

hypoxaemia: oxygen deficit in arterial blood (lower than 10 kPa)

hypoxia: oxygen deficit in the tissues

immunocompetence: ability of cells to distinguish antigens from substances that belong to the body and to launch an immune response

immunodeficiency disorder: disorder caused by a deficiency of the immune response due to hypoactivity or decreased numbers of lymphoid cells

immunoglobulin: serum protein synthesised by lymphocytes and plasma cells that has known antibody activity; main component of humoral immune response

intrinsic: naturally occurring electrical stimulus from within the heart's conduction system

ischaemia: decreased blood supply to a body organ or tissue

isotonic solution: solution that has the same concentration of solutes as another solution

leucocyte: white blood cell that protects the body against microorganisms that cause disease

lymph node: structure that filters the lymphatic fluid that drains from body tissues and is later returned to the blood as plasma; removes noxious agents from the blood

lymphocyte: leucocyte produced by lymphoid tissue that participates in immunity

macrophage: highly phagocytic cells that are stimulated by inflammation

metabolic acidosis: condition in which excess acid or reduced bicarbonate in the blood drops the arterial blood pH below 7.35

metabolic alkalosis: condition in which excess bicarbonate or reduced acid in the blood increases the arterial blood pH above 7.45

nephron: structural and functional unit of the kidney that forms urine

neuron: highly specialised conductor cell that receives and transmits electrochemical nerve impulses

nursing diagnosis: clinical judgement made by a nurse about a patient's responses to actual or potential health problems or life processes; describes a patient problem that the nurse can legally solve; may apply to families and communities as well as individual patients

nursing process: systematic approach to identifying a patient's problems and then taking nursing actions to address them; steps include assessing the patient's problems, forming a diagnostic statement, identifying expected outcomes, creating a plan to achieve expected outcomes and solve the patient's problems, implementing the plan or assigning others to implement it and evaluating the plan's effectiveness

nystagmus: involuntary, rhythmic movement of the eye

oliguria: low urine output, less than 400 ml/24 hours

orthostatic hypotension: drop in blood pressure and increase in heart rate that occur when the body changes position; can be caused by a loss of circulating blood volume

paroxysmal: episode of an arrhythmia that starts and stops suddenly

peristalsis: sequence of muscle contractions that propels food through the GI tract

petechiae: minute haemorrhagic spots in the skin

pH: measurement of the percentage of hydrogen ions in a solution; normal pH is 7.35–7.45 of arterial blood

phagocytosis: engulfing of microorganisms, other cells and foreign particles by a phagocyte

point of maximal impulse: point at which the upward thrust of the heart against the chest wall is greatest, usually over the apex of the heart

power of attorney for health care: legal document whereby a patient authorises another person to make medical decisions for them should they become unable to do so

practice guidelines: sequential instructions for treating patients with specific health problems

preload: stretching force exerted on the ventricular muscle by the blood it contains at the end of diastole

refractory period: brief period during which excitability in a myocardial cell is depressed

renin: enzyme produced by the kidneys in response to an actual or perceived decline in extracellular fluid volume; an important part of blood pressure regulation

repolarisation: recovery of the myocardial cells after depolarisation during which the cell membrane returns to its resting potential

respiratory acidosis: acid–base disturbance caused by failure of the lungs to eliminate sufficient carbon dioxide; partial pressure of arterial carbon dioxide above 6 kPa and pH below 7.35

respiratory alkalosis: acid–base imbalance that occurs when the lungs eliminate more carbon dioxide than normal; partial pressure of arterial carbon dioxide below 4.6 kPa and pH above 7.45

rhabdomyolysis: disorder in which skeletal muscle is destroyed; causes intracellular contents to spill into extracellular fluid

systole: phase of the cardiac cycle when both of the atria (atrial systole) or the ventricles (ventricular systole) are contracting

telangiectasis: permanently dilated small blood vessels that form a weblike pattern; may be the result of scleroderma, lupus erythematosus or cirrhosis or may be normal in healthy, older adults

thrombolytic: clot dissolving

Trousseau's sign: carpal (wrist) spasm elicited by applying a blood pressure cuff to the upper arm and inflating it to a pressure 20 mmHg above the patient's systolic blood pressure; indicates the presence of hypocalcaemia

vasopressor: drug that stimulates contraction of the muscular tissue of the capillaries and arteries

V̇/Q̇ ratio: ratio of ventilation (amount of air in the alveoli) to perfusion (amount of blood in the pulmonary capillaries); expresses the effectiveness of gas exchange

water intoxication: condition in which excess water in the cells results in cellular swelling

Selected references

Ashley, C., and Curry, A. *The Renal Drug Handbook*, 2nd ed. Oxford: Radcliffe Publishing Ltd, 2003.

Berston, A., and Soni, N. *Oh's Intensive Care Manual*, 6th ed. Edinburgh: Butterworth-Heinemann, 2008.

Bickley, L. S., and Szilagyi, P. G. *Bates' Guide to Physical Examination and History Taking*, 11th ed. Philadelphia: Lippincott, Williams and Wilkins, 2003.

British Association of Critical Care Nurses. British Association of Critical Care Nurses position statement on the use of restraint in adult critical care units. *Nursing in Critical Care* 9(5): 199–212, 2004.

British Thoracic Society Emergency Oxygen Guideline Group. Guideline for emergency oxygen use in adult patients. *Thorax* 63(Suppl VI), 2008. (Available at BTS.org).

British Thoracic Society Standards of Care Committee. Non-invasive ventilation in acute respiratory failure. *Thorax* 57: 192–211, 2002. (Available at BTS.org).

British Thoracic Society/Scottish Intercollegiate Guideline Network. *British Guideline on the Management of Asthma*. BTS/SIGN, 2008. (Available at BTS.org).

British Thoracic Society Standards of Care Committee. *Guidelines for the Management of Community Acquired Pneumonia in Adults*. BTS, in press. (Available at BTS.org).

Cutler, L., and Robson, W. *Critical Care Outreach*. Chichester: John Wiley & Sons Ltd, 2006.

Endacott, R., Jevon, P., and Cooper, S. *Clinical Nursing Skills*. Oxford: Oxford University Press, 2009.

Joint Formulary Committee. *British National Formulary*, 57th ed. London: British Medical Association and Royal Pharmaceutical Society of Great Britain, 2009.

Kumar, P., and Clark, M. *Clinical Medicine*, 6th ed. Oxford: Saunders Ltd, 2005.

National Institute for Health and Clinical Excellence. *Chronic Heart Failure: National Clinical Guideline for Diagnosis and Management in Primary and Secondary Care*. (*Clinical Guideline 5*). London: NICE, 2003.

National Institute for Health and Clinical Excellence. *Chronic Obstructive Pulmonary Disease: Management of Chronic Obstructive Pulmonary Disease in Adults in Primary and Secondary Care*. (*Clinical Guideline 12*). London: NICE, 2004.

National Institute for Health and Clinical Excellence. *Chronic Obstructive Pulmonary Disease: Management of Chronic Obstructive Pulmonary Disease in Adults in Primary and Secondary Care*. (*Clinical Guideline 12*). London: NICE, 2007.

National Institute for Health and Clinical Excellence. *Head Injury: Triage, Assessment, Investigation and Early Management of Head Injury in Infants, Children and Adults*. (*Clinical Guideline 56*). London: NICE, 2007.

National Institute for Health and Clinical Excellence. *Acutely Ill Patients in Hospital: Recognition of and Response to Acute Illness in Adults in Hospital*. (*Clinical Guideline 50*). London: NICE, 2007.

National Institute for Health and Clinical Excellence. *Rehabilitation after Critical Illness*. (*Clinical Guideline 83*). London: NICE, 2009.

Pocock, G., and Richards, C. D. *Human Physiology: The Basis of Medicine*, 3rd ed. Oxford: Oxford University Press, 2006.

Resuscitation Council (UK). *Advanced Life Support*, 5th edn. London: Resuscitation Council (UK), 2008.

Royal College of Physicians/British Thoracic Society Guideline Development Group. *Non-Invasive Ventilation in Chronic Obstructive Pulmonary Disease: Management of Acute Type 2 Respiratory Failure*. (*National Guidelines, Number 11*). London: Royal College of Physicians, 2008.

Sasada, M., and Smith, S. *Drugs in Anaesthesia and Intensive Care*, 3rd ed. Oxford: Oxford University Press, 2003.

Singer, M., and Webb, A. *Oxford Handbook of Critical Care*, 3rd ed. Oxford: Oxford University Press, 2009.

Siviter, B. *The Newly Qualified Nurse's Handbook: A Survival Guide*. London: Bailliere-Tindall, 2008.

UCLH Pharmacy Department. *UCL Hospitals Injectable Medicines Administration Guide*, 2nd ed. Oxford: Blackwell Publishing, 2007.

United Kingdom Clinical Pharmacy Association. *Detection, Prevention and Treatment of Delirium in the Critically Ill*. UKCPA, 2006.

Woodrow, P. *Intensive Care Nursing*, 2nd ed. London: Routledge, 2006.

Index

A

Abdomen, assessment of, 383–385, 385t
  auscultation, 384–385
  quadrant method for, 384i
Abdominal aortic aneurysm, 237
Abdominal palpation, 385, 386i
Abdominal sounds, abnormal, 385t
Abdominal x-rays, for GI disorders, 393
ABG. *See* Arterial blood gas analysis
ABO blood typing, 536
ACE inhibitors, 194–195
Acid-base balance
  renal system and, 436
  respiration and, 276
Acquired immunodeficiency syndrome, 557
  causes of, 559
  conditions associated with, 559
  diagnostic tests for, 560
  nursing considerations, 561–562
  opportunistic infections in, 561
  signs and symptoms of, 560
  treatment of, 560, 561
Acute coronary syndromes, 230–236
  causes of, 230
  diagnostic tests for, 232–233
  national framework for, 235–236
  signs and symptoms of, 231–232
  treatment for, 233–234
Acute idiopathic polyneuritis. *See* Guillain–
  Barré syndrome
Acute leukaemia, 549–550
  causes of, 549
  diagnostic tests for, 550
  nursing considerations, 550
  signs and symptoms of, 550
  treatment of, 550
Acute pain, 35
Acute renal failure, 460–466
  causes of, 460, 461–462t
  diagnostic tests for, 464
  nursing considerations, 465–466
  signs and symptoms of, 463–464
  treatment of, 464–465
Acute respiratory distress syndrome, 355–360
  alveolar changes in, C6–C7
  causes of, 355
  diagnostic tests for, 357, 358
  nursing considerations, 358, 359–360
  signs and symptoms of, 356–357, 357i
  treatment for, 358

Acute respiratory failure, 335–338
  causes of, 335–336
  diagnostic tests for, 337
  nursing considerations, 338
  signs and symptoms of, 336–337
  treatment for, 337
Acute tubular necrosis, 466–471, 468i
  causes of, 466–467
  diagnostic tests for, 469
  nursing considerations, 470–471
  signs and symptoms of, 469
  treatment of, 469–470
Addison's disease, 493–497, 494i
  causes of, 493, 495
  diagnostic tests for, 496
  nursing considerations, 496–497
  pathophysiology of, 495
  signs and symptoms of, 495–496
  treatment of, 496
Adenosine, 186–187, 186t
Adjuvant analgesics, for pain
  management, 40
Adrenal crisis, 494i
Adrenal glands, 477
Adrenal hypofunction, 493
Adrenergic blocking drugs, 203–205, 204t
  alpha-adrenergic blocking, 203,
    204, 204t
  beta-adrenergic blocking, 204t, 205
Adrenergic drugs, 199, 200–201t, 201–203
Advance decisions, 49
Advanced nurse practitioners, 13
Adventitious sounds, 290–291
Advocacy, critical care nurse and, 4
Agranulocytes, 518
AIDS. *See* Acquired immunodeficiency syndrome
Airways, 267–269, 268i
  lower, 268i, 269
  upper, 267, 268, 268i
Alimentary canal, 372
  large intestine, 375–376
  mouth, 373–374
  oesophagus, 374
  pharynx, 374
  small intestine, 374–375
  stomach, 374
Allen's test, 296i
Alpha-adrenergic blocking drugs, 203,
  204, 204t
Amines, 478
Anaemia, 550–551

causes of, 551
  diagnostic tests for, 551
  signs and symptoms of, 551
  treatment of, 551
Anaphylaxis, 551–553, C14–C15
  causes of, 552
  diagnostic tests for, 553
  nursing considerations, 553
  signs and symptoms of, 552
  treatment of, 553
Angina. *See also* Acute coronary syndromes;
    Antianginal drugs
  beta-adrenergic receptor
    blockers for, 188
  calcium channel blockers for, 188–189
  forms of, 231
Angiography, 80–81
  cerebral, 80–81
  digital subtraction, 81
Angiotensin II receptor antagonists, 195
ANP. *See* Advanced nurse practitioners
Antianginal drugs, 187–189
Antiarrhythmics, 183–187, 185–186t
  classes, 183–184, 186–187
Antibody screening test, 536
Anticoagulants, 195, 197i
  heparin, 195, 196, 197–198
  oral anticoagulants, 198
Antiglobulin test, 536–537
Antihypertensive drugs, 189, 191–195
Antiinflammatory agents, 322
Antilipemic drugs, 233
Antiplatelet drugs, 189, 191
Aortic aneurysm repair, 212i
Aortic aneurysms, 236–240
  causes of, 236
  diagnostic tests for, 238
  signs and symptoms of, 237
  treatment for, 238–239
Aortic insufficiency, 262, 263
  signs and symptoms of, 264
Aortic stenosis, 262, 263
  signs and symptoms of, 264
Apnoea, 283
ARDS. *See* Acute respiratory distress syndrome
Arterial blood gas analysis, 292, 293–294,
  295, 296i
Arterial blood pressure monitoring, 170–171
Arterial insufficiency, 149i
Arteries, 144
Arterioles, 144

i refers to an illustration; t refers to a table; and boldtype indicates colour pages

i refers to an illustration; t refers to a table; and boldtype indicates colour pages